CONCEPTUAL FOUNDATIONS

The Bridge to Professional Nursing Practice

CONCEPTUAL FOUNDATIONS

The Bridge to Professional Nursing Practice

FIFTH EDITION

JOAN L. CREASIA, PhD, RN
Professor and Dean
College of Nursing
University of Tennessee
Knoxville, Tennessee

ELIZABETH E. FRIBERG, DNP, RN
Assistant Professor
University of Virginia School of Nursing
Charlottesville, Virginia

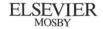

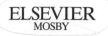

3251 Riverport Lane
St. Louis, Missouri 63043

CONCEPTUAL FOUNDATIONS:
THE BRIDGE TO PROFESSIONAL NURSING PRACTICE

ISBN: 978-0-323-06869-7

Copyright © 2011, 2007, 2001, 1996, 1991 by Mosby, Inc., an affiliate of Elsevier Inc.

Notice

Knowledge and best practice in this field are constantly changing. As new research and experience broaden our understanding, changes in research methods, professional practices, or medical treatment may become necessary. Practitioners and researchers must always rely on their own experience and knowledge in evaluating and using any information, methods, compounds, or experiments described herein. In using such information or methods, they should be mindful of their own safety and the safety of others, including parties for whom they have a professional responsibility.

With respect to any drug or pharmaceutical products identified, readers are advised to check the most current information provided (i) on procedures featured or (ii) by the manufacturer of each product to be administered to verify the recommended dose or formula, the method and duration of administration, and contraindications. It is the responsibility of practitioners, relying on their own experience and knowledge of their patients, to make diagnoses, to determine dosages and the best treatment for each individual patient, and to take all appropriate safety precautions.

To the fullest extent of the law, neither the Publisher nor the authors, contributors, or editors, assume any liabili-ty for any injury and/or damage to persons or property as a matter of products liability, negligence or otherwise, or from any use or operation of any methods, products, instructions, or ideas contained in the material herein.

Library of Congress Cataloging-in-Publication Data

Conceptual foundations : the bridge to professional nursing practice /
[edited by] Joan L. Creasia, Elizabeth E. Friberg. -- 5th ed.
    p. ; cm.
 Includes bibliographical references and index.
 ISBN 978-0-323-06869-7 (pbk. : alk. paper)
 1. Nursing--Practice. 2. Nursing. I. Creasia, Joan L. II. Friberg,
Elizabeth E.
 [DNLM: 1. Nursing--United States. 2. Nursing Care--United States.
WY 16 AA1]
 RT86.7.C66 2011
 610.73--dc22

2010034348

Editor: Maureen Iannuzzi
Senior Developmental Editor: Robin Richman
Publishing Services Manager: Anne Altepeter
Senior Project Manager: Cheryl A. Abbott
Design Direction: Amy Buxton

Printed in the United States of America

Last digit is the print number: 9 8 7 6 5 4 3 2

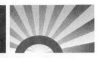

Contributors

Cathy L. Campbell, PhD, APN-BC
Assistant Professor
University of Virginia School of Nursing
Charlottesville, Virginia

Katharine C. Cook, PhD, RN, CNE
Chair and Professor of Nursing
College of Notre Dame of Maryland
Baltimore, Maryland

Joan L. Creasia, PhD, RN
Professor and Dean
College of Nursing
University of Tennessee
Knoxville, Tennessee

Sarah A. Delgado, RN, MSN, ACNP
Assistant Professor and Nurse Practitioner
University of Virginia School of Nursing
Charlottesville, Virginia

Elizabeth E. Friberg, DNP, RN
Assistant Professor
University of Virginia School of Nursing
Charlottesville, Virginia

Mattia J. Gilmartin, RN, MBA, PhD
Associate Professor and Graduate Coordinator,
    Clinical Nurse Leader™ Program
Hunter-Bellevue School of Nursing
New York, New York

Vicki S. Good, MSN, RN, CCNS, CENP
Director of Nursing Practice
Cox Health System
Springfield, Missouri

Pamela J. Grace, PhD, APRN
Associate Professor of Nursing and Ethics
Boston College William F. Connell School of Nursing
Boston, Massachusetts

Mary Gunther, PhD, RN, CNE
Associate Professor
Chair, MSN Program
College of Nursing
University of Tennessee
Knoxville, Tennessee

L. Louise Ivanov, DNS, RN
Associate Professor and Community Practice
    Department Chair
School of Nursing
University of North Carolina, Greensboro
Greensboro, North Carolina

Susan Kaplan Jacobs, MLS, MA, RN, AHIP
Health Sciences Librarian
Associate Curator
New York University Libraries
New York, New York

Arlene W. Keeling, PhD, RN, FAAN
Centennial Distinguished Professor of Nursing
Director, Center of Nursing Historical Inquiry
Charlottesville, Virginia

Kathryn Laughon, PhD, RN
Assistant Professor
University of Virginia School of Nursing
Charlottesville, Virginia

Dale Halsey Lea, MPH, RN, CGC, FAAN
Health Educator
Education and Community Involvement Branch
  and Genomic Healthcare Branch
National Human Genome Research Institute
National Institutes of Health
Bethesda, Maryland

Patricia McMullen, PhD, JD, CNS, CRNP
Associate Provost for Academic Administration
The Catholic University of America
Washington, DC

Brenda Morris, EdD, RN, CNE
Senior Director, Nursing Baccalaureate
  Programs
College of Nursing and Healthcare Innovation
Arizona State University
Phoenix, Arizona

Marilyn Grace O'Rourke, DNP, APHN-BC
Associate Professor
Department of Community, Systems, and Mental
  Health Nursing
Rush University Medical Center
Chicago, Illinois

Teresa L. Panniers, PhD, RN
Associate Professor
School of Nursing
College of Health and Human Services
George Mason University
Fairfax, Virginia

Nayna C. Philipsen, PhD, JD, RN, CFE, FACCE
Associate Professor
Director of Program Development
Helene Fuld School of Nursing
Coppin State University
Baltimore, Maryland

Kathryn B. Reid, PhD, RN
Coordinator, Clinical Nurse Leader Program
University of Virginia School of Nursing
Charlottesville, Virginia

Karen J. Saewert, PhD, RN, CPHQ, CNE
Clinical Associate Professor
Director, E3: Evaluation and Educational Excellence
Arizona State University
College of Nursing and Health Innovation
Phoenix, Arizona

Vickie H. Southall, MSN, RN
Assistant Professor of Nursing
University of Virginia School of Nursing
Charlottesville, Virginia

Jennifer Casavant Telford, PhD, ACNP-BC
Assistant Professor
University of Connecticut School of Nursing
Storrs, Connecticut

Sandra P. Thomas, PhD, RN, FAAN
Professor and Chair, PhD Program in Nursing
College of Nursing
University of Tennessee
Knoxville, Tennessee

Heather Vallent, RN, MS
Clinical Assistant Professor
Boston College William F. Connell School of Nursing
Boston, Massachusetts

Debra C. Wallace, PhD, RN
Associate Dean for Research
Director, Center for Health of Vulnerable Populations
Daphne Doster Mastroianni Distinguished Professor
School of Nursing
University of North Carolina at Greensboro
Greensboro, North Carolina

Ishan C. Williams, PhD
Assistant Professor
University of Virginia School of Nursing
Charlottesville, Virginia

Tami H. Wyatt, PhD, RN, CNE
Assistant Professor
College of Nursing
University of Tennessee
Knoxville, Tennessee

Elke Jones Zschaebitz, MSN, FNP-BC
Instructor, University of Virginia School of Nursing
Instructor, Healthy Appalachia Institute College
    at Wise, University of Virginia
Health Services Clinician, High Risk Breast
    and Ovarian Cancer Center
University of Virginia
Charlottesville, Virginia

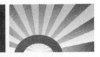

Reviewers

Barbara Camune, DrPH, MSN, RNC, CNM, WHNP-BC, FACNM
Clinical Associate Professor
Director, Midwifery and Women's Health Nurse
   Practitioner Programs
Women, Children, and Family Health Science
University of Illinois at Chicago
Chicago, Illinois

Karen Clark, PhD, RN, CCRN
Assistant Professor
School of Nursing, University of Maryland,
   Baltimore
Rockville, Maryland
Adventist Preferred Nursing
Silver Spring, Maryland

Kathleen Sanders Jordan, RN, MS, FNP-BC, SANE-P
Nurse Practitioner, Emergency Medicine
Mid-Atlantic Emergency Medicine Associates
Lecturer
Graduate School of Nursing, University of North
   Carolina, Charlotte
Charlotte, North Carolina

Arlene Kent-Wilkinson, RN, PhD
Assistant Professor
College of Nursing, University of Saskatchewan
Saskatoon, Saskatchewan, Canada

Joan M. Pryor McCann, PhD, RN, CNS, CNL
Professor of Nursing
Director of Undergraduate Studies
Department of Nursing
Otterbein College
Westerville, Ohio

Mary Beth Reid, PhD, RN, CNS, CCRN, CEN
Area Director, Education
Interim Director, Nursing and Clinical Services
Department of Nursing
Kindred Healthcare
Arlington, Texas

Sandra L. Siedlecki, RN, PhD, CNS
Assistant Professor
The Breen School of Nursing, Ursuline College
Pepper Pike, Ohio
Senior Nurse Researcher
Nursing Institute, Cleveland Clinic
Cleveland, Ohio

Diane Vail Skojec, RN, MS, CRNP, DNP(c)
Cardiac Transplant Nurse Practitioner
Department of Cardiac Surgery
The Johns Hopkins Hospital
Baltimore, Maryland

Barbara Weintraub, RN, BA, BSN, MSN, MPH, APN-AC, CE, FACN
Director, Emergency Department
Northwest Community Hospital
Arlington Heights, Illinois

Preface

The fifth edition of *Conceptual Foundations: The Bridge to Professional Nursing* brings a change in editors, several changes in chapter authors, and the addition of two new chapters. After more than 20 years of dedication to this text, Barbara J. Parker, PhD, RN, FAAN, has passed the editorial tasks to her colleague, Elizabeth E. Friberg, DNP, RN. Previous chapter authors are acknowledged at the beginning of chapters revised by new contributors. Their work provided a foundation on which new chapters were based, expanded, and revised. Our new authors have eagerly taken on the task of updating and verifying existing work while presenting the material in a creative or fresh format to encourage student engagement. We have added two new chapters, on genetics and genomics and on patient safety, both areas in which nursing has taken significant leadership. As we go to press, we have made every effort to integrate the most current information on the *Affordable Care Act of 2010* and *Healthy People 2020*. It is a period of dynamic change.

Since 2007 and the release of the fourth edition of this text, the profession and practice of nursing has faced many challenges, launched new initiatives, and taken leadership roles in various aspects of health care and health care service delivery. With the influence of the 1965 American Nurses Association (ANA) recommendation that the minimum educational preparation for professional nurses be at a baccalaureate level, educational pathways to increase the number of professional nurses and advanced practice nurses have created multiple models for professional entry and advancement. Nursing workforce shortages and other national agendas, such as patient safety and health care reform, have created a demand for professional nurses in a variety of health care delivery settings and academia. The demands of practice complexity, professional career advancement, and nurse/faculty shortages provide the stimulus for many associate degree and diploma program graduates to consider educational advancement.

The first edition of *Conceptual Foundations* targeted the RN-BSN student by focusing on the context, dimensions, and themes of professional nursing practice. The *context* of professional nursing practice sheds meaning on the nursing profession and the conditions that must be present for societal recognition of nursing as a profession. The *dimensions* of professional practice are the spatial influences on professional nursing practice that may change over time, such as the economy or the law. *Themes* in professional nursing practice reflect a sampling of nursing leadership areas of interest as the profession assumes its societal role as a recognized profession. Since the first edition, nursing programs other than completion programs have used this text in foundational courses at the baccalaureate and graduate levels. We believe that the content of this fifth edition remains relevant for use in these programs, but we have retained language targeted at a post-licensure audience seeking to advance professional careers.

APPROACH

The rapid changes in the health care delivery system continue to influence nursing education and practice. With the passage of a landmark health care reform initiative and the explosion of health care technology and informatics, professional nursing has provided extensive leadership and received public role recognition for its contributions. From planning and delivery to patient safety, consumer/patient–centric services, quality improvement, cost containment, community-based services, health promotion, and disease prevention, nursing has emerged as the pivotal coordinator to ensure high-quality care at reasonable cost. Now more than ever, nurses need strong foundations in the political, legal, economic, population, systems, and ethical aspects of health care in general and nursing care specifically. This text provides that foundation and relates those general concepts to the professional practice of nursing.

Nursing education programs have diverse student populations that span multiple ages and cultural and life experience parameters that bring a richness and depth to their educational advancement. Many are adult learners with increased capacity for critical thinking and self-directed learning. Others are advancing their education while working or raising a family. Some are pursuing their advanced education using distance learning pedagogies. *Conceptual Foundations* provides a meaningful and diverse conceptual approach to nursing practice that encourages exploration of original theorists, critical analysis of issues and concepts, and applicability to diverse client populations and clinical settings. The text frames the professional practice of nursing by using a variety of subject matter experts and reflective profiles of practicing professional nurses.

The reader will find both *client* and *patient* terminology used, at times interchangeably, to reflect changes in nursing practice and delivery settings. Although philosophically we believe a distinction exists, to maintain the flow of the content we allowed authors the liberty to use these terms interchangeably.

ORGANIZATION

The text is divided into three parts: **Part I, The Context of Professional Nursing Practice,** explores the historical development of professional nursing in the United States, pathways of nursing education, socialization to professional nursing, professional nursing roles, theories and frameworks for professional nursing practice, health policy and planning and the nursing practice environment, and economic issues in nursing and health care. The historical chapter engages students by flowing through issues, instead of using the typical timeline approach, and framing a future professional nursing vision. Nursing education includes current enrollment statistics and discussion of the most recent pathway changes. The chapter on roles addresses various professional roles as well as the dynamics of role stress in the work environment. Theories and frameworks provide links to the classic works of original theorists using their own words while updating these concepts with current research applications in nursing. The chapter on health policy includes a summary of the recent health care reform initiative passed as the Patient Protection and Affordable Care Act of 2010. Economic issues that currently drive health care reform and current nursing practice are presented in a manner that engages students in current economic climates.

Part II, Dimensions of Professional Nursing Practice, explores communication skills and techniques; critical thinking, clinical judgment, and the nursing process; challenges in teaching and learning; legal aspects of nursing practice; ethical dimensions of nursing and health care; health care informatics; and diversity in health and illness. The chapter on communications covers active listening and SBAR communication related to patient safety and interpersonal, group, and organizational dynamics of a high-reliability organization (HRO). The exploration of critical thinking and its relationship to clinical judgment and the nursing process includes a discussion of measureable behavioral outcomes, competencies, research measures, and application in evidence-based practice. The discussion of various learning principles and how they are used in teaching applications encourages students to identify their own learning styles by providing links to online learning style assessments and the distinctions between personal and professional beliefs in teaching various client populations. The chapter on legal aspects provides a basic understanding of statutory, public, and private law and covers topics such as licensure, delegation, and practice acts in a format that makes these legal aspects easily accessible to the student. The chapter on ethics includes values clarification and a framework for exploring moral dilemmas in practice. Health care informatics covers topics such as decision-support systems, telehealth, and nursing languages, and provides a framework and strategies for using a variety of library and Internet information resources to support evidence-based practice. The previous edition's chapter on cultural competency has been revised to cover diversity in health and illness by integrating new standards (CLAS Act) and other aspects of culturally relevant practice.

Part III, Themes in Professional Nursing Practice, explores subjects and topics in which professional nursing is demonstrating leadership, such as health and health promotion, genetics and genomics, rural health, intimate partner violence (IPV), vulnerable populations, and patient safety. The chapter on health and health promotion emphasizes the emerging interest in preventive services and the concepts of behavioral and lifestyle change, self-efficacy, and environmental influences. The new chapter on genetics and genomics provides a foundation for the rapid developments in this area and nursing's role, especially in the family history pedigree and referral for genetic testing and counseling. The discussion on rural health emphasizes the role of professional nursing in the delivery of services to rural populations. The chapter on intimate partner violence explores violence as a national health issue and the aspects of forensic nursing in the specific role of the sexual assault nurse examiner (SANE). The needs of vulnerable populations are explored within the framework of *Healthy People* 10-year assessment and the 2020 goals and objectives as defined to date. The new chapter on patient safety explores the critical role that nursing performs in providing a safe health care environment for the delivery of health care services in a variety of settings consistent with current national quality and safety initiatives.

PEDAGOGY

Each chapter is organized to direct the attention of the student or faculty reader and developed in a similar format. Chapters begin with learning **Objectives** followed by a reflective **Profile in Practice** related to the chapter topic. The text includes an opening **Introduction** to explain the approach of the chapter and closes with a **Summary** of the chapter content followed by **Key Points** that emphasize the major take-away concepts from the chapter. Chapter content flows from the general concept to application in nursing practice. **Key terms** are presented in italics, and **definitions** are embedded in the text for reading ease. The nature of the content creates the need for **cross-references** of topics that are addressed by multiple chapters. We provided those cross-references where we felt they were most useful to the reader. **Boxes, Tables,** and **Figures** are used throughout for emphasis and provide a visual reinforcement for important content. **Internet links** are embedded within the text or provided in **Additional Resources** when websites other than those referenced in the chapter may be useful for both the student and faculty. **Critical Thinking Exercises** are provided at the end of each chapter to expand the student's exploration of key concepts and stimulate group discussions.

References, either classic or current (within the past 5 years), are provided for all citations. The authors have chosen to reference classic works where appropriate to instill in students a sense of the richness of nursing's body of knowledge that supports current professional practice. Evidence- and research-based references are largely current except where a classic reference is better suited. We have retained our practice of providing classic references for major theorists and use of the actual theorist's language/words in describing their theories. This practice provides the opportunity for students and faculty to experience their work first-hand and refer to their original writings. Current research and evidence-based application are integrated throughout the content.

This format challenges the reader to discover new knowledge or reframe prior learning on a more conceptual and universally applicable level in professional practice. The contextual, dimensional, and theme-based approach provides a comprehensive source text for exploring foundational concepts of professional nursing practice targeted to transition or completion programs but applicable in a variety of educational programs. Nursing practice as it is today and will be in the future is supported by these foundational concepts and the ever-expanding nursing knowledge base that flows from them.

SPECIAL FEATURES

A website, http://evolve.elsevier.com/Creasia/bridge/, provides student resources as well as a faculty instruction manual, test bank, and PowerPoint presentations for each chapter.

Joan L. Creasia, PhD, RN
Elizabeth E. Friberg, DNP, RN

To
Barbara J. Parker, PhD, RN, FAAN,
for her dedication to this text
for more than 20 years

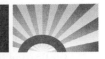

Contents

PART I
The Context of Professional Nursing Practice

Chapter 1 Historical Development of Professional Nursing in the United States, *1*
JENNIFER CASAVANT TELFORD
ARLENE W. KEELING

Introduction, *3*
The Historical Evolution of Nursing, *3*
Nursing in Institutions of Higher Education, *14*
Rise of Advanced Practice Nursing in Clinical
   Settings, *16*

Chapter 2 Pathways of Nursing Education, *22*
JOAN L. CREASIA
KATHRYN B. REID

Introduction, *23*
History of Nursing Education in the United
   States, *23*
Considerations in Selecting a Nursing Education
   Program, *30*
Observations and Analysis, *35*
Impact of Studies of the Profession, *37*
Looking Toward the Future, *38*

Chapter 3 Socialization to Professional Nursing, *42*
KAREN J. SAEWERT

Introduction, *44*
Nursing as a Profession, *44*
Professionalization of Nursing, *47*
Professional Nursing Practice, *49*
Socialization to Professional Nursing, *53*
Socialization and Career Development, *58*
Environmental Factors That Influence
   Socialization, *59*
Professional Governance, *63*
Professional Associations, *63*

Chapter 4 Professional Nursing Roles, *71*
SARAH A. DELGADO
ELKE JONES ZSCHAEBITZ
ELIZABETH E. FRIBERG

Introduction, *72*
Nursing Roles, Functions,
   and Characteristics, *72*
Professional Practice Roles, *81*
Role Dynamics, *83*

Chapter 5 Theories and Frameworks for Professional Nursing Practice, *95*
MARY GUNTHER

Introduction, *97*
Terminology Associated with Nursing
   Theory, *97*
Overview of Selected Nursing Theories, *100*
 Grand Theory, *100*

Midrange Theory, *106*
Practice Theory, *109*
Practice Theory Characteristics, *110*
Application to Nursing Practice, *110*

Chapter 6 Health Policy and Planning and the Nursing Practice Environment, *117*
DEBRA C. WALLACE
L. LOUISE IVANOV

Introduction, *118*
Politics, *118*
Understanding the Legislative Process, *123*
Budget Process, *126*
Health Programs, *128*
Leadership, *131*
Nursing, *133*
Health Policies, *133*
Nursing and Health Policy, *139*
Nurse Participation in Health Policy, *143*
Health Care Reform 2010, *144*

Chapter 7 Economic Issues in Nursing and Health Care, *151*
MATTIA J. GILMARTIN

Introduction, *152*
Health Economics, *153*
Economic Concepts Specific to the Nursing Profession, *156*
Economic Concepts for Advocacy and Professional Practice, *161*
Health System Reform: Emerging Models and Trends, *173*

PART II
Dimensions of Professional Nursing Practice *186*

Chapter 8 Communication Skills and Techniques, *186*
KATHARINE C. COOK

Introduction, *187*
Intrapersonal Communication, *188*
Interpersonal Communication, *189*
Organizational Communication, *194*

Chapter 9 Critical Thinking, Clinical Judgment, and the Nursing Process, *200*
BRENDA MORRIS

Introduction, *202*
Defining Critical Thinking, *202*
Critical Thinking in Nursing, *204*
The Nursing Process, *205*
Nursing Judgment Model, *211*
Characteristics of Critical Thinkers, *213*
Disposition Toward Critical Thinking, *213*
Strategies to Build Critical Thinking Skills, *214*
Research and Measurement Issues Associated with Critical Thinking, *216*
Research, *216*
Application of Critical Thinking in a Clinical Situation, *217*

Chapter 10 Challenges in Teaching and Learning, *223*
TAMI H. WYATT

Introduction, *224*
Teaching and Learning Theories, *225*
Teaching and Learning Principles, *228*
Characteristics of Effective Teachers, *229*
Characteristics of Effective Learners, *229*
Designing Teaching-Learning Plans, *233*
Evaluating the Teaching-Learning Experience, *237*
Future Trends in Teaching and Learning, *239*

Chapter 11 Legal Aspects of Nursing Practice, *242*
NAYNA C. PHILIPSEN
PATRICIA MCMULLEN

Introduction, *243*
Administrative Law in Nursing, *243*
Nursing and Employment Law, *247*
Tort Law in Nursing, *249*
Criminalization of Unintentional Error, *256*

Chapter 12 Ethical Dimensions of Nursing and Health Care, *260*

HEATHER VALLENT
PAMELA J. GRACE

Introduction, *261*
Overview of Ethics, *261*
Foundations of Ethical Nursing Practice, *262*
Ethical Nursing Practice, *265*
Contemporary Issues and Problems, *279*

Chapter 13 Health Care Informatics, *288*

TERESA L. PANNIERS
SUSAN KAPLAN JACOBS

Introduction, *289*
Health Care Informatics: A Driving Force for Nursing Practice, *289*
Library Information Resources to Support Nursing Practice, *299*
The Internet, *305*
Strategies for Managing Information, *306*

Chapter 14 Diversity in Health and Illness, *312*

CATHY L. CAMPBELL
ISHAN C. WILLIAMS

Introduction, *315*
Diversity and Health, *315*
Diversification of America, *322*
Resources, *323*
Cultural Assessment Strategies, *325*

PART III
Themes in Professional Nursing Practice

Chapter 15 Health and Health Promotion, *329*

SANDRA P. THOMAS

Introduction, *330*
Concept of Health, *330*
Evolving Conceptions of Health, *331*
Health Promotion and Disease Prevention, *332*

Modification of Health Attitudes and Behaviors, *332*
Evidence-Based Interventions to Promote Behavior Change, *341*
Environmental Factors That Affect Wellness, *344*
National Health Promotion Goals, *345*
Community Health Promotion, *346*

Chapter 16 Genetics and Genomics in Professional Nursing, *354*

DALE HALSEY LEA

Introduction: Why Genetics and Genomics? *356*
Essentials of Genetic and Genomic Nursing, *358*
Applying Genetics and Genomics in Nursing Practice, *359*
Tomorrow's Genetics and Genomics: Personalized Medicine, *362*
Ethical Issues in Genetics and Genomics, *363*

Chapter 17 Rural Health Concepts, *368*

VICKIE H. SOUTHALL

Introduction, *369*
What Is Rural? *370*
Health Status of Rural Residents, *372*
Characteristics of Rural Nursing Practice, *375*
Rural Nursing Theory, *376*
Rural Health Policy and Resources, *376*
Implications for Rural Nursing Practice, *377*

Chapter 18 Intimate Partner Violence as a Health Care Problem, *385*

KATHRYN LAUGHON

Introduction, *386*
Background, *386*
Consequences of Intimate Partner Violence, *387*
Pregnancy and IPV, *388*
Children and IPV, *388*
Missed Opportunities in the Health Care System, *388*
Assessment for Intimate Partner Violence, *389*
After a Positive Screen, *390*

Chapter 19 Vulnerable Populations, *394*
MARILYN GRACE O'ROURKE

Introduction, *396*
Key Concepts, *396*
Current Challenges to Health Equity, *401*
Working with Vulnerable Populations, *403*

Chapter 20 Patient Safety, *407*
VICKI S. GOOD

Introduction, *408*
Regulatory Overview, *409*
Patient Safety Culture, *411*
Key Processes, *413*

CONCEPTUAL FOUNDATIONS

The Bridge to Professional Nursing Practice

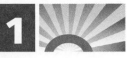

1

Historical Development of Professional Nursing in the United States

JENNIFER CASAVANT TELFORD, PhD, APN-BC
ARLENE W. KEELING, PhD, RN, FAAN

OBJECTIVES

At the completion of this chapter, the reader will be able to:

- Discuss the impact of Florence Nightingale's model and the American Civil War on mid to late–19th-century American nursing education.
- Describe the transition of nursing education from the hospital to collegiate programs.
- Discuss the role of nursing licensure in safeguarding the public and developing educational and clinical nursing standards.
- Discuss the development of advanced clinical practice nursing from the 1960s through the present.

PROFILE IN PRACTICE

Laura I. Robinson
Adult Primary Care Nurse Practitioner Student, University of Connecticut School of Nursing

Nursing history is important to me because it has provided me with the opportunity to fulfill my goal to advance my career as a nurse practitioner, a role that was not existent less than half a century ago. Ambitious nurses before me had to establish themselves in a new career, gain recognition, and succeed in order for the position to be present today. One person whom I particularly admire and who helped pave the way is my grandmother, Olive Shea.

Grandma Shea earned her RN diploma in 1944 after completing the 3-year certification program offered by Hartford Hospital in Hartford, Connecticut. After various nursing positions, she was employed by the University of Connecticut at the campus Infirmary in Storrs, Connecticut, beginning in 1968. At that time the facility was the home to physicians whose time was mainly devoted to scheduled appointments with their student patients, as well as two floors of inpatient beds where nurses provided individualized care.

Grandma Shea recounted that an integral part of her day as a nurse was the 20-minute back rubs she gave to all five of her patients after bathing each with a bar of soap and warm water from a basin. She took the time to familiarize herself with the patients, establish trust, and relate to their needs.

Soon patient volume in the infirmary exceeded what the physicians could possibly manage. Director of Nursing and nurse practitioner Sydney Ayotte proposed a more economical solution of adding more nurse practitioners to the office to tend to the needs of the students. The university paid for Grandma Shea to attend Northwestern University in Evanston, Illinois.

In the summer of 1977, my grandmother and nine other nurses from various parts of the country gathered at Northwestern for 3 months of intense learning. In the fall, they returned to their respective nursing jobs; they regrouped for another 6-week learning session in the winter and again for 6 more weeks the following summer. They lived in dormitories and then in the private homes of some generous host families. Classes, headed entirely by female physicians, were taught in the medical school with much didactic learning. She fondly recalled Dr. Yeager, who "did not miss a thing; each body system was covered in such great detail." The students practiced assessments on one another, learning the normal from abnormal findings with periodic testing and oral examinations. She remembered the training being particularly challenging, having been out of school for so long. "I wished I could have gone through the classes all over again; it was so difficult to take it all in," she stated after recalling each intensive semester. She could easily recollect the excitement of first looking in the eyes and ears of the patients and coming to know a different set of skills. She explained, "That was what the doctors did; we were doing a new job. It was wonderful to understand the reason for doing things in a more definitive way."

These nurses' symbol was the butterfly, starting out in a cocoon and emerging with wings, which represented their transformation from bedside nurse to nurse practitioner. At the close of the summer of 1978, a small informal graduation ceremony was held. There were no caps and gowns and no formal pinning ceremony. The graduates were each given a real butterfly and a certificate earning each nurse the title of College Health Nurse Practitioner. Grandma Shea returned to the University of Connecticut Infirmary with her own schedule of appointments and began to diagnose and treat patients. Not all the physicians were supportive of the nurse practitioners in their new role. Early on, Grandma Shea relied on the help of one mentor in particular, Dr. Don McLaughlin. She recalled, "If I knocked on his door and needed him, he was there." It did not

take long for her to gain confidence and become regarded as a gifted diagnostician.

Listening to Grandma Shea describe her nursing practice, particularly the importance of time spent with the patient at the bedside while providing morning care, has helped guide me in my own career practices as a nurse. I strive to uphold her values and give the best care and personal attention to my patients in a modern day setting, where many of the tasks that were once a nurse's job have now been delegated to aides. These values continue to direct my practice as I advance my career, just as these same values guided my grandmother.

Although my career path is following a course similar to that of my grandmother, some of the education procedures have changed in the past 32 years. One striking difference is that her advanced nursing training was taught by physicians, whereas my professors are experienced advanced practice RNs (APRNs). In Grandma Shea's era, there simply were not as many nurse practitioners who had the knowledge or skill to serve as educators and teach the medical components of the new role.

During my grandmother's era, many nurses were able to obtain an advanced degree after completion of a 3-year hospital-based program. Soon after this time, nurse leaders were successful in requiring that all nurses obtain a baccalaureate degree as the basic prerequisite to pursue an advanced nursing position. We continue to face the redefinition of our educational standards today as contemporary nurse leaders are striving to make a doctorate of nursing practice required for entry into advanced practice nursing. Currently, nurse practitioner certification requires a master's of science degree. Changes in nomenclature have also occurred; those once seeking to become college health nurse practitioners would now likely be enrolled as adult primary care or family nurse practitioner students.

Despite these differences in our education and in our titles, the fundamental emotions Grandma Shea experienced still resonate with me. Like my grandmother, I feel excitement in learning a new role and immense gratitude for the support of respected mentors. Although I often feel overwhelmed by the vast amount of knowledge I must acquire, I am always reassured by remembering to return to a solid commitment to patient care—just as my grandmother did. The symbol of starting from a cocoon and growing into a butterfly is an apt metaphor for each individual nurse practitioner student. Likewise, this metamorphosis appropriately fits the emergence of the role of the nurse practitioner as it has grown in acceptance among the medical population and the general public. We have people such as Sydney Ayotte and my grandmother to thank for preparing the way for subsequent generations of nurse practitioners.

Introduction

On September 21, 2001, the Board of Directors of the Association for the History of Nursing adopted a Position Paper wherein the authors make a substantial argument for the integration of the study of the history of nursing throughout all levels of nursing education. In this work, the authors argue that studying nursing history provides nursing students with a "sense of professional identity, a useful methodological research skill, and a context for evaluating information" (Keeling & Ramos, 1995). Therefore the purpose of this chapter is to provide the reader with a brief overview of the history of American nursing from the middle of the 19th century through present-day nursing practice. Because of the breadth and depth of the history of nursing in the United States, this chapter is not meant to be considered exhaustive but instead will focus on selected highlights and major historical events. Topics include Florence Nightingale's influential nursing practice and the spread of her ideas about nursing education from Britain to the United States; issues surrounding the development of professional and educational standards for nurses; the influence of science and technology on the development of nursing; and the rise of nurse practitioner programs and doctoral education for nurses.

These events and topics did not happen in isolation from the history of medicine and the health care system. Therefore that context is considered, as well as how nursing has shaped—and has been shaped by—a confluence of factors. Nursing has indeed evolved over the course of more than 150 years since the inception of the first Nightingale schools in the United States, but it has not done so without significant challenges along the way. In fact, many of these challenges persist today: issues surrounding gender, race, socioeconomic status, educational requirements for entry into practice, professional licensure, pandemic disease, war, and nursing shortages.

Historically, women have been recognized as belonging to the gender charged with providing physical care to those who are sick or injured. Women's role in society as mothers and caregivers coincided with their domestic duties and was accepted as a natural extension of the homemaker role. To assist mid–19th-century women with their caretaker role, Florence Nightingale published *Notes on Nursing: What It Is and What It Is Not*. In the preface of this book, first published in 1859, Nightingale explained that her notes on nursing were "meant simply to give hints for thought to women who have personal charge of the health of others. Every woman … or at least almost every woman has, at one time or another of her life, charge of the personal health of somebody, whether child or invalid—in other words, every woman is a nurse" (Nightingale, 1859, p. 8). Although more than 150 years have passed since Nightingale wrote her book, and today's nurses are professionals, many of her notes on nursing continue to be relevant to contemporary nursing practice.

The Historical Evolution of Nursing

THE BEGINNING OF NURSING TRAINING PROGRAMS

Florence Nightingale is well known for her work during the Crimean War (1853 to 1856). Her wartime experience shaped her ideas about the value of the trained nurse and was later the impetus for the creation of the Nightingale Training School for Nurses at St. Thomas's Hospital in London in 1860. Just as Nightingale's work in the Crimea was an impetus for instituting a training school for nurses in England, the provision of nursing care by American women during the United States Civil War (1861 to 1865) demonstrated the effectiveness of skilled nursing on improving outcomes for sick and injured soldiers. Women from both the North and South volunteered *en masse* to care for the injured, sick, and dying soldiers in hospitals and infirmaries and on battlefields. Their success in reducing morbidity and mortality in the camps provided evidence that the use of trained nurses could benefit the military and society as a whole. Thus in the years following the war, philanthropic women in the United States devoted their energies to establishing nurse training schools that were based on the Nightingale model (Woolsey, 1950; Dock, 1907).

The apprenticeship model of nursing advocated by Nightingale provided physicians and hospitals with an inexpensive and skilled workforce. It also gave working-class women an opportunity for employment outside the home that was an alternative to factory and domestic work. Skilled nursing also helped reform the care of the sick. In 1873 the first three training schools were established: one at Bellevue Hospital in New York City, one at the Connecticut Hospital in New Haven, and one at Massachusetts General Hospital in Boston. In exchange for 2 to 3 years of intense work, pupil nurses acquired the necessary knowledge and skills to find employment as graduate private duty nurses following graduation. In addition, working-class women who graduated from these programs quickly acquired an elevated social status as a "trained nurse."

In 1873 fewer than 200 hospitals existed in the entire United States. In a relatively short time, training schools gained in popularity, and by 1900 the United States had 432 such schools (Roberts, 1954). By 1910 there were more than 4000 hospitals in existence (Melosh, 1982). The training in these hospital-based schools was arduous, requiring long days of patient service. Classes were held at the end of the day on the wards. Aside from patient care, students' duties included housekeeping, meal preparation, and assisting physicians. A 1902 textbook of nursing describes

the relationship between physicians and nurses during this era: "To the doctor, the first duty [of the nurse] is that of obedience—absolute fidelity to his orders, even if the necessity of the prescribed measures is not apparent to you. You have no responsibility beyond that of faithfully carrying out the directions received" (Weeks-Shaw, 1902, p. 4).

NURSING SUPERINTENDENTS AND THE BEGINNING OF PROFESSIONALISM THROUGH ORGANIZATION

Obedience to the physician and long days on the wards did not create an environment conducive to learning, nor did it promote nursing as a profession. Superintendents of nursing, responsible for student learning within nurse training schools, expressed their concern about the demands on students to staff

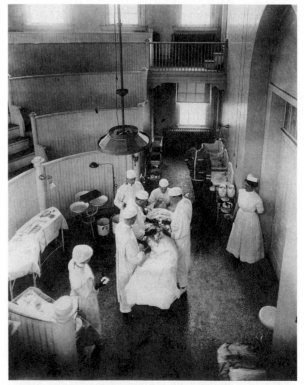

FIGURE 1-1 1913 Operating room, University of Virginia. (Courtesy Center for Nursing Historical Inquiry, The University of Virginia, School of Nursing, Charlottesville, VA.)

hospitals. In 1893 Isabel Hampton, Superintendent of the Johns Hopkins Hospital School of Nursing, assembled superintendents of America's largest schools at the World's Fair in Chicago to discuss nursing education problems. Discussions among these women resulted in a movement to raise and standardize the training of nurses (Billings & Hurd, 1894).

In January 1894 these superintendents created the Society of Superintendents of Training Schools for Nurses of the United States and Canada (later renamed the National League for Nursing Education [NLNE] in 1912). The goals of the Society of Superintendents were "to promote fellowship of members, to establish and maintain a universal standard of training, and to further the best interests of the nursing profession" (American Society of Superintendents of Training Schools for Nurses, 1897, p. 4). Along with the difficulties nursing superintendents faced with the education of nurses, data released by the national census revealed to the public that there were almost 109,000 "untrained nurses and midwives competing with 12,000 graduate nurses," for nursing positions (U.S. Bureau of Census, 1900, p. xxiii). While the NLNE was concerned with the educational standards for nurses, the Nurses' Associated Alumnae of the United States and Canada (renamed the American Nurses Association [ANA] in 1912) focused on achieving legal recognition for trained nurses.

To protect the public from nurses who lacked formal training, the Nurses' Associated Alumnae began to pursue legal registration for trained nurses. Superintendent Isabel Hampton argued in support of this measure, because at that time a trained nurse meant "… anything, everything, or next to nothing" (Hampton, 1893/1949, p. 5). Securing legal recognition was seen as a way to counter the prevailing belief in society that "an ignorant woman, who was not fit for anything else, is good enough for a nurse" (Draper, 1893/1949, p. 151). The Nurses' Associated Alumnae, composed of alumnae associations from schools of nursing, quickly moved to establish associated state organizations so that nurses could undertake the necessary political lobbying for the enactment of state registration laws. Their mission was to "strengthen the union of nursing organizations, to elevate nursing education, [and] to promote ethical standards" for the profession

(Nurses' Associated Alumnae, 1902, p. 766). The two substantive issues that concerned this group were the establishment and maintenance of a journal, the *American Journal of Nursing*, and securing state registration for nurses. The latter was of major importance because it "would achieve legal recognition of nursing as a profession and provide a means for distinguishing trained nurses from those who purported to be but whose preparation for the practice of nursing fell short of standards (Daisy, 1996, p. 35).

The efforts of the Associated Alumnae resulted in nursing registration legislation in March 1903 in North Carolina, followed by New Jersey, New York, and Virginia later that same year. These acts defined for the public that a "registered nurse" had attended an acceptable nursing program and passed a board evaluation examination. Still lacking, however, were universal educational standards and an agreed-upon definition of professional nursing practice. Following the enactment of nurse licensure, leaders of the profession created state nursing boards and empowered them to use their legal authority to protect the public from unfit nurses. Ironically, women who lacked the legal right to vote in 1910 aided 27 states in enacting nurse registration laws. By 1923 all the states in the nation, along with Hawaii and the District of Columbia, possessed nurse registration laws (Bullough, 1975). Although many nursing leaders praised the accomplishment of the passing of registration laws for nurses, Annie Goodrich, Inspector of Nurses Training Schools for the New York State Education Department (and later dean of the Yale School of Nursing), noted that the boards were "conspicuously weak and inefficient in every state" (Goodrich, 1912, p. 1001).

NURSING PRACTICE IN EARLY 20TH-CENTURY AMERICA

Employment opportunities for graduate nurses in the early 20th century were, for the most part, limited to caring for ill persons in their own homes; hospitals were seen as places to care for those who had no one else to care for them. Nursing students staffed the hospital, under the direction of the head nurse, who was usually a training school graduate. Therefore after graduation, graduates eagerly donned their white uniforms, caps, and nursing pins and joined a "registry," allowing them to practice as private duty nurses in patients' homes. Nurse registries, operated by hospitals, professional organizations, or private businesses, provided sites where the public could acquire the services of these private duty nurses. Families could contract for the services of a nurse for a day or a few hours to care for their loved ones either at home or in the hospital (Whelan, 2005). Although physicians' orders were required, private duty in the home provided graduate nurses with the venue and the opportunity to break away from the rigid hospital routine and allowed for a more autonomous practice. These nurses provided care to patients with contagious diseases such as pneumonia and typhoid fever, aided women in childbirth, and supported those with fractures, infected wounds, strokes, and mental diseases. Private duty nurses lived with and worked for their patients, providing 24-hour care, often for weeks at a time (Stoney, 1919).

Private duty nurses were usually employed only by middle- and upper-class households. Graduate nurses were generally pleased with their role as private duty nurses, but their employment was seasonal and sporadic. Because of the onslaught of contagious diseases in the cold months of the year, winters were busy and summers slow. Average annual income of a private duty nurse in the late 1910s was approximately $950, a sum that sustained her but left little savings for future needs (Reverby, 1987). Nonetheless, the trend toward private duty prevailed. By the 1920s, 70% to 80% of graduates worked in private duty.

During the early 20th century, however, new medical discoveries led the public to hospitals for the latest in scientific care. Hospitals could provide blood and urine tests and x-rays, as well as perform surgery in modern surgical amphitheaters equipped with anesthetics (Howell, 1996). To deal with the increasing hospital census in the 1920s, nursing superintendents were pressured to admit more students into school programs. In turn, the increase of nursing students resulted in an increase of graduate nurses, thus creating a surplus. In 1926 the ANA and NLNE grew concerned about the economic plight of graduate nurses and authorized a comprehensive study of the working conditions of graduate nurses. The study, later known as the *Burgess Report,* documented that registered nurses faced widespread underemployment and harsh working conditions (Burgess, 1928). Another survey, conducted by Janet Geister, underscored the private duty nurses' economic plight. According to Geister, 80% of nurses' patient cases lasted only 1 day. This level of employment earned them approximately $31.26 a week, or 49 cents an hour—less than the income of scrubwomen, who earned 50 cents an hour (Geister, 1926). A few years later, with the collapse of the stock market and the subsequent economic depression that enveloped the country, even the lowest-paying jobs for private duty nurses disappeared. Private duty nursing became a "luxury" few could afford. This combined with the fact that patients preferred the scientific medical care offered in hospitals created a gloomy occupation outlook for private duty nurses.

Despite the increasing complexity of hospital work, administrators and physicians simply could not justify hiring large numbers of graduate nurses when they had an inexpensive nursing student workforce readily available. Employing registered nurses would increase overhead costs immensely; moreover, physicians were afraid that graduate nurses would get involved with decision making in the hospital. As noted by one physician-hospital administrator, nursing was "only a differentiation of domestic duty" and the graduate nurse a "half-baked social product thrust into the fulfillment of an uncertain social need" (Howard, 1912). Although private duty nurses outnumbered other professional nurses, and many were members of the ANA Private Duty Nurses Section, they lacked leaders at both the national and state levels. Without leaders, private duty nurses failed to unite or develop effective strategies to upgrade their clinical standards or improve their economic conditions. However, many private duty nurses, who diligently upgraded their medical knowledge and skills, did achieve individual distinction and respect in their communities. These nurses fared much better economically than other graduates because physicians and families requested their services. For most graduates, however, job opportunities would not improve until the late 1930s when hospitals began to add registered nurses to their staffs (Roberts, 1954).

SOCIAL REFORM THROUGH COMMUNITY HEALTH NURSING

During the same time period in which nursing was establishing itself, the United States was undergoing social changes that would also affect the profession. Urbanization, industrialization, and the influx of European immigrants, especially into the northeastern section of the country, soon resulted in overcrowded tenement slums, filthy streets, and poor working conditions. Communicable diseases ran rampant. One young nurse, Lillian Wald, saw the conditions in New York City as her opportunity to care for the poor and to establish a role for nursing in the community. According to Wald, the needs of these New York City residents were limitless.

There were nursing infants, many of them with the summer bowel complaint that sent infant mortality soaring during the hot months; there were children with measles, not quarantined; there were children with ophthalmia, a contagious eye disease; there were children scarred with vermin bites; there were adults with typhoid; there was a case of puerperal septicemia, lying on a vermin-infested bed without sheets or pillow cases; a family consisting of a pregnant mother, a crippled child and two others living on dry bread ...; a young girl dying of tuberculosis amid the very conditions that had produced the disease (Wald, quoted in Duffus, 1938, p. 43).

Thus in 1895 Wald and her colleague Mary Brewster founded the Henry Street Settlement House and Henry Street Visiting Nurse Services (Wald, 1938; Keeling, 2007). Wald's work promoting health and preventing disease made an enormous impact on the lives of the poverty-stricken immigrants on New York City's Lower East Side. The visiting nurses' work quickly expanded to new services, including school nursing, industrial nursing, tuberculosis nursing, and infant welfare nursing. Later, Wald joined forces with the Metropolitan Life Insurance Company to send nurses into the homes of the company's customers when they became ill (Struthers, 1917; Hamilton, 1989). In 1912 Wald founded the National Organization for Public Health Nursing (NOPHN)—nursing's first specialty organization. That year there were approximately 3000 public health nurses working throughout the

United States (Gardner, 1936). The major goals of NOPHN were to develop adequate numbers of public health nurses to meet the needs of the public and to link the emerging field of public health nursing to preventive medicine (Brainard, 1922).

The creation of the federally based Children's Bureau, also in 1912, as well as the passage of the Maternal and Infant Act (Sheppard-Towner) in 1921, reflected the federal government's growing concern for the health of women and children. Public health nurses served as the backbone of this program as they traveled to remote areas in their states to bring clinics and health services to those most in need. Although the federal programs experienced opposition, especially from physicians, in the 8 years of their existence, the programs demonstrated the effectiveness of nurses in the screening of ill patients and referring those patients to physicians. The programs also brought health education to thousands of American families (Meckel, 1990).

The development of community health nursing was important to the nation and to the nursing profession because it brought essential health services to the public. It also provided nurses with unique opportunities to integrate epidemiological knowledge and sanitation practices—as well as medical science—into the care and education of the public. Community nurses, using their hospital training, expanded the domain of nursing practice to include individuals, families, and communities. Their pioneering activities in health promotion and disease prevention, along with their stand on health and welfare issues, have proven vital in shaping America's health system and the discipline of nursing (Bullough & Bullough, 1978).

THE NURSE'S ROLE IN WAR

As noted earlier, during the American Civil War (1861 to 1865), both the Union and the Confederate leaders sought the services of women to care for sick and wounded soldiers. Providing aid through Ladies' Aid societies and the U.S. Sanitary Commission, numerous white middle-class women volunteered to nurse. In the South, many elite women brought along their black female slaves to help, and throughout the Confederacy hundreds of black men (both slave and free)

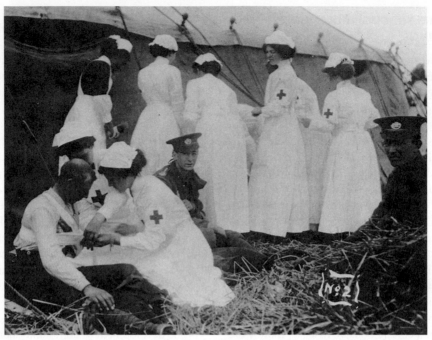

FIGURE 1-2 Nursing in World War I. (Courtesy Center for Nursing Historical Inquiry, The University of Virginia, School of Nursing, Charlottesville, VA.)

also served. In addition, Catholic nuns and Lutheran deaconesses provided care to the soldiers. However, there were no trained nurses and no military nurses at this time. In 1898, during the Spanish-American War, trained nurses volunteered to serve in the army to care for soldiers suffering from yellow fever. This experience helped to convince military physicians and Congress that trained female nurses should become permanent members of the nation's defense forces. It set the stage for the creation of the Army Nurse Corps in 1901 and the Navy Nurse Corps in 1908 (Sarnecky, 1999).

Both the Army Nurse Corps and the Navy Nurse Corps would serve in the Great War during the next decade. Although the United States' formal involvement in World War I (1917 to 1919) was short, it was important in documenting the ability of trained nurses to work effectively in war. Nursing leaders cooperated with the federal government in a major recruitment and mobilization campaign to remedy the profound shortage of nursing personnel that existed in the spring of 1917. As part of that effort, the American Red Cross,

led by Jane Delano, conducted an ambitious campaign to draw women into the war effort. Meanwhile, nursing leaders debated the issue of who was qualified to serve in the war. In the existing environment of patriotic fervor, many women of higher society, as well as numerous minimally trained nurses' aides, wished to serve by performing the work of trained nurses; however, leaders of the nursing profession insisted on the use of properly trained nurses. A dual solution was reached: the creation of an innovative program at Vassar College and the establishment of an Army School of Nursing, both designed to increase the supply of trained nurses for the military (Clappison, 1964). During the war, even those who were properly trained faced extreme challenges. Tested by harsh conditions on the European front, severe nursing shortages, and the occurrence of a devastating influenza pandemic, white female nurses demonstrated their effectiveness (Telford, 2007). Because of the segregated nature of American society at the time, black nurses, both male and female, were for the most part, denied the opportunity to participate.

HOSPITALS BECOME BUSINESSES

After World War I, hospitals continued to grow in both number and size. Between 1925 and 1929, $890 million was spent on the construction of hospitals. Modern obstetrics, with its promise of "twilight sleep" to reduce the pain of childbirth, brought women, who previously had their babies at home, into hospitals. The addition of pediatric, psychiatric, and physical therapy services, as well as private patient rooms, enhanced the hospital's image and attracted thousands of new patients into hospitals (Roren, 1930). Indeed, the early 20th-century saw America's appreciation of the benefits of scientific medicine (Howell, 1996). Many new hospitals were erected, and the social and economic status of staff physicians and hospital directors increased. Nursing educators, on the other hand, continued their long struggle to convince hospitals that graduate nurses, rather than nursing students, should be responsible for patients' care. This struggle continued even after the Goldmark Report revealed shocking deficiencies in the education of nursing students (Goldmark, 1923).

It would take the profound national emergency caused by the stock market crash of 1929 and the subsequent economic depression of the 1930s to change the situation. Indeed, the economic depression that gripped the country drastically altered the life of Americans. The sharp decline in the world's economy caused serious financial, social, and health problems for the nation. Business failures and unemployment spread; by 1932, 25% of working Americans had lost their jobs (Blum, 1981). The Social Security Act of 1935, with its financial aid for the elderly and its Title V health care benefits for disabled children, extended the government's mandate for the well-being of its citizens. Meanwhile, as fewer and fewer patients were able to pay for health care services, hospital administrators were forced to examine the costs of providing care. The cost of maintaining nursing schools proved too expensive for many small hospitals, and 570 training programs were closed during the decade (Roberts, 1954). To keep the remaining nursing schools intact, their budgets were seriously curtailed and students' education was further compromised. At the same

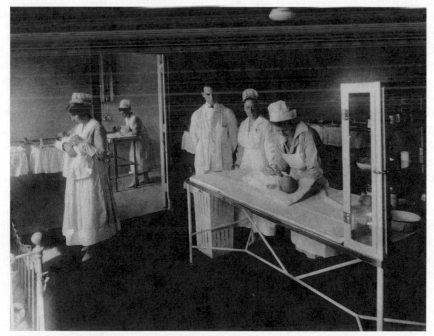

FIGURE 1-3 Newborn nursery, Columbia Women's Hospital, Washington, D.C. (Courtesy Center for Nursing Historical Inquiry, The University of Virginia, School of Nursing, Charlottesville, VA.)

time, large hospitals, especially municipal hospitals, experienced a large influx of patients seeking charitable care. In the mid-1930s, to help rectify hospitals' serious economic distress, hospital administrators developed Blue Cross, a revolutionary prepaid health insurance plan (Numbers, 1978). Selling health plans to workers able to pay for future hospitalizations proved to be an engaging idea because it helped to ensure the financial stability of hospitals that became Blue Cross associates. The public was demanding hospital care, and Blue Cross could pay for it.

Members of the American Medical Association (AMA), however, rejected the new Blue Cross health plan, characterizing it as "economically unsound, unethical and inimical to the public interests" (Kimball, 1934, p. 45). In spite of the AMA's opposition, Blue Cross proved to be attractive to patients and hospitals, and because it filled the beds of hospitals with paying patients, it was formally endorsed by the American Hospital Association in 1937. As a hospital official noted, "Blue Cross was sired by the Depression and mothered by hospitals out of desperate economic necessity" (Sommers & Sommers, 1961). Despite the opposition of many physicians, more than 1 million people participated as members of Blue Cross in 1937, providing hospitals with adequate incomes to remain open and to plan for their futures.

As the economy slowly improved in the late 1930s, training school costs continued to be viewed as a burden to hospital budgets. Hospitals that closed their schools substituted untrained attendants for student workers, but it soon became evident, especially to physicians, that additional staff graduate nurses were needed to provide patients with safe and effective nursing care. This recognition, coupled with the availability of unemployed graduate nurses willing to work for minimum wages and the new sources of income from health insurance and government relief programs, encouraged administrators to add graduate nurses to their staffs gradually (Fitzpatrick, 1975). The increase of registered nurses on hospital staffs—from 4000 positions in 1929 to 28,000 in 1937 and to more than 100,000 by 1941—helped improve the quality of patient services. Paradoxically, graduate nursing staffs also introduced a new professional tension within the hospital system (Cannings & Lazonick, 1975).

Hospital administrators, accustomed to a docile and inexpensive student workforce, considered graduate nursing services costly and only partially necessary. In addition, registered nurses were seen as potential threats to administrators and physicians because they were far less compliant than students, and their clinical judgments were based on their professional knowledge and experiences rather than hospital routines.

Registered nurses, although welcoming the steady hospital employment and the opportunity to develop new clinical skills, experienced professional conflicts when they worked as staff nurses. As independent, private duty nurses, they had possessed the power to give the quality of care they believed patients needed. Now, as staff members, they were part of a bureaucracy that demanded loyalty to the hospital itself and staff physicians rather than to patients. The hospitals' employment of subsidiary nursing and housekeeping staff added managerial tasks to their responsibilities. For many nurses these new tasks were not considered in the sphere of nursing, and the strict institutional control of their clinical practice reminded them of the exploitation, harsh discipline, and regimentation they had experienced in their training schools (Flood, 1981).

Given the economic realities of the Depression, graduate nurses and hospitals began an uneasy working alliance. Learning how to interact successfully with professional graduates rather than a student workforce challenged hospital administrators and nursing superintendents for decades. Hospitals struggled to establish personnel policies that befitted professional nurses. For years hospitals offered registered nurses "low pay, long hours, split shifts, authoritarian supervision, and rigid rules" (Reverby, 1987, p. 192). Nonetheless, hospitals became the major employers of nurses by the 1950s. As such, they gained the power to set nursing wages and working conditions and often thwarted nurses in their quest for adequate compensation and the right to participate in hospital decisions regarding patient care (Reverby, 1987). Likely fueled by their lack of autonomy and their plight as subservient members of a hierarchical hospital system, nurses identified education as a potential pathway to leadership.

COLLEGIATE NURSING EDUCATION: THE EARLY YEARS

Although nursing training was firmly entrenched in hospital schools of nursing, many believed that the profession's superintendents, faculty, and public health nurses must have postgraduate education in institutions of higher learning. As early as 1899, Teachers College at Columbia University offered a post-diploma hospital economics program. Mary Adelaide Nutting and Isabel Stewart directed this program and offered innovative programs in administration, education, and public health nursing to thousands of nurses from the United States and abroad (Christy, 1969).

The first permanent undergraduate university nursing program in the United States was established at the University of Minnesota in 1909. Students found the investments of time and finances prohibitive; thus enrollment in these institutions remained extremely low compared with diploma programs. By 1923, only 17 collegiate schools nationwide offered 5-year degree programs. Although the profession had made some progress toward collegiate status, it still lacked the social endorsement and financial support that had paved the way for medical education to move into universities. Indeed, medical education experienced a very different trajectory from nursing. Large financial endowments, primarily from the Rockefeller, Carnegie, and Commonwealth foundations, had propelled medical education into the mainstream of university education. Data from the famous 1910 Abraham Flexner Report had demonstrated inadequacies in medical education, acting as a catalyst for reform. The Rockefeller General Education Board alone funneled more than $91 million into medical schools (Starr, 1982). Although nursing leaders sought similar assistance for nursing education. only the Rockefeller Foundation was persuaded to endow the establishment of two university-based nursing schools—Yale in 1924 and Vanderbilt in 1930 (Abram, 1993). Annie Goodrich, a noted nursing educator, directed the first independent nursing collegiate school at Yale University. This baccalaureate program was based on the premise that nursing concepts pertinent to acute illness, the psychosocial dimensions of illness, and public health principles were essential to professional nurses (Sheahan, 1979).

By 1935 sufficient numbers of collegiate programs provided the catalyst for the organization of the Association of Collegiate Schools of Nursing, an organization whose mission was to establish collegiate nursing programs in American universities. Its early members strongly maintained that nursing could not develop into a profession until it could generate scientifically sound nursing knowledge that could sustain the practice of nursing (Stewart, 1943). Although this group later disbanded, in 1969 a small group of deans of collegiate and university programs established the Conference of Deans of Colleges and University Schools of Nursing, known today as the American Association of Colleges of Nursing (Keeling, Kirchgessner, & Brodie, 2009). The AACN continues to play a vital role in nursing education, research, and health policy. Ironically, though, nursing continues to allow many pathways into practice and has yet to reach a consensus about the educational qualifications needed by entry-level practicing nurses.

WORLD WAR II

The United States' entry into World War II in 1941 immediately increased the demand for skilled nurses to care for sick and injured soldiers, while the supply of nurses needed to meet the nation's military and civilian needs remained inadequate. To meet the increased demands, the federal government created two new programs: the American Red Cross volunteer nurse's aides program (1941) and the Cadet Nurse Corps in 1943 (Johnston, 1966). The loss of professional and nonprofessional staff to the military and defense industry left hospitals and public health agencies in need of auxiliary help to care for citizens at home. Through a joint venture with the Office of Civilian Defense and the American Red Cross, more than 200,000 women volunteered to become certified nurse's aides and work under nursing supervision to provide nursing services. This venture proved to be an important step in the stratification of nursing into registered, practical, and aide levels, which still exists today. Its success encouraged hospitals to continue to use auxiliary nursing personnel after the war to ease the nation's postwar shortage of nurses (Bullough & Bullough, 1978).

In 1943 Frances Payne Bolton, a congresswoman from Ohio, sponsored a bill that authorized the U.S. Public Health Service to establish the Cadet Nurse Corps. This was the most significant federally sponsored program to increase the supply of professional nurses in the 1940s. The bill subsidized the education of students who agreed, upon graduation, to serve in military or civilian health agencies for the duration of the war. Students were provided tuition, fees, and books, plus a monthly stipend throughout their training. Participating schools also received funds for instructional facilities and postgraduate education for their nursing faculty.

Although the cadet corps accepted students for only 2 years (July 1943 to October 1945), almost 170,000 cadets entered 1125 participating schools, and two thirds of them graduated. The program recruited a large number of graduates to the profession and led to major changes in nursing education. The government's requirements of a modified program, including removing policies that discriminated on the basis of race and marital status, allowed an opportunity to redesign nursing education. In addition, because nursing school directors rather than hospital administrators were required to administer the federal funds, the actual costs of the nursing program and the services provided to hospitals by students became known. Armed with this information, nursing directors were better equipped to negotiate with administrators for funds to upgrade their programs after the war (Brueggemann, 1992).

AFRICAN AMERICAN AND MALE NURSES

Unlike their predecessors, nursing leaders during World War II attempted to remedy the shortage of nursing personnel by employing people belonging to two groups that had been previously excluded from mainstream nursing: men and African American women. Since their inception in the late 19th century, most nursing schools had excluded men and African American women from admission, based on discriminatory and restrictive policies. To ensure that African American patients received medical care and that

African American physicians and nurses had opportunities to become professionals, separate African American hospitals and schools were created in the late 1800s (Gamble, 1989). African American graduates of these programs faced further discrimination as registered nurses because many hospitals and community health agencies refused to employ them, citing objections from white patients to being cared for by African American nurses. African American nurses faced additional discrimination when they attempted to join most of the state associations of the ANA. To overcome such overt and covert forms of discrimination, the National Association of Colored Graduate Nurses (NACGN) was formed in 1908. The NACGN fought valiantly for almost 50 years to end the social, economic, and professional injuries inflicted on African American graduate nurses (Staupers, 1951).

The bias against male nurses was based on society's belief that nursing was a feminine skill and therefore men should not be nurses (O'Lynn & Tranbarger, 2007). Although a few nursing schools were coeducational, most male nurses attended all-male programs sponsored by religious groups or affiliated with psychiatric hospitals. Many hospitals were willing to hire male graduate nurses but often treated them as orderlies rather than as nursing professionals (Craig, 1940).

Stirred by patriotism, many young African American women entered the Cadet Nurse Corps because that program prohibited discrimination based on race. African American nurses, denied entry into the military, were recruited to work in white hospitals to fill the vacancies of white nurses who had left for war (Hine, 1989). Throughout the war, the Army Nurse Corps maintained restrictive racial quotas, and the Navy Nurse Corps excluded all African Americans. These restrictions, combined with the willingness of Congress to consider drafting nurses in 1944, turned public opinion against the armed services' discriminatory policies. As a result, in January 1945, both corps lifted their racial restrictions and accepted African American female nurses.

Male nurses, however, faced a more entrenched form of military discrimination than did their African American female nurse counterparts. Tradition and sentiment had long dictated that nursing was a woman's field, and Congress, in establishing the nurse corps, ruled that only women could be appointed as military nurses. Male nursing students and graduates were subject to the Selective Service Act draft, and most volunteered for military service rather than wait to be drafted. Although their military assignments varied, male nurses were denied professional nursing status, but most served as enlisted personnel in health-related positions (Rose, 1947). Congress did not pass legislation that allowed the appointment of male nurses as reserve officers in the Army, Navy, and Air Force Nurse Corps until 1955, after the Korean conflict (Sarnecky, 1999).

When World War II came to an end, the presence of many more African American registered nurses, many of whom were graduates of the Cadet Nurse Corps, caused many nursing state nurses associations to remove racial barriers to membership. General integration into the ANA was hastened in 1948, when its House of Delegates granted individual membership to African American nurses barred from their state associations and called for the establishment of biracial integration at district and state levels. In 1950 only two state associations retained racial restrictions,

allowing the NACGN to announce its dissolution. By 1952 all state nurses associations had removed racial restrictions for ANA membership. Unfortunately, the end of overt professional discrimination against African American nurses and male nurses did not eradicate the more subtle and entrenched forms of prejudice. For black nurses the struggle to be fully accepted as professionals by patients, hospitals, and fellow heath care colleagues continued to be a problem. This deep-seated discrimination led to the emergence of the National Black Nurses Association in 1971. As was its predecessor (the NACGN), the National Black Nurses Association is committed to acting as an advocate for improvement of the health care of blacks and removing the barriers against black nurses so that they might fully participate in the profession and the health care system (Carnegie, 1995).

POST–WORLD WAR II ERA

America emerged from World War II profoundly changed as a people, society, and country. After years of war, with its rationing of resources and lack of

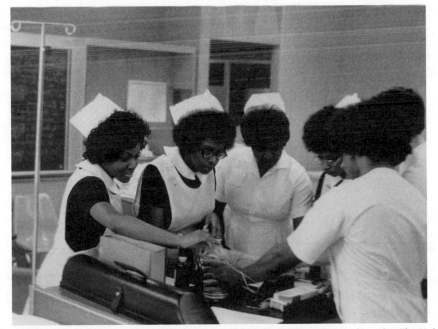

FIGURE 1-4 University of Virginia nursing students, 1971. (Courtesy Center for Nursing Historical Inquiry, The University of Virginia, School of Nursing, Charlottesville, VA.)

individual choices, Americans wanted better lives for themselves and their families, including health care and educational opportunities. In response to citizens' needs, the federal government formulated new health priorities and policies and funded health initiatives. One of the first of these was the Hospital Survey and Reconstruction Act (the Hill-Burton Act) of 1946, which began to provide federal funds for hospital construction and new health centers. For years these funds significantly expanded and updated the nation's hospitals, increased bed capacity, and transformed hospitals into scientific and technical medical centers (Risse, 1999).

The public's growing trust in the power of modern medicine was sustained by impressive advances in pharmacology, medicine, and surgery. Penicillin, one of the earliest "miracle drugs," successfully treated serious infections and, in preventing postoperative infections, it opened the door to radically new surgical procedures. The dramatic advances in pharmacology, medical sciences, and technology enticed health professionals and patients alike to believe in the possibility that humans might conquer all diseases. The public encouraged the federal government to continue its large appropriations for medical research, education, and services (Stevens, 1989).

Post–World War II Nursing Shortages. The nation's demand for nurses increased dramatically after World War II, as 78 million children were born between 1946 and 1964 (eventually known as *baby boomers*). This phenomenon was coupled with a rise in chronic disease among a growing elderly population. Unfortunately, although hospitals were now recipients of massive federal financial aid and patients with health insurance were seeking admission, administrators were forced to restrict admissions because of a severe shortage of registered nurses. Initiatives to remedy the nursing shortage focused primarily on acquiring more nurses, rather than on creating ways to improve the education of nurses (Lynaugh & Brush, 1996). Other strategies to decrease the urgency posed by the nursing shortage included many of the same methods used today, including employing ward clerks, practical nurses, and aides to help nurses provide patient care; changing the way that patient care was

given (team nursing was initiated); importing foreign nurses; and attempting to improve nurses' salaries and working conditions.

Federal funding for nursing education remained modest until 1964, when Congress enacted the Nurse Training Act, in response to pressure from the American Medical Association and the American Hospital Association about the need for nurses. This landmark legislation awarded $242.6 million for nursing student scholarships, loans, recruitment, school construction and maintenance, and special educational projects (Kalisch & Kalisch, 1995). The success of the many initiatives helped diminish the nation's shortages of nurses. Between 1950 and 1967 the number of registered nurses rose by 67%, the number of practical nurses rose by 134%, and the number of nursing aides/assistants rose by 244% (U.S. Public Health Service, 1976).

Nursing in Institutions of Higher Education

BACCALAUREATE PROGRAMS

In addition to other legislation after the war, in 1946 Congress passed the GI Bill of Rights, enabling veterans to acquire vocational training or a college education (Kiester, 1994). Nurse veterans took advantage of the opportunity to enroll in college programs and earned degrees in nursing education and administration. The increased enrollment gave a new direction to collegiate nursing programs. Beginning in the 1950s, entry-level baccalaureate nursing programs were opened to high school graduates throughout the nation. In 1962, 178 colleges offered undergraduate degrees in nursing, and the pool of baccalaureate-educated nurses, essential to the creation of advanced nursing educational programs, had dramatically expanded (Brown, 1978).

COMMUNITY COLLEGE PROGRAMS

The severity of the nursing shortage in the postwar years encouraged faculty to develop new entry-level nursing programs. In 1951 nurse educator Mildred Montag proposed a new program to prepare nurse technicians in 2-year associate degree (AD) community colleges. After completing a 5-year study of these graduates, the program was deemed successful because the AD graduates were able to pass state nursing licensure examinations, demonstrated an adequate level of clinical nursing competency, and were employed as graduate nurses (Haase, 1990). The results of this study launched the AD educational movement. Securing funding from the Nurse Training Act of 1964, community colleges opened AD programs at a phenomenal rate. From 1952 to 1974, the number of AD programs in the country doubled every 4 years. During one period, new programs opened at the rate of one per week (Rines, 1977).

Several important goals were attained by the AD programs' success. A new pool of students, including men, married women with children, and older-than-typical undergraduates, were now able to choose nursing careers. The AD graduates helped minimize the nursing shortages of the 1970s and 1980s; this encouraged hospital directors to close their expensive programs and let colleges and universities educate nurses. Soon diploma education disappeared in most states (Lynaugh & Brush, 1996). Today AD programs are the major point of entry into nursing; as reflected by a recent survey of nursing programs and graduates, AD programs prepared more graduates than did the combined baccalaureate and diploma programs (National League for Nursing, 2003). Although AD education opened nursing education to a broader student population, the existence of three entry-level educational programs—diploma, associate, and baccalaureate degree, all leading to registered nurse licensure and beginning positions—has led to confusion among the public and the profession as to the exact requirements for a credential as a professional nurse.

GRADUATE PROGRAMS

In the mid-1950s, the need for nurses prepared at the graduate level to direct nursing service departments and teach in baccalaureate programs encouraged faculty to develop more master's-level programs. These earlier programs focused on preparing educators and administrators rather than clinicians. However, in the 1960s, as the pace of medical innovation increased and new clinical subspecialties such as cardiology, nephrology, and oncology came into existence, master's programs shifted their focus to preparing clinical nurse specialists and nurse practitioners.

Although nurses have earned doctoral degrees since the mid-1920s, most of them acquired their education in related disciplines such as education and sociology. In the late 1960s, aided by funds from the federal government, doctoral nursing programs began to appear (Grace, 1978). Nursing doctoral programs provided the profession the rigorous academic environment it needed to develop its unique disciplinary knowledge and prepare its future researchers and scholars. Questions about the nature of nursing, its mission and goals, and the scope of nurses' roles drove nurse educators in the 1950s to consider the answers to these questions and present them in a more coherent whole. These questions grew out of an interest in changes in the educational preparation of nurses from diploma to baccalaureate programs, as well as concerns about what to include or exclude in curricula and what nurses needed to learn to function as nurses (Meleis, 2004).

To begin to answer questions about the philosophy of nursing, schools and colleges of nursing were incorporated into institutions of higher education devoted to scholarly inquiry and research, including Columbia University Teachers College. Many of the prominent nursing leaders of the 1950s took courses in education and administration at Teachers College. Some of these nursing leaders received a doctoral degree in education (EdD). Teachers College can also be credited with the birth of nursing theory (Omery, Kasper, & Page, 1995). The earliest nursing theories were similar to system and physiologic models. These models reflected the paradigm that was strongly supported by the field of education at the time: the received view of science. Other disciplines considered these tenets to be *one* way of gaining knowledge in the sciences; however, education—and therefore nursing—believed that these tenets were the *only* way. Nurses then adopted this paradigm as truth. This view was not without its problems; as nurses restricted themselves mainly to the use of quantitative methods of inquiry, they simultaneously restricted knowledge development in the discipline (Telford, 2004). Only later did the profession's leaders incorporate other ways of knowing, including clinical expertise, qualitative methods, and others. Further discussion of this topic occurs in Chapter 2.

Rise of Advanced Practice Nursing in Clinical Settings

ACUTE CARE NURSE SPECIALIST

Advances in medical science and technology through the latter half of the 20th century radically changed the practice of medicine and the treatment of hospitalized patients. However, the newly constructed hospitals, with their private rooms and long hallways, caused new problems for an already short-handed nursing staff, as patients could no longer be seen from a central nurses' station. Moreover, many nurses were unskilled and unfamiliar with the new treatments and new technologies. As a result, nurse and physician teams initiated the concept of the intensive care unit (ICU), a large room in which the hospital's most experienced and competent nurses could work with critically ill patients. Within these new units, the care of the critically ill was changed in every hospital in the United States. Their success paved the way for the creation of acute care nurse specialist roles (Fairman & Lynaugh, 1998; Lynaugh & Brush, 1996).

An example of one of these units was the coronary care unit (CCU). Influenced by research on the success of cardiopulmonary resuscitation and cardiac defibrillation, and interested in using electronic monitoring technology for improving the care of cardiac patients, physicians and nurses opened CCUs to manage patients with acute myocardial infarction. Supported by federal appropriations for medical research, CCUs proliferated. Central to the coronary care specialist movement was the nurses' drive toward independent practice, nurse-derived standards of care, and a collegial relationship with the units' physicians. Working together, nurses and physicians shared the emerging clinical knowledge for managing critically ill patients. They mastered new medical technology and wrote standard "order sets," educating nurses to identify changes in cardiac rhythms and to treat patients without waiting for physicians' orders. Gaining acceptance as essential members of the CCU team, nurses stretched

the boundaries of nursing practice and laid the foundation for a more autonomous practice for other master's-prepared nurses (Keeling, 2004).

As these highly specialized nurses realized their need for continuing education, ICU nurses quickly formed national specialty organizations, including the American Association of Cardiovascular Nurses (AACN) in 1969, renamed the American Association of Critical Care Nurses in 1972. These organizations established practice standards and developed continuing education programs and certification for their respective emerging clinical specialties. The success of ICU nurses paved the way for the creation of many subspecialty units (including units for neonatology, burns, renal dialysis, and oncology) and marked a

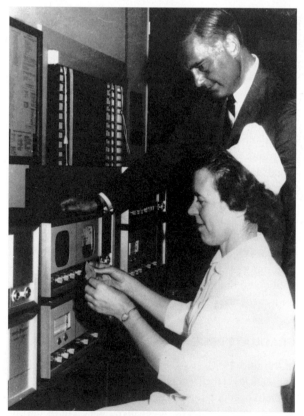

FIGURE 1-5 Rose Pinneo, RN, and Lawrence Meltzer, MD, in the CCU at Presbyterian Hospital in Philadelphia, Pennsylvania, circa 1963. (Courtesy Center for Nursing Historical Inquiry, The University of Virginia, School of Nursing, Charlottesville, VA.)

significant advancement of the discipline (Fairman & Lynaugh, 1998; Keeling, 2004).

PRIMARY CARE NURSE PRACTITIONERS

At the same time that acute care specialist roles were emerging in hospitals, the primary care nurse practitioner movement, which had started with the Frontier Nursing Service in the 1920s, crystallized and "took off" in the community setting (Keeling, 2007). The idea of an advanced practice role for community nurses, the rise of medical specialization, the concurrent shortage of primary care physicians (especially in rural areas), and the public's demand for improved access to health care all helped foster the movement. In 1965 Loretta Ford and Henry Silver opened the first pediatric nurse practitioner program at the University of Colorado. This collaborative project, designed by a nurse and a pediatrician, prepared professional nurses to provide well child care and manage the care of children with common childhood illnesses. Its success would lead to federal funding for the education of nurse practitioners (NPs) in many clinical areas. Similar to acute care specialists, primary care NPs developed organizations that created certification requirements and clinical standards. However, because NPs assumed diagnostic and treatment responsibilities outside the confines of the hospital, they set in place legal certification at the state level and also obtained prescriptive authority (Fairman, 1999; Keeling 2007; Fairman, 2008).

By the 1970s NPs were employed in a variety of primary care settings, including physicians' offices, clinics, and schools. In addition, some practiced in hospitals in subspecialty areas such as nephrology, oncology, and neonatology. In the early 1990s, in response to the growing shortage of medical residents in subspecialty areas and the need to manage patients with increasingly complex medical needs (e.g., heart and lung transplants), acute care nurse practitioner (ACNP) programs began to develop across the nation. Today numerous ACNPs work in acute care hospitals in various subspecialties—some as "nurse hospitalists." In addition, states are beginning to require that NPs have the proper educational requirements (e.g., ACNP versus primary care NP) for the setting in which they hope to practice.

CLINICAL NURSE LEADER AND DOCTOR OF NURSING PRACTICE

The recent development of a new role for nurses, clinical nurse leader (CNL), came about as a response to growing patient care needs and to the changing health care delivery environment. In February 2004, the American Association of Colleges of Nursing Board approved the development of a new model of nursing practice and nursing education at the master's level— the CNL (AACN, 2004). The CNL, a generalist master's-prepared clinician, provides care in all health care settings at the point of care and assumes accountability for client care outcomes by coordinating,

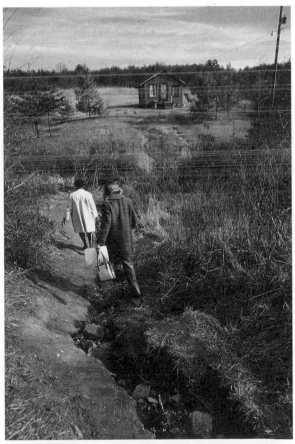

FIGURE 1-6 Nurse practitioner in rural Virginia, circa 1970s. (Courtesy Center for Nursing Historical Inquiry, The University of Virginia, School of Nursing, Charlottesville, VA.)

delegating, and supervising the care provided by the health care team. The CNL is not considered to be an advanced practice nurse. As the education of the generalist nurse is elevated to the master's-degree level, it is reasonable to assume that specialty education and the education of those individuals prepared for the highest level of nursing practice would occur at the doctoral level.

The last several years have seen an increased interest in developing a viable alternative to the research-focused degrees, including the doctor of philosophy (PhD) and the doctor of nursing science (DNS, DNSc, DSN) degrees. The practice-focused doctoral degree programs in nursing, however, are not a recent development. The first such program, offering the doctor of nursing (ND), was established at Case Western Reserve University in 1979 and offered an entry-level nursing degree. Since then, numerous practice-focused doctoral programs have been initiated throughout the country (AACN, 2004). By 2015, it is anticipated that the doctor of nursing practice (DNP) will be the requisite preparation for all advanced practice nursing roles, including the NP, CNS, certified nurse midwife, and certified registered nurse anesthetist (CRNA).

SUMMARY

This chapter provides a brief overview of the progression and advancement of American nursing from the middle of the 19th century to present-day nursing practice. Because of the breadth and depth of the history of nursing in the United States, the chapter is not meant to serve as a definitive discussion of nursing history. Some of the topics covered include Florence Nightingale's influential nursing practice and the way her model for nursing education was adopted in the United States, issues surrounding the development of professional and educational standards for nurses, and the development of nurse practitioner programs and doctoral education for nurses. These events and topics did not happen in isolation; rather they occurred in the context of the development of the practice of medicine and the health care system. Therefore the chapter discusses how nursing was influenced by these events, as well as how nursing has also shaped its own progress. Although it is important to recognize the ways in which nursing has evolved over the course of more than 150 years since the inception of the first Nightingale schools in the United States, this chapter also discusses the challenges the profession has faced. Many of the contentious issues that occurred in the past persist today. Among these are questions of equality of opportunity for all races, genders, and classes and the issue of consensus by the profession's leaders about the educational requirements for entry into practice. The context in which the nursing profession exists is also still a consideration as the world faces the implications of a global society and the challenges of potential pandemic diseases, persistent wars, and continuing nursing shortages. The future of nursing will likely continue to demand nursing care that is innovative, efficient, cost effective, and responsive to human needs in all settings. As in the past, the decisions made by nursing leaders today in response to these forces are already shaping the near future for the profession and influencing the nation's health system. To find the paths that nursing must travel to meet its responsibilities to society in the future, the history of the profession must be carefully examined.

KEY POINTS

- The first hospital-based nurse training schools, built on the apprenticeship model of learning, had the dual task of providing care to patients and educating students to become professional nurses.
- Nursing state licensure, begun in 1903, is important because it protects the public and defines the role and scope of nursing practice.
- Nurses have played a major role in providing essential health services to the community for more than a century, especially for the poor and chronically ill.
- During World War II, the U.S. Public Health Service Cadet Nurse Corps attracted thousands of students to the profession and provided essential nursing services in civilian hospitals.
- Discrimination against men and African American women in nursing has existed for many years.
- Associate degree programs, begun in 1952, opened the nursing profession to a more diverse population than had existed with diploma and baccalaureate education.
- Advanced clinical practice nurses, as acute care nurses and nurse practitioners, expanded the boundaries of the profession.

● Graduate programs prepared nursing educators, directors, clinical specialists, researchers, and administrative leaders needed by the health care system and society. The clinical nurse leader and the doctorate of nursing practice degrees continue to evolve.

CRITICAL THINKING EXERCISES

1. Why do many consider professional nursing less intellectually demanding than medicine?
2. How did community health nursing expand the domain of nursing?
3. How do the education and practice of primary and acute nurse practitioners blur the boundaries between nurses and physicians?
4. How did the federal government influence the development of the nursing profession? What are the positive and negative implications of this influence?
5. Does discrimination against male nurses and ethnic minorities still exist? If so, how does it influence the profession? How does it influence patient care?
6. How has the development of medical and nursing clinical specialization influenced patient care, the professions, and the hospital?

REFERENCES

Abram, S. (1993). Brilliance and bureaucracy: Nursing and changes in the Rockefeller Foundation. 1915–1930. *Nursing History Review, 1,* 119–138.

American Association of Colleges of Nursing (AACN) (2004, October). AACN position statement on the practice doctorate in nursing. 2004, p. 4. Retrieved from http://www.aacn.nche.edu/DNP/DNPPositionStatement.htm.

American Society of Superintendents of Training Schools for Nurses. (1897). *First and second annual reports.* Harrisburg, PA: Harrisburg Publishing.

Billings, J. S., & Hurd, H. M. (Eds.), (1894). *Hospitals, dispensaries, and nursing: Papers and discussions in the International Congress of Charities, Correction and Philanthropy, Section III, Chicago, June 12th to 17th, 1893, Part III, Nursing of the Sick.* Baltimore: Johns Hopkins Press.

Blum, J. (1981). The end of an era. In J. Blum (Ed.), *The national experience* (pp. 652–669). New York: Harcourt Brace Jovanovich.

Brainard, A. (1922). *The evolution of public health nursing.* Philadelphia: Saunders.

Brown, J. (1978). Master's education in nursing, 1945-1969. In M. L. Fitzpatrick (Ed.), *Historical studies in nursing* (pp. 104–130). New York: Teachers College.

Brueggemann, D. (1992). *The United States Cadet Nurse Corps 1943–1948: The Nebraska experience.* Unpublished master's thesis, University of Nebraska at Omaha.

Bullough, B. (1975). The first two phases in nursing licensure. In B. Bullough (Ed.), *The law and the expanding nurse's role* (pp. 7–21). New York: Appleton-Century-Crofts.

Bullough, V., & Bullough, B. (1978). *The care of the sick: The emergence of modern nursing.* New York: Prodist.

Burgess, M. (1928). *Nurses, patients and pocketbooks.* New York: National League for Nursing Education, Committee on the Grading of Nursing Schools.

Cannings, K., & Lazonick, W. (1975). The development of the nursing labor force in the United States: A brief analysis. *International Journal of Health Services, 5,* 185–217.

Carnegie, M. (1995). *The path we tread: Blacks in nursing 1854–1984.* Philadelphia: Jones & Bartlett.

Christy, T. (1969). *Cornerstone for nursing education.* New York: Teachers College.

Clappison, G. B. (1964). *Vassar's rainbow division 1918.* Lake Mills, IA: Graphic Publishing. (Original work published 1918).

Craig, L. (1940). Opportunities for men nurses. *American Journal of Nursing, 40,* 667–670.

Daisy, C. (1996). *Keeping the flame: The influence of Agnes Ohlson on licensure and registration for nurses: 1936-1963.* Unpublished doctoral dissertation.

Dock, L. (1907). *A history of nursing* (Vol. 2). New York: G.P. Putnam's Sons

Draper, E. A. (1893/1949). Necessity of an American Nurses' Association. In J. S. Billings & H. M. Hurd (Eds.), *Nursing of the sick* (pp. 149–153). New York: McGraw-Hill.

Duffus, R. L. (1938). *Lillian Wald, neighbor and crusader* (pp. 40–46). New York: McMillan.

Fairman, J., & Lynaugh, J. (1998). *Critical care nursing: A history.* Philadelphia: University of Pennsylvania.

Fairman, J. (1999). Delegated by default or negotiated by need? Physicians, nurse practitioners, and the process of clinical thinking. *Medical Humanities Review, 13*(1), 38–58.

Fairman, J. (2008). *Making room in the clinic: Nurse practitioners and the evolution of modern health care.* New Brunswick: Rutgers University Press.

Fitzpatrick, M. L. (1975). Nurses in American history: Nursing and the great depression. *American Journal of Nursing, 75,* 2188–2190.

Flood, M. (1981). *The troubling expedient: General staff nursing in United States hospitals in the 1930s: A means to institutional, educational, and personal ends.* Unpublished doctoral dissertation, University of California—Berkeley.

Gamble, V. (1989). *Making a place for ourselves.* New York: Oxford University.

Gardner, M. (1936). *Public health nursing* (3rd ed.). New York: Macmillan.

Geister, J. (1926). Hearsay and fact in private duty. *American Journal of Nursing, 26,* 515–528.

Goldmark, J., & the Committee for the Study of Nursing Education. (1923). *Nursing and nursing education in the United States.* New York: Macmillan.

Goodrich, A. W. (1912). A general presentation of the statutory requirements of the different states. *American Journal of Nursing, Vol. 12,* 1001–1008.

Grace, H. C. (1978). The development of doctoral education in nursing: A historical education perspective. *Journal of Nursing Education, 17,* 17–27.

Haase, P. (1990). *The origins and rise of associate degree nursing education* (pp. 10–35). Durham: Duke University Press.

Hamilton, D. (1989). The cost of caring: The Metropolitan Life Insurance Company's Visiting Nurse Service, 1909-1953. *Bulletin of the History of Medicine, 63,* 414–434.

Hampton, I.A. (1893/1949), Educational standards for nurses. In *Nursing of the sick* (pp. 1–12). New York: McGraw-Hill. Reprinted from Billings, J.S. & Hurd, H.M. (Eds.), (1894). *Hospitals, dispensaries and nursing: Papers and discussions in the International Congress of Charities, Correction and Philanthropy, Section III, Chicago, June 12th to 17th, 1893, Part III, Nursing of the Sick.* Baltimore: Johns Hopkins University Press.

Hine, D. (1989). *Black nurses in white* (pp. 186–192). Bloomington: Indiana University.

Howell, J. (1996). *Technology in the hospital: Transforming patient care in the early twentieth century.* Baltimore: Johns Hopkins University Press.

Howard, H.B. (1912). The medical superintendent (section on hospitals). *American Medical Association Transactions, 76.*

Johnston, D. F. (1966). *History and trends of practical nursing* (pp. 96–98). St. Louis: Mosby.

Kalisch, P., & Kalisch, B. (1995). *The advance of American nursing* (3rd ed.). Philadelphia: Lippincott.

Keeling, A. (2004). Blurring the boundaries between medicine and nursing: Coronary care nursing, 1960s. *Nursing History Review, 12,* 139–164.

Keeling, A. (2007). *Nursing and the privilege of prescription, 1893-2000.* Columbus: Ohio State University Press.

Keeling, A., Kirchgessner, J., & Brodie, B. (2009, in press). *Suite 530, One DuPont Circle: A History of the American Association of Colleges of Nursing.* Washington, DC: AACN.

Keeling, A., & Ramos M. C. (1995). The role of nursing history in preparing nursing for the future. *Nursing and Health Care, 16*(1), 30–34.

Kiester, E. (1994). The GI Bill may be the best deal ever made by Uncle Sam. *Smithsonian, 25*(8), 128–139.

Kimball, J. F. (1934). Prepayment plan of hospital care. *American Hospital Association Bulletin, 8,* 45.

Lynaugh, J., & Brush, B. (1996). *American nursing: From hospitals to health systems.* Cambridge, MA: Blackwell.

Meckel, R. (1990). *Save the babies* (pp. 175–180). Baltimore: Johns Hopkins University Press.

Meleis, A. I. (2004). *Theoretical nursing development & progress.* Philadelphia: Lippincott Williams & Wilkins.

Melosh, B. (1982). *The physician's hand.* Philadelphia: Temple University.

National League for Nursing (2003). Annual Report, 2003. Nursing data review, academic year, 27.

Nightingale, F. (1859). *1860 Notes on nursing: What it is and what it is not* (p. 8). New York: D Appleton and Company.

Numbers, R. (1978). The third party: Health insurance in America. In J. Leavitt, & R. Numbers (Eds.), *Sickness and health in America* (pp. 142–145). Madison, WI: University of Wisconsin.

Nurses' Associated Alumnae of the United States. (1902). Proceedings of the fifth annual convention. *American Journal of Nursing, 3,* 743–809.

O'Lynn, C., & Tranbarger R. E. (Eds.), (2007). *Men in nursing: History, challenges, and opportunities.* New York: Springer.

Omery, A., Kasper, C. E., & Page, G. G. (1995). *In search of nursing science.* Thousand Oaks, CA: Sage.

Reverby, S. (1987). *Ordered to care* (p. 192). New York: Cambridge University.

Rines, A. (1977). Associate degree nursing education: History, development and rationale. *Nursing Outlook, 25,* 496–501.

Risse, G. B. (1999). *Mending bodies, saving souls: History of hospitals.* New York: Oxford University.

Roberts, M. (1954). *American nursing: History and interpretation* (pp. 222–240). New York: Macmillan.

Roren, R. (1930). *The public's investment in hospitals (Committee on the Costs of Medical Care, Publication No. 7).* Chicago: University of Chicago.

Rose, J. (1947). Men nurses in military service. *American Journal of Nursing, 47*, 147–148.

Sarnecky, M. (1999). *History of the Army Nurse Corps.* Philadelphia: University of Pennsylvania.

Sheahan, D. (1979). *The social origins of American nursing and its movement into the university.* Unpublished doctoral dissertation, New York University.

Sommers, H., & Sommers, A. (1961). *Patients and health insurance.* Washington, DC: Brookings Institution.

Starr, P. (1982). *The social transformation of American Medicine.* New York: Basic Books.

Staupers, M. (1951). Story of the NACGN. *American Journal of Nursing, 51*, 221–222.

Stevens, R. (1989). *In sickness and in wealth.* New York: Basic Books.

Stewart, I. (1943). *The education of nurses.* New York: Macmillan.

Stoney, E. (1919). *Practical points in nursing* (pp. 20–23). Philadelphia: Saunders.

Struthers, L. (1917). *The school nurse.* New York: G.P. Putnam's Sons.

Telford, J. (2004). *The liberation of the minds and practices of nurses: The evolution and adoption of the Received View to enlightenment in nursing science, circa 1873-present.* Unpublished doctoral dissertation.

Telford, J. (2007). *American Red Cross nursing during World War I: Opportunities and obstacles.* Unpublished doctoral dissertation.

Taylor, P. (1971). *The distant magnet* (pp. 188–191). London: Eyre & Spottiswoode.

U.S. Bureau of Census. (1900). *Special reports: Occupation roles, and gender* (p. xxiii). Washington, DC: U.S. Government Printing Office.

U.S. Public Health Service. (1976). *The consumer and health planners.* Washington, DC: U.S. Government Printing Office.

Wald, L. (1938). *The house on Henry Street.* New York: Henry Holt.

Whelan, J. (2005). A necessity in the nursing world: Chicago Nurses Professional Registry 1918-1950. *Nursing History Review, 13*, 49–76.

Weeks-Shaw, C. (1902). *A text-book of nursing, for the use of training schools, families, and private students.* New York: Appleton.

Woolsey, A. H. (1950). *A century of nursing, with hints toward the organization of a training school* (originally published 1876), and Florence Nightingale's historic letter on the Bellevue School, September 18, 1872. Hospitals and training schools; report to the Standing Committee on Hospitals of the State Charities Aid Association, New York, May 24, 1876. To which is added: "Founding of the Bellevue Training School for Nurses," Chapter 6 of *Recollections of a Happy Life,* by E. Christophers Hobson (originally published 1916). New York: Putnam.

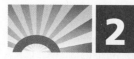

2

Pathways of Nursing Education

JOAN L. CREASIA, PhD, RN
KATHRYN B. REID, PhD, RN

OBJECTIVES

At the completion of this chapter, the reader will be able to:

- Trace the history of nursing education from its inception to the present.
- Compare nursing education programs for similarities and differences.
- Classify nursing education programs according to role preparation, scope of practice, eligibility for licensure, and eligibility for specialty certification.
- Identify and analyze trends in nursing program development, including eligibility for admission, career mobility and advancement opportunities, and program accessibility.
- Evaluate the effectiveness of mechanisms to ensure program quality.
- Analyze the merits and shortcomings of the current nursing education system.

PROFILE IN PRACTICE

Mary Gunther, PhD, RN
Associate Professor, University of Tennessee College of Nursing, Knoxville, Tennessee

I was never one of those little girls who wanted to be a nurse. In fact, if early favorite toys and after-school activities had been a predictor, I now would be a truck driver or a librarian. The high school I attended did not provide academic counseling to educate families about tuition assistance or scholarships. My grandmother, who was raising me, made it clear that a college education was beyond our financial means. It was her fervent wish that I always be able to take care of myself (that is, be able to get a well-paying job) without relying on anyone else. She gave me two choices: become a nun or study nursing. I chose the latter.

I completed a 2-year nursing diploma program at a community hospital in Chicago. It was the type of program common at the time: students staffed the hospital around the clock 5 days a week and worked weekends for pay. The opportunity for hands-on clinical experience was unsurpassed. When it came time to look for a job, I chose to specialize in pediatrics, since children were less intimidating to me than adults. Furthermore, they were easier to physically move! Over the first 10 years of my career, I became "a good nurse," developing both my intuitive and technical skills. I could recognize what needed to be done and when. What I did not know was why. I decided to take advantage of working at a university hospital and returned to school. It took me 15 years of on-again, off-again study to get my BSN. (Obviously, I was not exactly driven; it's more like I meandered through the undergraduate program.) By that time, I was a head nurse and had a whole new set of skills to learn.

Flushed with the success of being the first one in my family ever to graduate from college, I went back for a master's degree in nursing administration. What a difference! Almost everyone in my class had worked as a nurse for several years. Everyone had a story to tell about where they had been and where they wanted to go. The classes were not necessarily harder than those in the undergraduate program—just more interesting because they were directly applicable to our various jobs. I fell in love with nursing all over again. I finished my MSN degree in 18 months, just in time to become the director of a large pediatric nursing department. Within a few years, I was the budget director for the entire division of nursing. Suddenly, I was explaining to administrators just what it is that

nurses do that makes them irreplaceable and invaluable. It was a very challenging and stressful (although not necessarily intellectually stimulating) job. I was homesick for the College of Nursing. There were so many more things I wanted to know. So back I went.

My days as a doctoral student were among the happiest in my life. It was both the hardest and the most rewarding program I had undertaken. I also found out that I enjoy teaching, mainly because I like to talk about nursing and its place in the real world. Over the past several years, I have become increasingly interested in nursing conceptual models and theories and their role in guiding nursing research, practice, and education. Studying the various models has given me an appreciation of the values and philosophies of nursing, while enabling me to answer clearly the question, "What is it that nurses do, and why do they do it?" I hope the fascination never wanes.

Introduction

For individuals seeking a career in nursing, deciphering the various types of educational programs and the relationship of each program type to future nursing practice can be daunting. Many types of programs at all levels provide multiple pathways to one or more nursing credential. Chapter 1 described the social, political, and economic forces that influenced the evolution of nursing as a profession and the system of nursing education. This chapter analyzes the various educational opportunities with some considerations for selecting among the options. A brief historical overview of each type of program helps build greater understanding of the factors influencing nursing education. More important, this chapter highlights the contributions each type of program provides for contemporary health care systems, advancement of the nursing profession, and promotion of a professional workforce dedicated to lifelong learning.

In 1965, the American Nurses Association (ANA) designated the baccalaureate degree as the educational entry point into professional nursing practice (ANA, 1965). Now, more than 40 years later, three educational pathways for RN licensure still exist: baccalaureate,

associate degree, and diploma programs (Figure 2-1). The existence of multiple pathways contributes to a confusing landscape of nursing education and creates challenges for aspiring nurses as they try to choose the most appropriate type of program in which to enter the profession. No matter which type of entry into practice program one chooses, "the demands placed on nursing in the emerging health care system are likely to require a greater proportion of RNs who are prepared beyond the associate degree or diploma level" (Pew Health Professions Commission, 1998, p. 64). The nursing education system is challenged to balance the goal of providing adequate numbers of baccalaureate-prepared nurses while simultaneously advancing the educational level of nurses prepared at the associate degree or diploma level.

History of Nursing Education in the United States

DIPLOMA PROGRAMS

The first formal nursing education program in the United States was a 4-month hospital-based diploma program at the Boston Training School for Nurses at

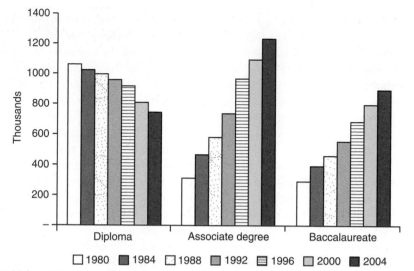

FIGURE 2-1 Initial nursing preparation of the registered nurse population, 1980 to 2004. (From U.S. Department of Health and Human Services, Health Resources and Services Administration. [2006]. Preliminary findings: 2004 national sample survey of registered nurses. [Online]. Retrieved from http://bhpr.hrsa.gov/healthworkforce/reports/rnpopulation/preliminaryfindings.htm.)

Massachusetts General Hospital. That program, established in 1873, was originally intended to emulate the model put forward by Florence Nightingale when she established collegiate nursing in London in 1860. Anticollegiate forces prevailed, however, and the hospital-based diploma program became the predominant model for nursing education in the United States. The model, in fact, flourished for nearly a century and still exists today.

At their peak in 1958, diploma programs numbered 944. At that time and during the decade that followed, diploma graduates constituted nearly the entire registered nurse (RN) workforce. In 1963 the Surgeon General's Report indicated that 86% of working nurses were diploma graduates. The decline in the number of programs began in earnest in the 1960s and 1970s and continues even today. By 1993, 126 diploma programs existed in 26 states, with more than half of the programs in three states: Ohio, New Jersey, and Pennsylvania. In 2010, 54 accredited diploma programs remained in 16 states, and half of them were located in two states: Pennsylvania with 20 programs and New Jersey with 13 programs (National League for Nursing Accrediting Commission [NLNAC], 2010).

Diploma programs are typically 2 to 3 years in length, and graduates are eligible to take the RN licensure examination (NCLEX-RN). As the length of diploma programs increased over the years from 4 months to 3 years, nursing students were increasingly used to meet hospital staffing needs rather than function in the student role. This exploitation of nursing students was addressed in several landmark studies of nursing and nursing education, and student life eventually became more compatible with sound educational practices. Many of these same studies also encouraged the profession to move its programs into collegiate settings (e.g., Brown, 1948; Goldmark & the Committee for the Study of Nursing Education, 1923) and to abandon the apprenticeship model. Ultimately, the high cost of these programs to students and to the hospitals that offered them, coupled with an increasing number of collegiate options, brought about the closure of many diploma programs.

Some diploma programs, rather than closing outright, began to align themselves with academic institutions. Others actually joined forces with academic institutions and began to offer joint degrees. Some became freestanding degree-granting institutions in their own right and now grant associate or baccalaureate degrees in nursing. These programs have been accredited by the regional accrediting body and have also achieved professional nursing accreditation from one of the specialized accrediting agencies.

BACCALAUREATE DEGREE EDUCATION

The first baccalaureate nursing program was established in the United States at the University of Minnesota in 1909. The baccalaureate phenomenon caught on slowly and did not gain much momentum until after World War II. Until the mid-1950s many baccalaureate programs were 5 years in length and consisted of 2 years of general education followed by 3 years of nursing. The main difference between the 3 years of nursing in baccalaureate and diploma programs was the inclusion of public health nursing as part of the baccalaureate curriculum. Eventually, the nursing content in baccalaureate programs was strengthened and expanded.

The proliferation of baccalaureate programs was slowed by the paucity of faculty members qualified to teach in these programs. Although this was understandable given the relative youth of nursing in academic centers, it created reluctance on the part of college and university administrators to establish baccalaureate nursing programs. Those that were established were often forced to hire nursing faculty who would not otherwise qualify for university faculty appointments. This deficit has taken several decades to correct itself, but nursing faculty teaching in baccalaureate programs today are for the most part bona fide members of their respective academic communities.

Most baccalaureate programs are now 4 academic years in length, and the nursing major is typically concentrated at the upper division level. Graduates are prepared as generalists to practice nursing in beginning leadership positions in a variety of settings, and they are eligible to take the NCLEX-RN. To prepare nurses for this multifaceted role, several components are essential for all baccalaureate programs. These components are liberal education, quality and patient safety, evidence-based practice, information management, health care policy and finance, communication/collaboration, clinical prevention/population health,

and professional values (American Association of Colleges of Nursing [AACN], 2008a). The number of BSN programs has continued to increase over the past several years. In 2004, 674 baccalaureate programs existed in the United States and its territories; in 2008 the number was 748 (AACN, 2005a, 2009a). After a worrisome decline in enrollment in the late 1990s, trend data for a select group of 488 schools indicate that traditional baccalaureate student enrollment had increased an average of 6869 students per year from 2004 to 2008 (AACN, 2009a).

Accelerated BSN Programs. As the nursing shortage has gained national recognition, accelerated BSN programs have emerged to hasten the time to graduation for select groups of students. Some programs accept nonnurse college graduates, and the curriculum is designed for completion in less time than the traditional BSN program through a combination of "bridge" and transition courses (AACN, 2009a). These programs are especially attractive for individuals desiring a career change. In the fall of 2008, 209 colleges and universities offered accelerated BSN programs for nonnurse college graduates (AACN, 2009a).

RN-BSN Track. The majority of baccalaureate programs admit both prelicensure students and RNs who are graduates of diploma and associate degree nursing programs, but some programs admit only RNs. The general education requirements are the same for all students. Although some content in the RN track may be configured differently, both RN and prelicensure students meet the same program objectives. Licensed practical nurses (LPNs) may also be given credit for prior learning when they enroll in baccalaureate programs. The baccalaureate in nursing degree is the most common requirement for admission to graduate nursing programs, but it is not the only route to graduate nursing education.

The RN-BSN track or option in the baccalaureate program is designed to recognize and reward prior learning and to capitalize on the characteristics of the adult learner. Several models of awarding academic credit to RNs for prior education and experience exist to facilitate educational mobility. These include direct transfer of credits, credits awarded by examination, variable credits awarded after portfolio review of educational and professional experiences, the holding of lower division nursing credits in "escrow" until completion of the program, and a number of other innovative models. This reflects the AACN's assertion that "educational mobility options should respect previous learning that students bring to the educational environment . . . and build on knowledge and skills attained by learners prior to their matriculation" (AACN, 1998, p. 1). More than 600 RN-BSN programs are offered nationwide (AACN, 2009a).

VOCATIONAL EDUCATION

Practical/vocational nurse programs were begun in 1942 in response to the acute shortage of licensed nurses in the United States created by World War II. Because of the dramatic influx of RNs into the various military branches, U.S. hospitals were largely staffed by nurse's aides, volunteers, and other unlicensed personnel. Practical/vocational nurse programs were established to provide some formal training for those who were entering the nursing workforce with little or no knowledge about nursing and few, if any, nursing skills. The programs eventually led to a new kind of licensure for nurses, namely, licensed practical nurse/licensed vocational nurse (LPN/LVN). The license is awarded by the state board of nursing after the graduate has passed the NCLEX-PN examination.

LPN/LVN programs are typically located in technical or vocational education settings. Programs are 9 to 15 months long, require proof of high school graduation or its equivalent for admission, and are designed to prepare graduates to work with RNs and be supervised by them. Programs lead to a certificate of completion and eligibility to take the NCLEX-PN. More than 1500 state-approved practical/vocational nursing programs currently exist in the United States (Education-Portal, 2009). Because many courses taken by practical nurse students do not carry academic credit, these programs do not always articulate well with collegiate nursing programs. Associate degree programs, however, often have procedures for accommodation of practical nurses into their programs by way of advanced placement.

ASSOCIATE DEGREE EDUCATION

In 1952 the associate degree in nursing (ADN) became another program option for those desiring to become RNs. Designed by Mildred Montag, these programs were intended to be a collegiate alternative for the preparation of technical nurses and a response to the nursing shortage (Haase, 1990). In 1958 the W. K. Kellogg Foundation funded a pilot project at seven sites in four states. The success of the pilot project led to a phenomenal growth of associate degree programs in the United States. These programs multiplied in community colleges and also began to appear at 4-year colleges and universities. By 1973 approximately 600 associate degree programs existed in the United States. Today, NLNAC states that nearly 1000 state-approved associate degree nursing programs exist (Associate Degree Nursing, 2009), of which 652 are accredited (S. Tanner, personal communication, February 10, 2010).

Associate degree nursing programs are designed to be 2 years in length and consist of a balance between general education and clinical nursing courses, all of which carry academic credit. ADN programs prepare technical bedside nurses for secondary care settings, such as community hospitals and long-term health care facilities. Montag's intent was that nurses with associate degrees would work under the direction of registered professional nurses who were prepared at the baccalaureate level. Some confusion arose about roles and relationships, so that by the time the first groups of students had graduated from ADN programs, they were declared eligible for the RN licensure examination, an eligibility that graduates of these programs retain today. The degree most often awarded on completion of the associate degree program is the ADN. A few institutions award the associate of arts in nursing (AAN) degree.

MASTER'S DEGREE EDUCATION

While the establishment of associate and baccalaureate degree nursing programs was proceeding, master's programs were beginning to emerge on university campuses. The need for nursing faculty to teach in all the new and developing nursing education programs was apparent. Interest in master's-prepared nurses also surged in the service sector as the roles of clinical nurse specialists, nurse practitioners, nurse anesthetists, nurse midwives, and nurse administrators became more clearly defined.

Master's education in nursing traces its origins to 1899, when Teachers College in New York began to offer graduate courses in nursing management and nursing education. However, master's programs did not begin to escalate and become nationally visible until the late 1950s and early 1960s. The first programs were strong on role preparation and light on advanced nursing content. This was not surprising because the nurses teaching in these programs did not themselves hold graduate degrees in nursing. As advanced nursing content became more clearly defined, and as increasing numbers of nursing faculty became proficient at teaching it, strong advanced nursing content became the prevailing characteristic of master's programs in nursing. Role preparation received somewhat less attention as clinical emphasis increased, and by the 1990s advanced practice had become the predominant focus for most master's degree programs. The expanding authority of advanced practice nurses (APNs) to serve as autonomous providers of care requires that the education of the clinicians be sound and that the consumers of APN care be able to have confidence in the quality of the educational experience (Booth & Bednash, 1994, p. 2).

Master's programs in nursing are typically 1 to 2 years of full-time study and are built on the baccalaureate nursing major. The program content includes a set of graduate-level foundational (core) courses, including a research component, and clinical specialty courses. Other recommended core content areas include theoretical foundations of nursing practice, health care financing, human diversity and social issues, ethics, health promotion, health care delivery systems, health policy, and professional role development. For specialty tracks that prepare APNs, an additional clinical core consists of advanced pathophysiology, pharmacology, and advanced health/ physical assessment (AACN, 1996).

Master's degree programs in nursing have experienced phenomenal growth over the past several decades. In 1973 only 86 such programs existed. By 1983 the number had increased to 154, and in 2008 there were 475 (AACN, 2009a). During the late 1980s and early 1990s, enrollment in master's degree programs increased rapidly as the demand for APNs escalated, but a slight decline (1.9%) was evident in 1999 (AACN, 2000). The decline in enrollment reversed itself in the early 2000s, and master's program enrollment increased by an average of 5993 students per year from 2004 to 2008 in a select group of 391 schools for which trend data were available (AACN, 2009a). Master's degree programs currently are offered in all states and territories of the United States.

RN-MSN and Nonnurse Master's Entry Options. The bachelor of science in nursing (BSN) degree or its equivalent is usually a requirement for admission to a master's program in nursing, but several interesting models that accommodate other types of students have emerged. Some master's programs admit RNs without a baccalaureate degree or with a baccalaureate degree in another field into a streamlined track that includes both baccalaureate and master's level courses. Other programs admit students who are not nurses at all. Approximately 158 RN-MSN programs are in existence nationwide (AACN, 2009a).

The impetus for opening admissions to other types of students was the recognition of the kinds of students who were applying in significant numbers to associate degree and baccalaureate nursing programs. Frequently nonnurses with baccalaureate or graduate degrees in other fields were seeking admission to basic nursing programs. RNs from associate degree and diploma programs who had completed baccalaureate degrees in fields other than nursing were applying for admission to baccalaureate nursing programs to present the appropriate credential for admission to a master's program in nursing. These students brought a rich and diversified background to their educational programs and were highly motivated, self-directed adult learners with a strong and clearly defined career orientation. Some of these students were well served by an accelerated second baccalaureate degree offered by several institutions, but master's programs could clearly accommodate them and take them to the master's level in educationally sound and cost-effective ways.

Master's programs in nursing that admit nonnurse college graduates and RNs without a baccalaureate degree in nursing take the necessary steps to ensure that both groups complete whatever undergraduate or graduate prerequisite courses are needed to acquire the equivalent of a baccalaureate nursing major. They then pursue the same graduate-level foundational, specialty, and cognate courses required of master's students; thus they exit the program having met the same program objectives that all graduates of both programs must meet. Nonnurses are eligible to take the NCLEX-RN examination on completion of the generalist or baccalaureate equivalent portion of the program or at program completion. In 2008, 55 nonnurse master's entry programs and nearly 300 programs that offered RN-MSN options existed (AACN, 2009a).

Dual Degree Programs. Another option regarding master's programs in nursing is the joint program leading to two master's degrees awarded simultaneously. This type of program is especially relevant for nurses seeking administrative positions that require both advanced nursing knowledge and business management skills. Several joint program models now exist across the country, reflecting nursing's responsiveness to documented student need and interest and also demonstrating nursing's ability to collaborate with other academic disciplines. Among the available programs in conjunction with the master's degree in nursing are the master's degree in business administration (MSN/MBA), master's degree in public administration (MSN/MPA), and master's degree in hospital administration (MSN/MHA). Degree candidates must be admitted to both programs and must fulfill requirements for both programs. However, requirements common to both programs may be consolidated. More than 130 such programs are currently in existence, with several more in development (AACN, 2009a).

Clinical Nurse Leader Program. A relatively new nursing role is that of the clinical nurse leader (CNL), a master's-prepared nurse who "oversees the care coordination of a distinct group of patients and actively provides direct patient care in complex situations" (AACN, 2005b, p. 1). The concept was developed in collaboration with leaders from education and practice settings. The AACN (2003) further describes the CNL role: "Along with the authority, autonomy,

and initiative to design and implement care, the CNL is accountable for improving individual care outcomes and care processes in a quality cost-effective manner" (p. 7). The CNL role differs from advanced practice nursing roles in that the CNL is a generalist and not a specialist, as are nurse practitioners and clinical specialists. A more in-depth presentation of the role and expectations of the CNL can be found in the White Paper on the Role of the Clinical Nurse Leader (AACN, 2007). Approximately 100 schools of nursing partnering with almost 200 health care delivery organizations in 35 states and Puerto Rico were involved in a pilot project to develop the CNL role, integrate it into the health care system, and evaluate the outcomes. Currently, 77 schools of nursing are admitting students into CNL programs, and more programs are being developed (AACN, 2009b).

A number of master's programs in nursing across the United States have multiple entry options such as those described here, and more are being developed as adult learners from diverse backgrounds migrate toward nursing. The degree most often awarded on completion of a master's degree program is the master of science in nursing degree (MSN). At least 90% of nursing master's degrees are MSN degrees. Other degree designations include the master's degree in nursing (MN), master of science degree with a major in nursing (MS), and master of arts degree with a major in nursing (MA). The degree designation is more a matter of institutional policy than a reflection of program type or content. In fact, no substantive distinction can be made among these various degree designations for master's-level nursing programs.

DOCTORAL EDUCATION

As might be expected, given nursing's relative youth in academe, the profession has only recently carved out a major doctoral presence in the academic community. Until 1970 fewer than a dozen doctoral programs with a major in nursing existed across the country. Most nurses who earned doctoral degrees did so in related disciplines such as sociology, anthropology, education, psychology, or physiology. In 1983, 27 doctoral programs in nursing existed. By 1990, only 7 years later, their number had nearly doubled.

As the movement toward the practice doctorate gained momentum, the number of doctoral programs in nursing increased rapidly. In 2004, 93 programs existed (AACN, 2005a), and in 2008 the number of doctoral programs had increased to 158 (AACN, 2009a).

Two pathways to the doctoral degree in nursing can be taken: research-focused programs and practice-focused programs. As is evident from their titles, these programs have different emphases.

Research-Focused Programs. The degree most commonly awarded for the research-focused doctorate in nursing is the doctor of philosophy (PhD) with a major in nursing. Other degrees awarded include the doctor of nursing science (DNS or DNSc) and the doctor of science in nursing (DSN), although with the advent of the doctor of nursing practice (see the following section), these are slowly being phased out. The varying degree designations do not necessarily distinguish one program from another in terms of content, rigor, or research emphasis, but some programs may have a heavier clinical emphasis than others. In most instances, the degree designation is that specified for the discipline by the institution that awards the degree. Although some are still questioning nursing's readiness to join the doctoral community of scholars, the profession is quietly preparing an array of scholars and researchers whose contributions to the health and nursing literature are qualitatively and quantitatively impressive.

Most research-focused doctoral programs admit students with an MSN degree, but a few admit students with a BSN. These programs range in length from 3 to 5 years of full-time study or that equivalent in part-time work. The curriculum includes advanced content in concept and theoretical formulations and testing, theoretical analyses, advanced nursing, supporting cognates, and in-depth research. The culminating requirement for the degree is the completion and defense of the doctoral dissertation. In 2008, 116 research-focused doctoral programs existed in 42 states (AACN, 2009c), awarding degrees to an average of 35 students per year from 2004 to 2008 (AACN, 2009a).

Practice-Focused Programs. The clinical practice doctorate in nursing is the doctor of nursing practice (DNP). Conceptualized as the highest degree for

nursing practice, the DNP program prepares graduates to identify emerging clinical patterns and problems within a practice setting; synthesize data, information, and knowledge for developing evidence-based practice care regimens; demonstrate advanced levels of clinical judgment, cultural sensitivity, and systems thinking; and work collaboratively with other health professionals, consumers, and policy makers (AACN, 2005c). As noted by Edwardson (2004), "the graduates of these programs will not represent a point on a continuum between researchers and practitioners but rather will be highly specialized practitioners of the profession engaged in either direct or indirect clinical activities" (p. 44).

Rather than focusing on the generation of new knowledge, practice-focused doctoral programs emphasize the translation and application of new knowledge to practice. Thus students in these doctoral programs are encouraged to develop projects grounded in clinical practice as opposed to conducting dissertation research. In 2005 only 10 DNP programs existed; by 2009, 91 schools offered such programs, with 50 additional schools planning to do so in the future (AACN, 2009d). The rapid increase in the number of DNP programs is a response to the AACN position that by 2015 the education of advanced practice nurses should be moved from the master's to the doctoral level (AACN, 2009e).

An earlier model of practice-focused doctoral education was the nursing doctorate (ND). First conceptualized by Rozella Schlotfeldt as analogous to medical, dental, and legal models of education, the ND program was designed to prepare graduates for licensure and professional practice in their field (Schlotfeldt, 1978). According to Jones and Lutz (1999), "an ND is a clinically focused degree that emphasizes research utilization (not generation) in patient care and health care policy. The goal for ND programs is to produce highly specialized practitioners for practice, teaching, consultation, and management" (p. 246).

The first ND program was established in 1979 at the Frances Payne Bolton School of Nursing, Case Western Reserve University. This 4-year program admitted students with a baccalaureate degree in another field; on completion of the generalist component of the program they were eligible to take the NCLEX-RN.

As part of the academic program, students also acquired an advanced practice specialty. This program model did not enjoy much growth, and by 2004 just four programs existed in four states (Colorado, Illinois, Ohio, and South Carolina) (AACN, 2005a). With the emergence of the DNP described above, ND programs made the transition to the DNP model.

To put the various educational programs in perspective, a comparison of their characteristics is presented in Table 2-1. The changes in the highest educational preparation of the nursing workforce from 1977 to 2004 are presented in Figure 2-2.

Considerations in Selecting a Nursing Education Program

A number of considerations influence an individual's choice in selecting either a basic or a graduate-level nursing program. Perhaps among the most important are cost to the student, quality of the program, and accessibility. Refer to www.allnursingschools.com and www.aacn.nche.edu for more information.

COST

Colleges, national summary documents, and public libraries provide relevant cost information on public and private institutions that offer nursing education programs. From this information some generalizations can be made. First, state-supported community or junior colleges tend to be less expensive than state-supported 4-year colleges and universities. Second, state-supported institutions of higher education usually give a substantial tuition reduction to in-state students. Third, state- or government-supported higher education is almost always significantly less expensive than private education, but this fact should not deter investigation of private institutions because of the availability of financial aid.

Financial Assistance. Financial aid packages at most institutions are somewhat commensurate with actual costs. Assistance can take the form of scholarships, loans, work-study appointments, employment opportunities within the institution, assistantships, tutoring assignments, or some combination of these or other options. Many of these options are no longer limited to full-time students. Financial assistance awards may be based on scholarship alone, need alone, competitive performance alone, or a combination of two or more of these factors. Financial support may be, and in most cases should be, sought from more than one source. Although most financial assistance awards are administered and awarded by the institution, a variety of packages are available from community- or government-based agencies and organizations. Examples of such agencies include state and local governments, the military, chambers of commerce, minority organizations, churches, community clubs, and local or state chapters of health-related organizations (e.g., March of Dimes, American Red Cross, American Heart Association). Local banks frequently have attractive student loan packages. Local hospitals and other health care agencies often sponsor or support nursing students in exchange for a commitment from the student to work for the sponsoring agency for a specified period of time after graduation.

To determine how entry-level nursing students financed their education, a study was conducted with a national sample of 496 students (Norman, Buerhaus, Donelan, McCloskey, & Dittus, 2005). Financial aid was the major source of funding for 32% of the students, followed by parental support (18%), personal savings (16%), government loans (15%), institutional scholarships (8%), and bank loans (5%). Many students also held part-time jobs. The researchers postulated that nursing students may not be aware of or have a full understanding of the benefits of federal student loan programs, which may forgive a portion of the balance each year in exchange for working in an underserved area or teaching in a school of nursing.

QUALITY

Issues of program quality relate to the quality of the educational program itself, as well as the eligibility of its graduates to become licensed or certified. Regarding program quality, how are prospective students protected from program mediocrity? And how is the public protected from low-quality nursing practice, which can frequently be traced to low-quality programs?

TABLE 2-1	Comparison of Nursing Education Programs						
	Diploma Programs	Baccalaureate Programs	Practical/ Vocational Nurse Programs	Associate Degree Programs	Master's Programs	Research-Focused Doctoral Programs	Practice-Focused Doctoral Programs
Year established	1873	1909	1942	1952	Late 1950s	1960s	1979 (ND) 2004 (DNP)
Location	Hospitals	4-year colleges and universities; a few in community colleges	Vocational/ technical schools	Community, junior, or 4-year colleges and universities	Universities and colleges	Universities and colleges	Universities and colleges
Accessibility	Limited to 54 accredited programs in 16 states, with half of programs in 2 states—New Jersey and Pennsylvania	Universal; all states, most cities; 748 programs; some are RN-BSN only	Universal; all states, most cities; more than 1500 programs	Universal; all states, almost all cities; 980 programs	Very good; 475 programs with at least 1 in every state	Somewhat limited; 116 programs in 41 states	Limited but increasing rapidly; 91 programs with several more under development
Length	2-3 years	4 years	9-15 months	2 years	1-2 years for full-time post-baccalaureate BSN-prepared nurses; additional work for other types of students	3-5 years post-master's; 4-5 years post-baccalaureate	3-4 years post-baccalaureate; 2-3 years post-master's
Cost	A few hundred dollars per term	Highly variable; a few thousand to several thousand dollars per year	Minimal; mostly books and cost of living	Reasonable in state or other public colleges; a few hundred to a few thousand dollars per year	Variable; several hundred to several thousand dollars per term	Several thousand dollars per term	Several thousand dollars per term

Continued

TABLE 2-1	Comparison of Nursing Education Programs—cont'd						
	Diploma Programs	Baccalaureate Programs	Practical/Vocational Nurse Programs	Associate Degree Programs	Master's Programs	Research-Focused Doctoral Programs	Practice-Focused Doctoral Programs
Purpose	Prepare clinically competent bedside nurses	Prepare professional nurse generalists for acute care settings, community-based practice, and beginning leadership/management positions	Prepare assistive licensed nurse workers	Prepare competent technical bedside nurses for secondary care settings	Prepare nurse generalists (CNLs) or APNs in a clinical specialty	Prepare leaders for education, administration, clinical practice, and research	Prepare clinically adept APNs for leadership positions in clinical settings
Advanced placement or acceleration opportunities	For LPNs or LVNs	For LPNs/LVNs or RNs from diploma and associate degree nursing programs	None	For LPNs or LVNs	For nonnurse college graduates, RNs with degrees in other fields, some RNs without degrees	For BSNs (limited number of programs)	Varies by program
Degree/certificate	Diploma	BSN	Certificate of completion	ADN (usually) or AAN	MSN (most common) or MN, MS, MA	PhD (most common) or DSN, DNS, DNSc, EdD	DNP
License eligibility	RN	RN (if not already licensed)	LPN/LVN	RN	RN if unlicensed at entry	Not applicable	Not applicable
Certification eligibility	None	Limited	None	None	Multiple	None	Multiple
Program growth pattern	Significant decline; 944 programs in 1958; 126 in 1993; 86 in 2000; 67 in 2005; and 54 in 2010	Gradual increase; 420 programs in 1983; 507 in 1993; 695 in 2000; 680 in 2005; and 748 in 2008	Stable, then sharp increase; 1200 programs in 1994; 1100 in 2000; 1150 in 2005; and 1500 in 2009	Sharp increase, then plateau; 600 programs in 1973; 900 in 1993; 885 in 2000; 880 in 2005; and 980 in 2009	Gradual increase; 150 programs in 1983; 300 in 1993; 358 in 2000; 417 in 2005; and 475 in 2008	Gradual increase; 27 programs in 1983; 56 in 1993; 75 in 2000; 93 in 2005; and 116 in 2008	Sharp increase; 10 DNP programs in 2005; 91 in 2008 with several more under development

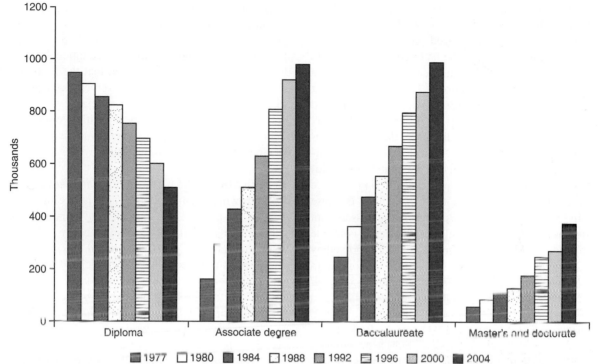

FIGURE 2-2 Highest educational preparation of registered nurses, 1977 to 2004. (From U.S. Department of Health and Human Services, Health Resources and Services Administration. [2006]. Preliminary findings: 2004 National sample survey of registered nurses. [Online]. Retrieved from http://bhpr.hrsa.gov/healthworkforce/reports/rnpopulation/preliminaryfindings.htm)

The public is protected by licensure and certification procedures that ensure a standardized level of competence. The student is protected from marginal programs by institutional accreditation through regional accrediting bodies, specialized accreditation of the nursing program(s) by the National League for Nursing Accrediting Commission (NLNAC) or the Commission on Collegiate Nursing Education (CCNE), and approval from the legal regulatory body for programs preparing for licensure, specifically the respective state boards of nursing. Appropriate questions to ask about the quality of nursing programs include the following:

- Is the parent institution accredited by the appropriate regional accrediting body?
- Is the nursing program unconditionally approved by the state board of nursing and fully accredited by a professional accrediting agency (if eligible)?

- What is the usual pass rate for first-time writers of the licensure examination from the school or program of interest?
- Is the faculty appropriately credentialed for the area of responsibility?
- Is each faculty member certified in his or her clinical specialty, if appropriate?
- Are graduates of the program eligible for the appropriate certification examination for the program being pursued?
- Does the program have a troubled history regarding licensure examination performance, accreditation, or state approval?

Specialized Accreditation. The NLNAC (2009) defines accreditation as "a voluntary self-regulatory process by which nongovernmental associations recognize educational institutions or programs that have been found to meet or exceed standards and criteria for educational quality." Some developments are occurring regarding specialized accreditation of nursing programs that need to be factored into the assessment of program quality, especially at the master's level. Until 1999 the National League for Nursing (and subsequently, the NLNAC) was the specialized accrediting body for all nursing programs, LPN/LVN through master's degree. In 2000 the CCNE was approved by the Department of Education as an official accrediting agency for baccalaureate and graduate nursing education programs, thus offering a choice of accrediting agencies for those programs. Because accreditation is a voluntary process, programs are not required to seek professional accreditation to continue to operate (although all programs must be approved by their respective state boards of nursing). According to NLNAC (2010), 652 associate degree and 153 LPN/LVN programs are accredited, representing 65% and 10%, respectively, of existing programs (S. Tanner, personal communication, February 10, 2010). Virtually all baccalaureate and master's programs are accredited by either CCNE or NLNAC. Students should recognize that attending a nonaccredited program may limit access to federal loans and scholarships. In addition, most graduate schools will accept only students who have earned degrees from accredited schools.

In the past, when a master's program was accredited by a specialized accrediting body, the accreditation covered all specialties that were offered within the master's program. However, when a nurse-midwifery program was one of the options in the master's program, even though it was covered by master's program accreditation, separate specialized accreditation for the nurse-midwifery program was sought from the American College of Nurse Midwives so that graduates of that program could take the midwifery license/certification examination and therefore practice as nurse-midwives. Now nurse anesthesia programs have been upgraded from diploma or certificate programs (which most of them were) to master's-level programs. Although many nurse anesthesia programs are accredited as one of the offerings within the master's program, these programs also seek and receive specialized accreditation from their specialty organization, the American Association of Nurse Anesthetists.

This practice will continue so that nurse anesthetists are eligible for the credentials that enable them to practice their specialty. Other nursing specialties may possibly seek programmatic accreditation that goes beyond the broader accreditation that the NLNAC or CCNE makes available. This movement is closely tied to the increasing emphasis on specialty certification and the organizations in the best position to provide it. Persons pursuing advanced specialty preparation need to monitor this issue with vigilance.

Certification. The certification of individual nurses is a growing quality-control activity being implemented by a variety of nursing and nursing-related organizations. Certification is directed toward attesting to or endorsing the demonstrated knowledge base and clinical practice behaviors associated with high-quality performance in an area of specialization.

Certification protects the public by enabling anyone to identify competent people more readily. Simultaneously it aids the profession by encouraging and recognizing professional achievement. Certification also recognizes specialization, enhances professionalism and, in some cases, serves as a criterion for financial reimbursement (American Nurses Credentialing Center [ANCC], 2009a). This movement is a very important one for the profession. Initiatives are in place to make eligibility and certification requirements more uniform, reduce duplicate or similar certification requirements among organizations, and match certification programs with the specialties being practiced.

Currently, ANCC (an arm of the American Nurses Association) offers nearly 40 certification examinations, 18 of which are for advanced practice in a variety of specialties. Eleven baccalaureate level certification examinations and six associate degree/diploma level examinations in selected clinical specialties are also available. In addition, examinations for nursing case management, ambulatory care nursing, and pain management are offered (ANCC, 2009b). The Commission on Nurse Certification, an autonomous arm of AACN, offers the certification exam for the CNL.

Other certification examinations are offered by a variety of nursing specialty organizations. Some certifications are highly specialized in such areas as addiction, diabetes, neuroscience, nephrology, ophthalmology, perioperative nursing, oncology, critical care, and occupational health. Many nursing specialty organizations that offer certification examinations are members of the American Board of Nursing Specialties. This board has a national peer-review program that sets standards for certification and approves certification programs. All certification efforts are designed to recognize the competence of nurses in specific areas and to protect the public from unsafe or uninformed nursing practice.

ACCESSIBILITY: DISTANCE EDUCATION

To improve accessibility in terms of geographic location and scheduling of classes, some nursing programs offer all or part of their curriculum through distance education technologies. Distance or distributive education is a method of teaching and learning that takes place outside the traditional classroom setting. Often students are in locations that are remote from the site where the course is taught. A variety of technologies are used to deliver education at a distance, including interactive television, e mail and facsimile transmissions, and Internet-based courses with real-time interactive chat rooms. Less-sophisticated and readily available technologies include audiocassettes, videotapes, and CD-ROM media. The potential benefits of distance education were recognized by the AACN in 1999: "Careful use of technology in education may well enhance the profession's ability to educate nurses for practice, prepare future nurse educators, and advance nursing science in an era when the number of professional nurses, qualified nurse faculty, and nurse researchers is well below national need" (p. 3).

As this movement gains momentum in nursing education, a number of issues need to be addressed, including the following:

- What is the effect of distance education on the cost and quality of the program?
- What equipment is needed by both the teacher and learner to maximize distance learning?
- What impact does distance education have on the process of professional socialization?

- How can teaching strategies best match learner needs?
- What policies exist to clarify intellectual property rights and the use of copyrighted material in distance education courses?
- What effect, if any, does distance education have on student financial aid support?

The answers to these questions will likely challenge traditional assumptions about the effectiveness of various teaching-learning strategies and their relationship to program quality. A further discussion of distance learning occurs in Chapter 10.

Observations and Analysis

Many have argued that regardless of the reasons, the system of nursing education that has been created is chaotic, confusing, and redundant. Some hold out for the day when there will be only one way to become a nurse, only one degree to be obtained, only one license to be acquired, and only one way to be approved and recognized as a specialist. That, after all, is the way medicine, dentistry, pharmacy, and law do it. Can nursing look to any more likely professions for modeling and emulation? Probably not.

But consider for a moment how different the evolution of medicine has been. Consider the venerable age of the profession. Consider how readily and completely the European model for medical education was transplanted unchanged to the United States. Consider the unquestioned dominance of the medical profession in the United States from the time the health care system was first defined until it began to crumble. And now that it is crumbling, consider the serious criticism being leveled at the medical profession—criticism about education, practice, costs, and societal insensitivities. Medical reform is being demanded by the federal and state governments, by consumers, and by the profession itself. And this reform must be conducted and completed by those who entered that profession in good faith and with a set of information-based expectations that they thought would last a lifetime. This state of affairs is by no means an indictment of the medical profession or the majority of its members.

It is, instead, an example of what can happen when the status quo is unquestioned, when a service profession loses touch with its constituencies, and when hard questions are not answered because they are not asked.

Wherever the nursing education system is right now, it is clearly in a better place than many of its other health profession counterparts. Nursing does not necessarily need to look to other health professions to take the right cues or develop the right models. Rather, it needs to look within itself to examine what has been created; to retain, build on, and reconfigure as needed that which is good; to abandon or revamp that which is no longer germane; to clarify ambiguities; to underline uniqueness; to stay in touch with its consumers; and to continue the trend of the profession to embrace and participate fully in the higher-education academic community, enjoying and benefiting from all the collegial and professional relationships that accrue from that participation. Those, after all, are relationships that can only get better.

With those observations as a backdrop, an analysis of strengths, weaknesses, and areas needing attention is presented. The information is organized around program types and educational level.

PRACTICAL/VOCATIONAL NURSE PROGRAMS

Strengths. Programs are short, economical, and accessible. Programs prepare assistive nurse workers who are eligible to take the NCLEX-PN.

Weaknesses. Programs are not collegiate based. Graduates are not prepared to do what they are often called on to do in the workplace. Practical nurses are exploited and are frequently called on to perform functions beyond their legally defined scope of practice.

Recommendations. Elevate these programs to the community college level and award the ADN. Adjust enrollments downward to reflect market demands.

DIPLOMA PROGRAMS

Strength. Programs prepare competent bedside nurses who are eligible to take the NCLEX-RN.

Weaknesses. Programs, for the most part, are not collegiate based, and nursing courses may not be readily transferable for educational advancement. In addition, they are expensive to operate.

Recommendation. Continue admirable and effective efforts to align with degree-granting institutions or become degree-granting as newly established academic institutions.

ASSOCIATE DEGREE PROGRAMS

Strengths. Programs are offered in academic/collegiate settings and are affordable and accessible. Programs prepare competent technical bedside nurses who are eligible to take the NCLEX-RN.

Weaknesses. Some programs may require as many as 75 course credits and take 3 years or longer to complete (Nelson, 2002). Programs and their graduates go beyond the purposes and scope of the practice envisioned by the program founder. When combined with practical nurses, the total number of technical nurse types being produced is excessive given current and future market demands (Benner et al., 2000).

Recommendations. Collaborate with the LPN/LVN leadership to develop one program type that prepares the technical nurse, using what is most effective from both programs to bring about this outcome. Once the two programs have become one, assess the marketplace and consumer needs for this type of nurse and adjust the program output accordingly. Some states are exploring transitioning associate degree programs to the baccalaureate level. Community colleges are encouraged to partner with baccalaureate programs whenever possible to achieve this goal (AACN, 2005d).

BACCALAUREATE PROGRAMS

Strengths. Programs provide a solid liberal education and a substantive upper-division nursing major. Both components are combined in ways that prepare a nurse generalist who is able to provide professional nursing services in beginning leadership positions in a variety of settings and who is eligible to take the NCLEX-RN. Programs are accessible and accommodate RNs who are graduates of associate degree and diploma programs. Baccalaureate programs in nursing have been designated by the ANA as the entry point for professional practice (ANA, 1965).

Weaknesses. The legal scope of practice for associate degree–prepared and baccalaureate-prepared nurses is undifferentiated because both groups are awarded the same license. This limits differentiated roles in work settings and hinders the reward system for leadership responsibilities.

Recommendations. Consider a different license for baccalaureate-prepared nurses. Give additional emphasis to health care costs, evidence-based practice, management/delegation, health promotion/wellness care, and informatics in the curriculum (Speziale & Jacobson, 2005). Strive to reach the goal recommended by the National Advisory Council for Nursing Education that at least two thirds of the nursing workforce hold a baccalaureate or higher degree (Division of Nursing, 1996). Currently, only 47.2% of the nursing workforce hold degrees at the baccalaureate level or above (AACN, 2008b).

MASTER'S PROGRAMS

Strengths. Programs are accessible and prepare graduates for advanced practice in a clinical specialty. Some of the programs admit nonnurse college graduates, RNs with baccalaureate degrees in other fields, and some RNs without baccalaureate degrees. Graduates of these programs are prepared to function as clinical nurse leaders or engage in advanced practice nursing as nurse practitioners, clinical nurse specialists, nurse anesthetists, or nurse-midwives as well as in other specialty practices.

Weaknesses. Nonnurses take the same licensure examination (NCLEX-RN) as associate degree and baccalaureate graduates. Certificate programs for master's-prepared nurses are not uniformly consistent in terms of eligibility requirements and examination rigor.

Recommendations. Collaborate with baccalaureate nurse educators and other interested professionals in bringing to fruition a different examination for professional nurses. Bring greater uniformity and meaning to certification programs. Monitor the status of transitioning advanced practice nursing education to the DNP.

DOCTORAL PROGRAMS IN NURSING

Strengths. Programs prepare leaders and clinicians for responsible advanced positions in nursing education, nursing administration, nursing research, nursing practice, or some combination of these roles. Programs are fairly accessible compared with doctoral programs in other disciplines.

Weakness. Proliferation of research-focused programs may result in the use of some unqualified faculty members for program delivery.

Recommendations. Stabilize growth of research-focused programs at the current level so that faculty can fine-tune their qualifications and participate more fully in the life of scholarship. Market the practice-focused doctorate as the preferred route to preparation for advanced practice nursing

Impact of Studies of the Profession

Throughout this chapter the history of nursing education has been traced from professional, organizational, regulatory, and institutional perspectives. The system has been described, analyzed, compared within itself, and presented for what it is and what it is becoming. One frame of reference that has not been formally considered from the standpoint of impact or programmatic direction is that provided by the multiple studies published about nursing and nurses. Many such studies have been conducted—some by nurses, some by the federal government, and some by human behavior experts from other disciplines (e.g., sociology, anthropology). The findings and recommendations from these studies have not been ignored by the profession. The best of them have been used to bring about improvements and needed change.

To analyze these studies and their impact on the developments that have occurred would constitute a book in its own right. The analysis of nursing education that completes this chapter is presented without direct reference to these studies, while recognizing fully that the studies are quite directly related to what is and what will be in nursing education. The following studies are recommended to the reader for serious review:

- The Goldmark Report: Nursing and Nursing Education in the United States (1923)
- The Brown Report: Nursing for the Future (1948)
- The Lysaught Report: An Abstract for Action (1970)
- The Institute of Medicine reports: Nursing and Nursing Education: Public Policy and Private Actions (1983); Crossing the Quality Chasm: A New Health System for the 21st Century (2001); Health Professions Education: A Bridge to Quality (2003)
- The Pew Health Professions Commission reports: Healthy America: Practitioners for 2005 (Sugars, O'Neil, & Bader, 1991) and Recreating Health Professional Practice for a New Century (Pew, 1998)
- Educating Nurses: A Call for Radical Transformation (Benner, Sutphen, Leonard, & Day, 2009).

Looking Toward the Future

However nursing education programs are configured for the future, facets of the system must be retained that ensure continued and growing representation of the gender and cultural diversity that exists in American society. Efforts to attract ethnic and racial minorities and men to nursing must be intensified. Ethnic and racial minority enrollment in baccalaureate and graduate programs is showing a slight increase, but at approximately 18% it does not adequately reflect the diversity of the population. African Americans represent the largest minority group (11%) in all levels of nursing education (AACN, 2009a). Male nurses are

still a minority, but their ranks are also increasing. In 2008 approximately 10% of baccalaureate students, 8.5% of master's students, and 7.9% of doctoral students were male (AACN, 2009a).

Historically, transformations in nursing and nursing education have been driven by major socioeconomic factors, developments in health care, and professional issues unique to nursing. Trends to watch in terms of their potential impact on nursing education for the future are the following (Heller, Oros, & Durney-Crowley, 2000):

- The changing demographics and increasing diversity of society
- The technological explosion
- The globalization of the world's economy and society
- The era of the educated consumer, alternative therapies, genomics, and palliative care
- The shift to population-based care and the increasing complexity of client care
- The cost of health care and the challenge of managed care
- The impact of health policy and regulation
- The growing need for interdisciplinary education for collaborative practice
- The current nursing shortage and opportunities for lifelong learning and workforce development
- Advances in nursing science and research

A system of nursing education that is responsive to society and that maximizes career development of nurses and advancement of the profession must be maintained. Greater clarity and meaning must be brought to licensure and certification programs. And the kinds and numbers of nurses we educate to meet societal and professional needs must be monitored and controlled (Bellack & O'Neil, 2000).

As these goals are pursued, the extent to which the profession attracts and uses the people who earn the most respected advanced degrees and then gives those people the opportunity to be role models and spokespersons for nursing will determine how the profession will grow in viability, usefulness, and esteem.

If this chapter conveys a message of endorsement and enthusiasm for the nursing profession and most components of its educational enterprise, a major outcome has been realized. Every reason exists to believe that our successes will continue and that our problems can be solved. Nursing is a profession in which exciting things are happening and the best is yet to come.

SUMMARY

This chapter has analyzed the various pathways to several types of nursing credentials and has offered considerations for choosing among those educational opportunities. The various pathways are linked to the historical social, political, and economic forces that influenced the development of nursing as a profession. The contributions of each pathway to our contemporary health system, the profession of nursing, and the professional workforce are highlighted. The existence of multiple educational pathways contributes to the confusion of aspiring nurses and the public. The health care system of the future will require a greater proportion of RNs prepared at beyond the diploma or associate–degree level. This creates a challenge for the nursing education system to meet the demand for adequate numbers of baccalaureate-prepared nurses while advancing the educational level of nurses prepared at the diploma or associate-degree level. Additionally, nursing education programs must address the shifting demographics and diversity of our society; advances in science, technology, and care practices (e.g., genomics, palliative care, alternative therapies, collaborative practice, population-based practice); globalization; health policy impacts; educated consumers; workforce shortages and lifelong learning needs; as well as advances in nursing, science, and research.

KEY POINTS

- Health care needs in society, along with certain historical events, influenced the development of multiple tracks of nursing education.
- Hospital-based diploma programs were the predominant model of nursing education in the United States for nearly 100 years.
- Although the first baccalaureate program in nursing was established in 1909, the development of significant numbers of these programs progressed slowly.
- Practical/vocational nursing programs were established to provide formal training for unlicensed personnel who, in large numbers, staffed U.S. hospitals during World War II.

- As a reaction to the vocational model of practical nursing, associate degree programs were established to educate technical nurses in collegiate programs.
- Master's programs prepare advanced practice nurses, other nurse specialists, and clinical nurse leaders to assume significant roles in a variety of health care settings.
- Practice-focused doctoral programs are designed to prepare graduates for the highest level of clinical nursing practice.
- Research-focused doctoral programs in nursing are designed to prepare scholars and researchers to expand the body of nursing knowledge.
- Cost and quality are two major considerations in selecting educational programs in nursing.
- Indicators of academic program quality include the status of program accreditation and approval, pass rates on licensure examinations, and pass rates on certification examinations.
- Although each nursing education program has unique strengths, each also has weaknesses to which attention must be given.
- The tapestry of nursing education has the potential to be affected by societal and professional trends and issues.

CRITICAL THINKING EXERCISES

1. Defend or refute the following statement: Nurses with baccalaureate and/or master's degrees should take a different licensing examination than the one taken by nurses educated in associate degree or diploma programs.
2. What is your career goal in nursing? What, if any, further education will you need to fully achieve your goal?
3. How does the certification of advanced practice nurses and nurse specialists protect the public?
4. Consult your state nurse practice act to determine the scope of practice of advanced practice nurses and other nurse specialists. What are the constraints on advanced practice nursing in your state?
5. Clarify the differences between practice-focused and research-focused doctoral programs in nursing.
6. Discuss the validity of licensure examination pass rates, regional and specialized accreditation status, and pass rates on certification examinations as indicators of the quality of a nursing education program.
7. What changes must be made in nursing education to ensure a culturally diverse nursing profession, career advancement opportunities, and credibility in the higher education community?
8. Analyze the potential impact on nursing education and nursing practice of each trend identified on p. 38.

REFERENCES

American Association of Colleges of Nursing. (1996). *Essentials of masters education for advanced practice nursing.* Washington, DC: Author.

American Association of Colleges of Nursing. (1998). *Position statement on educational mobility.* Washington, DC: Author.

American Association of Colleges of Nursing. (1999). *Distance technology in nursing education.* Washington, DC: Author.

American Association of Colleges of Nursing. (2000). *1999-2000 Enrollments and graduations in baccalaureate and graduate nursing programs.* Washington, DC: Author.

American Association of Colleges of Nursing. (2003). Working paper on the role of the clinical nurse leader. [Online]. Retrieved from http://www.aacn.nche.edu/Publications/WhitePapers/ ClinicalNurseLeader.htm

American Association of Colleges of Nursing. (2005a). *2004-2005 Enrollments and graduations in baccalaureate and graduate nursing programs.* Washington, DC: Author.

American Association of Colleges of Nursing. (2005b). Fact sheet: The clinical nurse leader. [Online]. Retrieved from http://www.aacn.nche.edu/Media/FactSheets/CNL FactSheet.htm

American Association of Colleges of Nursing. (2005c). The essentials of doctoral education for advanced nursing practice. [Draft] [Online]. Retrieved from http://www.aacn.nche.edu/DNP/pdf/Essentials5-06.pdf

American Association of Colleges of Nursing. (2005d). Position statement on baccalaureate programs offered by community colleges. [Online]. Retrieved from http://www.aacn.nche.edu/Publications/positions/ccbsn.htm.

American Association of Colleges of Nursing. (2007). White paper on the education and role of the clinical nurse leader. [Online]. Retrieved from http://www.aacn.nche.edu/Publications/WhitePapers/ClinicalNurseLeader07.pdf.

American Association of Colleges of Nursing. (2008a). *Essentials of baccalaureate education for professional nursing practice.* Washington, DC: Author.

American Association of Colleges of Nursing. (2008b). Nursing fact sheet. [Online]. Retrieved from http://www.aacn.nche.edu/Media/FactSheets/nursfact.htm

American Association of Colleges of Nursing. (2009a). *2008-2009 enrollments and graduations in baccalaureate and graduate programs.* Washington, DC: Author.

American Association of Colleges of Nursing. (2009b). [Online]. Retrieved from http://www.aacn.nche.edu/CNL/cnlweblinks.htm

American Association of Colleges of Nursing. (2009c). *Institutions offering doctoral programs in nursing.* [Online]. Washington, DC: Author. Retrieved from http://www.aacn.nche.edu/IDS/pdf/DOC.pdf

American Association of Colleges of Nursing. (2009d). Doctor of nursing practice programs. [Online]. Retrieved from http://www.aacn.nche.edu/DNP/DNPProgramList.htm

American Association of Colleges of Nursing. (2009e). Doctor of nursing practice. [Online]. Retrieved from http://www.aacn.nche.edu/Media/FactSheets/dnp.htm

American Nurses Association. (1965). *Educational preparation for nurse practitioners and assistants to nurses: A position paper.* New York: Author.

American Nurses Credentialing Center. (2009a). Frequently asked questions about ANCC certification. [Online]. Retrieved from http://www.nursecredentialing.org/FunctionalCategory/FAQ/CertiticationFAQs.aspx

American Nurses' Credentialing Center. (2009b). ANCC nurse certification. [Online]. Retrieved from http://www.nursecredentialing.org/certification.aspx

Associate Degree Nursing. (2009). Associate degree nursing schools and programs—your path to becoming a nurse! [Online]. Retrieved from http//www.associatedegreenursing.com

Bellack, J., & O'Neil, E. H. (2000). Recreating nursing practice for a new century: Recommendations and implications of the Pew Health Professions Commissions final report. *Nursing and Health Care Perspectives, 21*(1), 14–21.

Benner, P., Sutphen, M., Leonard, V., & Day, L. (2009). *Educating nurses: A call for radical transformation.* San Francisco: Jossy-Bass.

Booth, R. Z., & Bednash, G. (1994). *Syllabus: The newsletter of the American Association of Colleges of Nursing, 20*(5), 2.

Brown, E. L. (1948). *Nursing for the future.* New York: Russell Sage Foundation.

Division of Nursing. (1996). *National Advisory Council on Nurse Education: Report to the Secretary of the Department of Health and Human Services.* Washington, DC: U.S. Government Printing Office.

Education-Portal. (2009). LPN/Licensed practical nurse education/LPN training. [Online]. Retrieved from http//education-portal.com/lpn.html

Edwardson, S. R. (2004). Matching standards and needs in doctoral education in nursing. *Journal of Professional Nursing, 20*(1), 40–46.

Goldmark, J., & the Committee for the Study of Nursing Education. (1923). *Nursing and nursing education in the United States*. New York: Macmillan.

Haase, P. (1990). *The origins and rise of associate degree nursing education*. Chapel Hill, NC: Duke University Press.

Heller, B. R., Oros, M. T., & Durney-Crowley, J. (2000). The future of nursing education: 10 trends to watch. *Nursing and Health Care Perspectives*, *21*(1), 9–13.

Institute of Medicine. (1983). *Nursing and nursing education. Public policies and private actions*. Washington, DC: National Academy Press.

Institute of Medicine. (2001). *Crossing the quality chasm: A new health system for the 21st century*. Washington, DC: National Academy Press.

Institute of Medicine. (2003). *Health professions education: A bridge to quality*. Washington, DC: National Academy Press.

Jones, K. D., & Lutz, K. F. (1999). Selecting doctoral programs in nursing: Resources for students and faculty. *Journal of Professional Nursing*, *15*, 245–252.

Lysaught, J. (1970). *An abstract for action*. New York: McGraw-Hill.

National League for Nursing Accrediting Commission. (2005). *Directory of accredited nursing programs*. New York: Author.

National League for Nursing Accrediting Commission. (2009). NLNAC Mission. [Online]. Retrieved from http://www.nlnac.org/About%20NLNAC/AboutNLNAC.htm#RECOGNITION

National League for Nursing Accrediting Commission. (2010). About NLNAC. [Online]. Retrieved from http://www.nlnac.org/About%20NLNAC/whatsnew.htm

Nelson, M.A. (2002). Education for professional nursing practice: Looking backward into the future. [Online]. Retrieved from http://www.nursingworld.org/ojin/topic18/ tpc18_3.htm

Norman, L., Buerhaus, P. I., Donelan, K., McCloskey, B., & Dittus, R. (2005). Nursing students assess nursing education. *Journal of Professional Nursing*, *21*(3), 150–158.

Pew Health Professions Commission (1998). *Recreating health professional practice for a new century*. San Francisco: Author.

Schlotfeldt, R. M. (1978). The professional doctorate: Rationale and characteristics. *Nursing Outlook*, *26*, 302–311.

Speziale, H. J. S., & Jacobson, L. (2005). Trends in registered nurse education programs 1998-2008. *Nursing Education Perspectives*, *26*(4), 230–235.

Sugars, D. A., O'Neil, E. H., & Bader, J. D. (Eds.). (1991). *Healthy America: Practitioners for 2005. An agenda for action for U.S. health professional schools. A report of the Pew Health Professions Commission*. Durham, NC: Author.

U.S. Department of Health and Human Services, Health Resources and Services Administration. (2006). Preliminary findings: 2004 national sample survey of registered nurses. [Online]. Retrieved from http://bhpr.hrsa.gov/health workforce/reports/rnpopulation/preliminaryfindings.htm

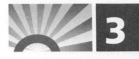

3

Socialization to Professional Nursing

KAREN J. SAEWERT, PhD, RN, CPHQ, CNE

The author acknowledges the important foundational work for this chapter developed by Mary L. Killeen, PhD, RN, in previous editions of this book.

OBJECTIVES

At the completion of this chapter, the reader will be able to:

- Evaluate the current status of nursing as a profession.
- Describe the barriers that slow the professionalization of nursing.
- Discuss factors that influence professional socialization.
- Differentiate accountability, autonomy, and shared governance as characteristics of professional practice.
- Describe the relationship between professional socialization and participation in professional nursing associations.

PROFILE IN PRACTICE

Cynthia Ann Holcomb, BSN, MS, RN, BC
BSN and MS Graduate, College of Nursing and Healthcare Innovation, Arizona State University, Phoenix, Arizona

"Do you have passion?" a sign stated in my church gift shop. It reminded me of a topic in my human development class. It was a discussion of how people defined what they did for a living. Was it a job, a career, or a passion? I am fortunate to have two: a career and a passion. I have been a nurse for 28 years, and I have never regretted it. I cannot imagine my life without this passion I feel in my heart. I explored a different avenue for a year when I painted wall murals and realized that I could not do without nursing in my life. How does a person decide what he or she will do in life? If asked why I went into nursing, I could not pinpoint a specific reason or initial thought of wanting

to be in a professional career. The decision could have come from the impression a kind nurse gave me when I had an appendectomy. On the other hand, my desire to take care of people could have begun, as my husband points out, when I saw my mother live through her illnesses.

My high school counselor challenged me, but not in the way he thought. He informed me that I was not smart enough to be a registered nurse, that I should consider a different career. Did I set out to prove him wrong, or did I truly want to take care of someone's mother, father, or child? Whatever the reason, I chose to go to a community college, and I was the first member of my family to seek a college degree. College was not talked about at home. My mother graduated from high school and became a mother of six children. My father quit school when he was 16 and joined the Navy, earning his GED while serving. I do not know what drove me to become a nurse, but I certainly do not regret my choice of careers. As I was going through my associate degree program, I came to realize that being a nurse took perseverance and dedication.

Pediatrics has been the focus of most of my nursing career. I worked in the hospital setting in general pediatrics, rehabilitation, and pediatric intensive care. I helped a pediatrician open her office, worked in the school setting, and found myself wanting something more. I applied for a position as a regional nurse in a school district and another as a parish nurse. Both required a bachelor's degree in nursing. I felt as if I had hit a wall.

So, after 20 years of nursing I returned to obtain my BSN. It took me 2 years to fulfill prerequisites before entering the RN-BSN program. In the RN-BSN program I needed to learn what I would learn: the reasons for mastering the nursing skills I had used in my career. Who were the nurses who walked before me, and what were their contributions to this profession? I finally began to feel connected to the profession of nursing. Nursing was much more than knowing the technical aspects of taking care of a patient, running the machines that kept them alive in the intensive care units, memorizing the five rules of medications, and knowing the signs and symptoms of different diseases. It was increasing my knowledge of nursing research, understanding theorists in nursing and interdisciplinary fields, and improving my critical thinking skills. I felt renewed and anxious to pursue my passion.

My professional journey continued in a different direction as I began work in a hospice setting. This was a new area for me: instead of curing someone, the focus was to giving comfort and support during the dying process. An experience with one of my patients motivated me to continue on my quest to learn more about my profession. She was a woman in her forties, and she had Lou Gehrig's disease, or amyotrophic lateral sclerosis. The night nurse was in the process of

giving report when a patient's alarm light activated. The night nurse said, "Oh, there she is again. I don't know how many times I have been with her tonight. She continues to insist on having water in her mouth when she can't even swallow!" I was taken aback by this nurse's response. Was she here for her agenda or for her patients? When I met the patient, she wrote a note to me on her wipe board, since she no longer could speak: "I was the president of a human relations company and taught this at the college level. The nurse last night did not have people skills." I apologized not only for the night nurse but for the nursing profession. She then wrote, "What I wouldn't give to be able to drink a cold glass of water!" I saw my patient as a mom, a professional, a human being who could not fulfill a basic human need because her disease took away her ability to swallow. We worked together on a plan that would allow her to feel the cold water in her mouth and not choke on it.

I was also fortunate to be given the opportunity to help teach a pediatric competency course for nurses who came in contact with our pediatric hospice patients. This experience ignited another flame inside me: I loved teaching. I have mentored others throughout my career, but I loved the idea of teaching. If I was to pursue teaching, I knew I had to return to college for a higher degree.

What had changed for me in the hospice setting was the partnership I felt with my patients. I cherish all that they have taught me. I wanted to pass on to future nurses the need to look at our patients individually and to partner with them on a course of care. During this time I had stayed in contact with my advisors from my RN-BSN program, and they encouraged me to return to the academic setting to reach for another star, my master's degree in community health nursing.

Two years later I am an advanced practice nurse in community health. Advanced practice nursing means more than obtaining advanced education in nursing. Earning a master of science degree was part of the goal, but developing a higher level of critical thinking skills, taking on greater responsibility, and refining professional judgment were motivations as well. My education included gaining an understanding of the nurse paradigm and nursing theories, including their importance in changing the direction of nursing practice. Being an advanced practice nurse also affords me the opportunity to influence and teach nursing students in the art of nursing. I can impress upon students that nursing encompasses not only the important technical skills we need to provide our patients with effective care, but also the roles of teacher, advocate, and resource for preventing disease and promoting health.

The grandmother of one of my patients told me, "You are a good nurse because you have compassion and heart for what you do." I want to strengthen these aspects of nursing and the voice of the nursing profession. Nurses are a critical resource for insight into the holistic world of the human being and health care. Nurses bring empathy and emotion to the experience of health and illness, balancing knowledge with a deep understanding of who their patients are as people and as members of families and communities.

☼ Introduction

How does someone go from being a regular person—student, son, daughter, employee—to being a professional nurse? Each person must acquire values, skills, behaviors, and norms appropriate to nursing practice. The process of learning and incorporating these aspects of a profession into individual professional identity is termed *socialization*. Socialization to professional nursing is an interactive process that begins in the educational setting and continues throughout one's nursing career.

The first socialization occurs in the basic nursing program. The socialization process is again activated at each of the following junctures: (1) when the new graduate leaves the educational setting and begins professional practice; (2) when the experienced nurse changes work settings, either in a new organization or within the same organization; and (3) when the nurse undertakes new roles, such as assuming a leadership role or returning to school. Socialization, whether the first time it is experienced or as a later change in practice setting or role, involves personal changes as a new professional self-identity is formed or redefined. These changes, as with other kinds of change, can be both exciting and stressful and may evoke strong emotional reactions and inner conflict as old patterns are replaced with new perspectives, values, behaviors, and skills.

To better understand the process of socialization to professional nursing practice, examination of the status of nursing as a profession is helpful.

☼ Nursing as a Profession

The roots of nursing are firmly anchored in service to others: individuals, groups, and communities. Since the days of Florence Nightingale, nurses have entered nursing to help people and serve the health care needs of society. This service orientation is evident in the Nightingale Pledge, which has been spoken by millions of nurses since the late 1800s. Dedication to duty is reflective of nursing's evolutionary links from holy orders (Birchenall, 1998). The pledge concludes with "devote myself to the welfare of those committed to my care" (American Nurses Association, Nursing World: Media resources, n.d.). But are devotion and caring sufficient for nursing to call itself a profession? This question has stimulated discussion, debate, and controversy within health care and related disciplines. The ongoing debate about what nursing *is* and *is not* is timely and essential as the profession delineates its place within the emerging new order of health care delivery (Gordon, 2005).

Social scientists and leaders in nursing have worked for several decades to define what constitutes a profession. A *profession* is defined as an occupation that meets specified criteria beyond that of an occupation. Although the terms *occupation* and *profession* are often used interchangeably, the critical differences between the two concepts must be understood. A *profession* is characterized by prolonged education that takes place in a college or university and results in the acquisition of a body of knowledge based on theory and research. Values, beliefs, and ethics relating to the profession are integral parts of the educational preparation. By definition, a professional is *autonomous* in decision making and is *accountable* for his or her own actions. Personal identification and commitment to the profession are strong, and individuals are unlikely to change professions. In contrast, craft and trade *occupations* are characterized by technical skills learned through on-the-job apprenticeships. The training does not incorporate, at least as a prominent feature, the values, beliefs, and ethics of the occupation. Workers are supervised, and ultimate accountability rests with the employer. Thus commitment from individuals may vary, and job changes are more common.

CHARACTERISTICS OF A PROFESSION

In response to concerns about the quality of educational programs in medical schools, particularly admission standards and curriculum, the Carnegie Foundation issued a series of papers. Abraham Flexner's classic paper (1910) was part of this series and served as the catalyst for reform of medical education in the United States and Canada. Flexner's recommendations were supported by the American Medical Association and the American Public Health Association. Their collective efforts, along with the willingness of members of the medical community to embrace a major reorientation of medical education, led to changing the face of medicine within a 10-year period, strengthened medicine as a profession, and raised its status in the eyes of the public (Schwirian, 1998).

Flexner also studied other disciplines, and in 1915 he published a list of those criteria he believed were characteristic of all true professions. He viewed the intellectual aspect as central to professions. According to Flexner, a true profession includes the following characteristics:

- It is basically intellectual (as opposed to physical), with high responsibility.
- It is based on a body of knowledge that can be learned.
- It is practical (applied) rather than theoretical.
- It can be taught through the process of professional education.
- It has a strong internal organization of members.
- It has practitioners who are motivated by altruism (the desire to help others).

Since Flexner's work in 1915, additional authors have modified and amplified the criteria of a profession. The works of Greenwood (1957), Bixler and Bixler (1959), Houle (1980), and Joel (2003) are summarized in Table 3-1. The cluster of characteristics that emerges include (1) relevance to social values and needs, (2) a lengthy and required education, (3) a code of ethics, (4) a mechanism for self-regulation, (5) research-based theoretical frameworks for practice, (6) common identity and distinctive subculture, and (7) members motivated by altruism and commitment to the profession.

A specified body of knowledge and altruism are the most widely acknowledged characteristics of a profession. A professional possesses unique knowledge, and members of the profession acquire this knowledge through a significant period of training. Group members profess to be knowledgeable in an area that is not known by most people but which society needs. Members also are invested with a service ideal, *altruism*. Nursing actions convince the public that members are not self-serving but use knowledge to benefit the public. Society then grants autonomy or control to the profession to set its standards and regulate practice (McCloskey & Maas, 1998).

What society sees as nursing has, to a large extent, influenced nursing's public image: "The manner in which the public thinks of nurses will strongly influence the destiny of nursing and the contributions that nurses can make to better health care" (Kalisch & Kalisch, 2005, p. 16). Members of the public play an important role as they are called on to participate in decision-making processes in health care by voting, organizing, and exercising influence on government. For public citizens to do this responsibly and to make intelligent judgments, they need a clear awareness of nursing activities; however, the public more typically holds an "obsolete, one-dimensional image of nurses and their roles" (Kalisch & Kalisch, 2005, p. 16). Benner (2005), in a commentary to the Kalisch and Kalisch article, indicates that "nurses' voices are still relatively silent in the newspapers" (p. 14). She continues saying that nurses do much but say little in public arenas. However, outsiders cannot be expected to be the major champions of the visibility of nursing; nurses must move from "silence to voice" through public communication about nurses and nursing (Buresch & Gordon, 2000).

TABLE 3-1	Characteristics of a Profession			
Characteristic	**Joel (2003)**	**Houle (1980)**	**Bixler & Bixler (1959)**	**Greenwood (1957)**
Knowledge	Uses well-defined and well-organized body of knowledge that is intellectual and describes phenomena of concern	Mastery and use of theoretical knowledge Role distinctions that differentiate professional work from that of other vocations	Uses well-defined body of specialized knowledge at the intellectual level of higher learning	Uses a systematic body of knowledge
Mission	Enlarges body of knowledge and subsequently imposes on its members the lifelong obligation to remain current	Concept of mission open to change Capacity to solve problems	Continuously enlarges body of knowledge; uses scientific method to improve education and service	
Education	Entrusts the education of its practitioners to institutions of higher education	Formal training	Prepares practitioners in institutions of higher learning	
Social construct	Applies body of knowledge in services that are vital to human welfare	Service to society Public acceptance	Applies knowledge through services that are vital to human and social welfare	Sanctions of the community
Autonomy	Functions autonomously in formulation of professional policy and in monitoring of its practice and practitioners	Autonomous practice Credentialing system to certify competence	Functions autonomously in formulating professional policy and controlling professional activity	Professional autonomy
Accountability	Guided by a code of ethics that regulates the relationship between professional and client	Ethical practice Legal reinforcement of professional standards Penalties against incompetent or unethical practice		Ethical codes of conduct
Culture	Distinguished by presence of specific culture, norms, and values that are common among its members Attracts individuals of intellectual and personal qualities who exalt service above personal gain and who recognize their occupation as their life work	Creation of subculture	Attracts individuals who exalt service above personal gain and who recognize their chosen occupation as their life work	Professional culture
Compensation	Strives to compensate its practitioners by providing freedom of action, opportunity for continuous professional growth, and economic security	Continued seeking of self-enhancement by its members	Compensates practitioners by providing freedom of action, opportunity for continuous professional growth, and economic security	

Professionalization of Nursing

Professionalization is the process through which an occupation achieves professional status. The status of nursing as a profession is important because it reflects the value society places on the work of nurses and the centrality of this work to the good of society (Strader & Decker, 1995). Guided by the descriptions of what constitutes a profession, how does nursing measure up? At the time those criteria were being developed, nursing fell short of professional status in a number of areas. For example, most nursing education programs were based in hospitals and reflected an apprenticeship model rather than being in institutions of higher education. Nursing research was in its infancy, thereby offering little toward the identification of a unique body of knowledge that would improve nursing practice and education. In addition, autonomous nursing practice was relatively uncommon, and no formalized code of ethics existed.

In contrast, today most nursing education programs are based in institutions of higher education. An expanding body of knowledge derived from systematic research provides frameworks to guide evidence-based practice. Opportunities for autonomous practice are expanding, and a well-defined code of ethics has been developed. Areas still needing attention include nursing's control of policies and activities that affect the delivery of nursing care. This has become more evident as health care delivery has undergone dramatic organizational, financial, and personnel changes that individually and collectively affect how, what, and where nursing is practiced. In this redesigned health care environment, nurses are challenged to engage in practice that embodies the social service ideal, where clients rather than tasks are given the highest level of importance.

An analysis of nursing's placement along the occupation-profession continuum reveals strengths and challenges. Strengths include (1) a service-to-society mission, (2) the provision of services that are vital to human welfare, and (3) a well-defined code of ethics. Challenges include (1) limited development of nursing theory and a unique body of nursing knowledge, (2) lack of standardization of nursing education, with university preparation still not the minimum entry requirement, (3) variation in members' commitment to their work, and (4) minimal cohesive culture within the nursing community (Schwirian, 1998).

BARRIERS TO PROFESSIONALISM

Autonomy, the freedom to act, is a key characteristic present in all definitions of a profession and is clearly linked to achieving professional status. But autonomy is linked to other characteristics as well. A limited body of scientific knowledge and an incomplete articulation of phenomena unique to nursing are cited as major contributors to the lack of autonomy in nursing practice. Nursing is still viewed by many as a lower level of medical knowledge that should be under the jurisdiction of medicine (Wurst, 1994). In contrast, Gordon (2005) compares the difference between nurses and physicians to that of a ship's captain and its pilot. She identifies similarities between a physician and the captain, suggesting that their knowledge is more abstract, with general skills needed to manage a vessel in open waters. In contrast, the nurse is similar to the ship's pilot, possessing more particular knowledge that is highly contextual. She describes nurses as piloting patients into ports of health, coping, cure, and death.

The development of nursing knowledge is fundamental to the professionalization of nursing. The science of nursing is concerned with developing a unified body of knowledge that includes skills and methods for applying that knowledge (Chinn & Kramer, 1999). Until the 1980s knowledge, by definition, was empirically based, focusing exclusively on objective, observable data and an analytical, linear line of reasoning. Since that time awareness has been growing that exclusive reliance on empirical data provides only a partial view of the world and that knowledge can best be expanded by using multiple approaches to scientific inquiry. Carper's classic publication (1978) describes four fundamental and enduring patterns of knowing:

- *Empirics*—the science of nursing
- *Ethics*—the component of moral knowledge in nursing
- *Aesthetics*—the art of nursing
- *Personal*—the component of personal knowledge in nursing

According to Chinn and Kramer (1999), "the fundamental patterns of knowing remain valuable in that they conceptualize a broad scope of knowing that accounts for a holistic practice" (p. 4). Thus nursing knowledge is derived from theoretical formulations and scientific research, as well as an analysis of personal experiences that contributes to clinical knowledge and expertise. The continued development of a distinct body of knowledge will aid in differentiating nursing from other health professions and provide a stronger basis for practice.

Other factors identified as limiting nursing's autonomy include gender stereotypes and public image. Historically, women have been socialized to shy away from power and assume more subservient roles. Gordon (2005) cites the fusion of nursing and moral virtues as one of the building blocks of this 19th-century secularization and professionalization of nursing. If nursing is viewed as a calling, a form of penance, or a hobby, then education and experience will not seem relevant. The typical emphasis on the emotional aspects of nursing rather than on the required intelligence and skill returns attention to nurses as self-sacrificing and silent. Unfortunately, some of the current language being used in public relations efforts keeps nursing in this emotional state. Use of phrases such as "the noble profession," "lifting spirits, touching lives," or identifying rewards of nursing as being "big doses of public affection" and "a job where people will love you" returns nursing to that 19th-century stereotype. In sharp contrast, nursing is a profession with a high level of specificity. Aiken, Clarke, Sloane, and Sochalski (2001) describe nurses as the early warning and intervention systems; Gordon (2005) views nursing as creating order out of chaos and protecting patients from risk without making them feel at risk.

Presentation of self may also act as a barrier to advancing the professional status of nursing. For example, "nurses' verbal informality with patients is linked to persistent stereotypic themes that diminish the professional image, shroud the cognitive nature of their work, perpetuate hierarchical relationships between physicians and nurses, and even threaten nurses' therapeutic effectiveness" (Campbell-Heider, Hart, & Bergren, 1994, pp. 212-213). However, attempts to elevate the language of nurses must be balanced with

clarity in meaning. Gordon (2005) points to the confusion by the official-sounding statements used in nursing diagnoses. Use of this language is "an understandable attempt to give status to nursing work but ends up concealing it from those who have a need to know" (p. 217). She goes on to say that speaking English rather than "code" would help everyone better understand what nurses do. Gordon asserts that it would be far "more productive if nurses professionalized their appearance rather than their jargon" (p. 438).

Indeed, clothing styles seem to diminish the professional status of nursing. The current style of dress may make nurses seem more accessible, but Gordon (2005) asserts that today's common attire also makes nurses more forgettable, stating that the "new uniforms" make nurses look immature and silly, signaling that they are not a threat to anyone's power or authority. In contrast, physicians continue to dress for status as well as easy identification. Nurses today tend to dress in "pajama-like outfits with heart, flower, and angel designs or in pastels. Nurses blend into an undifferentiated mass of people whose outfits signal an asymmetrical power relationship" (Gordon, 2005, p. 34), whereas most physicians wear lab coats or business suits. In response to an editorial on appropriate nursing attire in *NurseWeek* (Ulrich, 2005), comments from patients focused on the importance of being able to tell who the nurses are; they were less interested in color of uniform. In this article a nurse reader commented, "If nurses cannot agree on what image they present to their clients and the public, then how can nurses come together concerning nursing as a profession?" (p. 3).

In addition to uniforms that do little to distinguish a nurse from a janitor, failure to allow nurses to use their last names and titles further adds to a lack of professional status. To fully appreciate this effect, consider that a nurse with a name tag that says "Kristen, Nursing" would be comparable to a physician being referred to as "Eric, Geriatrics." The medical field recognizes that this familiarity would diminish a physician's status. Nursing has not yet reached such a consensus.

Takase, Kershaw, and Burt (2002) focused on nurses' perceptions of common public stereotypes and identified that these perceptions were related to the development of self-concept, collective self-esteem, and job satisfaction. To counter these public stereotypes, nurses must be less modest about taking credit for what they know and do. Too often, nurses do not take ownership, but instead assign the credit to others.

Other groups that attempt to control nursing, such as organized medicine and health services administration, are well organized, have clearly defined their unique content and roles, and are viewed as having control of professions that enjoy high status. However, the occupation-profession distinction is largely artificial. The designation of what is professional versus what is occupational is based on tradition and existing mechanisms (unions and academic departments) in an effort to maintain the status quo (McCloskey & Maas, 1998).

Taking a different approach to professionalization, Adams, Miller, and Beck (1996) focus on the individual nurse. Their approach reflects the view of Styles (1982), who maintained that the individual and her or his personal presentation fosters the collective image of nursing.

A MODEL FOR PROFESSIONALISM

Citing lack of consensus among nurses on what behaviors exemplify professional status, Miller (1985) and Miller, Adams, and Beck (1993) drew from common definitions of a profession and added behaviors expressed in key nursing documents, such as early versions of the American Nurses Association's *Social Policy Statement* and *Code of Ethics for Nurses*. Miller's "wheel of professionalism" is presented in Figure 3-1. The basic education of a professional, occurring in a university setting with emphasis on the scientific basis of nursing, is at the hub of the wheel. The eight spokes extending from the hub represent behaviors deemed essential to achieving, maintaining, and expanding professionalism in the individual nurse.

Professional Nursing Practice

Florence Nightingale (1860), in her clear and direct manner, stated that the goal of nursing is to "put the patient in the best condition for nature to act upon

him" (p. 133). This essence of nursing practice continues to be reflected in contemporary nursing. In the revised *Social Policy Statement* developed by the ANA (2003), six essential features of contemporary nursing practice are identified (p. 5):

1. Provision of a caring relationship that facilitates health and healing
2. Attention to the full range of human experiences and responses to health and illness within the physical and social environments
3. Integration of objective data with knowledge gained from an appreciation of the patient's or group's subjective experience
4. Application of scientific knowledge to the processes of diagnosis and treatment through the use of judgment and critical thinking
5. Advancement of professional nursing knowledge through scholarly inquiry
6. Influence on social and public policy to promote social justice

VALUES OF THE PROFESSION

Knowledge, skills, and ethical grounding of the nurse directly affect the quality of care provided. The profession's values give direction and meaning to its members, guide nursing behaviors, are instrumental in clinical decision making, and influence how nurses think about themselves. Although skills change and evolve over time, core values of nursing persist and are communicated through the ANA's *Code of Ethics for Nurses* (ANA, 2001). With licensure as a registered nurse, each nurse accepts responsibility for practicing nursing consistent with these values. The *Code of Ethics for Nurses* with associated ethical principles is summarized in Table 3-2 and discussed further in the chapter on ethics (Chapter 12). Note that philosophical ethical principles and concepts of interpersonal relationships are reflected, either directly or indirectly, in all the canons. The ethical principles are those most directly reflected in the respective canons.

Weis and Schank (2000) developed and tested an instrument based on the ANA's *Code of Ethics for Nurses* that measured professional nursing values. Included were 44 short descriptive phrases (each

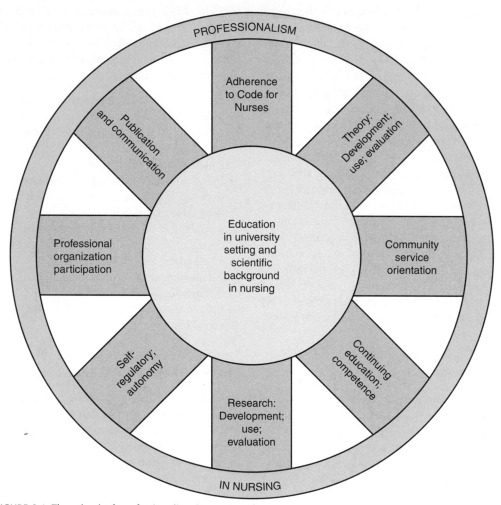

FIGURE 3-1 The wheel of professionalism in nursing. (Reprinted with permission: Wheel of Professionalism in Nursing. © 1984, Barbara Kemp Miller.)

reflecting a specific code statement), along with interpretive commentary for each phrase. With a sample of 599 respondents, *caregiving* was the predominant professional nursing value identified.

When nurses were asked to provide a description of a patient care situation that would exemplify what was meaningful in nursing, *altruism* (unselfish concern for or devotion to the welfare of others) was identified as the overall philosophy that guided nursing practice. Human dignity was further identified as a core value, with linking values of recognition of the client as an individual, empathetic understanding, and reciprocal trust.

Examining professional values held by baccalaureate and associate degree nursing students, Martin, Yarbrough, and Alfred (2003) found that the student groups did not differ significantly. However, significant differences were found for both gender and ethnicity. Men scored lower on all subscales and on the total scale. Ethnic groups differed on responses to three subscales representing respect for human dignity, safeguarding the client and public, and collaborating to meet public health needs.

Service to society has remained a central value of nursing, and nursing's consistent provision of service

TABLE 3-2	Code of Ethics for Nurses*	
Code Provisions	**Ethical Principles**	**Ethical/Therapeutic Concepts Addressed**
The nurse, in all professional relationships, practices with compassion and respect for the inherent dignity, worth, and uniqueness of every individual, unrestricted by considerations of social or economic status, personal attributes, or the nature of health problems.	Autonomy (client) Veracity Justice (distributive)	Dignity and worth of client Respect Advocacy for client rights Interpersonal connectedness Therapeutic relationships Compassion
The nurse's primary commitment is to the patient, whether an individual, family, group, or community.	Confidentiality Fidelity Veracity	Trustworthiness Therapeutic boundaries Conflict resolution
The nurse promotes, advocates for, and strives to protect the health, safety, and rights of the patient.	Confidentiality Beneficence Nonmaleficence	Advocacy Obligations (legal; professional)
The nurse is responsible and accountable for individual nursing practice and determines the appropriate delegation of tasks consistent with the nurse's obligation to provide optimum patient care.	Beneficence Nonmaleficence Fidelity Autonomy (nurse)	Responsibility/accountability Scope of practice Clinical competency Collaboration
The nurse owes the same duties to self as to others, including the responsibility to preserve integrity and safety, to maintain competence, and to continue personal and professional growth.	Beneficence	Self-respect Integrity Trustworthiness
The nurse participates in establishing, maintaining, and improving health care environments and conditions of employment conducive to the provision of quality health care and consistent with the values of the profession through individual and collective action.	Fidelity Autonomy	Advocacy Integrity Standards of practice Change
The nurse participates in the advancement of the profession through contributions to practice, education, administration, and knowledge development.	Autonomy	Professionalism Standards of practice Patterns of knowing** Scholarship/research
The nurse collaborates with other health professionals and the public in promoting community, national, and international efforts to meet health needs.	Justice Beneficence Nonmaleficence	Collaboration Health policy
The profession of nursing, as represented by associations and their members, is responsible for articulating nursing values, for maintaining the integrity of the profession and its practice, and for shaping social policy.	Justice Beneficence	Social policy Collaboration Patterns of knowing**

*Based on the American Nurses Association. (2001). *Code of ethics for nurses with interpretative statements*. Washington, DC: Author.
**Carper, B. A. (1978). Fundamental patterns of knowing in nursing. *Advances in Nursing Science, 1*(1), 13-23. Courtesy B. P. Fargotstein, Tempe, AZ.

to benefit the public has earned the public's trust. A key component in preserving this trust is accountability. *Accountability* is the state of being responsible and answerable for one's own behavior. This is explicit in the ANA's *Code of Ethics for Nurses* (2001): "Nurses are accountable for judgements made and actions taken in the course of nursing practice irrespective of health care organizations' policies or providers' directives" (p. 16). Accountability extends to self, the client, the employing agency, the profession, and the public. The ANA's *Scope and Standards of Clinical Nursing Practice* (2004) describe both the "what" and "how" of professional nursing. *Standards of practice* are the "what" and describe a competent level of nursing care through use of the nursing process. *Standards of professional performance* are the "how" of nursing, with nine standards describing a competent level of behavior in the professional role. Each standard is accompanied by criteria that permit measurement of performance and characterize competent, professional practice. These standards are listed in Box 3-1. Further elaboration of professional nursing responsibilities can be found in the standards of care for the various specialty practices.

RESPONSIBILITY

Areas of responsibility within nursing's role are constantly being affected by changes in the larger health care arena. Johnson, Friend, and MacDonald (1997) describe a "sense of displacement" as nurses experience a shift to new areas of responsibility while relinquishing some of the more traditional ones. They identify emerging professional nurse responsibilities as:

- Establishing and maintaining partnership relationships with client and family
- Caring and creating healing space by spending non–task-related time with clients
- Using time and skills to build trust and work collaboratively
- Understanding and appreciating client stories and experiences with health and illness as these experiences affect their lives
- Learning through reflection on self and practice
- Encouraging the active collaboration of client and family in choosing their own care

---

BOX 3-1	Standards of Clinical Nursing Practice

Standards of Practice
- Assessment
- Diagnosis
- Outcome identification
- Planning
- Implementation
- Evaluation

Standards of Professional Performance
- Quality of care
- Practice evaluation
- Education
- Collegiality
- Collaboration
- Ethics
- Research
- Resource utilization
- Leadership

Modified from American Nurses Association. (2004). *Nursing: Scope and standards of clinical nursing practice.* Washington, DC: Author.

- Sharing work responsibilities in a mindful way
- Informing clients of treatment choices and teaching self-care and responsibility for their own health
- Serving as a mentor to different levels of health care providers

With a strong emphasis on the emotional aspects of nursing, the above list does not adequately capture the nurse's responsibilities in the areas of science and technology, critical thinking and decision making, and skillful management of risk. This is of limited use in better informing the public of nursing's role and may not attract the next generation of young adults to select nursing as their career choice. Recently, Utley-Smith (2004) identified more specific competencies for new baccalaureate graduates. Using a cross-sectional survey design, she queried 363 nurse administrators from three health care settings. Competency areas included (1) health promotion, (2) supervision, (3) interpersonal communication, (4) direct care, (5) computer technology, and (6) caseload management. The delineation of skill items within each of the competency areas provides a more explicit description of the cognitive aspects of nursing (Utley-Smith, 2004, p. 168), providing a better balance to the frequently overemphasized emotional aspects of nursing.

ACCOUNTABILITY

By virtue of the ANA's *Standards of Clinical Nursing Practice* and the state nurse practice acts, society holds nurses and those under their supervision accountable for their actions. The nurse has a responsibility to demonstrate sound judgment, critical thinking, and competence in the caregiver role. In the supervisory role, the nurse must ensure that only competent health care workers be allowed to care for clients and is obligated to take action in response to inappropriate or questionable practice. Although a task can be delegated, accountability remains with the nurse.

Another demonstration of nursing's accountability is through formulating policies, controlling its activities, and advocating professional issues in the political system. Nursing organizations have developed standards of practice for general and specialty nursing care, with each set of standards addressing *professional accountability*. *Legal accountability* occurs through licensing procedures, certification, and disciplinary actions that are established and implemented by state boards of nursing. These measures support the public trust that safe, effective practice will be the standard of practice. In the political arena, nurses demonstrate their commitment to service to others by becoming increasingly involved in advocating for health care legislation that strengthens nursing practice, protects the public, and offers choice to consumers. A more in-depth discussion of the legal aspects that influence professional nursing practice is provided in Chapter 11.

AUTONOMY

A further reflection of the public's trust in the nursing profession is the responsibility to be self-governing or autonomous. *Autonomy* is independence or the freedom to act. It implies control over practice and is exemplified by the profession being invested with responsibilities for nursing education, development of policies and standards that guide practice, and oversight to ensure competent practice.

Autonomy involves independence on the part of the nurse, as well as a willingness to take risks and be accountable for actions. MacIntosh (2003) asserts that "the context of the workplace is influential in nurses' development as autonomous professionals" (p. 726). Gordon (2005) questions nurses' autonomy, indicating that control over education, licensure, and nursing service in hospitals gives the appearance of autonomy, but concluding that the work that nurses perform remains in many ways subject to another occupation. Autonomy in nursing practice must be balanced with interdependence (not dependence) because health care is a multidisciplinary endeavor and several disciplines contribute to total client care.

Socialization to Professional Nursing

Socialization is the process of becoming—acquiring knowledge and skills and internalizing attitudes and values specific to a given social group. Much of the literature on socialization has focused on child development and the influence of the family on the child's socialization. This process occurs through role modeling and the reinforcement of socially relevant behaviors. Increased attention is now being given to *adult socialization*, the process by which individuals develop new behaviors and values associated with roles they assume as adults. With assistance from others, individuals learn necessary behaviors, values, norms, and skills to assume new roles successfully.

Socialization to professional nursing is the process of learning the skills, roles, and values of the profession, with the outcome being the development of a professional identity. It represents a complex process by which a student or practicing nurse acquires the knowledge, skills, and a sense of occupational identity. This process involves the internalization of the values and norms of the profession in the individual's own behavior and self-concept. It is the process of taking the values and norms and making them part of who the person is as a nurse. The individual's conception of what it means to be a nurse and to act as a nurse initially occurs through education and is then extended into the work setting.

SOCIALIZATION THROUGH EDUCATION

Learning any new role can be a challenging and anxiety-producing task. As adults, individuals have developed competencies in various previously learned roles. The choice to learn a new role returns the adult to novice status, one of limited or no knowledge of new role expectations.

Initial Socialization. Professional socialization through education is the pathway to learning new roles within the culture of nursing. Initial socialization to nursing occurs in the educational setting and is subsequently transferred to the practice setting. Howkins and Ewens (1999) sought to understand how nursing students make sense of the socialization process. Through their research, they identified three themes relating to how a student's role identity changes and develops during his or her education. The first theme, *development of the graduate practitioner,* focuses on awareness of having more knowledge, perspective, confidence, reflective thinking, political awareness, and being able to think critically. The second theme, *gaining a better understanding of own role,* focuses on continuing refinement of role components. The third theme, *adopting a less-polarized view,* is characterized by no longer seeing roles as having rigid boundaries and reveals "the development of graduate practitioners who understand their own role while becoming less rigid in their thinking" (Howkins & Ewens, 1999, p. 47).

The socialization process experienced by baccalaureate nursing students was described by Reutter, Field, Campbell, and Day (1997). The setting for the study was a large university that offered a 4-year baccalaureate nursing program. The development of the students was tracked longitudinally, and their experiences were described as follows:

Year 1: Learning the Ideal. Students begin to internalize new values, focusing on caring and holistic individualized practice. Students are more passive as learners, and although they can delineate professional values, they are unable to describe how these values play out in the practice setting.

Year 2: Confronting Reality. Students place greater emphasis on the application of theory and are more aware of their limited knowledge base and scope of responsibilities. This results in greater feelings of inadequacy but increased appreciation of organizational skills, time management, and the uniqueness of patient situations. With limited confidence they seek validation and are vulnerable to feedback.

Year 3: Becoming Comfortable with Reality. Students' activities are focused on fine-tuning their art of nursing, role making and role taking, modifying behaviors of the role, and moving from "ideal" to "optimal" care delivery.

Year 4: Extending Beyond Reality of Student Practice. Increasing focus is placed on skills of the real world, greater initiation in seeking out experiences to increase confidence, and a broadening of their view of nursing to include political action strategies, the health care system, and public awareness of nursing's expanding role (Reutter et al., 1997).

Meyer and Xu (2005) consider whether nursing education is guilty of "failure to rescue." They contrast the educational environment with the reality of work and describe education as being "black and white," whereas the work setting consists of shades of gray. They assert that nursing students are "naive and, without benefit of interventions from the faculty, are at peril of maladaptive change, either reinforcing their belief in the academic ideal and becoming disillusioned, or devaluing the academic ideal to a well-meant but clinically irrelevant concept" (Meyer & Xu, 2005, p. 77). They maintain that students must engage both the academic ideal and the clinical reality. To assist students in managing these seemingly opposite perspectives, they developed primary, secondary, and tertiary interventions. *Primary interventions* focus on preparing the student before clinical experience by openly discussing these different realities. Benner's *Novice to Expert* (1984) can assist students in understanding that as novices they are learning the rules before learning the exceptions, and that "ideal procedural techniques be precluded by less than ideal circumstances" (Meyer & Xu, 2005, p. 78). The goal of *secondary interventions* is early identification of dissonant stress and a reduction of the impact of negative responses. Secondary intervention should occur during clinical experiences and include prompt discussions of any dissonant experiences. Finally, through *tertiary interventions*, benefit is obtained from engaging students in reflective practice during postclinical discussions.

MacIntosh (2003) identified a similar dissonance problem for nurses in the workplace. She indicated that "new graduates assume that they are professional, competent, and respected, but soon realize that there is more to being professional than completing their initial education" (p. 739) and earning the legal title of nurse. MacIntosh identified an interactive three-stage process described as "reworking professional identity." Stage 1, *assuming adequacy*, is characterized by nurses' diminished awareness of others' opinions and of their own practice. This occurs through neglecting reflection on one's own practice and concentrating on more technical skills and recognizes stress as leading nurses to focus on tasks. Stage 2 is *realizing practice*. In this stage nurses become aware of discrepancies between expectations and experiences and values and practice. Then, through the use of critical thinking, they attempt to balance these discrepancies. With this comes a gradual realization that their skills and attitudes may be limited. MacIntosh identified three strategies nurses use to attempt this balance: (1) they develop response patterns to protect themselves from critics, (2) they make connections with a mentor to aid in their development, and (3) they work to build their own credibility. In this second stage nurses also make a decision on whether to pursue professional development and begin to notice that they are accepted as team members. They have stronger self-esteem and an increased sense of confidence and competence as they struggle with the idea of what being professional means to them. Finally, Stage 3 is *developing a reputation*. This requires intentional effort and is achieved through actions directed toward the goal. During this stage nurses establish practice patterns that reflect a consistent way of managing their practice and approaches to learning. They also select standards that will guide their practice and how their work will be done. MacIntosh (2003) concludes that "at the end of this stage, nurses have developed professional identities that reflect reputations for expertise, interest in learning, active contributions to the profession, and interest in assisting new nurses" (p. 737).

Resocialization. Returning to school represents a role transition and triggers a new socialization process as new role expectations are synthesized and a new professional identity is established. Knowles' classic work on adult education (1970) defined what he termed *andragogy* as the "art and science of how adults learn" (p. 43). According to Knowles, adult learners:

- Exhibit self-direction and self-responsibility
- Demonstrate acquired experience that serves as a resource for learning
- Have shifted from learning with postponed application to learning with immediate application
- Strive for self-esteem and self-actualization

This model is particularly applicable to the nurse who returns to school for an additional degree. Most RNs who return to school continue their employment and must balance concurrent roles of nurse, student, parent, and significant other, to name a few. Although challenging, multiple roles can provide new rewards and a positive synergy that might not be experienced from a single role (Curry, 1997).

Historically, educational programs have not been known for their accommodation of the nurse as student. RN students came with a nursing role identity, but little recognition was given to the expertise the nurse possessed. Returning nurses were frustrated when they were expected to repeat and validate their clinical knowledge and competencies; their licenses and clinical practice were seemingly ignored. The perception was one of questioning the nurse's legitimacy in holding a license to practice. The friction produced by such activities could serve as a barrier to learning and a hindrance to socialization into the new role of a BSN graduate. Fortunately, returning nurses today are more likely to be recognized for the experience and knowledge they bring. The focus has turned to building on their existing foundation, emphasizing new learning to support the transition to the baccalaureate role.

Learning any new role requires the ability to embrace change. The struggle between the old and new may cause anxiety and tension related to being a novice again or experiencing fear of failure and fear of the unknown. Although nursing has not been successful in reaching agreement about the education needed for entry into professional practice, developing educational models that facilitate movement from one level of preparation to another in a relatively user-friendly way has been successful (McBride, 1999). With increased recognition and appreciation of what the RN student brings to the educational setting, and working to provide program structures that acknowledge the need to balance multiple roles, the RN educational experience can be positive and growth producing. If resocialization through education is fully effective, the student (basic and RN) leaves the educational program with changes in attitudes and behavior that reflect an integration of the values and norms of the expanded scope of the professional practitioner.

SOCIALIZATION TO THE WORK SETTING

Education is only the initial process in socialization. The professional nursing role learned in the educational setting must now be transferred and modified to fit the workplace. Thus the continuum of socialization extends as resocialization begins.

The socialization process is built around role theory. Individuals learn behaviors that accompany each role by two simultaneously occurring processes: (1) interaction involving groups and significant others in a social context, and (2) learning through role playing, identification, modeling, instruction, observation, trial and error, and role negotiation (Hardy & Conway, 1988). Adding to the complexity of this process is the "should be," or ideal presented in the educational setting, and the "what is," or reality of the actual practice environment. Faculty and staff have the obligation of helping students understand the logic and rationale for any discrepancies that may exist (Coudret, Fuchs, Roberts, Suhrheinrich, & White, 1994).

Kramer's Socialization Model. One of the best-known models of socialization in nursing is Kramer's *Reality Shock: Why Nurses Leave Nursing* (1974). She describes fears and difficulties new graduate nurses experience in adapting to the work setting and refers to feelings of powerlessness and ineffectiveness as *reality shock*. Reality shock results from a conflict between a new graduate's knowledge and skills acquired in the educational program and the reality of the behaviors

required in the actual work setting. New graduates progress through four stages before feeling comfortable in the professional role.

Phase 1 focuses on *mastery of skills and routines*. New graduates feel inadequate and frustrated and, as a result, tend to focus on the mastery of essential skills. A potential problem here is that the nurse may become fixated on technical skills and fail to see other important aspects of client care, such as emotional needs.

Phase 2 is *social integration*. The new nurse's major concern is getting along with co-workers and fitting into the work group. Conflict occurs when a new nurse strives to maintain high ideals and standards learned in the educational setting and at the same time avoid alienating co-workers.

Phase 3 is *moral outrage*. During this stage incongruities among roles in the work setting cause the new nurse to feel angry, frustrated, and inadequately prepared. Determining priorities is a challenge.

In Phase 4, *conflict resolution*, new nurses either give up or compromise their values and behaviors or successfully integrate them into the professional and bureaucratic systems. This results in one of four possible outcomes. The new nurse (1) finds work situations that are more compatible with her or his beliefs or leaves nursing altogether; or (2) accepts the values of the bureaucracy and gives up values gained in the educational program and simply tries to fit into the organization; or (3) yields to the organization, with the focus on survival; or (4) learns to use values of both the profession and the organization to influence positive change in the system. Kramer calls this fourth outcome *biculturalism* and considers it the healthiest and most successful resolution.

After the publication of Kramer's work, educational programs and employers, primarily hospitals, began to examine methods that could reduce reality shock in the transition from student to professional. For example, students were encouraged to gain experience outside school settings as nursing assistants or nurse externs during the summer, school breaks, and weekends. In addition, educational programs began to pair students with preceptors so they could work closely with a practicing RN. In the work setting, longer orientation programs provided an opportunity for smoother transitions. Preceptor programs were also offered to allow the new nurse to work alongside an experienced nurse. In recent years, formal nurse residency programs were established by some hospitals. Commitment, creativity, and collaboration among educational programs and employers are key factors in facilitating the new graduate's successful socialization into the professional nursing role.

SOURCES OF LEARNING: SOCIALIZING AGENTS IN EDUCATION AND PRACTICE

Educational programs and employers can assist in clarifying role expectations and decreasing conflict through the use of role models, preceptors, and mentors. If these socializing agents were placed along an involvement continuum, one end would be anchored by role models (least involvement) and the other end would be anchored by mentors (most involvement). Despite the somewhat blurred boundaries and functions of these roles, each has an important part to play in the nurse's socialization process.

A *role model* is someone to copy, emulate, and admire. Role models are usually experienced, competent nurses who exemplify excellence in practice. Qualities of role models may include a skillful, intelligent, empathetic approach to care delivery, compassion, accessibility, approachability, flexibility, professional competence, and power (Thomka, 2001). Learning through role modeling occurs primarily through observation and then is followed by emulation. Little contact is needed, and it is usually viewed as a passive process—the student or new nurse observes the behaviors of the role model and incorporates selected behaviors into his or her own professional identity. The availability of role models in practice is a key influence on professional socialization. Thomka reported a lack of consistency in the way new nurses were assisted in their first positions. This inconsistency, combined with the variability of role models in practice, may have a significant impact on nurses' socialization and professional development.

Students may also adopt one another as role models and differentiate between peers who are becoming "good" nurses and those who are less effective in their care delivery. These peer role models facilitate learning by sharing experiences, knowledge, and clinical expertise; providing emotional support; and assisting with psychomotor skills. Students are most influenced by a combination of positive and negative versus positive-only modeling. Nonexemplars (negative role models) are used to reaffirm their own ideals about what they want (and do not want) to become (Reutter et al., 1977). Observing, judging, and developing the ability to differentiate between effective and ineffective care delivery are critical skills for competent professional practice (Parathian & Taylor, 1993). New graduates are also aware of both positive and negative role models and consciously structure their interactions after positive role models (Benner, Tanner, & Chelsa, 1996). Role models may also be preceptors and mentors.

Preceptors are experienced members of a clinical staff who work one-on-one with students or new graduates to provide guidance and supervision for a predetermined amount of time. More specifically, a *preceptor* models behavior, fosters independence and skill development, aids in application of theory, promotes socialization to the work setting, and helps build competence and confidence in the student or new graduate (Letizia & Jennrich, 1998; McGregor, 1999). Preceptors may function in more than one role. Roles identified include change agent, educator, mentor, consultant, supervisor, and resource person (Ellerton, 2003). Lockwood-Rayermann (2003) stated that the most effective mode of leadership in a preceptor is one that complements the organizational environment, the task, and the characteristics of the person being precepted. She described two primary styles to be used with followers: directing and coaching. *Directing*, which involves specific instruction and close supervision, is most useful when the follower is unable or unwilling to complete the task. This approach is described as "high directive and low supportive" (Lockwood-Rayermann, 2003, p. 248). *Coaching* includes explaining decisions while providing opportunities for clarification. Lockwood-Rayermann emphasized that successful matching of preceptors with students or new graduates can influence their perceptions of the organization and the profession of nursing.

Benefits are evident for preceptors as they build knowledge and skills through teaching, learn with students or new graduates, and feel they are making a contribution to the profession. These benefits contribute to preceptors voicing a renewed sense of pride in nursing (McGregor, 1999). However, stress may result from demands on preceptors that exceed their available time and resources. Typically, nurses add the preceptor role to their other regular clinical responsibilities. In addition, some preceptors may not have preparation in teaching and evaluation, which are key responsibilities of the role. With recent nursing program expansions, demand is growing for quality clinical placements. This demand is taxing available clinical sites and placing greater demands on preceptors. Active agency and educational support is essential in recognizing preceptors' contributions to nursing education and in sustaining preceptor involvement in socialization of new nurses into the practice setting (Greenberg, Colombraro, DeBlasio, Dolan, & Rich, 2001).

Mentors take on an even more powerful role in the socialization process. *Mentoring* is defined as a "planned pairing of a more experienced person with a lesser skilled individual for the purpose of achieving mutually agreed upon outcomes" (Dorsey & Baker, 2004, p. 260). It is described as a partnership in which both individuals share in the personal growth process and development of one another. Mentoring serves two functions: (1) a career function and (2) a psychosocial function. The *career function* includes such activities as teaching, coaching, protecting, and challenging work assignments. The *psychosocial function* may include providing emotional support and helping build self-confidence and self-worth (Dorsey & Baker, 2004). A mentor takes a personal interest in helping an individual over a period to develop the knowledge and skills needed to realize the full potential and major life goals of the person being mentored.

Identification of a mentor does not occur automatically but requires a proactive approach from both the potential mentor and the protégé in search of a mentor. Certain individual characteristics are necessary before mentoring can occur. These include a mutual attraction with sharing of similar views and common interests; respect; altruism; belief in the other's potential; capacity to work hard; integrity; mastery of concepts and ideas; unselfish gifts of time, energy, and trust; and a willingness for self-disclosure (Stewart & Krueger,

1996). "Successful mentoring requires active participation in the relationship with equal responsibility for its success on both mentor and protégé, along with institutional and collegial support" (Owens, Herrick, & Kelley, 1998, p. 22).

A review of the literature confirmed six essential features of mentoring. First is a teaching-learning process in which the protégé can benefit from the mistakes and successes of the mentor and avoid adverse situations. Second, a reciprocal role exists, with the protégé gradually shifting from dependence on the mentor in the beginning to increasing independence and autonomy with a balanced, two-way give and take between mentor and protégé. Third, nurses who have been mentored experience greater career development, position advancement, productivity, and development of a "nursing gestalt." Fourth, a knowledge or competence differential exists between mentor and protégé. Fifth, mentoring has a duration of several years. Sixth, a resonating phenomenon occurs—those who have been mentored will mentor others in the future as a way of expressing gratitude for their own experience (Stewart & Krueger, 1996). Factors such as time with the mentor, the mentor's experience, and choice in selection of a mentor provide positive benefit for role socialization and, ultimately, patient care outcomes. Age differences and the tone of the clinical setting can either facilitate or hinder the development of mentoring (Hayes, 2001). The benefits of mentoring are significant and make the demands on time and energy worthwhile. Unfortunately, not every nurse has the benefit of having a mentor during each career change.

Socialization and Career Development

Career development extends over time, with the process beginning when the new graduate enters the work setting and proceeding at varied rates along a career path. Two models of career development in nursing are presented. The stages of one model lead to an increased level of responsibility (Dalton, Thompson, & Price, 1977); the stages of the other lead to a higher level of clinical expertise (Benner, 1984).

DALTON'S LONGITUDINAL MODEL

Dalton and colleagues described a four-stage model of career development that builds on prior knowledge and experience:

Stage 1. The nurse learns to perform routine duties competently and to use both formal and informal channels of communication. Ideally, the nurse works with an experienced preceptor who also serves as a role model. A problem occurs when the organization does not permit enough time to master this stage.

Stage 2. The individual develops a reputation as a competent nurse, often in an area of clinical specialty. Again, adequate time is needed in this stage to master this level of expertise.

Stage 3. The nurse assumes responsibility for others. The nurse may take on multiple roles, such as informal mentor, manager, supervisor, or coordinator.

Stage 4. The nurse assumes the roles of manager and innovator of ideas to influence the direction of the organization. Relationships are developed inside and outside the organization. Individuals in Stage 4 think more broadly about the organization and feel comfortable in exercising power and taking a position with which others may disagree. Only a small percentage of nurses achieve this level of career development, either by choice or because of limits on the number of positions available.

BENNER'S NOVICE-TO-EXPERT MODEL

Five stages or levels of proficiency in nursing care delivery are identified in the novice-to-expert model (Benner, 1984). These stages reflect changes in three general aspects of skilled performance. First, movement from reliance on abstract principles to the use of past concrete experiences as paradigms occurs. Second, the learner's perception of the demand situation changes, in which the situation is seen less as a compilation of equally relevant bits and more as a complete whole in which only certain parts are relevant. Third, a change from being a detached observer to an involved performer engaged in the situation takes place. Benner also identified 31 different competencies that are evident in clinical practice. She organized the competencies into the following seven domains of nursing practice:

1. The helping role
2. The teaching-coaching function
3. The diagnostic and patient monitoring function
4. Effective management of rapidly changing situations
5. Administration and monitoring of therapeutic interventions and regimens
6. Monitoring of (and ensuring the quality of) health care practices
7. Organizational and work role competencies

This classic model addresses changes that occur across the seven domains of nursing practice as the inexperienced nurse moves from being a novice (Stage 1) to an expert practitioner (Stage 5). Characteristics of each of the five stages are presented in Box 3-2.

Environmental Factors That Influence Socialization

Recall that socialization is the adaptation to changing roles and is a continuing, interactive, lifelong process. Each role change may produce stress and conflict, regardless of whether the nurse is experienced. To facilitate successful socialization to nursing roles in the workplace, nurses need to have an awareness and understanding of environmental factors that may enhance or constrain professional nursing practice.

PROFESSIONALS IN A BUREAUCRATIC ENVIRONMENT

Nursing education focuses on the knowledge, skills, behaviors, and values of the profession. Once in the work setting, the nurse's goal is to put the profession's values into practice. This may be a significant challenge if the setting is highly bureaucratic and not supportive of professional practice. In a bureaucratic organization, decision making takes place above the level of the practitioner. Under these circumstances, conflict between the practitioner and the bureaucracy is inevitable.

BOX 3-2	**From Novice to Expert**

Stage 1: Novice (No Experience)
- Learns objective information; tasks are broken down into steps.
- Knowledge is free of context and can be understood without experience.
- Practice is based on theoretical knowledge, rules, and procedures.
- Rules determine actions that are limited and inflexible.
- Dependent on and has total confidence in those with greater expertise.
- Unable to use discretionary judgment.

Stage 2: Advanced Beginner
- Clinical situation presents as set of tasks that must be completed.
- Patient appears as perplexing collection of problems/conditions for action.
- Work is shaped by concern to organize, prioritize, and complete tasks.
- Assessment is more a task rather than a structure to direct clinical care.
- Has a fragmented or partial grasp of patient condition; absorbed in biological needs and feels unable to attend to psychosocial needs of patient/family.
- Attention and energies are focused on inventory of things to do, all of which are relevant.
- Respects and relies on judgment of nurse experts and defers complex clinical observations and decision making to those with greater expertise.
- Aware of his or her partial grasp; anxiety makes the advanced beginner more vigilant in providing care.
- Preceptor involvement helps to fit disjointed pieces together, see patterns, validate observations, weigh and balance competing concerns, appreciate immense variation in individual responses and tailoring of care, and analyze situations that did not go well.

Stage 3: Competent (1-2 Years in Similar Job Situation)
- Checklist approach now seen as inadequate.
- Struggles to learn to "read" the situation.
- Has improved time management, efficiency, organizational ability, and technical skills; performance is more fluid and coordinated.
- Able to prioritize and anticipate demands and to engage in anticipatory planning.
- Able to mesh theoretical and clinical knowledge.

- Able to alter protocols and standards of care to meet particular patient/family needs.
- Suffering of patient is more apparent; "conscious repersonalization" of patient/family.
- Increased diagnostic reasoning with ability to make a clinical case for action to physicians.
- Emotional responses become more informative and guiding.
- Co-workers now recognized as fallible.
- Preceptor role by proficient to expert nurse very beneficial for refining ability to "read" situation.

Stage 4: Proficient (3-5 Years with Similar Patient Populations)
- Increasingly accurate grasp of situation; when grasp is missing, nurse has a vague sense of uneasiness/discomfort.
- Actively interprets direction of change.
- Able to recognize when the situation is not normal.
- Able to recognize early warning signs and notice when patient condition is sufficient to warrant redefinition and change in actions.
- Knows what things can wait and what cannot.
- Has a growing sense of nursing concerns and difference from medical concerns.
- Learning to be engaged in clinical situation and be connected with patient/family in ways that are helpful.
- Challenges information given but does not take into account all variations that might occur.
- Greater trust in emotional responses to guide attentiveness and consultation with others.
- Most likely will progress to Stage 5.

Stage 5: Expert
- Management of multiple tasks simultaneously with skill in performance, timing, and anticipation evident; "thinking in action."
- Grasp of the big picture with ability to go beyond immediate clinical situation with sense of future and recognition of anticipated trajectories.
- Attuned to situation that allows responses to be shaped by mindful reading of patient responses without recourse to conscious deliberation.
- Recognition and assessment language are so linked with actions and outcomes that they become obvious; may have difficulty explaining how they know something.

BOX 3-2	From Novice to Expert—cont'd

Stage 5: Expert, cont'd

- Expanded "peripheral vision"—sensing the needs of other patients in area and capabilities of nurses assigned to their care.
- Concern for revealing and responding to patients as persons, respecting their dignity, caring in ways that preserve personhood, protecting when vulnerable, helping patients to feel safe in alien environment.
- Working to preserve integrity of close nurse-patient relationship.

- Learning to orchestrate actions in relation to working with others to minimize being overburdened and seeing that all possible resources are brought to bear in difficult situations.
- Expert mastery of technology and expert caring provide prudent and critical view of technology.
- Compelled to take strong positions/moral stands with other nurses and physicians to provide what the expert believes a patient needs.

Modified from Benner, P. A., Tanner, C. A., & Chelsa, C. A. (1996). *Expertise in nursing practice: Caring, clinical judgement, and ethics.* New York: Springer.

TABLE 3-3	Characteristics of Professional and Bureaucratic Organizations

Bureaucratic	Professional
Hierarchical power with centralized decision making	Knowledge-based power with decentralized decision making
High formalization	Low formalization
Work performed according to division of labor	Work performed according to professional norms
Uniformity of product emphasized; work standardized	Uniqueness of client emphasized; work not standardized
Service to organization	Nonroutine tasks
Achievement of organizational goals	Loyalty to profession

Providing care to clients is complex and requires individuals with differing areas of expertise. An essential dimension is the concept of collegial teams. Outcomes can be improved with shared decision making and mutual trust for the clinical abilities of doctors and nurses. However, the use of titles for physicians while overlooking titles of other care providers in an organizational culture may contribute to status discrepancies. Gordon (2005) refers to nurse-doctor relationships as a kind of chronic illness to which the profession may have adapted but nevertheless causes persistent dysfunction. She describes a "sobering picture of disruptive behaviors" (p. 24) to the point that The Joint Commission (TJC) has called for a voluntary policy of zero tolerance in the workplace. Gordon advocates for explicating the full role of nursing, which will bring understanding of the scope of nursing practice and transform the typically hierarchical hospital organization into more engaging structures that encourage professional advancement and empowerment of nurses.

In an organization where decision making occurs at the level of the practitioner, conflict is reduced. Characteristics of professional and bureaucratic organizations are summarized in Table 3-3. The nurse must learn how to balance the values of both the profession and the organization. Successful blending of these role conceptions will facilitate the socialization process and decrease the amount of perceived stress and conflict. The strong service ideal inherent in nursing sometimes helps mediate the effects of clashes between professional and bureaucratic values.

SUCCESSFUL NURSING ORGANIZATIONS: MAGNET HOSPITALS

During the nursing shortage of the 1980s, some hospitals were successful in attracting and retaining professional nurses when most hospitals were having great difficulty recruiting sufficient nursing staff (Scott, Sochalski, & Aiken, 1999). These facilities were referred to as "magnets" because of their ability to attract and retain professional nursing staff. *Magnet hospitals* are described as model patient care facilities that typically employ a higher proportion of baccalaureate-prepared nurses (American Association of Colleges of Nursing, 2008). Because of the significant nurse shortage, a formal study was conducted to identify what made these hospitals so successful. Three areas were examined: (1) leadership characteristics of nursing administrators, (2) professional attributes of staff nurses, and (3) the environment that supported professional practice. Hospitals were selected by these criteria: nurses considered them a good place to practice nursing, they had low turnover and vacancy rates, and they were located in a region where significant competition for nursing services was present.

Leadership is critical to the establishment and maintenance of a cohesive and efficient work culture. In their review of the research on magnet hospitals, Scott and colleagues (1999) extracted nursing administrator attributes that were most prevalent in the studies. Their research found that a successful nursing administrator:

- Is visionary and enthusiastic
- Is supportive and knowledgeable
- Maintains high standards and high staff expectations
- Values education and professional development
- Is highly visible to staff nurses; has a presence
- Is responsive to concerns and maintains open communication
- Is actively involved in state and national professional organizations

Staff nurses working within magnet hospitals were also studied. Professional practice attributes of the staff nurses included the following:

- Ability to establish and maintain therapeutic nurse-patient relationships
- Nurse autonomy and control
- Presence of collaborative nurse-physician relationships at the level of patient care units

To practice as professionals, nurses must have control over the practice environment so that clinical judgments and interventions can reflect the uniqueness of each client. Scott and colleagues defined *autonomous nursing practice* as "full command of expert knowledge and allow[ing] for accountability and authority in decision making" (1999, p. 11). They address two dimensions of autonomy: organizational and clinical. *Organizational autonomy* relates to the environment in which nurses participate in clinical decision making that guides the unit and organization. *Clinical autonomy* relates to the nurses' scope of practice for which they are accountable. Among the most significant factors in explaining job satisfaction and productivity were autonomy and staff involvement in decision making.

The complexity of care delivery makes collaboration essential: "Twenty-first century learning in nursing may not be about competition as much as coalition building, resource acquisition, and transforming expectations" (Pesut, 1998, p. 37). Open communication and dialogue among peers and other health care providers allow nurses to validate clinical judgments according to standards of professional practice. Collaborative nurse-physician relationships at the level of patient care units are fostered when nurses and doctors have mutual respect for each other's knowledge and competence and a shared concern for provision of quality patient care (Scott, Sochalski, & Aiken, 1999).

In assessing job satisfaction of nurses in magnet and nonmagnet hospitals, Upenieks (2002) found significant differences. The magnet hospitals employed a greater number of baccalaureate-prepared nurses, and magnet nurses rated their job satisfaction higher than the nonmagnet nurses across the following five areas:

- Sufficient autonomy to influence others and distribute needed resources for patient care (their contributions were acknowledged and appreciated)
- Positive nurse-physician relationships
- Participatory management structure with enhanced self-governance
- Greater support with more responsiveness to their concerns and a more visible chief nurse
- More availability of professional development opportunities

Passion about nursing was described as a vital feature of the nurse leader. Magnet nurses spoke of supportive attributes of the leader and professional attributes of their colleagues. With major transformations in health care, nurse leaders must "maintain a panoramic view of the world to discern the direction their efforts should take. Their ability to see intersections, relationships, and themes is what ensures that the organization will undertake the activities it needs to in order to survive" (Porter-O'Grady & Malloch, 2002, p. 20).

Professional Governance

The magnet hospital findings are consistent with earlier work by Porter-O'Grady (1986), who identified five key issues involved in creating a professional practice climate. The nurse must have the following:

- The freedom to function effectively
- A sense of support from peers and leaders
- Clear expectations of the work environment
- Appropriate resources to practice effectively
- An open organizational climate

A number of contemporary client care delivery models have been developed to facilitate the practice of nursing as a professional discipline. Specific organizational designs may vary, but all can be classified as professional governance models when they have a focus on autonomy of, and accountability for, nursing practice.

Three structural approaches to professional governance have been proposed (Porter-O'Grady, 1987). The *councilor model* uses elected councils to structure the governance processes of staff and management. Councils on practice, quality assurance, and education are composed primarily of practicing nurses, with management having minority representation. These councils make decisions related to clinical practice. Management has a management council, with clinical staff having minority representation. This council makes decisions regarding system operations.

The *congressional model* consists of a president and cabinet of officers who are elected from the staff of the organization and who oversee the operations. Cabinet members are a mixture of clinical and management representatives. There may be equal representation from each group or, consistent with the belief that the organization is a clinical service, it may be weighted with more clinical representatives. Committees, often chaired by cabinet officers, are empowered with certain responsibilities and accountabilities and report back to the cabinet.

The *administrative model* is perhaps the least professionally structured. Although a management and clinical forum are the basic structural units, each forum is more typically aligned in a hierarchical fashion, and the nurse executive often has a mechanism for vetoing considerations of the various decision-making groups.

Shared governance models are effective in empowering staff nurses with increased responsibility for clinical decisions (Ludemann, Lyons, & Block, 1995). In addition, in successful system integration, commitment to shared governance and point-of-service decision making contribute to the success of systems that have been redesigned (Aikman, Andress, Goodfellow, LaBelle, & Porter-O'Grady, 1998).

Additional research is needed on factors related to socialization of nurses in today's health care environment. The diverse needs of the learner, multiple roles of students, processes and strategies that best facilitate role transition, effectiveness of role models and preceptors in the socialization process, and resocialization for RNs returning to school are some issues deserving attention.

Professional Associations

A *professional association* is "an organization of practitioners who judge one another as professionally competent and have banded together to perform social functions which they cannot perform in their separate capacity as individuals" (Merton, 1958, p. 50). Professional organizations provide a structure for the exercise of autonomy and accountability to ensure that quality services will be provided by competent professionals.

Associations can be classified as one of two main types: broad-purpose associations and specialty associations. The ANA and its affiliation with the International Council of Nursing (ICN), the National League for Nursing (NLN), and the National Student Nurses Association (NSNA) are examples of broad-purpose associations.

AMERICAN NURSES ASSOCIATION (ANA)

Mission. By caring for nurses who care for America, the ANA works to unite all registered nurses to advance the profession. Areas of focus include improving health, promoting standards and availability of health care services for all people, fostering high standards for nursing and professional practice advocacy, lobbying on health care issues affecting nurses and the public, stimulating and promoting the professional development of nurses, projecting a positive and realistic view of nursing, and advancing the economic and general welfare of nurses in the workplace. Core values include leadership, standard of excellence, integrity/honesty, stewardship, knowledge, response to change, and the right to health care.

Origin. Founded in 1896 by a group of representatives from nursing school alumnae associations and originally named the Nurses' Associated Alumnae of the United States and Canada; became the ANA in 1912.

Membership. Professional association for RNs in the United States, with 54 constituent state and territorial associations and more than 150,000 members. Because the ANA represents every RN, all nurses should become active, contributing members.

Programs
- Promotes collective bargaining rights and workplace advocacy for all nurses
- Provides specialty certification of RNs
- Accredits continuing education programs
- Maintains government relation activities
- Develops standards for nursing practice
- Promotes economic and general welfare, research, and priorities for human rights
- Publishes scope and standards for 26 areas of nursing practice (cardiovascular, corrections, faith community, forensic, genetics/genomics, HIV/AIDS, home health, hospice/palliative, intellectual and developmental disabilities, legal nurse consulting, neonatal, nursing administration, nursing informatics, pain management, pediatrics, plastic surgery, psychiatric-mental health, public health, radiology, school, addiction, diabetes, gerontology, neuroscience, nursing professional development, vascular)
- Publishes *Code of Ethics for Nurses*
- Publishes *Nursing's Social Policy Statement*

Official Journal. *The American Nurse*

Website. www.nursingworld.org

INTERNATIONAL COUNCIL OF NURSES (ICN)

Mission. To lead societies of the world toward better health through working together to harness the knowledge and enthusiasm of the entire nursing profession. Committed to advocacy for patients, helping people help themselves, and doing for people what they would do unaided if they had the necessary strength. Determined that science will remain the servant of compassion and ethical caring that includes meeting emotional needs.

Origin. Founded in 1899 as a federation of national nurses' associations. Was the first and widest-reaching international organization of health professionals. Currently represents a federation of 129 national associations representing nurses worldwide.

Membership. There is no individual membership to ICN. Nurses who are a part of their national nurses' association automatically are a part of ICN.

Programs
- Works in professional practice, regulation, and social economic welfare areas to represent nursing internationally and influence health policy worldwide
- Serves as a hub for international exchange of ideas, experience, and expertise through established networking mechanisms
- Offers a student network to individuals currently enrolled in an education program leading to initial qualification as a nurse in their country or who have qualified within the last 2 years
- Focuses on leadership for change and negotiation

- Ongoing initiative for development of the International Classification for Nursing Practice (ICNP), a common language to be used worldwide for practice, education, research, and management that would permit comparison of nursing data among clinical populations, settings, and geographic areas to document outcomes of nursing interventions
- Sets and enforces standards for nursing education through member associations to ensure that nursing is recognized as a profession
- Has proposed universal guidelines for basic and specialty practice to aid professionals working in different regions of the world
- Focuses on fair and equitable compensation and other work benefits for nurses worldwide
- Serves as resource to member associations; represents nurses and nursing within the International Labor Organization
- Publishes the ICN *Code of Ethics* to serve as the basis for national codes worldwide

Official Journal. *International Nursing Review*

Website. www.icn.ch

NATIONAL LEAGUE FOR NURSING

Mission. To advance quality nursing education that prepares the nursing workforce to meet the needs of diverse populations in an ever-changing health care environment.

Origin. Begun in 1893 as the American Society of Superintendents of Training Schools for Nurses. Formed to establish and maintain universal standards of training for nursing. Became the National League of Nursing Education (NLNE) in 1912 and, along with two other organizations, formed the National League for Nursing in 1952. At that time, the organization assumed responsibility for accrediting nursing education programs. Currently offers its programs and services to 28,000 individual and 1200 institutional members.

Membership. Offers individual, educational agency (schools of nursing), and associate memberships.

Programs
- Accredits practical, diploma, associate, baccalaureate, and master's nursing programs in the United States and its territories through the National League for Nursing Accrediting Commission (NLNAC)
- Provides testing services for nursing schools ranging from preadmission through graduation as well as certification examinations for specialty nursing groups and health care institutions
- Publishes books and journals and presents workshops and conferences related to nursing education and practice
- Offers faculty development opportunities, networking opportunities, nursing research grants, and public policy initiatives

Official Journal. *Nursing Education Perspectives*

Website. www.nln.org

NATIONAL STUDENT NURSES ASSOCIATION (NSNA)

Mission. To provide nursing students practice in self-governance, advocate for student rights and rights of patients, and take collective, responsible action on vital social and political issues.

Origin. Begun in 1952 with the assistance of the ANA and NLN to prepare students for eventual participation in professional nursing organizations.

Membership. Open to students enrolled in associate, baccalaureate, diploma, and generic graduate nursing programs.

Programs
- Provides opportunities to learn and practice leadership skills through self-governance model, MidYear Career Planning Conference, and Annual Convention
- Offers discounts on products and services designed especially for nursing students

Official Journal. *Imprint*

Website. www.nsna.org

Examples of specialty-focused professional organizations are the American Association of Colleges of Nursing (AACN) and The Honor Society of Nursing, Sigma Theta Tau International (STTI).

AMERICAN ASSOCIATION OF COLLEGES OF NURSING (AACN)

Mission. The national voice for baccalaureate and graduate-degree nursing education, AACN serves the public interest by providing standards and resources, and by fostering innovation to advance professional nursing education, research, and practice.

Origin. Begun in 1969 with 121 member institutions. Today, represents more than 600 schools of nursing at public and private universities and senior colleges nationwide, representing a mix of baccalaureate, graduate, and postgraduate programs.

Membership. Schools of nursing offering a mix of baccalaureate, graduate, and postgraduate degree programs, with the nursing dean or other chief administrative nurse serving as representative to the AACN.

Programs
- Publishes and disseminates essentials of baccalaureate, graduate, and practice doctorate education; core standards for master's degree curricula for advanced practice nursing; core standards for and guidelines defining essential clinical resources for nursing education, research, and faculty practice
- Maintains government relations focusing on advancing public policy on nursing education, research, and practice; secures federal support for nursing education and research; shapes legislative and regulatory policy affecting nursing school programming; and ensures continuing financial assistance for nursing students
- Created the Commission on Collegiate Nursing Education (CCNE) in 1996; CCNE accredits baccalaureate degree nursing programs, master's degree nursing programs, and clinical nursing doctorates that are practice-focused and have the title Doctor of Nursing Practice (DNP)

- Operates the AACN Institutional Data System, a comprehensive national databank reporting statistics, trends, and conditions in baccalaureate and graduate nursing education

Official Journal. *Journal of Professional Nursing*

Website. www.aacn.nche.edu

THE HONOR SOCIETY OF NURSING, SIGMA THETA TAU INTERNATIONAL

Mission. A international nursing honor society that fosters, develops, and connects nurse scholars and leaders in practice, education, and research to improve health care worldwide.

Origin. Founded in 1922 by six nursing students at Indiana University to advance the status of nursing as a profession through recognition of the value of scholarship and importance of excellence in practice. The name Sigma Theta Tau is formed from the first letter of the three Greek words *storge*, *tharsos*, and *time*, meaning "love," "courage," and "honor."

Membership. By invitation to baccalaureate (prelicensure and registered nurse) nursing students; by application for graduate (master's and doctoral) nursing students who demonstrate excellence in scholarship, have the potential for leadership, and meet the expectation of academic integrity; and to nurse leaders who demonstrate exceptional achievements in nursing. More than 405,000 members have been inducted worldwide. Currently has 130,000 active members in 463 chapters located at more than 570 college and university campuses around the world. Members reside in 86 countries.

Programs
- Funds nursing research through grants and scholarships and holds annual research-oriented educational programs
- Provides programs to foster and enhance career advancement, leadership development, and community service and to reward professional competence and integrity in health care

- Maintains an electronic library that includes online services of *The Online Journal of Knowledge Synthesis for Nursing* and the *Registry of Nursing Research* (RNR)
- Houses the International Leadership Institute (ILI), which seeks to develop and advance nurses as leaders

Official Journal. *Journal of Nursing Scholarship*

Website. www.nursingsociety.org

SUMMARY

The ANA's *Code of Ethics for Nurses* (2001) reminds nurses of their obligation to participate in knowledge development, implementation and improvement of standards, establishment and maintenance of conditions of employment, and protection of the public from misinformation and misrepresentation. Nursing associations provide a structure for participation and empower nurses to engage in the advancement of nursing and improve health care services to the public.

As nursing continues to expand and specialize, many nurses have chosen to join a specialty practice organization that most closely represents their clinical area of expertise. These include organizations representing maternal-child, community, medical-surgical, and mental health nursing specialties. Other specialty organizations focus on the areas where nurses work, such as the emergency department, operating room, and critical care.

What are the benefits of belonging to a professional organization? Membership in the ANA and specialty practice organizations provides nurses with the opportunity to play an active role in the present and future of nursing. Through these professional organizations, nurses are elected to represent their peers as standards of practice are revised, policies are formulated, and issues affecting nursing practice and the public's health are addressed. Membership in professional associations benefits both the individual nurse and the profession of nursing. Recognition of expertise through certification, collective bargaining to improve salary and working conditions, lobbying to influence laws affecting nursing, and promoting state laws that will ensure quality care are some of the initiatives undertaken by these organizations. To increase the effectiveness of professional associations as official representatives of nurses, more nurses must become active by becoming members, attending meetings, and participating in organizational activities. Through active participation, nurses become a powerful collective of professionals. Nurses can amplify their impact on nursing care delivery and the health of the nation by participation in and support of professional associations.

KEY POINTS

- Socialization is an interactive, dynamic, lifelong process.
- Socialization to professional nursing includes internalizing its attitudes, behaviors, skills, and values.
- The ANA's *Code for of Ethics for Nurses* identifies the professional values of nursing; these should be evident in the delivery of nursing care.
- The status of nursing as a profession can be analyzed by using criteria for professions as indicators.
- Actions of individual nurses contribute to the public's collective image of nursing.
- Accountability is the cornerstone to maintaining the public's trust in nursing.
- Models of socialization identify the progression that occurs when learning new roles in professional practice.
- Nurses in practice and education serve as role models, preceptors, and mentors to guide new practitioners in their socialization to roles and responsibilities and assist in the development of career paths.
- Environmental factors influence the delivery of professional nursing care.
- Autonomy is a critical factor in attracting and retaining nurses in work settings.
- Participation in professional organizations is one of the defining attributes of being a professional nurse.
- Professional organizations benefit the individual nurse, the profession, and the public.

CRITICAL THINKING EXERCISES

1. Select one set of criteria for a profession from Table 3-1 and use it to analyze nursing's status as a profession. Give concrete examples of how nursing fulfills each criterion, or identify improvements that must be made.

2. List five ways to advance your own level of professionalism.
3. Identify characteristics of what you want to be and don't want to be as a nurse and compare these with the values in the *Code of Ethics for Nurses*.
4. Describe your nursing role model and explain why you have selected that nurse. How did this role model influence your nursing practice? What, if any, impact did this role model have on your decision to return to school for further nursing education?
5. Talk with a nursing faculty member, a hospital nurse recruiter, and a clinical nurse administrator about strategies they use to address reality shock.
6. Use the Internet to compare the mission, purpose, and services of two professional organizations.

REFERENCES

Adams, D., Miller, B. K., & Beck, L. (1996). Professionalism behaviors of hospital nurse executives and middle managers in 10 western states. *Western Journal of Nursing Research*, *18*(1), 77–88.

Aikman, P., Andress, I., Goodfellow, C., LaBelle, N., & Porter-O'Grady, T. (1998). System integration: A necessity. *Journal of Nursing Administration*, *28*(2), 28–34.

Aiken, L. H., Clarke, S. P., Sloane, D. M., & Sochalski, J. (2001). Nurses' reports on hospital quality of care and working conditions in five countries. *Health Affairs*, *20*(3), 43–53.

American Association of Colleges of Nursing. (2008). Fact sheet: The impact of education on nursing practice. Retrieved April 26, 2009, from http://www.aacn.nche.edu/Media/FactSheets/ImpactEdNP.htm

American Nurses Association. Nursing World: Media resources - National Nurses Week Media Kit. (n.d.) *Florence Nightingale Pledge*. Retrieved January 16, 2010, from http://www.nursingworld.org/FunctionalMenuCategories/MediaResources/NationalNursesWeek/MediaKit/FlorenceNightingalePledge.aspx

American Nurses Association. (2001). *Code of ethics for nurses with interpretative statements*. Washington, DC, Author.

American Nurses Association. (2003). *Nursing's social policy statement* (2nd ed.). Washington, DC, Author.

American Nurses Association. (2004). *Nursing: Scope and standards of clinical nursing practice*. Washington, DC, Author.

Benner, P. A. (1984). *Novice to expert*. Menlo Park, CA: Addison-Wesley.

Benner, P. A. (2005). Commentary. *Nursing Education Perspectives*, *26*(1), 14–15.

Benner, P. A., Tanner, C. A., & Chelsa, C. A. (1996). *Expertise in nursing practice: Caring, clinical judgement, and ethics*. New York: Springer.

Birchenall, P. (1998). Professional and educational directions. In M. Birchenall, & P. Birchenall (Eds.), *Sociology as applied to nursing and health care* (pp. 174–194). London: Harcourt Brace.

Bixler, G. K., & Bixler, R. W. (1959). The professional status of nursing. *American Journal of Nursing*, *59*, 1142–1147.

Buresch, B., & Gordon, S. (2000). *From silence to voice*. Ottawa: Canadian Nurses Association.

Campbell-Heider, N., Hart, C. A., & Bergren, M. D. (1994). Conveying professionalism: Working against old stereotypes. In B. Bullough, & V. Bullough (Eds.), *Nursing issues for the nineties and beyond* (pp. 212–231). New York: Springer.

Carper, B. A. (1978). Fundamental patterns of knowing in nursing. *Advances in Nursing Science*, *1*(13), 13–23.

Chinn, P. L., & Kramer, M. K. (1999). *Theory and nursing: Integrated knowledge development* (5th ed.). St. Louis: Mosby.

Coudret, N. A., Fuchs, P. L., Roberts, C. S., Suhrheinrich, J. A., & White, A. H. (1994). Role socialization of graduating student nurses: Impact of a nursing practicum on professional role conception. *Journal of Professional Nursing*, *10*, 342–349.

Curry, B. D. (1997). Coping with returning to school. In R. K. Nunnery (Ed.), *Advancing your career: Concepts of professional nursing* (pp. 16–38). Philadelphia: Davis.

Dalton, G. W., Thompson, P. H., & Price, R. L. (1977). The four states of professional careers: A new look at performance by professionals. *Organizational Dynamics*, *6*, 9–42.

Dorsey, L. E., & Baker, C. M. (2004). Mentoring undergraduate nursing students: Assessing the state of the science. *Nurse Educator*, *29*, 260–265.

Ellerton, M. (2003). Preceptorship: The changing face of clinical teaching. *Nurse Educator*, *28*, 200–201.

Fargotstein, B. P. (1999). *Ethical foundations of the code for nurses*. AZ: Tempe, Unpublished manuscript.

Flexner, A. (1910). *Medical education in the United States and Canada*. New York: Carnegie Foundation for the Advancement of Teaching.

Flexner, A. (1915). Is social work a profession? *School Society*, *1*, 901.

Gordon, S. (2005). *Nursing against the odds: How health care cost cutting, media stereotypes, and medical hubris undermine nurses and patient care*. Ithaca, NY: Cornell University.

Greenberg, M., Colombraro, G., DeBlasio, J., Dolan, J., & Rich, E. (2001). Rewarding preceptors: A cost-effective model. *Nurse Educator, 26*, 114–116.

Greenwood, E. (1957). Attributes of a profession. *Social Work, 2*(3), 45–54.

Hardy, M. E., & Conway, M. E. (1988). *Role theory: Perspectives for health professionals*. New York: Appleton-Century-Crofts.

Hayes, E. F. (2001). Factors that facilitate or hinder mentoring in the nurse practitioner preceptor/student relationship. *Clinical Excellence for Nurse Practitioners, 5*(2), 111–118.

Houle, C. O. (1980). *Continued learning in the professions*. San Francisco: Jossey-Bass.

Howkins, E. J., & Ewens, A. (1999). How students experience professional socialization. *International Journal of Nursing Studies, 35*, 41–49.

Joel, L. A. (2003). *Kelley's dimensions of professional nursing* (9th ed.). New York: McGraw-Hill.

Johnson, B., Friend, S., & MacDonald, J. (1997). Nurses' changing and emerging roles with the use of unlicensed assistive personnel. In S. Moorhead, & D. G. Huber (Eds.), *Nursing roles: Evolving or recycled?* (pp. 78–89). Thousand Oaks, CA: Sage.

Kalisch, P. A., & Kalisch, B. J. (2005). Looking forward/looking back: Perspectives on improving nursing's public image… including commentary by Benner. Reprinted in *Nursing Education Perspectives, 26*(1), 10–17.

Knowles, M. (1970). *The modern practice of adult education: From pedagogy to andragogy*. Chicago: Follett.

Kramer, M. (1974). *Reality shock: Why nurses leave nursing*. St. Louis: Mosby.

Letizia, M., & Jennrich, J. (1998). A review of preceptorship in undergraduate nursing education: Implications for staff development. *Journal of Continuing Education in Nursing, 29*, 211–216.

Lockwood-Rayermann, S. (2003). Preceptors, leadership style, and the student practicum experience. *Nurse Educator, 28*, 247–249.

Ludemann, R. S., Lyons, W., & Block, L. (1995). A longitudinal look at shared governance: Six years of evaluation of staff perceptions. In K. Kelly (Ed.), *Health care work redesign* (pp. 234–250). Thousand Oaks, CA: Sage.

MacIntosh, J. (2003). Reworking professional nursing identity. *Western Journal of Nursing Research, 25*, 725–741.

Martin, P., Yarbrough, S., & Alfred, D. (2003). Professional values held by baccalaureate and associate degree nursing students. *Journal of Nursing Scholarship, 35*, 291–296.

McBride, A. B. (1999). Breakthroughs in nursing education: Looking back, looking forward. *Nursing Outlook, 47*, 114–119.

McCloskey, J. C., & Maas, M. (1998). Interdisciplinary team: The nursing perspective is essential. *Nursing Outlook, 46*, 157–163.

McGregor, R. J. (1999). A preceptored experience for senior nursing students. *Nurse Educator, 24*(3), 13–16.

Merton, R. (1958). The functions of the professional association. *American Journal of Nursing, 58*(1), 50–54.

Meyer, T., & Xu, Y. (2005). Academic and clinical dissonance in nursing education. *Nurse Educator, 30*, 76–79.

Miller, B. K. (1985). Just what is a professional? *Nursing Success Today, 2*(4), 21–27.

Miller, B. K., Adams, D., & Beck, L. (1993). A behavioral inventory for professionalism in nursing. *Journal of Professional Nursing, 9*, 290–295.

Nightingale, F. (1860). *Notes on nursing: What it is and what it is not*. New York: Appleton.

Owens, B. H., Herrick, C. A., & Kelley, J. A. (1998). A prearranged mentorship program: Can it work long distance? *Journal of Professional Nursing, 14*, 78–84.

Parathian, A. R., & Taylor, F. (1993). Can we insulate trainee nurses from exposure to bad practice: A study of role play in communicating bad news to patients. *Journal of Advanced Nursing, 18*, 801–807.

Pesut, D. J. (1998). Twenty-first century learning. *Nursing Outlook, 46*, 37.

Porter-O'Grady, T. (1986). *Creative nursing administration: Participative management into the 21st century*. Rockville, MD: Aspen.

Porter-O'Grady, T. (1987). Shared governance and new organizational models. *Nursing Economics, 58*, 50–54.

Porter-O'Grady, T., & Malloch, K. (2002). *Quantum leadership: A textbook of new leadership*. Gaithersburg, MD: Aspen.

Reutter, L., Field, P. A., Campbell, I. E., & Day, R. (1997). Socialization into nursing: Nursing students as learners. *Journal of Nursing Education, 36*, 149–155.

Schwirian, P. M. (1998). *Professionalization of nursing: Current issues and trends* (3rd ed.). Philadelphia: Lippincott.

Scott, J. G., Sochalski, J., & Aiken, L. (1999). Review of magnet hospital research. *Journal of Nursing Administration, 29*(1), 9–19.

Stewart, B. M., & Krueger, L. E. (1996). An evolutionary concept analysis of mentoring in nursing. *Journal of Professional Nursing, 12*, 311–321.

Strader, M. K., & Decker, P. J. (1995). *Role transition to patient care management*. Norwalk, CT: Appleton & Lange.

Styles, M. (1982). *On nursing: Toward a new endowment.* St. Louis: Mosby.

Takase, M., Kershaw, E., & Burt, L. (2002). Does public image of nurses matter? *Journal of Professional Nursing, 18,* 196–205.

Thomka, L. A. (2001). Graduate nurses' experiences of interactions with professional nursing staff during transition to the professional role. *Journal of Continuing Education in Nursing, 32,* 15–19.

Ulrich, B. (2005, March 14). Uniforms revisited. *NurseWeek, 3.*

Upenieks, V. (2002). Assessing differences in job satisfaction of nurses in magnet and nonmagnet hospitals. *Journal of Nursing Administration, 32*(11), 564–576.

Utley-Smith, Q. (2004). Five competencies needed by new baccalaureate graduates. *Nursing Education Perspectives, 25,* 166–170.

Weis, D., & Schank, M. J. (2000). An instrument to measure professional nursing values. *Journal of Nursing Scholarship, 32*(2), 201–204.

Wurst, J. (1994). Professionalism and the evolution of nursing as a discipline: A feminist perspective. *Journal of Professional Nursing, 10,* 357–367.

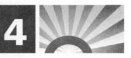

4

Professional Nursing Roles

SARAH A. DELGADO, RN, MSN, ACNP
ELKE JONES ZSCHAEBITZ, MSN, FNP-BC
ELIZABETH E. FRIBERG, DNP, RN

OBJECTIVES

At the completion of this chapter, the reader will be able to:

- Articulate the impact of culture on perceptions of the professional nursing role.
- Discuss the role and identity dyads in the framework of the nursing profession.
- Describe the roles commonly assumed by professional nurses and the associated identity characteristics.
- Discuss the impact of the multiple roles experienced by the professional nurse.
- Differentiate between common sources of role stress and resultant role strain.
- Identify strategies for managing role stress and strain.

PROFILE IN PRACTICE

Kristi D. Kimpel, MSN, RN, CCRN, CCNS
University of Virginia Health System, Charlottesville, Virginia

Each step in my health care profession has shaped my ability to better serve as the clinical nurse specialist (CNS) for the Surgical Trauma Burn Intensive Care Unit (STBICU) at the University of Virginia Health System. My student job in the Laboratory for Clinical Learning in nursing school gave me first-hand experience in developing and implementing effective processes to educate others. Working as a patient care assistant (PCA) allowed me the opportunity to learn to communicate and collaborate effectively with patients, families, and the interdisciplinary team. My first position as a new nurse sparked my interest in the care of the burn patient and subsequently my specialty in graduate school. A clinical nurse specialist's specialty may be defined by a population, care setting, or disease process. For me, this is the critical care setting as I care for patients with a diverse spectrum of conditions and needs: trauma, traumatic brain injury, burn, solid organ transplant, complex wounds and reconstructive surgery, and an array of other surgical diagnoses. An additional complexity is the care of patients across the care continuum from critically ill to acute care since the unit has designated beds for both ends of the care dichotomy. Tackling specialty knowledge in all of these patient populations is daunting; therefore my practice relies on effective utilization of resources and navigation of the health system.

A single day of practice provides a multitude of pivotal intersects to influence the care of a patient.

This may be as simple as collaboration with physician colleagues during patient rounds or empowering a patient and/or family member to be an active partner in establishing care goals. Or it may be as complex as ensuring effective glycemic control across the critical care division. It may include formally educating professional colleagues at surrounding hospitals in the care of the burn patient. Evaluating outcomes and implementing evidence-based strategies to prevent complications, shorten length of stay, and lower health care costs are some of the results that validate the role of the CNS.

The population within my care domain is not only patients and their families but also nursing and interdisciplinary colleagues—as well as the health care system as a whole. My day-to-day practice includes educating and mentoring clinical staff in care standards, health care technology, preventative care, and patient advocacy. The professional development of others is one of the most rewarding aspects of my role. I am expected to promote certification, to assist clinicians in furthering their career by challenging the clinical ladder, and to enable clinicians to contribute to nursing knowledge by creating clinical research. I often find myself explaining this aspect of my role to colleagues this way: *Simply put, I enable and empower you to better care for our patients.*

I believe the CNS or advanced practice nurse has the responsibility to influence nursing and medicine beyond one's immediate reach. This can be accomplished through a variety of mechanisms: active participation in one's professional organization, contributing to professional publications or presentations, or educating the next generation of nursing colleagues. Health care and health care systems are dynamic. The CNS, at any one moment of time, may focus on just one aspect of his or her arsenal of competencies, but it is the synthesis of all of these elements that allow the role to be effective and vital in health care excellence.

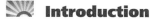 ## Introduction

In today's rapidly changing health care environment, the nursing role is becoming less traditional and increasingly diverse. As the professional disciplines are called on to provide expanded and more diverse health care services in a wide variety of settings, the traditional structure of provider roles is being challenged. Nursing is responding to this challenge by examining the nature of the professional role, exploring its underlying values and identity, and adapting it to better meet the needs of a dynamic health care system. This chapter focuses on role taking in nursing by examining stereotypes of nursing in the common culture, reviewing the historical development of nursing roles, identifying the types of roles nurses commonly assume and the associated identity characteristics, exploring the relevance of education and work environment to practice roles, and finally, addressing aspects of role dynamics, sources of role stress, and strategies for resolving role stress.

Nursing Roles, Functions, and Characteristics

NURSING ROLE STEREOTYPES

To examine the professional nursing role, first consider the kaleidoscope of media and culture and their impact in shaping the way society sees nurses. This is vital during a time in which there is a shortage of nurses and an emerging dissonance between nursing education and the experiences of nurses in health care. Research shows that representations of professional roles and gender in media and the arts can shape a society's view of that profession's work. Dr. Stanley, a lecturer in the School of Nursing and Midwifery at Curtin University of Technology in Perth, remarked, "Public perceptions of different professions are strongly influenced by the media, and in the past the way that nurses have been represented in featured films has often been at odds with the way nurses perceive their profession" (Stanley, 2008, para 3).

Nurses have often been portrayed in film and television as comedic sex kittens—from B-movie productions in the 1970s such as *Private Duty Nurses* (Armitage, 1971) to Hot Lips Houlihan in the acclaimed television series *M*A*S*H** (Hornberger, 1972) to contemporary productions such as the television series *ER* (Burns, 1994), *Scrubs* (Lawrence, 2001), *Nightingales* (Cramer, 1988), and *Grey's Anatomy* (Corn, 2005). In these portrayals, the nurse as caregiver is often twisted into an individual with uncontrolled libidinal impulse. Stanley (2008) noted, "Just over a quarter of the films I reviewed featured an overtly sexual representation of nurses ... an image that has negative implications for nursing professionals" (para 9).

In addition to sexualized roles, nurses have also been portrayed as harsh disciplinarians with an unyielding, even sadistic, worldview. Examples of these menacing roles include the ghoulish nurse in *The Lost Weekend* (Brackett & Wilder, 1945), the murderous caregiver in Stephen King's *Misery* (Reiner, Scheinman, Stott, & Nicolaides, 1990), and most notably, the sinister and terrifying Nurse Ratched, who provoked emotional breakdowns in her emasculated, unstable, male patients in the Oscar-winning movie, *One Flew Over the Cuckoo's Nest* (Douglas & Zaentz, 1975).

As nursing is often seen as a female profession, these portrayals reflect society's view of women, which shifted with the advent of the feminist movement, when women challenged sexist limitations on professional roles. Stanley believes, for instance, that the portrayal of nurses as sadistic coincided with the liberation of a repressed inner-self in line and the development of women's power (Stanley, 2008).

As women become more socially, professionally, and politically active, opportunities for women in the nursing field have also expanded. For example, military nurses are portrayed as heroes and heroines. The television show *China Beach* (Wells, 1988) was critiqued as "focusing on the women at the base, an emphasis fundamentally intended to undermine vainglorious heroism and to portray war instead, through women's eyes, as a vast and elaborate conceit. Contemporary critics divided between those applauding the program's feminine deflation of war, and those who regarded the characters and their orientations

toward war as wholly stereotypical invocations of femininity" (Saenz, 1988, para 3).

Recent films such as *Pearl Harbor* (Bruckheimer & Bay, 2001) and Ian McEwan's 2007 film from the honored book *Atonement* (McEwan, 2001) portray war nurses as heroines and self-sacrificing women. In the Academy Award–winning film *The English Patient* (Zaentz & Minghella, 1996), the nurse Hanna's selfless dedication to her craft and patient leads her to stay with him under desperate wartime conditions, her skilled compassion guiding her to assist him as he is dying.

Although recent films and television show improvements in the portrayal of nurses, such as Hanna in *The English Patient* (Zaentz, 1996) or actress Julianna Margulies' nursing role in *ER* (Spielberg, 1994), substantial obstacles and stereotypes still exist, driven by the gender-bound thinking attached to the nursing role. A major obstacle is demonstrated in the wildly successful film *Meet the Parents* (Tenenbaum, 2000), which reinforces how nursing struggles with its identity as gender-specific to women. Actor Ben Stiller's character, Greg Focker, is a nurse who comically raises our consciousness of the negative perceptions of men in nursing. In one critical scene Greg is staying at his new girlfriend's house in order to meet her father, Jack Byrnes, along with several other relatives, including two male physicians. When Greg arrives at the breakfast table—the only person in the house clad in pajamas—Jack introduces the bedraggled Greg to the group:

Jack Byrnes: Greg's a male nurse.

Greg Focker: Yes, thank you, Jack.

Kevin Rowley (surgeon): Wow, that's great. I'd love to find time to do some volunteer work. Just the other day I saw a golden retriever, he had like a gimp, and you know I wish I could have done something.

Greg Focker: Yeah, well I get paid too so it's sort of an "everyone wins" thing.

The stereotype that the male nurses are "less than male" and "do women's work" is still an image reflected in contemporary U.S. culture despite a long history of men in nursing. In fact, as early as the fourth and fifth centuries, men worked as nurses (Evans, 2004). Today, one of the little-known facts of military nursing is the high percentage of men performing nursing roles in all three service branches. In the Army, 35.5% of its 3381 nurses are men; in the Air Force, 30% of 3790 nurses are men; and in the Navy, 36% of the 3125 nurses are men. By contrast, men make up only 6% of the nursing workforce in the United States (Lucas, 2009).

Susan Wood, Associate Dean at the University of Washington School of Nursing, deplores the cultural bias against nurses and reflects the view of most nurses who see themselves played one-dimensionally with underlying stereotypes in culture when she writes, "I don't think that movies accurately portray nurse as they really are … I don't think there's anything in film that portrays the scope of what a nurse does" (Rasmussen, 2001, para 6). Right or wrong, public perceptions of nursing roles point to the importance of a comprehensive analysis of role identity in nursing.

ACTUAL NURSING ROLES

Distinct from the stereotypes portrayed in the media, including film and television, the actual roles nurses play are uniquely multifaceted. The scope of these roles to which Susan Woods refers is a provocative one that incites many opinions within and external to the profession since Florence Nightingale first examined the role of nursing in her publication *Notes on Nursing: What It Is and What It Is Not* (1860). The wisdom and vision of Nightingale were clear as she refrained from pigeonholing the profession in the context of time and space: "I do not pretend to teach her how, I ask her to teach herself, and for this purpose I venture to give her some hints" (Nightingale, 1860, p. 8).

Nightingale saw nursing as an art and, as such, the various roles in nursing as multilayered and fluid defined by the context and demands of the environment in which that nurse works. Professional nurses today function as researchers, administrators, community organizers, policy makers, clinicians, and educators, in a multitude of settings, with each context helping to set roles, expectations, and limitations. Furthermore, many nurses do not stop being a nurse when they leave the hospital, clinic, school, tent, office, lab, or mobile unit where they happen to work; many carry the identity of being a nurse into their personal lives.

Being a nurse is about executing a number of roles in service to health and health care that are intertwined with the identity, talents, and values of each individual. That is, nurses are defined by the roles they play and their personal identity, which provides the substance and motivation for their work. When this complex tangle of role and identity is bifurcated and nursing practice is industrialized, the meaning of being a nurse is diminished. Critically, this professional alignment of role and identity leads to personal and professional happiness; hence understanding the nature of role and identity and their interconnection is essential in evaluating the roles played by professional nurses.

Role is defined by the Merriam-Webster Online Dictionary as "a socially expected behavior pattern usually determined by an individual's status in a particular society" (2009). The word *role* may be interpreted as a set of behaviors and expectations, rights and obligations, as conceptualized by actors in a situation guided by individuals with social position who set these behaviors. Roles are associated with social positions (status, power) and are shaped by the expectations of others in an individual's workplace or social network (Biddle, 1979). Although structure and function are essential to an understanding of *role*, to define *nursing* in the context of expected behaviors would then interpret actions as solely prescribed by rules outlined in policy and procedure or a job description. From this functional perspective, the meaning of *role* is shallow and lacking the underpinnings of the individual's professional identity, which underscores the motivation for selecting the profession.

Identity is defined as "the distinguishing character or personality of an individual," and the word **identification** is defined as "a psychological orientation of the self in regard to something (as a person or group) with the resulting feeling of close emotional association" (Merriam-Webster Online Dictionary, 2009). There is no set identity in nursing, as the profession consists of individuals with unique values and experiences. Nursing roles are guided by a derived identity and sense of self gathered from the organizations or work groups to which nurses belong (Hogg & Terry, 2000). From this perspective, identity can be understood as how a person sees himself or herself in a particular role; what a person believes about the world, moral choices, and social justice; and a person's sense of profession in relationship to a work role.

According to one paradigm model, an individual's sense of identity is determined mostly by the explorations and commitments that she or he makes regarding certain personal and social traits (Marcia, 1966). In this framework, the identity of a nurse is determined by how that individual sees and experiences nursing.

PRAXIS AND THE NURSING META-DYAD

The fusion of role and identity set in an understanding of the cultural context of nursing represents **praxis**, the integration of action and reflection, which is essential to any transformative helping profession. To better understand this complex interplay of role and identity and the harmony and disunity it can create, it is helpful to use the theoretical construct of a dyad. The word **dyad** comes from the Greek *dyas*, which stands for the number two and represents the principle of "two-ness" or otherness. The Merriam-Webster Online Dictionary defines *dyad* as "a pair maintaining a sociologically or physically significant relationship" (2009). This can serve as a model for holding together, by way of exploration, the critical functions of nursing with personal identity that then make up the individual nurse's professional role identity.

Bringing together role and identity integrates nursing into the surrounding culture and opens up a broader understanding of the profession. For example, whereas role is about health and the interaction of person and disease, identity is about individualistic values and approaches concerning illness and wellness. When these concepts are combined, the result represents the fullness of nursing praxis. In terms of the individual nurse, this integration of role and identity brings balance. The nursing identity embraces wellness; the nursing role manages health and disease.

What infuses the art and practice of nursing is a single overarching dyad, a **meta-dyad** of the professional nurse role, driven by an intrinsic personal identity of being other-centered (other-centeredness). For the professional nursing role, the core identity is that of caring for others, or other-centeredness—the conscious movement of care directed to and with another human being or a community of human beings.

When one explores the meaning of the professional nursing role, most definitions lead to dyads that mate expressions of highly educated, highly skilled professionals with definitions of individuals who care for others with great empathy and compassion. Nurses couple scientific principle with people skills. A frequent expression is that nursing is both high tech and high touch.

These definitions invariably go on to indicate that professional nurses are educators as well as managers, colleagues, mentors, researchers, and advocates for health. An understanding of all of these roles and their parallel identity characteristics is essential for a nurse to be successful. The nurse must also be grounded in the concept of other-centeredness as opposed to being egocentric. An exceptional demonstration of this other-centeredness is nursing's central ethical doctrine, which holds that a nurse's first obligation is to the patient (Siefert, 2009).

Moral theorist and feminist thinker Carol Gilligan's work speaks to the morality of care defining the preservation of relationships as the highest level of moral reasoning. From her perspective of the nature of moral development, nursing based on other-centeredness represents the final stage in moral development. What underlies the skill and knowledge of professional nursing is caregiving, empathy, and compassion (McFadden, 2006).

ESSENTIAL ROLE FUNCTIONS AND CHARACTERISTICS

Embedded within this overarching construct of the role of the nurse with an identity of other-centeredness are seven key dyads that are essential to any exploration of nursing. These roles and the corresponding identity characteristics that infuse these roles (Figure 4-1) constitute an overlapping mosaic that is not exclusive but is foundational to the professional role of nurse. This mosaic of nursing role and identity dyads can be viewed as role progression as professional experience ensues.

Caregiver—Caring, Compassion, and Empathy

Compassion is that which makes the heart of the good move at the pain of others. It crushes and destroys the pain of others.
Buddha

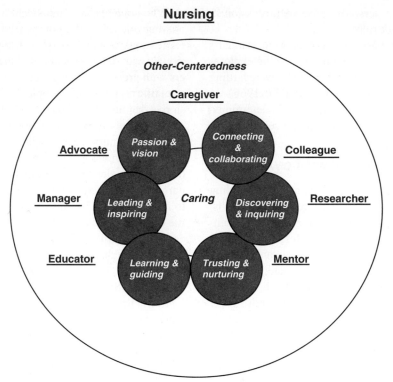

FIGURE 4-1 The nursing role identity dyads. Functions and internal characteristics.

If the act of caregiving drives the health care delivery role, compassion is an essential identity characteristic that guides the actions of assessment, planning, intervention, and evaluation. When asked about the most important role of a nurse, most nurses respond with one word: caregiving. The nursing profession is grounded in the phenomenon of caring (Leininger, 1988). Leininger discovered that patients from diverse cultures valued care differently than nurses did. Gradually, Leininger became convinced of the need for a theoretical framework to discover, explain, and predict dimensions of care and developed culture care theory, the only nursing theory that focuses on culture, (Leininger & McFarland, 1997). This theory defines caring behaviors on the part of a caregiver as those that are congruent with the beliefs, values, and expressions of the care recipient. Similarly, Jean Watson's theory of caring describes the scientific basis of nursing as extending beyond human interaction, to a moral concern for preserving human dignity and respect for the

wholeness of the care recipient (Childs, 2006). Both of these theories demonstrate the link between the caregiver role and the identity characteristics of compassion and empathy.

Caring is an essential feature of the profession, one that is central to a nurse's identity and that serves to facilitate health and healing: "The culture of caring, as a fundamental part of the nursing profession, characterizes both concern and consideration for the whole person, a commitment to the common good and health of all, and outreach to those who are vulnerable." (National League for Nursing, 2009, para 1).

Because of this fundamental maxim, preparing the nurse for the caregiving role is an established practice in nursing education. What is more difficult to engender, however, but nonetheless as fundamental, is fostering caring through compassion. Although "teaching" identity is a complex process, nurses need to be awakened to and evaluated on the emotions prompted by the pain and suffering of others. Grounded in the development of empathy, caring is the vigorous attempt not only to feel another's pain but to take steps to alleviate suffering and to seek the wellness within that person. Covington (2005) states, "Caring presence is mutual trust and sharing, transcending connectedness, and experience. This special way of being, a caring presence, involves devotion to a client's well-being while bringing scientific knowledge and expertise to the relationship" (p. 169). Kathy Robinson (2003), former president of the Emergency Nurses Association, writes, "No technology in health care replaces the critical thinking of a human mind, the caring of a human soul, the proficiency and skill of a human hand, and the warmth of a human heart in healing the sick and injured. That is nursing, esteemed colleagues; that is you" (p. 200).

Colleague—Collaborating and Connecting. The role of nurse as colleague is not only essential to collaborative clinical and research practices, but integral to the team process in dynamic health care. Working together toward common purposes, improving health, respecting shared strengths, caring and compassion—these are fundamental to the profession. For example, in 2009, 90% of American Association of Critical-Care Nurses (AACN) members responding to a survey reported that they were colleagues with physicians and administrators and that they believed this was among the most important elements in creating a healthy work environment (Morton & Fontaine, 2009). At the heart of being a colleague is the ability not only to cooperate, but to *actively* collaborate. Collaboration is a multifaceted process of working together to accomplish a common goal; it involves a mix of differing viewpoints to better comprehend a challenging issue. Arising between true colleagues, collaboration is the ability to be innovative in achieving consensus to achieve shared goals.

According to Gardner, there are 10 lessons in collaborations: (1) know thyself; (2) learn to value and manage diversity; (3) develop constructive conflict resolution skills; (4) use personal power to create win-win situations; (5) master interpersonal and process skills; (6) recognize that collaboration is a journey; (7) leverage all multidisciplinary forums; (8) appreciate that collaboration can occur spontaneously; (9) balance autonomy and unity in collaborative relationships;

and (10) remember that collaboration is not required for all decisions (Gardner, 2005, Section 3).

Interprofessional collaboration is a vital aspect of plans designed to increase the effectiveness of delivery of health care (Morton & Fontaine, 2009). According to Dorrie Fontaine, RN, PhD, FAAN, former president of the AACN, "Escalating financial pressures and alarming workforce shortages make it imperative that physicians and nurses actively work together to establish new patient-focused practice models. The combined efforts of the AACN and the American College of Chest Physicians (ACCP) will establish a strong leadership force in effecting meaningful change in our hospitals and health systems on behalf of the critically ill patients we serve" (Robinson, 2003, para 6). From initiatives to promote interdisciplinary education in health care to institutes focusing on fostering dynamic international collaboration involving nursing, medical and allied health researchers, clinicians, academics, and quality managers, collaboration among colleagues has emerged as vital to professional nursing.

An example of an important new arena for collaborative practice for nursing is the rapid advance of telehealth as a critical vehicle for health care delivery, especially in rural underserved communities. Telehealth is the exchange of medical and other health information via electronic communications from one site to another with the intent of addressing patient needs. Through telehealth, colleagues provide medical, nursing, or other health care to a remote location. The remote site almost always requires a nurse to be present with the patient to present the history and physical, provide clinical interventions, offer health education, and ensure follow-up. This is collaborative practice in its highest form, because the role of the nurse in this setting is to leverage technology and nursing expertise to provide quality health care (Cattell-Gordon, 2009).

Manager—Leading, Inspiring, Thinking Critically. Fundamental to nursing practice—whether it is an individual nurse directing patient care, an administrator of a nursing unit, or a chief nursing officer for a health system—is the role of nurse leader as manager. In this role, the nurse recognizes the identity of manager as the caregiver of the caregivers. In short, nurse manager is the role of pulling together people with the common goal of caregiving.

Although the role of manager or administrator of a nursing unit is not one that every nurse will assume, understanding managing as a primary nursing function is essential. All nurses essentially assume the role of manger every day in their work when they care for their patients. The role of manager requires a systematic way of providing care, a precise tending to details, and working from a comprehensive assessment and plan, as well as engaging colleagues in compassionate, collaborative, interdisciplinary practice.

A nurse, for example, in caring for a dying patient, needs to know the critical point when the family should be called, how to manage the medications, when to touch and not to touch, when to be silent, and when not to do anything but be present. This role calls for the nurse to manage care and demonstrate leadership, seeing the whole and the part—the individual patient and the whole of the process of dying.

A leader is someone grounded in the core value of compassion with the capacity to inspire mentorship, collaboration, creativity, and critical thinking. To communicate this leadership, the leader must provide the framework from which complex problem solving evolves. A core element of managing and leading is understanding the nature of servant leadership and possessing emotional intelligence (Triola, 2007). Nurse leaders demonstrate these identity characteristics when they set priorities based on the needs of those they are leading and are committed to the professional growth of others. Effective leadership is vital to creating healthy work environments that are conducive to promoting quality patient outcomes and health for staff. Authentic leadership, according to Kathleen McCauley, former president of the AACN, is the "glue" needed to hold together a healthy work environment.

In some settings, a nursing culture with a focus on task orientation, rigid hierarchical structures, and the possible disempowerment of staff is an impediment to delivery of compassionate patient-centered care. As a nurse leader, if one sets the tone of joining with the patient in a process of compassionate collaboration, outcomes in health will be more optimally achieved (Jonsdottir, Litchfield, & Dexheiner, 2004).

Educator—Learning and Guiding. The role of the educator is essential to the overall function and identity of the nurse. In the complex world of contemporary health care, as patients seek to manage their disease and cope with illness, the nurse assumes the primary role of educator. At every level, the patient educator role exists within the scope of practice because it significantly affects a patient's health and quality of life. The process of providing education parallels the nursing process, with the first step being an assessment of the learner's needs, readiness to learn, and learning style, followed by an individually designed intervention, and completed only when the outcome has been evaluated (Bastable, 2007). The ability of nurses to effectively provide health education is essential in addressing local and global health problems.

To be effective as a teacher requires a commitment to be a learner; to see teaching and learning as the act of guiding; and to understand the essence of the phrase "to educate." As John Dewey posits, learners grow in concert with others: "Every experience lives on in further experiences. Hence, the central problem of … education … is to select the kind of present experiences that develop fruitfully and creatively in subsequent experiences" (Dewey, Kilpatrick, Hartmann, & Melby, 1937, p. 45). The role of educator in the profession of nursing is based on the desire to help individuals and communities grow. The nurse educator is in essence nurturing a relationship, sharing knowledge, and empowering individuals, families, and communities. The nurse in this role can actively teach and guide patients, families, and communities about health/wellness and illness—about living and dying.

This role of the nurse as educator is further optimized by fostering personal knowing. It is the ability to be empathetic, to see an event from the perspective of another, and to recognize the other as a subject rather as an object. Personal knowing is the discovery of self and others, which is arrived at through reflection, synthesis of perceptions, and connecting with that which is known (Kaminski, 2006, p. 14).

In addition to empathy, nurse educators strive to foster critical thinking skills in their students. Lemire (2002, p. 69) notes that in educating nurses for leadership, the educator must emphasize the cognitive and disposition aspects of critical thinking in order to promote active and sequential learning. Critical thinking and problem-solving skills are acquired over time through lifelong learning and experience.

From this place of learning and knowing comes the ability to be a caring person who seeks to collaborate to achieve a common purpose for health and wellness. This same posture applies to the role of nurse educator—whether it is within a school of nursing, a community college, or with fellow nurses on a unit or in a clinic. The critical pedagogy of nursing requires a fundamental understanding of the dyads, an ability to guide and teach others a whole understanding of the profession, and an evaluation of the sociopolitical context of learning and care. In short, professional nurse educators teach role and nurture identity.

Mentor—Sharing and Role Modeling. *Mentoring* refers to a formal or informal process in which a mentor and a mentee establish a relationship with the mutual goal of meeting the career goals of the mentee (Bally, 2007). One role of the mentor—to be true to oneself and guide another to greater personal awareness and skill—is crucial to retaining and encouraging nurses in the workplace. According to the literature, the initial 3 months of a newly graduated nurse's transition is vital to long-term success in the profession (Winfield, Mclo, & Myrick, 2009). This initial transition involves an all-encompassing transformation of roles and responsibilities, an acceptance of the differences between the theoretical orientation of the nurse's education and the practical focus of professional work, and an integration into an environment that emphasizes teamwork as opposed to individually based care provision. The role of the professional nurse as caregiver, leader, teacher, colleague, and mentor is a critical one in helping newly graduated nurses or any nurses who change roles to feel successful in their new environment (Schumacher & Meleis, 1994).

Because nursing excellence is embodied in the combined competency of skills and practice, the experienced mentor, grounded in the spirit of nurturing, is crucial to the development of careers, collaborative networks, and a contagious enthusiasm within the profession. For this enthusiasm to take hold, the mentor must be a person whom the mentee can trust. The mentor acts as a "role model and advocate to pass

on life experiences and knowledge in order to motivate, support and enhance their mentee's personal and career development" (Kuhl, 2005, p. 9). Building on this, the key qualities in an effective nurse mentor reflect the identity characteristics of the role modeling and sharing.

The National League for Nursing (NLN), one of the membership organizations for nurse faculty and leaders in nursing education, states, "Experienced nurses everywhere have the opportunity to become mentors for other nurses. Mentoring another nurse is a professional means of passing along knowledge, skills, behaviors and values to a less experienced individual" (NLN, 2006, p. 10). The NLN further asserts that in a positive sense, the act of mentoring gives nurses an opportunity to create a legacy. By sharing information and insights with members of their own profession, experienced nurses can enable others to maximize their potential, thereby improving patient care and ultimately strengthening the profession of nursing (Henk, 2005).

Researcher—Inquiring and Discovering

Nothing in life is to be feared. It is only to be understood.
Marie Curie

The role of researcher in the nursing profession is vital for generating new knowledge to underpin nursing practice, clinical care, and public health. As both a caring art and scientific enterprise, nursing has an obligation to provide care that is continually examined through research (International Council of Nurses, 2009). Nurses working as independent investigators or in multidisciplinary research teams offer new insights and unique perspectives to the process. According to Patricia Munhall from the NLN, nurses change in "how" they believe in something rather than "what" they believe and states, "The sands of science itself are shifting, as more and more scientists, including nurse scientists, realize that science cannot be a field of absolute and final truth but is an endeavor focused on illuminating an ever-changing body of ideas" (Munhall, 2007, p. 12). Nursing research, in fact, is critical to the emergence of community-based participatory research, an approach in which the scientific process is applied to a collaborative process with the community of interest.

One way to illustrate the importance of the researcher role is to describe a misalignment between the role and identity of a nurse who works on an oncology unit who is not aware of research or curious about the discovery of new treatments for cancer. This dissonance in an area where so many die from the disease is likely to cause frustration and burnout. Thus at the most basic level, the role of the nurse requires a comfort with research and a curiosity with clinical investigation. At the next level, the nurse applies research at the bedside by providing interventions that are based on current evidence. At an advanced level, the role of nurse as a researcher is fundamental to improving patient care and public health by defining research questions and designing scientific studies to answer them. This process includes writing grants, analyzing data, and sharing findings with the larger health care community.

To be successful in the role of nurse researcher, the identity of the researcher must be grounded in curiosity and the desire for discovery driven by compassion for human suffering. This identity, in turn, empowers patients because it is not proprietary knowledge but rather is about sharing and inspiring new knowledge. Further, curiosity creates an interest in learning and guiding that helps break down barriers between cultures. The curious nurse researcher asks important "how" and "why" questions and builds essential stepping stones toward awareness, appreciation, and understanding of other cultures. Through curiosity, people can gain new perspectives, unparalleled learning and growth, and a chance for interesting conversation and reflection at every interaction (Kaminski, 2006).

Advocate—Passion and Vision

An individual has not started living until he can rise above the narrow confines of his individualistic concerns to the broader concerns of all humanity.
Martin Luther King, Jr.

The purpose of advocacy is change, and true change requires vision, passion, and agitation. This role and spirit has been part of nursing since its inception, although it has not been without contention. Florence Nightingale, for instance, despite being a strong advocate for the improvement of care and conditions in British military hospitals, taught nurses to be unquestioningly obedient to doctors (Hewitt, 2002). References to nurses maintaining loyalty and obedience to doctors were not removed from the ICN's code until 1973 (Snowball, 1996).

Over the past two decades, the word *advocacy* has appeared in nursing literature with increasing frequency (Malik, 1997). Snowball (1996) speaks to the evolution of nurses as advocates. As nursing began to develop its professional identity in the late 1960s, it became more patient-focused and less institution-directed. Since then, with an emphasis on human rights, social justice, equality, and self-determination; the rise of nurse-led advocacy for the Patient's Bill of Rights; and the need for global and national health care reform, the role of nurse as advocate for patients, families, and communities has become essential to the future of health care.

Advocacy has become even more critical in our current high-technology health care environment. Patient autonomy may be limited by the imbalance of power and information in the physician-patient relationship and by the bureaucratic health care system with an emphasis on scientific and technological expertise. This may result in patients surrendering their independence and welfare to an institutional care system with tendencies toward opportunist behaviors such as overutilization of high-cost but low-benefit procedures or treatments. Tuxhill (1994) states patient advocacy as one of the roles that separates nursing ethics from medical ethics. Moral and ethical reasoning, autonomy, and patient empowerment have become inextricably linked with the triad of nurse, patient, and advocacy.

Benner and Wrubel (1989) states that advocacy is the base of nursing as a caring practice, arguing that to be with patients in such a way acknowledges a shared humanity because nursing is a discipline with an active compassion at its core. In the role of patient advocate, the nurse is demonstrating the value of other-centeredness to advance the health of an individual. In the University of Pennsylvania's Health System

Nursing Annual Report, Sharon Fitzpatrick, a critical care nurse, speaks to the difficulty of end-of-life care and her role as advocate for patients during stressful times: "Most relatives can't bring themselves to authorize the removal of life-sustaining equipment … in the meantime, however, they do not see the patient's suffering" (2005, p. 11).

The role of nurse advocate is also essential to ensure universal access to care and for the improvement of public health. Despite an exceptional health care system in the United States, there are well-documented disparities in access to care that result in needless suffering and death. To be a nurse grounded in the value of other-centeredness requires action to promote social justice and equal access to health care. As an example of advocacy in public policy, in May 2009, on the day after the anniversary of Florence Nightingale's birthday (May 12, 1820), a group of 30 nurses wearing red scrubs stood up in a Senate hearing on health care reform and turned their backs to reveal signs that read, "Nurses Say: Stop AHIP, Pass Single Payer." (AHIP stands for "America's Health Insurance Plans," a lobbying group for the health insurance industry.) After standing for a few minutes in silent protest, the nurses walked out of the hearing to applause. In the role of advocate for health for all, the nurse is demonstrating, for example, the characteristics of leading, caring, serving, and connecting (California Nurses Association, 2009).

Professional Practice Roles

The dyads above describe the common elements in professional nursing roles, but roles are also shaped by educational preparation and by the environments in which nurses practice. The mix of skills and knowledge among professional nurses and the diversity of nursing roles expand the profession's impact on health care. In addition, nursing roles fluctuate with changes in the needs of individual patients, the systems of health care delivery and availability of health care technology. For all nurses, other-centeredness remains the core, while the other role-identity dyads dictate the role functions and characteristics.

EDUCATIONAL PREPARATION

All nurses entering the profession must demonstrate competency by passing a state board examination. By passing this exam, the nurse earns the title of registered nurse and demonstrates the ability to practice as a generalist nurse. Although the state board examination is the same for all persons entering the profession, there are several different educational programs that prepare nurses to sit for the state board examination and enter the practice of nursing. As discussed in Chapter 2, these educational programs include diploma, associate degree (AD), bachelor of science in nursing (BSN), and master of science in nursing (MSN) programs, as well as clinical nurse leader (CNL) generalist track. Diploma programs are scarce today, and most of them are hospital based. Associate degree programs focus on nursing theory and skills and require 2 or 3 years of study. The bachelor's degree programs are 4 years in length, and the first 2 years are usually focused on general education at the collegiate level. Although AD-prepared nurses and BSN-prepared nurses often function with the same job descriptions, they bring unique skill sets that often complement each other in clinical practice. The greater focus on skills in AD preparation contrasts to the greater focus on evidence-based practice in BSN preparation, offering each the opportunity to contribute to the other's practice. Many programs are available today for AD-prepared nurses seeking to transition to BSN preparation. Education programs are discussed in more detail in Chapter 2.

In 2003, the American Association of Colleges of Nursing (AACN-East) introduced the CNL as a new generalist nursing role requiring master's preparation. This role was a response to increasing complexity in the health care system, increased patient acuity, and a recognition that other members of the health care team were entering with postgraduate education. Although CNL graduates sit for the same state board exam as AD- and BSN-prepared nurses, additional certification is available to CNL graduates through AACN. The CNL may be viewed as an advanced generalist role, because the master's degree emphasizes systems thinking and leadership skills with the intent of increasing nursing's involvement at a health care systems level.

Nurses with specialty master's preparation or doctoral-level preparation often assume roles as advanced specialists. Although the dyads are the foundation for these nursing roles, advanced specialists offer additional skills and knowledge in a particular clinical area. For example, a community public health nurse designs and implements programs to address the health problems of a population, whereas a health systems specialist manages groups of nurses or other professionals within a health care system. The meta-dyad, other-centeredness, remains the focus of these roles, although the "other" is not a single patient but an entire group, population, or system. Postgraduate education allows nurses in these roles to refine the application of the role-identity dyads to the population of concern.

Advanced practice nurses (APN) are also categorized as advanced specialists. Figure 4-2 is taken from the leading text on advanced practice roles and shows the central aspects of clinical practice, certification, and master's preparation, along with seven core competencies (Hamric, Spross, & Hanson, 2008). The outer ring of the figure represents how the APN role interacts with the environment. All APNs apply the core competencies, but to varying degrees, and with particular emphasis on certain competencies over others depending on the setting in which they work. Currently, four different roles of advanced practice nursing are recognized: the nurse practitioner, who provides a blend of nursing and medical care in primary or acute care settings; the clinical nurse specialist, who provides specialized nursing care to a selected

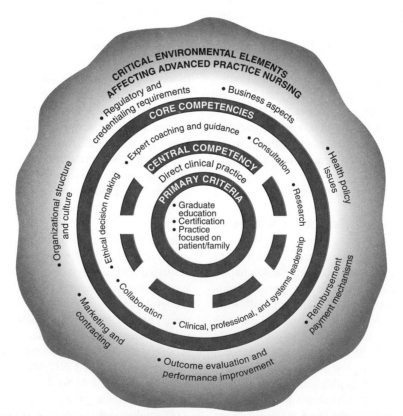

FIGURE 4-2 Critical elements in advanced nursing practice environments. (From Hamric, A. B. [2004]. A definition of advanced practice nursing. In A. B. Hamric, J. A. Spross, C. M. Hansom [Eds.], *Advanced practice nursing: An integrative approach* [4th ed., p. 89]. Philadelphia: Elsevier.)

population; the certified nurse midwife, who provides gynecological and obstetrical care; and the certified registered nurse anesthetist, who provides anesthesia and monitoring of patients during surgery. Although these four categories are distinct, they share the model in Figure 4-2 as the foundation of their practice.

WORK ENVIRONMENT

More than half of generalist nurses practice in hospitals, and the remaining 44% work in home care, outpatient clinics, or nursing homes (American Nurses Association, 2007). The practice settings of the advanced specialist nurse are also diverse and may include schools of nursing, policy work groups, professional organizations, outpatient clinics, state or local health departments, and acute care settings. In every case, nurses' roles are shaped by the environment in which they work. This occurs because of policies set in place by the administrators of the employing organization and the structure by which care is provided. For example, in the past, a short supply of nurses lead hospitals to apply a team nursing model, in which one registered nurse (generalist) is assigned to care for a larger number of patients with the assistance of one or more unlicensed care providers. The tasks performed by that nurse are confined to those that require a license, such as medication administration and assessment, whereas all other tasks are performed by other members of the team under the nurse's supervision. In contrast, the primary nurse model of care assigns one nurse a smaller group of patients with the expectation that most of the required tasks are performed by that nurse (Kerfoot, 1997). In both cases, the system of care shapes the implementation of the nursing role.

Many hospitals and health systems also differentiate nursing roles through a clinical ladder. Nurses are identified as practicing on different levels (or rungs) of the ladder and therefore face different role expectations (Fusilero et al., 2008). A new graduate from a BSN program is usually hired to the lowest level on the ladder and expected to demonstrate, within the first one or two years, the ability to practice at the next level and apply for promotion. Functioning as the charge nurse by applying the leader-managing and critical thinking dyad, precepting students or new nurses by

applying the mentoring-sharing and role modeling dyad, and participating in unit-based research projects by applying the researcher-inquiring and discovering dyad are all specific examples of activities associated with different levels in a clinical ladder. The work environment will also be explored later in this chapter in regard to how it relates to the creation of role stress.

Role Dynamics

MULTIPLE ROLES AND ROLE BALANCE

As the role-identity dyads suggest, professional nurses assume multiple roles. Context dictates which of the role dyads are predominant. When caring for a patient who is grieving after hearing a terminal diagnosis, the caregiver-compassion dyad takes precedence, whereas caring for the same patient on the day he is being discharged may bring the educator-learning and guiding dyad to the forefront. Similarly, nurses may change their role because they have advanced their education or develop an interest in a different clinical setting; in these transitions, the same role-identity dyads are called on in new ways and to different degrees. In a given work setting, the professional nurse is cognizant of the role-identity dyads, selecting among them as the situation demands, and moving fluidly between them.

Professionals also assume roles outside the work setting, and nurses are no exception. In addition to professional roles such as the role of a health care provider, there are personal roles such as the role of partner, parent, team member, or friend. People also may participate in religious or civic organizations by assuming membership or leadership roles that demand a different set of role behaviors. Often, multiple roles are assumed within different contexts. For example, when a professional nurse is at home with family, her primary role as a member of the family is clearly indicated by her physical location. When she walks through the doors of the hospital, a new physical environment suggests a new role.

Balancing multiple roles occurs along a continuum that involves the dynamics of both segmentation and integration. Possessing clear boundaries between roles is referred to as **role segmentation**. Practicing strict role segmentation means avoiding any blending of personal and professional roles (Olson-Buchanan & Boswell, 2005). For instance, role segmentation would mean avoiding checking an employment-related e-mail account from home or avoiding making a personal phone call at work. Role integration is the other end of the spectrum from role segmentation. Practicing **role integration** means that the movement between multiple roles is fluid (Olson-Buchanan & Boswell, 2005). Such professionals might use a cell phone or pager to stay in touch with work during a day off, or they might do volunteer work with co-workers, incorporating both collegial and community roles.

Few people practice roles that are fully segmented or fully integrated; most are somewhere in the middle. The balancing of roles along this continuum fluctuates over time. For instance, a professional nurse's role may be highly segmented with days off to spend with friends and family and days on when the professional role takes precedence. However, during a work shift, that same nurse may receive a call that a family member is ill or be asked to work overtime after making a commitment to attend a community event. In these instances, juggling multiple roles is more challenging.

ROLE STRESS

Role stress occurs when situations or aspects of the environment affect an individual's ability to carry out the perceived obligations of the role (Chen, Chen, Tsai, & Lo, 2007). In the situations described above, the nurse may feel obligated to stay and fulfill her professional role but also feel obligated to meet the needs of the sick family member or to follow through on the commitment made to the community event. **Role strain** refers to an emotional reaction when role stress is not resolved (Chen et al., 2007). Role stress is a common phenomenon that, if appropriately managed, can lead to increased role satisfaction. Unresolved role stress that leads to role strain contributes to professionals leaving a work setting. The terms *role stress* and *role strain* are sometimes used interchangeably, but understanding the difference is important. Role stress has a variety of forms; the causes are multifactorial and can be exacerbated when role functions collide with identity characteristics.

Role stress and role strain are not unique to nursing but can arise in any profession. The impact of role strain on health and well-being can be significant. For example, one study found that depression and job strain were correlated, suggesting that job strain was responsible for mental health inequities (LaMontagne, Keegel, Vallance, Ostry, & Wolfe, 2008). Other research shows that job strain has a modest effect on systolic blood pressure and that lower social support increases that impact (Guimont et al., 2006). In a survey of adults with personal roles as caregivers, Fredrikson and Scharlach (1997) found that those who worked shifts reported higher levels of role strain than those in salaried positions, perhaps due to conflicts between work and personal obligations that are not easily resolved in the face of rigid work schedules. This last study is particularly pertinent to nurses, who are likely to work shifts and also be looked to by friends and family to serve as caregivers outside the professional setting.

The meta-dyad of nursing, other-centeredness, may in part contribute to role stress. Because external elements shape the nurse's role, conflict, ambiguity, and differing expectations about specific role obligations are more likely to arise. In a review of international literature, Lambert and Lambert (2001) noted that the phenomenon of role strain occurs in nurses throughout the world. This review also identified factors in the work environment that were consistently correlated to higher levels of role stress in nurses across a wide variety of cultures and settings. These factors included poor relationships with colleagues, perceived lack of control over the job, time demands, and lack of support from the employing organization.

In a national survey in the United States, Ulrich, Buerhaus, Donelan, Norman, and Dittus (2005) examined registered nurses' views on the work environment and compared their results with findings from a similar survey conducted 2 years earlier. Overall job satisfaction was slightly higher in the more recent survey. Nurses in 2004 reported greater satisfaction in relationships with colleagues than did those surveyed in 2002, suggesting that some improvement in work environments has occurred. The authors note three areas still to be improved: nurses in both surveys reported low decision-making authority, a lack of time to form relationships with patients, and inadequate respect and support from employing organizations. These factors, which represent an imbalance in the dyads, may continue to contribute to role stress among nurses.

Role Conflict. Sources: Role conflict refers to role stress that occurs when an individual feels required to meet the obligations of two different roles at once. As described above, role conflict can occur between professional and personal roles. For example, consider the nurse who also is a parent or a primary caregiver to an aging relative. Attending to the needs of the dependent while also meeting the professional expectation to be on time for a shift and free of personal distractions creates role stress and may progress to role strain. Nevidjon (2004) notes that some nurses work multiple shifts in a single day, waking up early to do household chores and coming home after the work shift to childcare or eldercare responsibilities. Similarly, the nurse who is actively involved in the community may face role stress when asked to rotate to different shifts, requiring a change in sleep pattern.

In a review of literature, Stanley (2006) notes role conflict occurring among nurses who provide direct bedside care and have managerial responsibilities. Although both roles place a high priority on patient care and safety, the obligations of the direct bedside role are determined by the needs of a particular group of patients, whereas the obligations of the managerial role are determined by the needs of the unit and the institution. In both cases, other-centeredness provides the foundation for the role; the conflict comes from having two "others" with different expectations. Efforts to honor clinical obligations, provide service to patients and simultaneously honor administrative obligations and the institution's mission leaves the individual feeling pulled in two directions.

Strategies: Nevidjon (2004) lists several strategies to help alleviate the role stress that results from conflict between professional and personal roles. She suggests combining efforts, which means finding ways to meet the obligations of two roles simultaneously, such as including friends in work-related events or inviting co-workers to community-based activities. These periods of greater role integration can alleviate

the stress that comes from having multiple obligations in different directions. The same author also suggests taking short breaks during work, exercising, and getting enough sleep to help alleviate role strain due to role conflict.

An innovative strategy for addressing conflict between personal and professional roles involves adjusting the hours of nursing shifts. Some institutions offer flexible work hours, identified by Young, Albert, Paschke, and Meyer (2007) as "the Parent Shift," to reduce the stress that can occur from family and work role conflicts. The stress of conflicting personal and professional roles is widely recognized within our society. In 1993, federal legislation in the form of the Family Medical Leave Act (FMLA) was passed by Congress to ensure that employees who need time off to provide care to family members are able to return to their existing employment. Although documentation is required for FMLA time, the act applies to any personal caregiving role—from driving a sick child to multiple doctors' appointments to staying home to care for a dying relative.

Role Overload. Sources: Role overload refers to situations in which the time and resources allotted for a given role are insufficient to meet the role expectations. Essentially, role overload occurs when there is too much to do and too little time in which to do it. As indicated in the description of the dyads, professional nurses often have multiple subroles, or separate sets of behaviors and expectations that make up the larger role. The wide range of activities that constitute a professional nursing role is very rewarding but can also become overwhelming, particularly because many nurses work in shifts, meaning that a set time interval is given to complete required tasks.

Role overload is documented as a source of role stress among nurses (Chang & Hancock, 2003) and advanced practice nurses (Chen et al., 2007). Given the rising number of patients with complex and chronic illness, the efforts to make health care delivery more efficient and affordable, and the increase in health care technology, the workload of professional nurses continues to expand. Although role overload is a real and concerning phenomenon, strategies can be used to reduce the strain it causes.

Strategies: Delegation is an essential strategy to prevent the stress of role overload. **Delegation** is defined by the American Nurses Association (ANA) as "the transfer of responsibility for the performance of a task from one individual to another while retaining accountability for the outcome" (American Nurses Association, 2005, p. 4). In this strategy, the nurse asks another member of the health care team to perform particular tasks, such as checking patients' vital signs. By delegating a task, the nurse is not required to observe the task's completion and thus can attend to other tasks. The nurse retains responsibility, however, for the result of the task, so follow-up action may be required. Appropriate delegation requires knowing the skill set and scope of practice of the person to whom tasks are delegated and effectively communicating with that person about the patient's needs, the time in which the task should be completed, and the follow-up action planned.

As an example of delegation, consider a staff nurse who is assigned to care for patients and also take the charge nurse role for her unit. At a given time during the shift, she may be called on to be a caregiver when one of her patients requires medication for pain and also called on to act in a managerial role to determine how to handle a staffing shortage on the next shift. To resolve this potential role overload, the charge nurse can delegate the task of providing the patient's pain medicine to one of her staff nurses or colleagues or contact the nursing supervisor to help address the staff shortage as advocate for all.

Prioritizing is also essential when role overload emerges. Creating a list of the tasks required and numbering them according to their importance helps some nurses negotiate a busy shift. Often it is tempting to skip a break or meal when the shift is busy, but tasks may actually be completed in a more efficient manner if a few moments are taken to have a snack and think through the next steps. Rushing can lead to errors, which actually consume *more* time and can be dangerous, particularly when medication administration is involved.

Another strategy to address role overload involves appropriate changes to the physical environment. For instance, if supplies are kept at a distance from the site of care delivery, the time required for each task will be unnecessarily lengthened (Christmas, 2008). Providing input to a unit manager about changes to the physical environment or joining a task force to examine what supplies are most often needed and so should be kept in a closer location can help resolve role stress due to role overload.

Role Ambiguity. Sources: Role ambiguity refers to role stress that occurs when the obligations and privileges of a given role are not clearly defined. This leaves the individual unsure how to act. There are two distinct periods in which role ambiguity is likely to occur: during role transition and in times of role extension. **Role transition** occurs when an individual enters a new role, and **role extension** occurs when the duties associated with a particular role expand. Ideally, both role transition and role extension are temporary causes of role stress that resolve when an individual achieves **role mastery**, a sense of clarity regarding the role expectations and a firm confidence in the ability to meet those expectations.

An example of role transition occurs when a new graduate begins a position as a professional nurse. The degree of stress that a new graduate nurse experiences with this transition will vary depending on the availability of mentoring, organizational support, and preparation from the educational experience. In a study of new graduate nurses, Chang and Hancock (2003) found a correlation between role ambiguity and lower ratings of job satisfaction, indicating that this is an important source of stress and strain. Similarly, in examining role stress among nurses working 8- and 12-hour shifts, Hoffman and Scott (2003) found significantly different levels among nurses based on years of experience. Regardless of the length of the shift worked, higher levels of stress were reported by newer nurses.

The potential for role stress due to role ambiguity is not confined to the new graduate. In interviews with nurses at different career stages, Deppoliti (2008) noted that there were discrete periods or "passage points" in which nurses reaffirmed their professional identity. At certain stages, such as transitioning to the charge nurse role or the preceptor role, the participants experienced role ambiguity. Similarly, Chen et al. (2007) noted that experienced nurses in Taiwan experienced role ambiguity when they transitioned to advanced practice roles and when those roles were extended by their employing institution. Their survey results also confirmed a significant correlation between role ambiguity and lower ratings of job satisfaction. As hospitals and clinics adapt to economic and technological changes, nurses at every career stage are likely to experience periods of role ambiguity due to role extension.

Strategies: Essential in resolving the stress of role ambiguity is the development of a clear definition of the role. As described by Young, Stuenkel, and Bawel-Brinkley (2008), role ambiguity among new graduates is best prevented with a comprehensive structured orientation program. A combination of clinical and classroom activities provides new graduates with the chance to observe nursing expertise and an opportunity to discuss and validate their own expectations. Authors also identify that support from peers is essential in the resolution of role ambiguity (Bally, 2007; Young et al., 2008). Orientation sessions in which new graduates interact with each other encourage the development of needed peer support networks.

Mentoring is also a key strategy for addressing the stress of role ambiguity. **Mentoring**, as described in the dyads above, refers to a formal or informal process in which a mentor and a mentee establish a relationship with the mutual goal of meeting the career goals of the mentee (Bally, 2007). Mentors are distinct from friends in that there is not an even give-and-take expected. Although both parties expect to gain from the mentorship, the benefits on each side are different. Seeking a mentor who is not the assigned clinical preceptor provides a transitioning nurse with a wider base of support. The mentor can validate or correct the mentee's expectations about the new or expanded role and review situations that the mentee encounters during the orientation process.

All professional roles have written job descriptions that can be reviewed to assist in the process of gaining role clarity. This can be especially helpful for transitions into roles that are newly created. In advanced specialist roles, nurses may be asked to write or edit the content of the job description. Review of existing descriptions for similar roles or advice from a mentor can be valuable to the process of creating a role description. When role transition or extension occurs, a nurse can craft a simple statement or inquiry response that reinforces "what I do in my current role." Recalling, repeating, or responding with a prepared statement is helpful in alleviating role ambiguity during times of role transition or extension. An exercise to consider when role transitions and extensions occur is developing a one- or two-sentence description of the role (Hamric, 2008). An example of such an exercise is provided in the Critical Thinking Exercises at the end of this chapter.

Role Discrepancy. Source: Role discrepancy refers to role stress that occurs when an individual's conception of a role is incompatible with the actual obligations of the role. This phenomenon is well documented in studies of nurses. In fact, the importance of this source of role stress is exemplified by the fact that some professional nurse authors define role stress and strain as role discrepancy (Hall, 2004; Lambert & Lambert, 2001). Past president of the ANA, Barbara Blackeney, referenced role discrepancy when she told a *New York Times* reporter, "Nurses love nursing. They just hate their jobs" (Corbett, 2003, para 20). This quote suggests that a predominance of nurses have a concept of what their role *ought* to be that is inconsistent with the content of their day-to-day work.

Results of a national survey of nurses working in the United States suggest that Blackeney's assessment is accurate. More than half of respondents reported spending too little time engaged in direct patient care and too much time on documentation (Buerhaus, Donelan, Ulrich, DesRoches, & Dittus, 2007). Several authors note that role discrepancy as a source of role stress for nurses contributes to job dissatisfaction and even to the intention to quit (Lambert & Lambert, 2001; Takase, Maude, & Manias, 2006). Hall (2004), in a small qualitative explorative study, confirmed what the national survey indicated: nurses identified the inability to meet their own expectations as an important source of stress and strain.

Strategies: Although role discrepancy is a significant source of role stress and strain among nurses, there are strategies for managing it. **Debriefing,** which involves reviewing the events of a particular situation with a colleague or group of colleagues, can be helpful for several reasons. First, debriefing offers the chance to articulate the role expectations that came into conflict in a given situation. Often, role expectations are taken for granted, and simply putting these thoughts into words allows the concerned nurse to make progress in understanding the source of her stress. Second, colleagues present during a debriefing session can validate the concerned nurse's views and share similar experiences and expectations. In this way, debriefing builds positive relationships within the clinical settings, a key factor in reducing role stress (Lambert & Lambert, 2001). Finally, debriefing is helpful in identifying the types of situations that contribute to role discrepancy so that strategies to prevent these situations can be implemented.

For example, consider a novice intensive care unit nurse whose elderly patient develops a change in his cardiac rhythm in the early morning hours. The doctor on call asks that the nurse to manage this change by calling a cardiology consult, an action usually taken by medical providers during daytime hours. On the same shift, the charge nurse asks the novice ICU nurse to cover a break and give report to the hospital's nursing supervisor if she calls. This nurse is at risk for role discrepancy in two directions. First, calling the cardiology team is not an expectation of the ICU nurse role in this institution. Second, having never been oriented to the charge role, this nurse did not expect to take responsibility for reporting to the supervisor.

In a debriefing session, the nurse in the above scenario describes the shift to the mentor and the mentor validates that the expectations placed on the nurse during that shift were not consistent with the nurse's own views of the role. Together, they review possible ways of managing this kind of situation. First, the mentor suggests that the nurse politely but firmly refuse to call consults because this is not an appropriate expectation of the ICU nurse role. The mentor, who is a member of the unit leadership, also offers to write an e-mail to the unit's medical director to be forwarded to all medical providers, clarifying that ICU nurses are not expected to call consults. With regard to the charge nurse role, the nurse decides, with the support of the mentor, to speak with the manager about requiring charge nurses to seek coverage for breaks only from other nurses

who are oriented to the charge role. In this way, the nurse and the mentor take specific actions to change the expectations of others (the doctor and the charge nurse) so that the conflict with the nurse's own view of the role is resolved.

A second strategy to consider in situations of role discrepancy is investigating the **role advancement program** at the employing institution. Many institutions offer clinical ladders or advancement programs for registered nurses though which clinical experience, requisite educational background, and demonstrated professionalism lead to promotion to a higher level (Fusilero et al., 2008). The benefits of promotion may include higher pay, input on shift assignment, and the opportunity to participate in additional professional development activities. Nurses who have not considered career advancement but are asked to perform in the charge role or to be clinical preceptors may experience role discrepancy because these subroles are not within the scope of a novice nursing role. If a nurse is comfortable assuming these roles, he or she ought to pursue career advancement in order to receive the full benefits of providing additional services to the institution.

A final strategy involves examining which tasks create role discrepancy and determining how these can be more efficiently completed (**task analysis**). For example, some nurses find that the time spent writing progress notes takes away from time interacting with patients, thus conflicting with their expectation that their primary role is to provide care. Approaching a manager, an advanced practice nurse, or unit leadership about strategies that make documentation more efficient can alleviate this source of role discrepancy. Is there a policy that could be changed to reduce the required documentation so that notes are written once every 24 hours rather than on every shift? Could a template for the required documentation be created so that this task can be completed more quickly? As in the example above, in which the mentoring nurse sought to communicate with medical providers, actions that promote positive change can go a long way to minimize and prevent role discrepancy.

Role Incongruity. **Sources:** A final source of role stress for nurses is **role incongruity.** This term refers to situations in which the obligations of a role come into conflict with an individual's values. Although situations of role incongruity are similar to role discrepancy, they are likely to engender a more severe strain because values, unlike perceptions about a role, are personally determined and deeply revered. **Values** guide behavior, direct priorities, and determine how information is perceived (McNeese-Smith & Crook, 2003). Personal values are formed early in life through family, education, and religious and cultural experiences. Professional values develop through the process of professional socialization. Because values are deeply held—and a fundamental part of identity—they are sometimes taken for granted and therefore hard to articulate (Raines, 1993). Related to role incongruity is **moral distress,** a phenomenon in which an individual feels compelled to act in a manner that she or he believes is morally wrong (Hamric, Davis, & Childress, 2006). Moral distress is discussed further in the chapter on ethics (Chapter 12).

Two recent studies describe role incongruity among nurses. Persky, Nelson, Watson, and Bent (2008) found that the nurses perceived by patients as most caring were also more likely to report frustration with the work environment. The authors explain these findings by noting that the high value placed on caring among these nurses was incongruent with the emphasis on efficient time management and judicious use of resources within the work environment. Similarly, in a national survey, Yarbrough, Alfred, and Martin (2008) identified the congruity of nurses' values across areas of practice (advanced practice, staff nurses, administrators, and educators) and suggested that dissonance with organizational values contributes to poor retention, or resigning. Their respondents identified privacy, respect for dignity, and accountability as top priorities that they felt were not highly valued by their institutions.

A striking example of role incongruity comes from studies of nurses working in New Orleans in 2005, after Hurricane Katrina. Nurses who valued their ability to provide care to vulnerable patients were required to do so without appropriate resources, without adequate rest, and in isolation from their families. Nurses interviewed about their experiences became tearful as they described making decisions about evacuating

with their families or staying at the hospital, because both options engendered distress due to conflicting values (Giarratano, Orlando, & Savage, 2008).

Strategies: An essential starting point in managing role incongruity is values clarification, an exercise in which an individual practices articulating existing values. A variety of exercises are available for **values clarification;** but all of them encourage participants to see how their choices, behaviors, and perceptions are determined by deeply rooted beliefs. By undergoing values clarification, a nurse will better articulate the role incongruity being experienced and begin to seek needed changes to the work environment. Values clarification is discussed further in the chapter on ethics (Chapter 12).

A second strategy in addressing role incongruity is **empowerment**. Manojlovich (2007) observes that empowerment develops when nurses are competent in their clinical practice, are providing nursing care autonomously, and are represented on hospital committees and at administrative decision-making levels within an institution. Nurses can seek empowerment through connections with those in leadership positions and by recognizing their own ability to influence the work environment and control their nursing practice. Although caring and power may at first seem mutually exclusive, in fact, nurses are empowered by the care that they uniquely provide to patients (Manojlovich, 2007).

In situations in which role incongruity occurs repeatedly to the extent that the work environment is unsafe, the nurse may consider a whistle-blowing approach. **Whistle-blowing** refers to situations in which unethical or illegal conduct by an organization is reported to an outside authority by a member of that organization. A recent example of whistle-blowing came when members of the U.S. Army reported the treatment of war criminals in prison camps to federal authorities (Shenon, 2004). Despite their lack of authority within the Army structure, the soldiers making this report recognized they were part of an unethical environment and took steps to make a change. Lachman (2008) observes that nurses have a similar ethical obligation to act when a lack of organizational accountability threatens patient safety. Box 4-1 lists five recommendations for an ethical organizational culture. In an ethical organizational culture, nurses and all

BOX 4-1	Recommendations for an Ethical Organizational Culture

- Develop a code of conduct that corresponds to the organization's values and that cannot be compromised.
- Develop an ethics committee whose mission is to create infrastructure to support organization's values.
- Provide educational forums on organizational ethics.
- Avoid passivity (the "bystander effect" and "diffusion of responsibility").
- Establish and publish an internal procedure for individuals to employ when they believe organizational values and "principles of care" are being violated.

Lachman, V. D. (2008). Whistleblowing: Role of organizational culture in prevention and management. *MedSurg Nursing, 17*(4), 265–267.

members of the health care team are benefited. In such an environment, role incongruity is seldom a source of role stress, because mechanisms for addressing values conflicts are firmly in place. Box 4-2 summarizes the stepwise approach to a role-related problem.

SUMMARY

Nursing's contribution to health care is illustrated by the nature and diversity of nursing roles. At its core, the nursing profession requires a renewed vision for patient wellness and a passion for a society in which health and wellness is a right for all. Nursing demands a role identity to preserve the relationship at the individual level and for humanity at a society level. We have reached a critical transformation point for both the nursing profession and the U.S. health care system. It is no longer sufficient simply to advocate for policy

BOX 4-2	Summary of a Stepwise Approach to Role-Related Problems

1. Identify the cause. Acknowledging and anticipating sources of role stress is the first step.
2. Develop internal role clarity. Use the following questions to assist in developing a clear definition of the role:
   What are the primary obligations of the role?
   What tasks are prioritized by persons in the role?
   What percentage of time is appropriate for each of the tasks above?
   What are the values of the organization in which you are employed?
   What personal values relate to this role?
3. Identify the key stakeholders. Role problems may create a sense of isolation and can affect family, co-workers, patients, and friends. Consider who else might be affected by this problem and who can facilitate the resolution. Identify the best time and manner in which to communicate with those involved; some co-workers may rely on e-mail and others may prefer face-to-face contact. Often, a unit manager or advanced practice nurse can provide guidance and support.
4. Develop specific interventions, based on the source of role stress. Consider the following specific strategies for different sources of role stress:
   Role conflict: Seek opportunities for integrating personal and professional roles; adjust the work schedule for personal needs.
   Role overload: Delegate, prioritize, make changes to the physical work environment.
   Role ambiguity: Identify and form relationships with mentors. Consider adjusting your job description and develop a one- or two-sentence statement that describes your role.
   Role discrepancy: Debriefing. Seek out support from co-workers and offer support to others. Identify strategies for making work processes more efficient.
   Role incongruity: Values clarification. Repeated role incongruity may indicate the need for a whistle-blowing approach or a change in roles.
5. Select a course of action and take it!
6. Evaluate. What impact did the action have on your satisfaction with your role?

change or ensure the care of an individual patient. Massive system change and practice paradigm shifts are required in both health care delivery and nursing education and practice. The integration of nursing roles into a nurse's core identity and practice is necessary. That work begins in a renewed examination of the central role of nursing's other-centeredness (metadyad) and of all of the role-identity dyads (functions and characteristics) to ensure they are woven into a "single quilt" that is *nursing*. Although the roles described in this chapter do not constitute an exhaustive list, they are representative of the roles nurses commonly assume. As the health care system continues to change, it is anticipated that new nursing roles will emerge.

KEY POINTS

- The practice of nursing involves assuming a number of diverse roles that have corresponding identity elements.
- Central to nursing is "other-centeredness" because all nursing roles are focused on addressing the needs of a specific person or population.
- Culture and history shape the way nursing roles are interpreted by society, whereas education and work environment affect how nursing roles are implemented.
- The need to assume multiple roles in nursing can result in role stress and strain.
- Strategies to modify role stress and strain are situation specific and essential to effective nursing practice.

CRITICAL THINKING EXERCISES

1. Select a nursing role of your choice and then do the following:
   a. Identify how the seven role-identity dyads come into play.
   b. Describe the role stressors that may be an integral part of the role.
   c. Identify strategies that can be employed to reduce role strain.
2. Identify the sources of role conflict that you may be currently experiencing. How can you reduce the impact of this conflict? What can others do?
3. Describe a situation in which you experienced role overload. What were the consequences? How did you resolve the situation? Formulate additional strategies that might have been useful.

4. Describe a situation related to the professional nursing role where role incongruity might be an issue for you. What alternatives can you identify that could result in a satisfactory resolution?
5. Speculate how advanced practice nurses might best be used in your clinical setting. What would be the benefits for the patients? How would the organization benefit from their practice?
6. Formulate a brief statement describing your current role that you could use as a response in a social situation when asked, "What do you do?"

REFERENCES

American Nurses Association. (2005). *Principles of delegation*. Silver Spring, MD: American Nurses Association.

American Nurses Association. (2007). *About nursing*. Retrieved from http://www.nursingworld.org/MainMenu Categories/CertificationandAccreditation/AboutNursing aspx.

Armitage, G. (Director). (1971). *Private Duty Nurses*. [Television series]. United States: New World Pictures.

Bally, J. M. G. (2007). The role of nursing leadership in creating a mentoring culture in acute care environments. *Nurse Economics, 25*(3), 143–148.

Bastable, S. (2007). *Nurse as educator: Principles of teaching and learning for nursing practice*. Sudbury, MA: Jones & Bartlett Publishers.

Benner, P., & Wrubel, J. (1989). *The primacy of caring*. California: Addison Wesley.

Bevin, T. (Producer), & Wright, J. (Director). (2007). *Atonement*. [Motion picture]. United Kingdom: Focus Features.

Biddle, B. J. (1979). *Role theory: Expectations, identities and behaviors*. New York: Academic Press.

Brackett, C. (Producer), & Wilder, B. (Director). (1945). *The Lost Weekend*. [Motion picture]. United States: Paramount Pictures.

Bruckheimer, J. & Bay, M. (Producers), & Bay, M. (Director). (2001). *Pearl Harbor* (Motion picture). United States: Touchstone Pictures.

Buerhaus, P. I., Donelan, K., Ulrich, B. T., DesRoches, C., & Dittus, R. (2007). Trends in the experiences of hospital-employed registered nurses: Results from three national surveys. *Nursing Economics, 25*(2), 69–80.

Burns, T. (Producer), & Chulack C. (Director). (1994). *ER*. [Television series]. United States: Amblin Entertainment & Warner Bros. Television Production, Inc.

California Nurses Association. (2009). *Nurses and doctors call for Florence Nightingale Day*. Protest: Against Max Baucus and health insurers: May 12, 2009. Retrieved from http://www.calnurses.org/media-center/press-releases/2009/may/nurses-and-doctors-call-for-florence-nightingale-day-protest-against-max-baucus-and-health-insurers-may-12.html

Cattell-Gordon, D. (2009). *(Personal interview). Telehealth and collaborative practice*. University of Virginia Health System Retrieved from http://www.healthsystem.virginia.edu/internettelemedicine

Chang, E., & Hancock, K. (2003). Role stress and role ambiguity in new nursing graduates in Australia. *Nursing and Health Sciences, 5*, 155–163.

Chen, Y., Chen, S., Tsai, C., & Lo, L. (2007). Role stress and job satisfaction for nurse specialists. *Journal of Advanced Nursing, 59*(5), 497–509.

Childs, A. (2006). The complex gastrointestinal patient and Jean Watson's Theory of Caring in nutrition support. *Gastroenterology Nursing, 29*(4), 283–288.

Christmas, K. (2008). How work environment impacts retention. *Nurse Economics, 26*(5), 316–318.

Corbett, S. (2003). (March 16). *The last shift*. Retrieved January 19, 2009, from http://query.nytimes.com/gst/fullpage.html?res=9E00E5D8163EF935A25750C0A9659C8B63&sec=health&spon=&pagewanted=2

Corn, R. (Director). (2005). *Grey's Anatomy*. [Television series]. United States: ABC Studios.

Covington, H. (2005). Caring presence: Providing a safe place for patients. *Holistic Nursing Practice, 19*(4), 169–172, Retrieved from https://www.ncbi.nlm.nih.gov/pubmed/16006831

Cramer, D. (Producer). (1988). *Nightingales*. [Television series]. United States: Aaron Spelling Productions.

Deppoliti, D. (2008). Exploring how new registered nurses construct professional identity in hospital settings. *The Journal of Continuing Education, 39*(6), 255–262.

Dewey, J., Kilpatrick, W. H., Hartmann, G. H., & Melby, E. O. (1937). *The teacher and society*. New York: Appleton-Century.

Douglas, M., & Zaentz, S. (Producers), & Forman, M. (Director). (1975). *One Flew Over the Cuckoo's Nest*. [Motion picture]. United States: United Artists.

dyad. (2009). In *Merriam-Webster Online Dictionary*. Retrieved September 15, 2009, from http://www.merriam-webster.com/dictionary/dyad

Evans, J. (2004). Men nurses: a historical and feminist perspective. *Journal of Advanced Nursing, 47*(3), 321–328.

Fredrikson, K. I., & Scharlach, A. E. (1997). Caregiving and employment: The impact of workplace characteristics on role strain. *Journal of Gerontological Social Work, 28*(4), 3–22.

Fusilero, J., Lini, L., Prohaska, P., Szweda, C., Carney, K., & Mion, L. C. (2008). The career advancement for registered nurse excellence program. *The Journal of Nursing Administration, 38*, 526–531.

Gardner, D. (2005). Ten lessons in collaboration. *Online Journal of Issues in Nursing*. Retrieved September 15, 2009 from http://www.nursingworld.org/ojin/topic26/tpc26_1.htm

Giarratano, G., Orlando, S., & Savage, J. (2008). Perinatal nursing in uncertain times: The Katrina effect. *The American Journal of Maternal Child Nursing, 33*(4), 249–257.

Guimont, C., Brisson, C., Dagenais, G. R., Milot, A., Vezina, M., Masse, B., et al. (2006). Effects of job strain on blood pressure: A prospective study of white-collar workers. *American Journal of Public Health, 96*(8), 1436–1443.

Hall, D. S. (2004). Work-related stress of registered nurses in a hospital setting. *Journal for Nurses in Staff Development, 20*(1), 6–14.

Hamric, A. B., Davis, W. S., & Childress, M. D. (2006). Moral distress in health care providers: What is it and what can we do about it? *The Pharos*, 17–23.

Hamric, A. B. (2008). A definition of advanced practice. In A. B. Hamric, J. A. Spross, & C. M. Hanson (Eds.), *Advanced practice nursing: An integrative approach* (pp. 75–94). St. Louis: Elsevier.

Henk, B. (2005). *Mentoring: What's it all about? Notes from a Navy leadership presentation held in Bremerton, WA*. Unpublished manuscript.

Hoffman, A. J., & Scott, L. D. (2003). Role stress and career satisfaction among registered nurses by work shift pattern. *Journal of Nursing Administration, 33*(6), 337–342.

Hogg, M., & Terry, D. (2000). *Attitudes, behavior and social context: The role of norms and group membership*. Mahwah, NJ: Lawrence Erlbaum Associates.

Hornberger, R.H. (Producer). (1972). *M*A*S*H*. [Television series]. United States: 20th Century Fox.

identity. (2009). In *Merriam-Webster Online Dictionary*. Retrieved September 15, 2009, from http://www.merriam-webster.com/dictionary.identity

International Council of Nurses. (2009). International Council of Nurses: Mission Statement. Retrieved September 15, 2009, from http://www.icn.ch/resnetbul_00.htm

Jonsdottir, H., Litchfield, M., & Dexheimer Pharris, M. (2004). The relational core or nursing practice as partnership. *Journal of Advanced Nursing, 29*(5), 1205–1212.

Kaminski, J. (March 14, 2006). *Nursing through the lens of culture: A multiple gaze*: Unpublished PhD. Vancouver: University of British Columbia.

Kerfoot, K. (1997). Role redesign: what has it accomplished? *Online Journal of Issues in Nursing, 2*(4), Retrieved from http://www.nursingworld.org/MainMenuCatagories/ANAMarketplace/Periodicals/OJIN/TableofContents/vol21997/No4Dec97/RoleRedesign.aspx

Kuhl, L. (2005). Closing the revolving door: A look at mentoring. *Chart: Journal of Illinois Nursing, 102*(2), 9.

Lachman, V. D. (2008). Whistleblowing: Role of organizational culture in prevention and management. *MEDSURG Nursing, 17*(4), 265–267.

Lambert, V. A., & Lambert, C. E. (2001). Literature review of role stress/strain on nurses: An international perspective. *Nursing and Health Sciences, 3*, 161–172.

LaMontagne, A. D., Keegel, T., Vallance, D., Ostry, A., & Wolfe, R. (2008). Job strain—Attributable depression in a sample of working Australians: Assessing the contribution to health inequalities. *BMC Public Health, 8*, Article 181. Retrieved June 5, 2009, from http://www.biomedcentral.com/1471-2458/8/181

Lawrence, B. (Producer). (2001). *Scrubs.* [Television series]. United States: ABC Studios.

Leininger, M. (1988). Leininger's theory of nursing: Cultural Care Diversity and Universality. *Nursing Science Quarterly, 1,*(4), 152–160.

Leininger, M., & McFarland, M. (1997). *Transcultural nursing: Concepts, theories, research and practice* (3rd ed.). New York: McGraw-Hill Professional.

Lemire, J. (2002). Leader as critical thinker. *Nursing Leadership Forum, 7*, 69–76.

Lucas, J. (2009). History of male nurses. *Male Nurse Magazine.* Retrieved September 15, 2009, from http://www.malenursemagazine.com/historyof malenurses.html

Malik, M. (1997). Advocacy in nursing—a review of the literature. *Journal of Advanced Nursing, 25*(1), 130–138.

Manojlovich, M. (2007). Power and empowerment in nursing: Looking backward to inform the future. *OJIN: The Online Journal of Issues in Nursing, Vol. 12,* No. 1, Manuscript 1. Retrieved from www.nursingworld.org/MainMenuCategories/ANAMarketplace/ANAPeriodicals/OJIN/TableofContents/Volume122007/No1Jan07/LookingBackwardtoInformtheFuture.aspx

Marcia, J. (1966). Development and validation of ego identity status. *Journal of Personality and Social Psychology, 3*, 551–558.

McCauley, K. (2005). Doing the right thing. *AACN News, 22*(2).

McEwan, I. (2001). *Atonement.* New York: Random House.

McFadden, E. (2006). Moral development and reproductive health decisions. *Journal of Obstetric, Gynecologic & Neonatal Nursing, 25*(6), 507–512.

McNeese-Smith, D. K., & Crook, M. (2003). Nursing values and a changing nurse workforce. *Journal of Nursing Administration, 33*(5), 260–270.

Morton, P. G., & Fontaine, D. (2009). *Critical care nursing: A holistic approach* (9th ed.). Philadelphia: Lippincott-Raven.

Munhall, P. (2007). Chapter 1: The landscape of qualitative research in nursing. In P. Munhall (Ed.). *Nursing: A qualitative perspective* (4th ed.). Boston: Jones and Bartlett.

National League for Nursing. Statement: Mentoring of Nurse Faculty. Position statement. New York: Author. Retrieved September 15, 2009, from http://www.nln.org/aboutnln/PositionStatements/mentoring_3_22_06.pdf

Nevidjon, B. (2004). Managing from the middle: Integrating midlife challenges, children, elder parents, and career. *Clinical Journal of Oncology Nursing, 8*(1), 72–75.

Nightingale, F. (1860). *Notes on nursing: What it is and what it is not* (First American Edition ed). New York: D. Appleton and Company.

Olson-Buchanan, J. B., & Boswell, W. R. (2005). Blurring boundaries: correlates of integration and segmentation between work and nonwork. *Journal of Vocational Behavior, 68*, 432–445.

Persky, G. J., Nelson, J. W., Watson, J., & Bent, K. (2008). Creating a profile of a nurse effective in caring. *Nursing Administration, 32*(1), 15–20.

Raines, D. A. (1993). Values: A guiding force. *AWHONN's Clinical Issues, 4*, 533–541.

Rasmussen, E. (May 7, 2001). Picture imperfect: From Nurse Ratched to Hot Lips Houlihan—Film, TV portrayals of nurses often transmit a warped image of real-life RNs. *Nurse Week: News and Trends,* Retrieved from http://www.nurseweek.com/news/features/01-05/picture.html.

Reiner, R. (Director), & Reiner, R., Scheinman, A., Stott, J., & Nicolaides, S. (Producers). (1990). *Misery* [Motion picture]. United States: Columbia Pictures and Castle Rock Entertainment.

Robert, T. (2003). Patient-focused care pledge adopted: *The American College of Chest Physicians takes an exemplary step*. Retrieved from http://headaches.about.com/cs/advocacy/a/pledge/htm

Robinson, K. (2003). Technology can't replace compassion in health care. *Journal of Emergency Nursing, 29*(3), 199–200.

role. (2009). In *Merriam-Webster Online Dictionary*. Retrieved September 15, 2009, from http://www.merriam-webster.com/dictionary/role

Rose, A. (2009). *Teaching as a performing art*. (Philosophical statement). Retrieved from http://www/distance.mun.ca/faculty/dossier_philosophy_rose.pdf

Saenz, M. (Director). (1988). *China Beach: U.S. war drama* [Motion picture]. Retrieved from http://www.museum. tv.archives/etc/C/htmlC/chinabeach/chinabeach.htm

Schumaker, K. L., & Meleis, A. I. (1994). Transitions: A central concept in nursing. *IMAGE: Journal of Nursing Scholarship, 26*(2), 119–127.

Shenon, P. (2004). Officer suggests Iraq jail abuse was encouraged [electronic version]. *New York Times*. Retrieved from http://www.nytimes.com/2004/05/02/international/middleeast/02ABUS.html?scp=1&sq=may%202004%20iraq%20prisoner&st=cse

Siefert, P. (2009). The ANA Code of Ethics and AORN. *Perioperative Nursing Clinics, 3*(3), 183–189, Retrieved from http://visiblenurse.com/nurseculture7.html

Snowball, J. (1996). Asking nurses about advocating for patients: 'reactive' and 'proactive' accounts. *Journal of Advanced Nursing, 24*(1), 67–75.

Stanley, D. (2006). Role conflict: Leaders and managers. *Nursing Management, 13*(5), 31–37.

Stanley, D. J. (2008). Celluloid angels: A research study of nurses in feature films 1900-2007. *Journal of Advanced Nursing, 64*(1), 84–95.

Takase, M., Maude, P., & Manias, E. (2006). The impact of role discrepancy on nurses' intention to quit their jobs. *Journal of Clinical Nursing, 15*, 1071–1080.

Tenenbaum, N. (Producer), & Roach, J. (Director). (2000). *Meet the Parents*. [Motion picture]. United States: Universal Pictures & Dreamworks Productions.

Triolo, N. (2007). Authentic leadership begins with emotional intelligence. *AACN Advanced Critical Care, 18*(3), 244–247.

Tuxhill, C. (1994). In B. Miller, & P. Burnard (Eds.). *Critical care nursing*. London: Balliere-Tindall.

Ulrich, B. T., Buerhaus, P. I., Donelan, K., Norman, L., & Dittus, R. (2005). How RNs view the work environment. *Journal of Nursing Administration, 35*(9), 20–38.

University of Pennsylvania Health System: Nursing Annual Report 2005. Retrieved September 15, 2009, from http://pennhealth.com/nursing/annual_report_2005.pdf

Wells, J. (Producer). (1988). *China Beach* [Television series]. United States: ABC Studios

Winfield, C., Melo, K., & Myrick, F. (2009). *Journal for Nurses in Staff Development, 25*(2), E7–E13, doi: 10.1097/NND.ob013e31819c76a3.

Yarbrough, S., Alfred, D., & Martin, P. (2008). Research study: Professional values and retention. *Nursing Management, 39*(4), 10–18.

Young, C. M., Albert, N. M., Paschke, S. M., & Meyer, K. H. (2007). The 'parent shift' program: Incentives for nurses, rewards for nursing teams. *Nurse Economics, 25*(6), 339–344.

Young, M. E., Stuenkel, D. L., & Bawel-Brinkley, K. (2008). Strategies for easing the role transformation of graduate nurses. *Journal for Nurses in Staff Development, 24*(3), 105–110.

Zaentz, S. (Producer), & Minghella, A. (Director). (1996). *The English Patient*. [Motion picture]. United States: Mirimax Films.

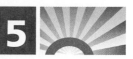

5

Theories and Frameworks for Professional Nursing Practice

MARY GUNTHER, PhD, RN, CNE

OBJECTIVES

At the completion of this chapter, the reader will be able to:

● Distinguish among a concept, a theory, a conceptual framework, and a model.
● Identify and define the four central concepts of nursing theories.
● Compare the main precepts of selected theories of nursing.
● Examine criteria for evaluating the utility of a specific nursing theory for its relevance to practice, education, or research.
● Identify selected theories from related disciplines that have application to nursing.

PROFILE IN PRACTICE

Jacqueline Fawcett, PhD, RN, FAAN
College of Nursing, University of Massachusetts—Boston, Boston, Massachusetts

I earned my baccalaureate degree in nursing from Boston University in 1964 and worked as an operating room staff nurse during that summer. My first exposure to a nursing discipline–specific theory occurred during my nursing coursework at Boston University. I learned Orlando's theory of the deliberative nursing process and have continued to find this simple yet elegant nursing theory of great utility in assisting patients, colleagues, and students to express their immediate needs for help.

I began teaching in a small hospital-based diploma nursing program in Connecticut in January 1965. I have continued to teach nursing since that time, first at the University of Connecticut for 6 years, with interruptions for my master's degree in parent-child nursing and my doctorate in nursing, then at the University of Pennsylvania for 21 years, and now at the University of Massachusetts in Boston.

During my master's program at New York University, I was introduced to theory-guided nursing practice. The clinical courses in parent-child nursing emphasized the application of theory to the nursing of childbearing women and their families, well children, and children with acute and chronic illnesses. At that time, knowledge about nursing discipline–specific conceptual models and theories was limited. The New York

University nursing faculty, my classmates, and I worked hard to adapt crisis theory to nursing situations and to explore the applicability of developmental theories and family theories to nursing situations. I immediately recognized the benefit of using theories to guide nursing practice—I had finally found a way to organize my thinking and my practice. Indeed, I finally knew what to say and do and the reasons for what I was saying and doing when I interacted with a patient!

When I returned to the University of Connecticut after earning my master's degree in 1970, my faculty colleagues and I began to design and implement a new curriculum based on crisis theory. We extended the original theory to encompass physiological as well as psychological events (White, 1983; Infante, 1982).

I returned to New York University 2 years later and entered the brave new world of Martha Rogers' conceptual system, now called the science of unitary human beings, which was my first exposure to a comprehensive nursing discipline–specific conceptual model. Given my strong interest in theory-guided nursing practice, I was very attracted to Rogers' work. I rapidly immersed myself in the coursework that led to my dissertation research, which was based on my extension of Rogers' conceptual system to the family (Fawcett, 1975, 1977). My coursework sensitized me to the need to use nursing discipline–specific conceptual models and theories to guide not only nursing practice but also nursing research. Furthermore, the coursework sensitized me to the reciprocal relationship between research and conceptual models and between practice and conceptual models. I realized that conceptual models inform research and practice and that research findings and the results observed in practice in turn inform revisions in the conceptual model.

I returned to the University of Connecticut in 1975 and completed all requirements for the doctoral degree in 1976. I began to teach nursing research courses and had the opportunity to develop courses in contemporary nursing knowledge and the relationship of theory and research. The latter two courses became the focus of my scholarly work and the underlying reason for my passion about nursing.

I was recruited by the University of Pennsylvania in 1978 and had the honor of teaching the subject matter of my scholarly work in a new nursing doctoral program. Throughout all the years at University of Pennsylvania and now at the University of Massachusetts in Boston, my teaching has informed my scholarly work and my scholarly work has informed my teaching. My books about analysis of nursing models and theories (Fawcett, 1989, 1993, 2000, 2005) and the relationship of theory and research (Fawcett, 1999) are the direct result of my students' requests for more information and more examples about the use of nursing discipline–specific conceptual models and theories.

Since 1979, I have used Roy's adaptation model to guide my empirical research, which has focused on women's responses to cesarean birth and on functional status in normal life transitions and serious illness. I have found Roy's model to be a very useful guide for my research and for the nursing practice that stems from the findings of the research.

Much of my current work focuses on helping nurses understand the connection between research and practice (Fawcett, 2000). I am firmly convinced that all nurse clinicians are also nurse researchers because the nursing practice process (assessment, labeling, goal setting, implementation, evaluation) is similar to the nursing research process (collection of baseline data, statement of the problem and hypotheses, experimental and control treatments, data analysis). I also am firmly convinced that the parallels between the nursing practice process and the nursing research process are most readily understood when both nursing practice and nursing research are guided by a nursing discipline–specific conceptual model or theory. The challenge is to assist nurses in practice to recognize that clinical information is research data and to report the effects of nursing practice in ways that will help other nurses and other health professionals and policymakers understand how nursing practice benefits the health of humankind.

Theory is the poetry of science. The poet's words are familiar, each standing alone, but brought together they sing, they astonish, they teach. (Levine, 1995, p. 14)

Introduction

Nursing is both a science and an art. The empirical science of nursing includes both the natural sciences (e.g., biology, chemistry) and the human sciences (e.g., sociology, psychology). The art of nursing is the ability to form trusting relationships, perform procedures skillfully, prescribe appropriate treatments, and morally conduct nursing practice (Johnson, 1994). Nursing is a knowledge-based discipline significantly different from medicine. Medicine focuses on the identification and treatment of disease, whereas nursing focuses on the wholeness of human beings (Fawcett, 1993). Nursing claims the health of human beings in interaction with the environment as its domain. *Knowledge* is commonly defined as a general awareness or possession of information, facts, ideas, truths, or principles and an understanding of the same gained through experience or study (Encarta World English Dictionary, 2009). Nursing knowledge is the organization of the discipline-specific concepts, theories, and ideas published in the literature (both print and electronic media) and demonstrated in professional practice. Nursing's desire to be regarded as a profession (e.g., law, medicine) was the impetus for building a substantial body of discipline-specific knowledge. Many of the existing theories emerged from the response to the simple question, "What is nursing?"

Theories and conceptual frameworks consist of the theorist's words brought together to form a meaningful whole. Theories and frameworks provide direction and guidance for structuring professional nursing practice, education, and research. They act as a "tool for reasoning, critical thinking, and decision-making" (Alligood, 2005, p. 272). In practice, theories and frameworks help nurses describe, explain, and predict everyday experiences. They also assist in organizing assessment data, making diagnoses, choosing interventions, and evaluating nursing care. In education, a conceptual framework provides the general focus for curriculum design. In research, the framework offers a systematic approach to identifying questions for study, selecting appropriate variables, and interpreting findings. The research findings may trigger revision and refinement of the theory. Figure 5-1 illustrates the relationships among theory, practice, education, and research.

Many nurse theorists have made substantial contributions to the development of a body of nursing knowledge. Offering an assortment of perspectives, the theories vary in their level of abstraction and their conceptualization of the client, health and illness, the environment, and nursing. From a historical perspective, nursing theories reflect the influence of the larger society and illustrate increased sophistication in the development of nursing ideas. Table 5-1 presents a chronology of events related to the development of nursing theories. While this chapter provides a comprehensive overview of nursing theory, other chapters in this text will make reference to specific nursing theories as they relate to individual chapter topics.

Terminology Associated with Nursing Theory

The most fundamental building block of a theory is a concept, which is defined as "a word or phrase that summarizes ideas, observations, and experiences" (Fawcett, 2005, p. 4). For a theory to exist, concepts must be related to one another. Theoretical statements, also called *propositions,* describe a concept or the relationship between two or more concepts (Fawcett, 2005). One theoretical statement, or several theoretical statements taken together, can constitute a theory. A theory, then, is a statement or a group of statements that describe, explain, or predict relationships among concepts.

A nursing theory is composed of a set of concepts and propositions that claims to account for or characterize the central phenomena of interest to the discipline of nursing: person, environment, health/illness, and nursing. Persons are the recipients of nursing care and include individuals, families, and communities. *Environment* refers to the surroundings of the client, internal factors affecting the client, and the setting where nursing care is delivered. *Health and illness* describe the client's state of well-being. *Nursing* refers

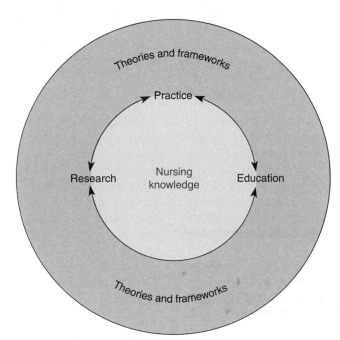

FIGURE 5-1 Relationships among theories and frameworks and nursing education, research, and practice.

TABLE 5-1	History of Nursing Theory Development	
Event	**Year**	**Nurse Theorists**
	1860	Florence Nightingale Described nursing and environment
	1952	Hildegard E. Peplau Nursing as an interpersonal process: patients with felt needs
Scientific era: nurses questioned purpose of nursing	1960	Faye Abdellah (also 1965, 1973) Patient-centered approaches
	1961	Ida Jean Orlando Nurse-patient relationship; deliberative nursing approach
Process of theory development discussed among professional nurses	1964	Ernestine Weidenbach (also 1970, 1977) Nursing: philosophy, purpose, practice, and art
	1966	Lydia E. Hall Core (patient), care (body), cure (disease)
	1966	Virginia Henderson (also 1971, 1978) Nursing assists patients with 14 essential functions toward independence
Symposium: theory development in nursing	1967	Myra Estrin Levine (also 1973) Four conservation principles of nursing

TABLE 5-1	History of Nursing Theory Development—cont'd		
Event	**Year**	**Nurse Theorists**	
Symposium: nature of science and nursing Dickoff, James, and Weidenbach published "Theory in a Practice Discipline" in *Nursing Research*	1968		
Symposium: nature of science in nursing First nursing theory conference	1969		
Second nursing theory conference	1970	Martha E. Rogers (also 1980) Science of unitary man: energy fields, openness, pattern, and organization	
Consensus on nursing concepts: nurse/ nursing, health, client/patient/individual, society/environment	1971	Dorothea E. Orem (also 1980, 1985) Nursing facilitates patients' self-care	
Discussion on what theory is: the elements, criteria, types, and levels and the relationship to research	1971	Imogene King (also 1975, 1981) Theory of goal attainment through nurse-client transactions	
National League for Nursing required conceptual frameworks in nursing education	1973		
Borrowed theories from other disciplines Expanded theories from other disciplines	1974	Sister Callista Roy (also 1976, 1980, 1984, 1989, 1999) Roy's adaptation model: nurse adjusts patient's stimuli (focal, contextual, or residual) Betty Neuman Health care systems model: a total person approach	
Recognized problems in practice and developed theories to test and use in practice	1976	Josephine Paterson and L. Zderad Humanistic nursing	
Second nurse educator conference on nursing theory	1978	Madeleine Leininger (also 1980, 1981) Transcultural nursing Caring nursing	
Articles on theory development in *ANS, Nursing Research,* and *Image*	1978 1979	Jean Watson (also 1985) Philosophy and science of caring; humanistic nursing	
Books written for nurses on how to critique and develop theory and describing application of nursing theories Graduate schools of nursing develop courses on how to analyze and apply nursing theories	1980	Dorothy E. Johnson Behavioral system model for nursing	
Research studies in nursing identified nursing theories as framework for study	1981	Rosemarie Rizzo Parse (also 1987) Man-living-health: a theory of nursing	
Numerous books published on analysis, application, evaluation, development, and expansion of nursing theories	1982–present		

Modified from Christensen, P. J., & Kenney, J. W. (1995). *Nursing process: Application of conceptual models.* (4th ed.). St. Louis: Mosby.

to the actions taken when providing care to a patient. These concepts, taken together, make up what is known as the *metaparadigm of nursing* (Fawcett, 1997). Most nursing theories define or describe these central concepts, either explicitly or implicitly. Because a concept is an abstract representation of the real world, concepts embedded in a theory represent the theorist's perspective of reality and may differ from that of the reader without invalidating the theory.

Theories represent abstract ideas rather than concrete facts (Alligood, 2005) and may be broad or limited in scope, thus varying in their ability to describe, explain, or predict. Theories may be categorized by their level of abstraction as grand theories, midrange theories, or practice theories. Grand theories (also known as *conceptual models* or *frameworks*) are representations of the broad nature, purpose, and goals of the discipline. Concepts and their relationships are very abstract, not operationally defined, and not empirically testable. Midrange theories, which may be derived from grand theories, are less abstract with relatively concrete concepts that address specific phenomena across nursing settings and specialties. Relationships between and among concepts can be defined explicitly and measured. Because they are narrower in scope, midrange theories appear more applicable to practice and remain abstract enough to allow a wide range of empirical research. Practice theories (sometimes called *situation-specific theories*) are limited further to a patient population or type of nursing practice (Im & Meleis, 1999; Meleis, 2005). Most practice theories are either descriptive (portraying an experience) or prescriptive (advocating specific nursing actions) in nature.

Descriptions of the theoretical perspectives presented in this chapter include a brief overview; the theory's basic assumptions about the individual and the environment; definitions of health and illness; a description of nursing, including the goal of nursing; and definitions of concepts and subconcepts specific to each theory. Some theories are more amenable to this scheme than others because of their degree of specificity or stage of development. When the needed information is not explicitly detailed by the theorist, inferences are made on the basis of what seems to be implicitly stated. Direct quotes from the theorists are used whenever possible to ensure that such interpretations are valid and reliable. The reader is encouraged to consult the primary source to gain a full appreciation of the depth, scope, and extent of the relationships put forth.

Overview of Selected Nursing Theories

Theories and frameworks selected for inclusion in this chapter are those that exemplify the different definitions of nursing along varying levels of abstraction.

> Exploring a variety of nursing theories ought to provide nurses with new insights into patient care, opening nursing options otherwise hidden, and stimulating innovative interventions. But it is imperative that there be variety—for there is no global theory of nursing that fits every situation. (Levine, 1995, p. 13)

Grand Theory

NIGHTINGALE'S ENVIRONMENTAL THEORY

Florence Nightingale conceptualized disease as a reparative process and described the nurse's role as manipulating the environment to facilitate and encourage this process. Her directions regarding ventilation, warmth, light, diet, cleanliness, variety, and noise are discussed in her classic nursing textbook *Notes on Nursing*, first published in 1859.

Brief Overview. The environment is critical to health, and the nurse's role in caring for the sick is to provide a clean, quiet, peaceful environment to promote healing. Nightingale's intent was to describe nursing and provide guidelines for nursing education.

Assumptions About the Individual. Individuals are responsible, creative, and in control of their lives and health.

Environment. The environment is external to the person but affects the health of both sick and well persons. As a chief source of infection, the environment must include pure air, pure water, efficient drainage, cleanliness, and light.

Health and Illness. *Health* is described as a state of being well and using one's powers to the fullest. Illness or disease is the reaction of nature against the conditions in which human beings have placed themselves. Disease is a reparative mechanism, an effort of nature to remedy a process of poisoning or of decay.

Nursing. Nursing is a service to humanity intended to relieve pain and suffering. Nursing's role is to promote or provide the proper environment for patients, including fresh air, light, pure water, cleanliness, warmth, quiet, and appropriate diet. The goal of nursing is to promote the reparative process by manipulating the environment.

Key Concepts. *Environment* refers to conditions external to the individual that affect life and development (e.g., ventilation, warmth, light, diet, cleanliness, noise). Nightingale (1860, 1946) identified three major relationships: the environment to the patient, the nurse to the environment, and the nurse to the patient. Examples of these follow:

- The need for light, particularly sunlight, is second only to the need for ventilation. If necessary, the nurse should move the patient "about after the sun according to the aspects of the rooms, if circumstances permit, |rather| than let him linger in a room when the sun is off" (Nightingale, 1946, p. 48).
- Nursing's role is to manipulate the environment to encourage healing. Nursing "ought to signify the proper use of fresh air, light, warmth, cleanliness, quiet, and the proper selection and administration of diet" (Nightingale, 1946, p. 6).
- The sine qua non of all good nursing is never to allow a patient to be awakened, intentionally or accidentally: "A good nurse will always make sure that no blind or curtains should flap. If you wait till your patient tells you or reminds you of these things, where is the use of their having a nurse?" (Nightingale, 1946, p. 27).
- Variety is important for patients to divert them from dwelling on their pain: "Variety of form and brilliancy of color in the objects presented are actual means of recovery" (Nightingale, 1946, p. 34).

ROGERS' SCIENCE OF UNITARY HUMAN BEINGS

First presented in *An Introduction to the Theoretical Basis for Nursing* in 1970, Martha Rogers' conceptualizations, dating back to the 1960s, evolved into the current science of unitary human beings. She posited that human beings are dynamic energy fields who are integral with the environment and who are continuously evolving. She viewed nursing as a science and an art that focus on the nature and direction of human development and human betterment.

Brief Overview. The individual is viewed as an irreducible energy field, integral with the environment. The nurse seeks to promote symphonic interactions between human beings and their environments (Rogers, 1970).

Assumptions About the Individual. The individual is a unified, irreducible whole, manifesting characteristics that are more than, and different from, the sum of his or her parts and continuously evolving, irreversibly and unidirectionally along a space–time continuum. Pattern and organization of human beings are directed toward increasing complexity rather than maintaining equilibrium. The individual "is characterized by the capacity for abstraction and imagery, language and thought, sensation and emotion" (Rogers, 1970, p. 73).

Environment. The environment is an irreducible, pandimensional energy field identified by pattern and integral with the human energy field (Rogers, 1994). The individual and the environment are continually exchanging matter and energy with one another, resulting in changing patterns in both the individual and the environment.

Health and Illness. Health and illness are value-laden, arbitrarily defined, and culturally infused notions. They are not dichotomous but are part of the same continuum. Health seems to occur when patterns of living are in harmony with environmental change, whereas illness occurs when patterns of living are in conflict with environmental change and are deemed unacceptable (Rogers, 1994).

Nursing. As both a science and an art, nursing is unique in its concern with unitary human beings as synergistic phenomena. The science of nursing should be concerned with studying the nature and direction of unitary human development integral with the environment and with evolving descriptive, explanatory, and predictive principles for use in nursing practice. The new age of nursing science is characterized by a synthesis of fact and ideas that generate principles and theories (Rogers, 1994). The art of nursing is the creative use of the science of nursing for human betterment (Rogers, 1990). The goal of nursing is the attainment of the best possible state of health for the individual who is continually evolving by promoting symphonic interactions between human beings and environments, strengthening the coherence and integrity of the human field, and directing and redirecting patterning of both fields for maximal health potential.

Key Concepts. The concepts describe the individual and environment as energy fields that are in constant interaction. The nature and direction of human development form the basis for the following principles of nursing science:

- *Energy field.* The fundamental unit of the living and nonliving. Energy fields are dynamic, continuously in motion, and infinite. They are of two types:
  - Human energy field: More than the biological, psychological, and sociological fields taken separately or together; an irreducible, indivisible, pandimensional whole identified by pattern and manifesting characteristics that cannot be predicted from the parts.
  - Environmental energy field: An irreducible, indivisible, pandimensional energy field identified by pattern and integral with the human field.
- *Openness.* Continuous change and mutual process as manifested in human and environmental fields.
- *Pattern.* The distinguishing characteristic of an energy field perceived as a single wave.
- *Principles of nursing science.* Principles postulating the nature and direction of unitary human development; these principles are also called *principles of homeodynamics:*

- Helicy: According to Rogers, helicy is "the continuous, innovative, probabilistic, increasing diversity of human and environmental field patterns characterized by repeating rhymicities" (1989, p. 186). Change occurs continuously.
- Resonancy: Rogers describes resonancy as "the continuous change from lower to higher frequency wave patterns in human and environmental fields" (1989, p. 186). Change is increasingly diverse.
- Integrality: Replacing the earlier concept of complementarity, integrality is "the continuous mutual human and environmental field process" (Rogers, 1989, p. 186). Field changes occur simultaneously.

OREM'S SELF-CARE DEFICIT THEORY

The foundations of Dorothea Orem's theory were introduced in the late 1950s, but the first edition of her work *Nursing: Concepts of Practice* was not published until 1971. Five subsequent editions (1980, 1985, 1991, 1995, 2001) show evidence of continued development and refinement of the theory. Orem focuses on nursing as deliberate human action and notes that all individuals can benefit from nursing when they have health-derived or health-related limitations for engaging in self-care or the care of dependent others. Three theories are subsumed in the self-care deficit theory of nursing: the theory of nursing systems, the theory of self-care deficits, and the theory of self-care (Orem, 2001).

Brief Overview. The individual practices self-care, a set of learned behaviors, to sustain life, maintain or restore functioning, and bring about a condition of well-being. The nurse assists the client with self-care when he or she experiences a deficit in the ability to perform.

Assumptions About the Individual. The individual is viewed as a unit whose functioning is linked with the environment and who, with the environment, forms an integrated, functional whole. The individual functions biologically, symbolically, and socially.

Environment. The environment is linked to the individual, forming an integrated system. The environment is implied to be external to the individual.

Health and Illness. Health, which has physical, psychological, interpersonal, and social aspects, is a state in which human beings are structurally and functionally whole or sound (Orem, 1995). Illness occurs when an individual is incapable of maintaining self-care as a result of structural or functional limitations.

Nursing. Nursing involves assisting the individual with self-care practices to sustain life and health, recover from disease or injury, and cope with their effects (Orem, 1985). The nurse chooses deliberate actions from nursing systems (see below) designed to bring about desirable conditions in persons and their environments. The goal of nursing is to move a patient toward responsible self-care or meet existing health care needs of those who have health care deficits.

Key Concepts. The concepts focus on self-care in terms of requisites, demands, and deficits and delineate the nurse's role in client care in the following manner:

- *Self-care.* This refers to "activities that individuals initiate and perform on their own behalf to maintain life, health, or well-being" (Orem, 1995, p. 104).
- *Self-care requisites.* Actions that are known or hypothesized to be necessary to regulate human functioning. Three types exist:
  - Universal: Common to all human beings; concerned with the promotion and maintenance of structural and functional integrity. These include air, water, food, elimination, activity and rest, solitude and social interaction, prevention of hazards, and promotion of human functioning.
  - Developmental: Associated with conditions that promote known developmental processes; occurring at various stages of the life cycle.
  - Health deviation: Genetic and constitutional defects and deviations that affect integrated human functioning and impair the individual's ability to perform self-care.

- *Therapeutic self-care demand.* Based on the notion that self-care is a human regulatory function; the totality of self-care actions performed by the nurse or self to meet known self-care requisites.
- *Self-care agency.* Acquired ability to know and meet requirements to regulate own functioning and development.
- *Self-care deficits.* Gaps between known therapeutic self-care demands and the capability of the individual to perform self-care.
- *Nursing systems.* Systems of concrete actions for persons with limitations in self-care. These actions are of three types (Orem, 1995):
  - Wholly compensatory: The nurse compensates for the individual's total inability to perform self-care activities.
  - Partly compensatory: The nurse compensates for the individual's inability to perform some (but not all) self-care activities.
  - Supportive-educative: With the individual able to perform all self-care activities, the nurse assists the client in decision making, behavior control, and the acquisition of knowledge and skill.
- *Subsystems of each nursing system:*
  - Social: The complementary and contractual relationship between the nurse and the client.
  - Interpersonal: The nurse-client interaction.
  - Technological: According to Orem, the "diagnosis, prescription, regulation of treatment, and management of nursing care" (1985, p. 160).

ROY'S ADAPTATION MODEL

Sister Callista Roy has continuously expanded her model from its inception in the 1960s to the present, building on the conceptual framework of adaptation. She focuses on the individual as a biopsychosocial adaptive system and describes nursing as a humanistic discipline that "places emphasis on the person's own coping abilities" (Roy, 1984, p. 32). The individual and the environment are sources of stimuli that require modification to promote adaptation.

Brief Overview. The individual is a biopsychosocial adaptive system, and the nurse promotes adaptation by modifying external stimuli.

Assumptions About the Individual. The individual is in constant interaction with a changing environment, and to respond positively to environmental change, a person must adapt. The person's adaptation level is determined by the combined effect of three classes of stimuli: focal, contextual, and residual. The individual uses both innate and acquired biological, psychological, or social adaptive mechanisms and has four modes of adaptation.

Environment. All conditions, circumstances, and influences surrounding and affecting the development and behavior of persons and groups constitute the environment. Having both internal and external components, the environment is constantly changing.

Health and Illness. According to Roy (1989), "health and illness are one inevitable dimension of a person's life" (p. 106). Health is "a state and process of being and becoming integrated and whole" (Roy & Andrews, 1999, p. 31). Conversely, illness is a lack of integration.

Nursing. As an external regulatory force, nursing acts to modify stimuli affecting adaptation by increasing, decreasing, or maintaining stimuli. The goal of nursing is to promote the person's adaptation in the four adaptive modes, thus contributing to health, the quality of life, and dying with dignity (Roy, 2009).

Key Concepts. The following concepts describe and define adaptation in terms of the individual's internal control processes, adaptive modes, and adaptive level:

- *Adaptation.* The individual's ability to cope with the constantly changing environment.
- *Adaptive system.* Consists of two major internal control processes (coping mechanisms):
  - Regulator subsystem: Receives input from the external environment and from changes in the person's internal state and processes it through neural-chemical-endocrine channels.
  - Cognator subsystem: Receives input from external and internal stimuli that involve psychological, social, physical, and physiological factors and processes it through cognitive pathways.

- *Adaptive modes.* The four ways a person adapts:
  - Physiological: Determined by the need for physiological integrity derived from the basic physiological needs.
  - Self-concept: Determined by the need for interactions with others and psychic integrity regarding the perception of self.
  - Role function: Determined by the need for social integrity; refers to the performance of duties based on given positions within society.
  - Interdependence: Involves ways of seeking help, affection, and attention.
- *Adaptive level.* Determined by the combined effects of stimuli:
  - Focal stimulus: That which immediately confronts the individual.
  - Contextual stimuli: All other stimuli present in the environment. These stimuli influence how the individual deals with the focal stimulus.
  - Residual stimuli: Beliefs, attitudes, or traits that have an indeterminate effect on the present situation.

NEUMAN'S SYSTEMS MODEL

Betty Neuman developed her systems model in 1970 in response to student requests to focus on breadth rather than depth in understanding human variables in nursing problems. First published in 1972 (Neuman & Young, 1972), the model was refined to its present form in *The Neuman Systems Model* (Neuman, 1995; Neuman & Fawcett, 2002). The Neuman systems model "is an open systems model that views nursing as being primarily concerned with defining appropriate actions in stress-related situations" (Neuman, 1995, p. 11). Neuman believes that nursing encompasses a wholistic client systems approach to help individuals, families, communities, and society reach and maintain wellness. Neuman's focus on the *whole* system explains her use of the term *wholistic*.

Brief Overview. This theory offers a wholistic view of the client system, including the concepts of open system, environment, stressors, prevention, and reconstitution. Nursing is concerned with the whole person.

Assumptions About the Individual. In this model, the client is a whole person, a dynamic composite of interrelationships among physiological, psychological, sociocultural, developmental, and spiritual variables: "The client is viewed as an open system in interaction with the environment" (Neuman, 1989, p. 68). The client is in "dynamic constant energy exchange with the environment" (Neuman, 1989, p. 22).

Environment. Both internal and external environments exist, and the person maintains varying degrees of harmony between them. The environment includes all internal and external factors affecting and being affected by the system (Neuman, 1995). Emphasis is on all stressors—interpersonal, intrapersonal, extrapersonal—that might disturb the person's normal line of defense.

Health and Illness. Neuman (1995) asserts that "health and wellness is defined as the condition or degree of system stability" (p. 12). Disharmony among parts of the system is considered illness: "The wellness-illness continuum implies that energy flow is continuous between the client system and the environment" (Neuman, 1989, p. 33).

Nursing. Nursing is a "unique profession in that it is concerned with all of the variables affecting the individual's response to stress" (Neuman, 1982, p. 14). The major concern of nursing is in "keeping the client system stable through accuracy in both the assessment of effects and possible effects of environmental stressors and in assisting client adjustments required for an optimal wellness level" (Neuman, 1989, p. 34). Nursing goals are determined by "negotiation with the client for desired prescriptive changes to correct variances from wellness" (Neuman, 1989, p. 73). This means that nursing interventions designed to improve health are accepted and approved by the individual client during communication with the nurse before implementation.

Key Concepts. The nurse is concerned with all the following variables affecting an individual's response to stressors:

- *Stressors.* Tension-producing stimuli that may alter system stability (Neuman, 1995):
  - Intrapersonal: Internal stressors (e.g., autoimmune response).

  - Interpersonal: External environmental forces in close proximity (e.g., communication patterns).
  - Extrapersonal: External environmental forces at distant range (e.g., financial concerns).
- *Concepts related to client system stability:*
  - Flexible line of defense: Outer boundary that ideally prevents stressors from entering the system.
  - Normal line of defense: A range of responses to environmental stressors when the flexible line of defense is penetrated; usual state of wellness (Neuman, 1995).
  - Lines of resistance: Protect the basic structure of the client and become activated when the normal line of defense is invaded by environmental stressors.
- *Interventions.* Purposeful nursing actions that help clients retain, attain, and/or maintain system stability. Three levels of intervention exist:
  - Primary prevention: Reduces the possibility of encounter with stressors and strengthens the flexible lines of defense.
  - Secondary prevention: Relates to appropriate prioritizing of interventions to reduce symptoms resulting from invasion of environmental stressors; protects the basic structure by strengthening the internal lines of resistance.
    - Tertiary prevention: Focuses on re-adaptation and stability. A primary goal is to strengthen resistance to stressors by reeducation to help prevent recurrence of reaction or regression: "Tertiary prevention tends to lead back, in a circular fashion, toward primary prevention" (Neuman, 1989, p. 73).

WATSON'S PHILOSOPHY AND SCIENCE OF CARING

Jean Watson's theoretical formulations focus on the philosophy and science of caring as the core of nursing. With the aim of reducing the dichotomy between nursing theory and practice, Watson's original theory draws from multiple disciplines to derive carative factors that are central to nursing and describes concepts as they relate to the pivotal theme of caring: "Caring is acknowledged as the highest form of commitment to self, to others, to society, to environment, and, at this point in human history, even to the universe" (Watson, 1996, p. 146). Watson (2007) states: "I consider my work more a philosophical, ethical, intellectual blue-print for nursing's evolving disciplinary/professional matrix, rather than a specific theory per se" (para 8).

Brief Overview. Caring, which Watson sees as a moral ideal rather than a task-oriented behavior, is central to nursing practice and includes aspects of the actual caring occasion and the transpersonal caring relationship. An interpersonal process, caring results in the satisfaction of human needs.

Assumptions About the Individual. Individuals (i.e., both the nurse and the client) are nonreducible and are interconnected with others and nature (Watson, 1985).

Environment. The client's environment contains both external and internal variables. The nurse promotes a caring environment, one that allows individuals to make choices relative to the best action for themselves at that point in time.

Health and Illness. Health is more than the absence of illness, but because it is subjective, it is an illusive concept: "Health refers to unity and harmony within the mind, body, and soul" (Watson, 1985, p. 48). Conversely, illness is disharmony within the spheres of the person.

Nursing. The practice of nursing is different from curing. It is a transpersonal relationship that includes but is not limited to the 10 carative factors described below. The goal of nursing is to help persons attain a higher degree of harmony by offering a relationship that the client can use for personal growth and development.

Key Concepts. The caring relationship forms the core of nursing, and the caritas processes (evolved from the original carative facotrs) delineate the domain of nursing practice:

- *Transpersonal caring.* An intersubjective human-to-human relationship in which the nurse affects and is affected by the other person (client). Caring is the moral ideal of nursing in which the utmost concern for human dignity and preservation of humanity is present (Watson, 1985).

- *Caritas processes* (Watson, 2007):
  - Practice of loving-kindness and equanimity within context of caring consciousness.
  - Being authentically present, and enabling and sustaining the deep belief system and subjective life world of self and the one-being-cared-for.
  - Cultivation of one's own spiritual practices and transpersonal self, going beyond ego self.
  - Developing and sustaining a helping-trusting, authentic caring relationship.
  - Being present to, and supportive of the expression of positive and negative feelings as a connection with deeper spirit of self and the one-being-cared-for.
  - Creative use of self and all ways of knowing as part of the caring process; to engage in artistry of caring-healing practices.
  - Engaging in genuine teaching-learning experience that attends to unity of being and meaning attempting to stay within other's frame of reference.
  - Creating a healing environment at all levels, physical as well as nonphysical, subtle environment of energy and consciousness, whereby wholeness, beauty, comfort, dignity, and peace are potentiated.
  - Assisting with basic needs, with an intentional caring consciousness, administering "human care essentials", which potentiate alignment of mind-body-spirit, wholeness, and unity of being in all aspects of care; tending to both embodied spirit and evolving spiritual emergence.
  - Opening and attending to spiritual-mysterious, and existential dimensions of one's own life-death; soul care for self and the one-being-cared-for.

Midrange Theory

PEPLAU'S INTERPERSONAL PROCESS

Hildegard Peplau published *Interpersonal Relations in Nursing* in 1952. The book described the phases of the interpersonal process in nursing, roles for nurses, and methods for studying nursing as an interpersonal process. Over the years the theory evolved, and in 1991 she published *Interpersonal Relations in Nursing: A Conceptual Framework of Reference for Psychodynamic Nursing.*

Brief Overview. The focus of Peplau's model is the goal-directed interpersonal process: "Psychodynamic nursing is being able to understand one's own behavior to help others identify felt difficulties and to apply principles of human relations to the problems that arise at all levels of experience" (Peplau, 1952, p. xiii). The interpersonal relationship "has a starting point, proceeds through definable phases, and, being time-limited, has an end point" (Peplau, 1992, p. 4). Peplau believed that once the problem that prompts the client to ask for nursing help has been resolved, the relationship ends.

Assumptions About the Individual. The individual is an organism that lives in an unstable equilibrium and "strives in its own way to reduce tension generated by needs" (Peplau, 1952, p. 82).

Environment. Although the environment is not explicitly defined, it can be inferred that the environment consists of "existing forces outside the organism and in the context of culture" (Peplau, 1952, p. 163).

Health and Illness. Health is a "word symbol that implies forward movement of personality and other ongoing human processes in the direction of creative, constructive, productive, personal, and community living" (Peplau, 1952, p. 12). By implication, illness is a condition that is marked by no movement or by backward movement in these human processes.

Nursing. Nursing is a therapeutic interpersonal process because it involves the interaction between two or more individuals who have a common goal. For individuals who are sick and in need of health care, it is a healing art. Six nursing roles emerge in the various phases of the nurse-patient relationship: stranger, resource person, teacher, leader, surrogate, and counselor.

Key Concepts. The nurse-patient relationship consists of four phases:

- *Orientation.* The patient seeks professional assistance with a problem. The nurse and patient meet as strangers and recognize, clarify, and define the existing problem.

- *Identification.* The patient learns how to make use of the nurse-patient relationship and responds selectively to people who can meet his or her needs; the patient and nurse clarify each other's expectations.

- *Exploitation.* The patient takes advantage of all available services. The nurse helps the patient in maintaining a balance between dependence and independence and using the services to help solve the current problem and work toward optimal health.

- *Resolution.* The patient is free to move on with his or her life as old goals are put aside and new goals are adopted. The patient becomes independent of the nurse, and the relationship is terminated.

KING'S THEORY OF GOAL ATTAINMENT

Although the foundation for Imogene King's theory was developed in 1964, she did not present her entire conceptual framework until the 1971 publication of her book *Toward a Theory for Nursing*. In it she identified the concepts of social systems, health, perception, and interpersonal relations. The midrange theory of goal attainment was refined in *A Theory for Nursing: Systems, Concepts, Process* (1981), in which King asserted that nursing is focused on people interacting with their environments. The goal of this interaction is a state of health, which King defines as the ability of people to function in their roles. The theory is derived from a systems framework and is concerned with human transactions in different types of environments (King, 1995a).

Brief Overview. The individual is viewed as an open system and as one component of a nurse-client interpersonal system whose interactions lead to the attainment of mutually agreed-upon goals.

Assumptions About the Individual. Human beings are open systems in transaction with the environment and are conceptualized as social, sentient, rational, perceiving, controlling, purposeful, action-oriented beings.

Environment. The theory implies that the open systems of the individual and the environment interact and that both the internal and external environments generate stressors.

Health and Illness. Health is described as an individual's ability to function in social roles. This implies optimal use of a person's resources to achieve continuous adjustment to internal and external environmental stressors. Illness is a deviation from normal, an imbalance in a person's biological structure, psychological makeup, or social relationships.

Nursing. In an interpersonal process of action, reaction, and interaction, the nurse and client communicate, set goals, and explore means to achieve those goals. According to King (1981), "the domain of nursing includes promoting, maintaining and restoring health, caring for the sick and injured and caring for the dying" (p. 4). Nursing's central goal is to help individuals maintain their health so that they can function in their roles. As King asserted, "The goal of the nursing system, as a whole, is health for individuals, health for groups, such as the family, and health for communities within a society" (King, 1995b, p. 24).

Key Concepts. Two sets of concepts are included in the theory, one relating to the parties involved in the nurse-client relationship and the other pertaining to the process of goal attainment, as follows:

- *Concepts related to the nurse-client relationship:*
  - Personal system: An individual.
  - Interpersonal system: Two or more interacting individuals.
  - Social system: Communities and societies.
- *Concepts related to goal attainment:*
  - Communication: The process of giving information from one person to another.
  - Interaction: The process of perception between the person and environment or one or more persons, represented by verbal and nonverbal behaviors that are goal directed.
  - Perception: An individual's representation of reality.
  - Transaction: Identification of mutual goals valued by persons interacting with each other.
  - Role: A set of behaviors displayed by the individual, who occupies a given position in a social system.

- Stress: A dynamic state of interaction with the environment to maintain balance for growth, development, and performance.
- Growth and development: According to King (1981), these are "continuous changes in individuals occurring at molecular, cellular, and behavioral levels" (p. 148).
- Time: A duration between one event and another.
- Space: Defined by "gestures, postures, and visible boundaries erected to mark off personal space" (King, 1981, p. 148).

LEININGER'S CULTURAL CARE THEORY

Drawing from a background in cultural and social anthropology, Madeleine Leininger's contribution to nursing knowledge is related to transcultural nursing and caring. Her book *Transcultural Nursing: Concepts, Theories, and Practice* (1978) presented her conceptual framework for cultural care and health. She continues to explicate the linkages between nursing and anthropology as she identifies and defines concepts such as care, caring, culture, cultural values, and cultural variations (Leininger, 1984, 1991, 1995; Leininger & McFarland, 2002, 2006).

Brief Overview. Transcultural nursing focuses on a comparative study and analysis of different cultures and subcultures in the world regarding their caring behavior, nursing care, health-illness values, and patterns of behavior, with the goal of developing a scientific and humanistic body of knowledge from which to derive culture-specific and culture-universal nursing care practices (Leininger, 1978).

Assumptions About the Individual. Clients are caring and cultural beings who perceive health, illness, caring, curing, dependence, and independence differently. The social structure, worldview, and values of people vary transculturally.

Environment. The environment is a social structure, the "interrelated and interdependent systems of a society which determine how it functions with respect to certain major elements, namely: the political (including legal), economic, social (including kinship), educational, technical, religious, and cultural systems" (Leininger, 1978, p. 61). The environment is the totality of an event, situation, or particular experience that gives meaning to human expression and interaction.

Health and Illness. Perceptions of health and illness are culturally infused and therefore cannot be universally defined: "Health refers to a state of well-being that is culturally defined, valued, and practiced, and which reflects the ability of individuals (or groups) to perform their daily role activities in culturally expressed, beneficial, and patterned lifeways" (Leininger, 1991, p. 48). Worldviews, social structure, and cultural beliefs influence perceptions of health and illness and cannot be separated from them. For example, some cultures perceive illness to be largely a personal and internal body experience, whereas others view illness as an extrapersonal or cultural experience. Another example is that many clients of Asian descent believe that health is a personal responsibility, a result of the individual maintaining balance. In Western society, health may be defined by the medical profession. As the Report of the Surgeon General (1999) noted: "Ten years ago a serum cholesterol of 200 was considered normal. Today, this same number alarms some physicians and may lead to treatment."

Nursing. Nursing is a learned humanistic and scientific profession that focuses on personalized (individual and group) care behaviors, functions, and processes that have physical, psychocultural, and social significance or meaning. The goal of nursing is to assist, support, facilitate, or enable individuals or groups to regain or maintain their health in a way that is culturally congruent or to help people face handicaps or death (Leininger, 1991).

Key Concepts. Among the core concepts of transcultural nursing theory are the following:

- *Care.* Phenomena related to assistive, supportive, or enabling behavior toward or for another individual with evident or anticipated needs to ease or improve a human condition.
- *Caring.* Actions directed toward assisting, supporting, or enabling an individual (or group) to

ameliorate or improve the human condition or "lifeway" (Leininger, 1991, p. 48).
- *Culture.* Values, beliefs, norms, and lifeway practices of a particular group that guides thinking, decisions, and actions in patterned ways.
- *Cultural care.* The cognitively known values, beliefs, and patterned lifeways that assist, support, or enable another individual or group to maintain well-being; improve a human condition or lifeway; or deal with illness, handicaps, or death.
  - Cultural care diversity: The variability of meaning, patterns, values, lifeways, or symbols of care that are culturally derived for health or to improve a human condition.
  - Cultural care universality: Common, similar, or uniform care meanings, patterns, values, lifeways, or symbols that are culturally derived for health or to improve a human condition.
- *Cultural-congruent care.* Assistive, supportive, facilitative, or enabling acts or decisions that fit individual, group, or institutional cultural values, beliefs, and lifeways (Leininger, 1995).
  - Cultural care preservation or maintenance: Professional actions and decisions that help people of a particular culture to retain and preserve relevant care values.
  - Cultural care accommodation or negotiation: Professional actions and decisions that help people of a designated culture adapt to or negotiate with others for a beneficial or satisfying health outcome.
  - Cultural care repatterning or restructuring: Professional actions and decisions that help a client change or modify his or her lifeway to improve health while still respecting the client's cultural values and beliefs.

Practice Theory

Being clinically specific, practice theories (also known as *situation-specific theories*) incorporate and reflect the actual provision of nursing care (McEwen, 2007), thus allowing the "incorporation of nurses' clinical wisdom" (Im & Meleis, 1999). They may be derived from existing theories, arise from practice, or emerge from research findings. The purpose of these theories is to describe or explain clinical problems or patient needs that nurses encounter daily within the boundaries of their specialty practices or settings. As such, they may prescribe specific nursing actions or lead to the in-depth analysis of such interventions. Practice theories may provide explanations about patient problems, describe therapeutic interventions, advocate specific approaches to a specified patient population, or identify nursing values that lead to a decision-making process (McEwen, 2007).

Examples of practice theories can be found in the nursing specialty–specific literature that discusses disease management and nursing interventions pertinent to a defined patient population.

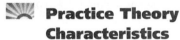

Practice Theory Characteristics

- A lower level of abstraction: limited in scope and focus; not developed to transcend time or place
- Focus on a single specific phenomenon of interest to nurses; developed to answer specific set of clinical questions
- Specific sociopolitical, cultural, and/or historical context
- Readily recognizable connection to both daily practice and clinical research
- Apparent respect for diversity, complexity, and context reflected in decreased generalizability (Im & Meleis, 1999; McEwen, 2007)

Application to Nursing Practice

The nursing theories and frameworks discussed here offer a variety of perspectives for application to clinical practice. For example, some are process oriented and dynamic, such as Peplau's interpersonal process, King's theory of goal attainment, and Rogers' science of unitary human beings. Others are more outcome oriented, such as Roy's adaptation model, Johnson's behavioral system model, and Orem's self-care deficit theory. The models of Rogers and Neuman focus

on the wholeness of the individual and conceptualize nursing as one component of the individual's life process. King's theory is directed toward the interaction between the nurse and the client, who are inseparable. Nightingale and Leininger developed humanistic perspectives, focusing on personalized, individualized care for all, and Roy conceptualizes the nurse as an external regulator whose function is to promote system balance or adaptation. Orem views the nurse as a person who assists the individual with self-care practices when the individual is unable to effectively care for himself or herself. A comparison of the theoretical perspectives discussed in this chapter is presented in Table 5-2.

Most of the nursing theories and frameworks presented in this chapter are too extensive to be used in their entirety in any one nursing care situation. For example, Orem describes three types of nursing systems, but for a client who is in the intensive care unit and on life support, only the wholly compensatory nursing system is relevant. Similarly, with Neuman's three levels of prevention, only clients with symptoms resulting from invasion of environmental stressors are appropriate recipients of secondary prevention. Despite these limitations, the theories can guide nursing assessment in terms of what questions to ask and what areas to assess. The type of client, the setting where care is delivered, and the goal of nursing are what influence the selection of an appropriate theoretical framework for practice. The more specific theories can be readily adapted for use in a practice setting. The more global theories may better serve as frameworks for research, the findings of which can then be applied to practice. Practice theories may best serve in the development of evidence-based nursing practice by providing valid and reliable substantiation of clinical guidelines.

EVALUATING THE UTILITY OF NURSING THEORIES

Not all theories and frameworks are equally comprehensive or equally useful in every situation, and they are not meant to be. The definition of the client and the setting in which care is delivered limit the usefulness of some of the theories and frameworks presented. To be useful in practice, a theory must work in a specific setting: "A nursing theory should structure

TABLE 5-2	Comparison of Theoretical Perspectives			
Theory/Model	**Nursing**	**Environment**	**Health**	**Person**
Nightingale's Environmental Theory	Intended to relieve pain and suffering and restore health by manipulating the environment	Conditions external to the person that affect both sick and well persons	State of well-being; using an individual's power to the fullest	An individual who is in control of his or her own life and health and desires good health
Peplau's Interpersonal Process	Therapeutic interpersonal process	Existing forces outside the organism	Forward movement of ongoing human processes and personality	An organism that lives in an unstable equilibrium and strives to reduce tension generated by needs
Rogers' Science of Unitary Human Beings	Science and art; the art of nursing is the creative use of science for human betterment	Pandimensional energy field integral with the human energy field	Patterns of living in harmony with the environment	A unified irreducible whole; more than and different from the sum of parts
Orem's Self-Care Deficit Theory	Involves assisting individuals with self-care practices	Linked to the individual, forming an integrated system	State in which human beings are structurally and functionally whole	A unity who functions biologically, symbolically, and socially and whose functioning is linked with the environment
King's Theory of Goal Attainment	Process of action, reaction, and interaction	Interactive with the individual	Ability to function in social roles	An open system in transaction with the environment who is social, sentient, rational, perceiving, controlling, purposeful, and action oriented
Roy's Adaptation Model	An external regulatory force that modifies stimuli affecting adaptation	Internal and external conditions that surround and affect individuals	State and process of being and becoming an integrated and whole person	A biopsychosocial adaptive system that is in constant interaction with a changing environment
Neuman's Systems Model	Concerned with variables affecting the individual's response to stress	Internal and external factors affecting and affected by the individual	Optimal system stability	A whole person; a dynamic composite of physiological, psychological, sociocultural, developmental, and spiritual variables
Leininger's Cultural Care Theory	Culturally congruent care behaviors, functions, and processes that have physical, psychocultural, or social significance	The interrelated, interdependent systems of a society	State of well-being that is culturally defined	Caring, cultural beings who perceive health, illness, caring, curing, dependence, and independence differently
Watson's Philosophy and Science of Caring	Transpersonal caring relationship that includes use of 10 caritas processes	Internal and external variables	Unity and harmony within mind, body, and soul	An entity that is nonreducible and is interconnected with others and nature

the work, giving the practicing nurse a frame of reference from which to view patients and from which to make patient care decisions" (Barnum, 1998, p. 80). Its concepts must be operationalized in ways that promote application and facilitate nursing activities in that setting. Examination of a theory's usefulness for its intended purpose and the consistency of its internal structure is important. The value and logical structure of a theory can be evaluated by asking questions proposed by Fawcett (2005) and Barnum (1998), such as the following:

1. Are the assumptions inherent in the theory clearly stated?
2. Does the model provide adequate descriptions of all four concepts of nursing's metaparadigm?
3. Are the relationships among the concepts of nursing's metaparadigm clearly explained?
4. Is the theory stated clearly and concisely?
5. Does the structure of the theory contain conflicting views?
6. Can relationships between concepts be tested in research (i.e., observed and measured) and applied to practice?
7. Does the theory lead to nursing activities that meet societal expectations (social congruence)?
8. Does the theory lead to nursing activities that are likely to result in favorable client outcomes (social significance)?
9. Does the theory include explicit rules for use in practice, education, or research (social usefulness)?

THEORIES FROM RELATED DISCIPLINES

Several nursing theories derived their conceptual basis from theories and frameworks developed by scholars from related disciplines and adapted to specific situations. Many of these theories are useful and relevant to nursing in their original form. A brief synopsis of selected theories from related disciplines follows.

One of the theories with wide applicability, general system theory, proposes that a system is a set of interrelated parts or subsystems that are in constant interaction with the environment working together toward a common goal (von Bertalanffy, 1956, 1968). Systems take in matter, information, and energy from the environment (input), process it (throughput), and release it back to the environment (output). Some of the output returns to the system as feedback in an attempt to return the system to a steady state (equilibrium) or, in the case of living systems, a condition of balance within the range of normal (homeostasis). A system is more than and different from the sum of its parts and, over time, becomes increasingly complex. The nurse who uses systems theory assesses the individual, family, or community as an aggregate and simultaneously considers the relationships among the subsystems, keeping in mind that a change in one part of the system changes the system as a whole.

Theories of change have been proposed by Lewin (1951) and expanded by Lippitt (1973) that view change as a goal-directed process. Lewin's theory includes three concepts: force field (driving and restraining forces for or against change), motivators (stimuli indicating the need for change), and stages of change (unfreezing, moving, refreezing). Lippitt focuses on the activities of the change agent to bring about the change. These theories provide a systematic method of planning, implementing, and evaluating change in individuals, organizations, and social systems.

Among the several theories of coping is one developed by Lazarus (1976) that views coping as a process that leads to adaptation. The major concepts in Lazarus' theory are stress caused by a lack of resources to cope with an environmental event, cognitive appraisal of the stressor to determine the perceived level of threat, and problem-focused coping (management of the stressor) or emotional-focused coping (management of the response) (Lazarus & Folkman, 1984). For clients experiencing an intense level of stress, nursing interventions designed to alter the perception of the threat level and promote and support the coping process can be derived from the relationships specified by this theory.

Aguilera (1998) provides a theory and framework for successful resolution of a crisis situation. She identifies three balancing factors (the perception of the event, the availability of situational supports, and usual coping mechanisms) that prevent an adverse reaction to a stressful situation. When a crisis or psychological disequilibrium occurs, the nurse can assess the balancing factors to establish a nursing diagnosis. Nursing interventions can then be designed to facilitate the return to equilibrium by assisting the client to establish a realistic perception of the event, providing situational supports, and identifying coping mechanisms.

Both coping and adjustment are embedded in Duvall's (1977) stages of family life and developmental tasks, which can serve as the framework for delivering age-specific or situation-specific nursing interventions to the family. Developmental stages are also specified in Erikson's theory (1963, 1982), which encompasses three major concepts: sequential developmental stages, developmental conflicts, and identity formation. Developmental tasks are associated with each stage, and a developmental conflict occurs if the tasks cannot be successfully accomplished. Identity formation is viewed as an ongoing process throughout the life span. Erikson's theory is useful as a framework for assessing an individual's psychosocial development and intervening when developmental conflicts are identified.

Selye's general adaptation syndrome, a theory of adaptation to stress, describes three phases of reaction to stress: stage of alarm, or immediate reaction to the stressor; stage of resistance, or adaptation to the stressor over time; and stage of exhaustion, or inability to adapt to the stressor (Selye, 1974, 1982). This theory can be applied to clients who are suffering not only psychological or social stress but physiological stress as well.

Maslow's theory of the hierarchy of needs is illustrated as a pyramid containing five broad layers of needs upon which human functioning is based. The bottom or first-level needs are physiological, followed by safety and security, love and belonging, self-esteem, and self-actualization (Maslow, 1970). The theory contends that basic needs, such as air, water, food, and safety, must be met before meeting higher-level needs such as self-esteem or self-actualization. The application of this theory to nursing practice can provide a framework for client assessment and assist in identifying nursing care priorities.

These theories are only a sample of those developed by related disciplines that have uses in nursing.

Others, such as Rotter's locus of control (1954) and Bandura's self-efficacy theory (1986), can be found in various chapters in this text. One or more of these theories can serve as a framework for designing interventions for clients throughout the life cycle, developing and implementing research studies, and framing educational curricula. In combination with nursing theories, a wide array of theoretical perspectives in various stages of development are available from which to choose.

SUMMARY

Nursing is a knowledge-based disciplines that is significantly different from medicine and focused on the wholeness of human beings. Nursing knowledge is the organization of discipline-specific concepts, theories, and ideas published in both print and electronic media and demonstrated in professional practice. Theories and frameworks provide direction and guidance for structuring professional nursing practice, education, and research. They provide a way to educate nurses; describe, explain, predict, organize, assess, diagnose, intervene, and evaluate nursing practice; and question, study, and interpret research. This chapter has provided a historical perspective and a comprehensive overview of some of the many nursing theorists who have made substantial contributions to the development of a body of nursing knowledge. The remainder of this text will introduce additional nursing theories that also contribute to the body of nursing knowledge.

KEY POINTS

- A theory is a group of statements that describe the relationship between two or more concepts.
- The main components of nursing theories are persons, environment, health/illness, and nursing.
- Nightingale's theory focuses on nursing's role in manipulating the environment.
- Peplau's theory centers on the interpersonal process in nursing.
- According to Rogers, the nurse seeks to promote coherence between individuals and their environments.
- As specified by Orem, when a client has a deficit in his or her ability for self-care, the nurse assists the individual with self-care practices.

- King conceptualizes the nurse and the client as components of an interpersonal system who seek to attain mutually agreed-upon goals.
- Roy's theory describes the client as a biopsychosocial adaptive system and the nurse as one who modifies stimuli to promote adaptation.
- Three levels of nursing intervention—primary, secondary, and tertiary prevention—are specified in Neuman's systems model.
- Leininger's theory centers on providing culturally congruent nursing care.
- Watson identifies the caring relationship and 10 carative factors that form the core of nursing.
- The more specific theories, in whole or in part, can be readily adapted for use in any practice setting.
- The more global theories may better serve as frameworks for research, the findings of which can then be applied to practice.
- Theories from related disciplines also have relevance to nursing practice, education, and research.
- All theories have the potential to make substantial contributions to the nursing profession by enhancing the development of a unique body of nursing knowledge.

CRITICAL THINKING EXERCISES

1. "An individual is in constant interaction with the environment." Apply this statement to the client in each of the following settings and discuss the implications for nursing practice:
   a. A community mental health clinic
   b. An intensive care unit
   c. An extended care facility
   d. A well-baby clinic
2. How do Florence Nightingale's ideas apply to nursing practice in the current health care system?
3. Defend or refute the following statement: "We should have only one nursing theory, rather than several, to guide education, practice, and research."
4. Compare the definitions of health and illness in two nursing theories, citing similarities and differences. Which one is most reflective of your own definitions of health and illness? Why?
5. What is your personal philosophy of nursing? Which of the theoretical perspectives of nursing presented in this chapter is most closely aligned with your philosophy of nursing? Why?
6. Identify the nursing theory or model that would be most useful to you in your practice and explain why.

7. Select a theory from a related discipline and apply it to a client for whom you have provided care. Use the major concepts to assess the client, identify the problem, design the plan of care, and evaluate the outcomes.

REFERENCES

Aguilera, D. C. (1998). *Crisis intervention: Theory and methodology* (8th ed.). St. Louis: Mosby.

Alligood, M. R. (2005). Nursing theory: The basis for professional nursing. In K. K. Chitty (Ed.), *Professional nursing: Concepts and challenges* (4th ed., pp. 271–294). Philadelphia: W.B. Saunders.

Auger, J. R. (1976). *Behavioral systems and nursing*. Englewood Cliffs, NJ: Prentice Hall.

Bandura, A. (1986). *Social foundations of thought and action: A social cognitive theory*. Englewood Cliffs, NJ: Prentice Hall.

Barnum, B. S. (1998). *Nursing theory: Analysis, application, evaluation*. Philadelphia: Lippincott.

Duvall, E. M. (1977). *Marriage and family development* (5th ed.). New York: Lippincott.

Encarta world English dictionary. (2009). New York: Bloomsbury Publishing.

Erikson, E. H. (1963). *Childhood and society* (2nd ed.). New York: Norton.

Erikson, E. H. (1982). *The life cycle completed: A review*. New York: Norton.

Fawcett, J. (1975). The family as a living open system: An emerging conceptual framework for nursing. *International Nursing Review, 22*, 113–116.

Fawcett, J. (1977). The relationship between identification and patterns of change in spouses' body images during and after pregnancy. *International Journal of Nursing Studies, 14*, 199–213.

Fawcett, J. (1989). *Analysis and evaluation of conceptual models of nursing* (2nd ed.). Philadelphia: Davis.

Fawcett, J. (1993). *Analysis and evaluation of nursing theories*. Philadelphia: Davis.

Fawcett, J. (1997). The structural hierarchy of nursing knowledge: Components and their definitions. In I. M. King & J. Fawcett (Eds.), *The language of nursing theory and metatheory* (pp. 11–17). Indianapolis: Sigma Theta Tau International.

Fawcett, J. (1999). *The relationship of theory and research* (3rd ed.). Philadelphia: Davis.

Fawcett, J. (2000). *Analysis and evaluation of contemporary nursing knowledge: Nursing models and theories*. Philadelphia: Davis.

Fawcett, J. (2005). *Analysis and evaluation of contemporary nursing knowledge: Nursing models and theories* (2nd ed.). Philadelphia: Davis.

Higgins, P. A., & Moore, S. M. (2000). Levels of theoretical thinking in nursing. *Nursing Outlook, 48,* 179–183.

Im, E., & Meleis, A. I. (1999). Situation-specific theories: Philosophical roots, properties, and approach. *Advances in Nursing Science, 22*(3), 11–24.

Infante, M. S. (Ed.). (1982). *Crisis theory: A frame-work for nursing practice.* Reston, VA: Reston Publishing.

King, I. (1971). *Toward a theory for nursing.* New York: Wiley.

King, I. (1981). *A theory for nursing: Systems, concepts, process.* New York: Wiley.

King, I. (1995a). A systems framework for nursing. In M. A. Frey & C. L. Sieloff (Eds.), *Advancing King's systems framework and theory of nursing* (pp. 14–21). Thousand Oaks, CA: Sage.

King, I. (1995b). The theory of goal attainment. In M. A. Frey & C. L. Sieloff (Eds.), *Advancing King's systems framework and theory of nursing* (pp. 23–32). Thousand Oaks, CA: Sage.

Lazarus, R. S. (1976). *Patterns of adjustment* (3rd ed.). New York: McGraw-Hill.

Lazarus, R. S., & Folkman, S. (1984). *Stress appraisal and coping.* New York: Springer.

Leininger, M. (1978). *Transcultural nursing: Concepts, theories and practice.* New York: Wiley.

Leininger, M. (Ed.) (1984). *Care: The essence of nursing and health.* Thorofare, NJ: Slack.

Leininger, M. (1991). *Culture, care, diversity and universality: A theory of nursing* (NLN Publication No. 15-2402). New York: National League for Nursing.

Leininger, M. (1995). *Transcultural nursing: Concepts, theories, research, and practice.* Columbus, OH: McGraw-Hill.

Leininger, M. M., & McFarland, M. R. (2002). *Transcultural nursing: Concepts, theories, research and practice.* New York: McGraw-Hill.

Leininger, M. M., & McFarland, M. R. (2006). *Culture care, diversity and universality: A worldwide nursing theory.* Sudbury, MA: Jones & Bartlett.

Levine, M. E. (1995). The rhetoric of nursing theory. *Image: Journal of Nursing Scholarship, 27*(1), 11–14.

Lewin, K. (1951). Defining the field at a given time. In D. Cartwright (Ed.), *Field theory in social science: Selected papers by Kurt Lewin* (pp. 43–59). New York: Harper and Brothers.

Lippitt, G. L. (1973). *Visualizing change.* La Jolla, CA: University Associates.

Maslow, A. (1970). *Motivation and personality* (2nd ed.). New York: Harper & Row.

McEwen, M. (2007). Application of theory in nursing practice. In M. McEwen & E. M. Wills (Eds.), *Theoretical basis for nursing* (2nd ed., pp. 411–433). Philadelphia: Lippincott, Williams & Wilkins.

Meleis, A. I. (2005). *Theoretical nursing: Development and progress* (3rd ed.). Philadelphia: Lippincott, Williams & Wilkins.

Neuman, B. (1982). *The Neuman systems model: Application to nursing theory and practice.* Norwalk, CT: Appleton-Century-Crofts.

Neuman, B. (1989). *The Neuman systems model* (2nd ed.). Norwalk, CT: Appleton & Lange.

Neuman, B. (1995). *The Neuman systems model* (3rd ed.). Norwalk, CT: Appleton & Lange.

Neuman, B., & Fawcett, J. (2002). *The Neuman systems model* (4th ed.). Upper Saddle River, NJ: Prentice Hall.

Neuman, B. M., & Young, R. J. (1972). A model for teaching total person approach to patient problems. *Nursing Research, 21,* 264–269.

Nightingale, F. (1860). *Notes on nursing: What it is and what it is not.* London: Harrison.

Nightingale, F. (1946). *Notes on nursing: What it is and what it is not.* (A facsimile of the first edition published in 1860.). New York: Appleton Century.

Orem, D. E. (1971). *Nursing: Concepts of practice.* New York: McGraw-Hill.

Orem, D. E. (1980). *Nursing: Concepts of practice* (2nd ed.). New York: McGraw-Hill.

Orem, D. E. (1985). *Nursing: Concepts of practice* (3rd ed.). New York: McGraw-Hill.

Orem, D. E. (1991). *Nursing: Concepts of practice* (4th ed.). St. Louis: Mosby.

Orem, D. E. (1995). *Nursing: Concepts of practice* (5th ed.). St. Louis: Mosby.

Orem, D. E. (2001). *Nursing: Concepts of practice* (6th ed.). St. Louis: Mosby.

Peplau, H. (1952). *Interpersonal relations in nursing: A conceptual framework of reference for psychodynamic nursing.* New York: Putnam.

Peplau, H. (1991). *Interpersonal relations in nursing: A conceptual framework of reference for psychodynamic nursing.* New York: Springer.

Peplau, H. (1992). Interpersonal relations: A theoretical framework for application in nursing practice. *Nursing Science Quarterly, 5,* 13–18.

Rogers, M. E. (1970). *An introduction to the theoretical basis of nursing.* Philadelphia: Davis.

Rogers, M. E. (1989). Nursing: A science of unitary man. In J. P. Reihl-Sisca (Ed.), *Conceptual models for nursing practice* (3rd ed., pp. 181–188). Norwalk, CT: Appleton & Lange.

Rogers, M. E. (1990). Nursing: Science of unitary, irreducible, human beings. Update 1990. In E. A. M. Barrett (Ed.), *Visions of Rogers' science-based nursing* (pp. 5–11). New York: National League for Nursing.

Rogers, M. E. (1994). Nursing science evolves. In M. A. Madrid, & E. A. M. Barrett (Eds.), *Rogers' scientific art of nursing practice* (NLN Publication No. 15-2610, pp. 3–9). New York: National League for Nursing.

Rotter, J. B. (1954). *Social learning and clinical psychology*. Englewood Cliffs, NJ: Prentice Hall.

Roy, C. (1984). *Introduction to nursing: An adaptation model* (2nd ed.). Englewood Cliffs, NJ: Prentice Hall.

Roy, C. (1989). The Roy adaptation model. In J. P. Reihl-Sisca (Ed.), *Conceptual models for nursing practice* (3rd ed., pp. 105–114). Norwalk, CT: Appleton & Lange.

Roy, C. (2009). *The Roy adaptation model* (3rd ed.). Upper Saddle River, N J: Prentice Hall.

Roy, C., & Andrews, H. A. (1999). *The Roy adaptation model* (2nd ed.). Stanford, CT: Appleton & Lange.

Selye, H. (1974). *Stress without distress*. Philadelphia: Lippincott.

Selye, H. (1982). History and the present status of the stress concept. In I. A. Goldberger, & S. Breznitz (Eds.), *Handbook of stress: Theoretical and clinical aspects*. New York: Free Press.

U.S. Department of Health and Human Services. (1999). *Mental health: A report of the Surgeon General*. Rockville, MD: U.S. Department of Health and Human Services, Substance Abuse and Mental Health Services Administration, Center for Mental Health Services, National Institutes of Health, National Institute of Mental Health.

von Bertalanffy, L. (1956). General systems theory. In B. D. Ruben & J. Kim (Eds.), *General systems theory and human communication* (pp. 7–16). Rochelle Park, NJ: Hayden.

von Bertalanffy, L. (1968). *General systems theory*. New York: Braziller.

Watson, J. (1979). *Nursing: The philosophy and science of caring*. Boston: Little, Brown.

Watson, J. (1985). *Nursing: Human science and health care*. Norwalk, CT: Appleton-Century-Crofts.

Watson, J. (1988). *Nursing: Human science and human caring—A theory of nursing*. New York: National League for Nursing.

Watson, J. (1994). *Applying the art and science of human caring*. New York: National League for Nursing.

Watson, J. (1996). Watson's theory of transpersonal caring. In P. Hinton Walker & B. Neuman (Eds.), *Blueprint for use of nursing models* (pp. 141–184). New York: NLN Press.

Watson, J. (1999). *Postmodern nursing and beyond*. Edinburgh: Churchill Livingstone.

Watson, J. (2007). Theory of Human Caring; Theory evolution. University of Colorado at Denver College of Nursing. Retrieved 2/1/2010 from http://www.nursing.ucdenver.edu/faculty/jw_evolution.htm

Watson, J. (2009). Assessing and measuring caring in nursing and health sciences (2nd ed.). New York: Springer.

Whall, A. L. (2005). The structure of nursing knowledge: Analysis and evaluation of practice, middle range, and grand theory. In J. J. Fitzpatrick & A. L. Whall (Eds.), *Conceptual models of nursing: Analysis and application* (4th ed., pp. 5–20). Upper Saddle River, N J: Prentice-Hall.

White, M. B. (Ed.) (1983). *Curriculum development from a nursing model: The crisis theory framework*. New York: Springer.

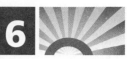

6

Health Policy and Planning and the Nursing Practice Environment

DEBRA C. WALLACE, PhD, RN
L. LOUISE IVANOV, DNS, RN

OBJECTIVES

At the completion of this chapter, the reader will be able to:

- Identify political, legislative, social, and economic factors affecting health policy and nursing.
- Describe the legislative, budgetary, and regulatory processes for developing, implementing, and evaluating policy.
- Discuss selected health programs mandated by federal health policy.
- Evaluate health policies for their impact on nursing practice, education, research, and the practice environment.
- Discuss strategies for nurse participation in health policy.

PROFILE IN PRACTICE

Maureen Nalle, PhD, RN
Assistant Professor, University of Tennessee College of Nursing, Knoxville, Tennessee

My professional career has spanned several decades and many professional opportunities and challenges, including military service, maternal-child health practice, and nursing education. As is the case with many professionals, questions and concerns regarding access to care, delivery systems, and the impact of health policy on nursing and patients were formulated as the result of encounters with the various dimensions of professional practice. Both clinical practice and doctoral studies in health promotion and health education promoted an in-depth appreciation of the social, economic, political, and policy factors that affected nursing education and practice.

The most important framework for understanding and contributing to health policy has been active participation in professional nursing organizations. Membership in the Tennessee Nurses Association and the Tennessee Association of Nurse Executives has provided an avenue for identifying state-level priorities, communicating needs, and collaborating with legislators to pursue a legislative agenda beneficial to patients, nurses, and the health care community. The American Nurses Association and policy work for the ANA Congress on Nursing Economics and Practice and the Center for American Nurses have created a remarkable framework of opportunities for partnership, collaboration, and contributions to health policy initiatives at the national level. I am currently involved with TNA, the Tennessee Center for Nursing, and a statewide coalition of nursing professionals focused on policy issues related to the professional shortage, quality and access to nursing education, and provision of continuing competence for nurses in the state.

As a faculty member, I promote student awareness and involvement in the policy process, including knowledge of current issues, participation in professional nursing organizations, and advocacy for clients. Instilling a belief in students' own capacity for influencing nursing practice and health care is crucial to sustained participation. Preparing future professionals to contribute to the development and implementation of effective health policy and an effective practice environment is not only an obligation but also a privilege that reflects commitment to this important process.

Introduction

Why should nurses be concerned with legislation regarding health? Health policy affects nursing at all levels of preparation, in all settings and specialties, and across all client groups. Policy decisions, allocations, and regulation dictate where care is delivered, to whom care is delivered, who delivers care, how care is delivered, and who pays for care. Specifically, policy determines or assists in decisions of every aspect of health care, including delivery modalities, settings of care, quality of care provider qualifications, payment level and mechanisms, type of services, and access to care. Additionally, practice environment, workplace safety, licensure, certification, accreditation, and educational funding are influenced by health policy and related regulation. Thus it is important for each nurse to have a working knowledge of health policy development, regulation, and evaluation in order to understand how members of the largest health care profession can influence policy to improve the health and well-being of society.

Before the 20th century, health care was typically an individual or private sector responsibility in most countries. Many health care facilities were affiliated with religious and civic organizations and groups or educational institutions. Physicians had private office practices with direct fee for service and out-of-pocket payment. The federal government in the United States became involved in the regulation, provision, and financing of health care primarily during the early 1900s. Government involvement, scientific developments, technology, social pressure, and increased costs associated with health care have resulted in the development of a health care industry that exceeds manufacturing and agriculture industries. The health care industry is often divided into subsystems that serve populations on the basis of payment decisions and condition specialties.

In industrialized countries in many parts of the world, such as the United Kingdom and Canada, centralized systems of care have been developed through socialized medicine models. In these countries, the infrastructure controls the number and location of health care delivery sites and the training, distribution, and reimbursement of providers, both physicians and nurses. The nursing practice environment is hospital and community based and is regulated by the types of services offered, payment decisions, and access points. Regardless of the nation, multiple factors affect the development, implementation, and evaluation of health policy, as well as its influence on nursing research, education, and practice.

Politics

One of the major factors influencing health policy is politics. Individuals, organizations, agencies, state, and federal processes are involved in developing health policy, the regulations for implementation, and the evaluation of outcomes. For example, a citizen writes a member of Congress and argues that certain needs are not being met for technology-dependent children. An organization such as the American Nurses Association (ANA) may be involved by writing, visiting, and lobbying state and congressional representatives for new and continuing needs of nurses and patients.

The need for educational and program grants in the Nurse Reinvestment Act is one example of a law that was passed to support nurses. Federal agencies such as the National Institutes of Health (NIH) and the Food and Drug Administration (FDA) invite members of Congress to attend administrative hearings and provide input on priority setting, program development, budgetary needs, and evaluation reports. For example, the Veterans Administration sought additional funding for care and research to improve care, resulting in the Veterans Mental Health and Other Care Improvements Act of 2008, which addresses postdeployment mental health. In addition, political leaders and legislators bring health-related agendas to congressional committees based on their constituents' values and priorities, as well as their own.

ORGANIZATIONS

Nurses are members of many organizations involved in and influencing the development of health policy and health care–related legislation. Nonlegislative citizens also play a political role in health policy development and implementation through participation in and support of civic organizations and activities, such as the American Association of Retired Persons (AARP), Mothers Against Drunk Driving (MADD), American Diabetes Association (ADA), the March of Dimes, the National Organization of Women (NOW), and the National Rifle Association (NRA). Most professional organizations (e.g., American Medical Association [AMA], American Hospital Association [AHA], American Academy of Nursing [AAN], Coalition for Patients' Rights [CPR]) develop legislative agendas, support political candidates, and employ lobbyists at state and federal levels. (See Box 6-1 for a list of government and health care organizations referred to in this chapter.) In 2004, the ANA moved its headquarters from Kansas City to Washington, D.C., to increase visibility and access to federal agencies and Congress. State nursing associations often have lobbyists to ensure state laws for advanced practice licensure, Medicaid benefits and coverage, and work environment protections. Lay, civic, and professional organizations, whether or not associated with a political party—such as the

AARP, the National Association for the Advancement of Colored Persons (NAACP), the NRA, the ANA, the National Home Care Association (NHCA), and the America's Health Insurance Plans (AHIP)—use grassroots activity, paid lobbyists, campaign support, advertisements, and organized rallies to make an impact on health policies affecting their members and special interest groups. Most health care professional organizations, including the ANA, have a paid lobbyist in each state capital and at least one in Washington, D.C. Because these organizations fund political and lobbying activity, a proportion of membership dues to these organizations are not tax deductible. For example, the ANA uses approximately 25% of its dues for lobbying activities and has a full-time lobbyist in Washington. Many state nursing associations have their own lobbyist or contract for this work in their state legislature.

POLITICAL PARTIES

Three major political parties have been involved in legislation: the Republican National Committee (RNC), the Democratic National Committee (DNC), and the Independent Reform Party (IRP). More recently, the Libertarian Party (LP) has become more involved. Political parties set forth the major issues of concern through party platforms during presidential conventions, website postings, and paid media advertisements. The party platforms consist of "planks" that delineate the party's philosophy and stand on issues of the day. Platforms are a consensus of the convention delegates, but they also mirror the presidential candidate's stand and arguments to be used during the campaign. Platform issues, then, often become the agendas for state legislatures and the U.S. Congress. Many of the issues during the 20th century were health related, such as gun control, abortion, and Medicare. In the early part of the 21st century, issues surrounding stem cell research, prescription drug coverage, bioterrorism, and electronic health records have emerged. The most recent platforms and priority issues can be reviewed on party websites or received from each party's national or state offices. The ANA has traditionally supported more of the Democratic Party's health issue planks.

BOX 6-1	Important Health Care Terms and Organizations

Administration on Aging (AOA)
Advanced Education Nursing Grants (AENP)
advanced practice registered nurse (APRN)
Agency for Healthcare Research and Quality (AHRQ)
American Academy of Nursing (AAN)
American Association of Colleges of Nursing (AACN)
American Association of Critical-Care Nurses (AACCN)
American Association of Retired Persons (AARP)
American Dental Association (ADA)
American Diabetes Association (ADA)
America's Health Insurance Plans (AHIP)
American Hospital Association (AHA)
American Medical Association (AMA)
American Nurses' Association (ANA)
American Nurses Credentialing Center (ANCC)
American Nurses Foundation (ANF)
American Public Health Association (APHA)
American Red Cross (ARC)
Association for Women's Health, Obstetrical and
    Neonatal Nursing (AWHONN)
Bureau of Census (BOC)
Bureau of Health Professions (BHP)
Centers for Disease Control and Prevention (CDC)
Centers of Excellence (COE)
Centers for Medicare and Medicaid Services (CMS)
certified registered nurse anesthetist (CRNA)
Children's Health Insurance Programs (CHIP)
Coalition for Patients' Rights (CPR)
colorectal cancer (CRC)
Commission on Collegiate Nursing Education (CCNE)
Comprehensive Geriatric Education Program (CGEP)
Congressional Budget Office (CBO)
Consolidated Budget Resolution (CBR)
Coordinating Office for Terrorism Preparedness and
    Emergency Response (COTPER)
Council for the Advancement of Nursing Science (CANS)
Culturally and Linguistically Appropriate Services (CLAS)
Democratic National Committee (DNC)
Department of Agriculture (DA)
Department of Education (DE)
Department of Homeland Security (DHS)
Department of Labor (DL)
Department of Veterans Affairs (DVA)
diagnostic related groups (DRG)
doctorate of nursing practice (DNP)
evidence based practice (EBP)

Federal Elections Commission (FEC)
Food and Drug Administration (FDA)
General Accounting Office (GAO)
gross domestic product (GDP)
Health Care Financing Administration (HCFA)
Health Insurance Portability and Accountability Act
    (HIPAA)
Health Resources and Services Administration (HRSA)
Homeland Security Act (HSA)
Independent Reform Party (IRP)
Institute of Medicine (IOM)
Interdisciplinary Nursing Quality Research Initiative
    (INQRI)
Internal Revenue Service (IRS)
Kaiser Family Foundation (KFF)
Libertarian Party (LP)
licensed practical nurse (LPN)
Magnet Nursing Services Recognition Program (MNSRP)
Mothers Against Drunk Driving (MADD)
National Academies of Science (NAS)
National Advisory Council (NAC)
National Advisory Council on Nurse Education and
    Practice (NACNEP)
National Association for the Advancement of Colored
    Persons (NAACP)
National Center for Chronic Disease Prevention and
    Health Promotion (NCCDPHP)
National Center for Health Statistics (NCHS)
National Center for Minority Health and Health
    Disparities (NCMHD)
National Center for Nursing Research (NCNR)
National Center on Minority Health and Health
    Disparities (NCMHD)
National Council Licensure Examination (NCLEX)
National Council of State Boards of Nursing (NCSBN)
National Database of Nursing Quality Indicators
    (NDNQI)
National Home Care Association (NHCA)
National Institute on Aging (NIA)
National Institute of Child Health and Human
    Development (NICHD)
National Institute of Mental Health (NIMH)
National Institute of Nursing Research (NINR)
National Institute of Occupational Safety and Health
    (NIOSH)
National Institutes of Health (NIH)

BOX 6-1	Important Health Care Terms and Organizations—cont'd

National League for Nursing (NLN)
National League for Nursing Accreditation Commission
  (NLNAC)
National Office of Public Health Genomics (NOPHG)
National Organization of Women (NOW)
National Rifle Association (NRA)
North Carolina Association of Nurse Anesthetists
  (NCANA)
Nurse Education, Practice and Retention (NEPR)
  program
Nurse Faculty Loan Program (NFLP)
nurse practitioners (NPs)
Nursing Care Quality Initiative (NCQI)
Nursing Home Quality Initiative (NHQI)
Nursing Research Initiative (NRI)
Nursing Workforce Diversity (NWD) grants
Nursing's Agenda for Health Care Reform (NAHCR)
Obstetrical and Neonatal Nursing (ONN)
Occupational Health and Safety Administration (OSHA)
Office on Management and Budget (OMB)
Office of Public Health and Science (OPHS)
Omnibus Budget Reconciliation Act (OBRA)
Oncology Nursing Society (ONS)
Pew Charitable Trusts (PCT)
Pew Health Professions Commission (PHPC)

political action committees (PACs)
Preadmission Screening and Resident Review (PASRR)
prescription drug plan (PDP)
Presidential Election Campaign Fund (PECF)
Republican National Committee (RNC)
registered nurse (RN)
Robert Wood Johnson Foundation (RWJF)
Safe Staffing Saves Lives (SSSL)
Senior Community Service Employment Program (SCSEP)
Sigma Theta Tau International (STTI)
Social and Rehabilitation Services (SRS)
Social Security (SS)
Society of Gastroenterology Nurses and Associates
  (SGNA)
State Children's Health Insurance Program (SCHIP)
Substance Abuse and Mental Health Services Adminis-
  tration (SAMHSA)
Surgeon General (SG)
Tennessee Bureau of TennCare (TBOT)
Tennessee Department of Health (TDH)
Templeton Foundation (TF)
United States Department of Health and Human
  Services (USDHHS)
vocational nurse (VN)
Women's Health Initiative (WHI)

POLITICAL ACTION AND 527 COMMITTEES

Registered *political action committees* (PACs) can be established independently or as a part of a formal organization to (1) raise, spend, and contribute money; (2) assist with campaigns; and (3) lobby on behalf of special interest groups, industries, or segments of society. PACs initiate much of the legislative activity or inactivity on both the state and federal levels. For example, *Roe v. Wade,* which legalized abortion, continues as a major PAC focus. PACs pay for television advertisements, hold public rallies and demonstrations, distribute literature, and invite political and other famous figures to events supporting their positions. Originally, PACs represented persons with specific needs who had been overlooked or not protected by society (e.g., those with AIDS, older adults, the homeless, poor children). In the late 1990s, PACs became more commonly representatives of particular groups of persons

that banded political, human, and financial resources to get policies initiated, funded, extended, or terminated for social and corporate agendas. For example, the ANA has a PAC to address issues related to the health and nursing workforce, including staffing, mandatory overtime, and supervision and delegation. The pharmaceutical industry also has multiple PACs to lobby Congress.

These focused activities, as well as financial support for and against politicians who have voted or will vote on bills relating to an issue, make PACs some of the most powerful entities influencing health policy decisions, especially those related to regulation and allocation of funds. The large amount of funding used for and against campaigns has changed how legislation is formed, what is passed, and the amount and type of appropriations approved. Legislators are finding it more difficult to meet the needs of one special interest group and not offend another group. For example, when political power shifts in state and federal legislatures, the influence of PACs change. The passage or failure of bills to protect the environment, reauthorize labor union and workers' rights and safety, change gun control, revise tort reform, cut or raise taxes, or increase the minimum wage may depend on which party is in power. One result of legislators trying to remain supportive of their funding sources is that a higher number of bills pass that require additional federal monies or require states to increase dollars allocated to programs or allow elected officials to vote for or against an issue with no simultaneous action. The No Child Left Behind legislation is an example of one unfunded mandate in which federal legislation required action but did not result in federal funding to states.

FINANCING

A major concern over the past two decades has been the influence of money on campaigns, resulting in increased access to legislators and greater influence on legislation by PACs and financial contributors. The Federal Elections Commission (FEC) regulates the type, amount, and reporting of such funds. State commissions handle funds within state, county, and municipal governments. Each candidate, political party, and PAC is required to register and submit quarterly, monthly, or annual financial reports. This is traditionally referred to as *"hard money." "Soft money"* is less regulated and refers to funds given to the party but for no specific purpose. Soft money is often used to support campaign activities but under a different guise. For example, instead of giving money to a senatorial campaign for travel to a state capital, the party supports a high school student workshop on a topic that invokes the candidate's position, thus averting the campaign finance rules constraining usage. Campaign finance reports, as well as documentation of PACs, corporate, and other large contributors to each party and candidate, are required by the FEC and are available to the public (see www.fec.gov). Monies spent on media, travel, and food by campaigns have increased tremendously in the past decade. Many of the organizations noted above—as well as many nurses, doctors, physical therapists, and patients—donated to these campaigns.

In federal campaigns in 2007 and 2008, individual contributions were limited to $2300 per candidate and $28,500 per national party, or a total of $42,700 to all candidates combined and $65,500 to all PACs or committees combined. In contrast, national, state, or local party committee contributions were limited to $5000 per candidate per election, unlimited to political parties yearly, and limited to a maximum of $39,900 to a U.S. Senate candidate per campaign (FEC, 2009a). However, in January 2010, the U.S. Supreme Court ruled that campaign contribution limits were an unconstitutional denial of free speech. It is unclear what effect this will have on future campaign financing.

Many state political contribution limits are similar to national levels or are based on population and candidate numbers each election cycle. In addition to funds raised by candidates, the government provides funds from the taxpayer-supported Presidential Election Campaign Fund (PECF). These monies are designated on federal income tax forms and then distributed to candidates after they raise a specified amount. A cap of $40 million is placed on what can be spent on primaries or preconvention efforts for presidential candidates who choose to accept these funds. In 2008, $103 million in federal funds were used in the presidential primaries and campaign. President (then Senator) Obama chose not to accept federal dollars; Senator McCain "opted in" to the system and received 84 million federal taxpayer dollars (FEC, 2009b). As was true in 2004, both candidates benefited greatly from the amounts the parties or PACS spent on advertisements and other media to support them. Before the 2000 election, the FEC reported that eight candidates for the presidency had raised a total of $181 million (FEC, 2000). In the 2004 election, presidential candidates Kerry and Bush both raised more than $298 million for their respective campaigns, and more than $1 billion was used by parties, candidates, and federal funds combined (FEC, 2005). Similarly, McCain, Obama, their rivals, and political parties raised more than $1.67 billion for the presidential primaries and campaign for the 2008 election (FEC, 2009b). This is more than the initial year of spending for the Medicare Prescription Drug Plan (PDP).

Two new modes of funding appeared in the 2004 presidential campaign. Howard Dean, MD, was the first candidate to formally use the Internet to solicit and receive contributions. Second, a new type of committee called *527 political groups* arose and altered political fundraising and campaign activities. These groups can engage in voter mobilization efforts, issue advocacy, and other activity short of expressly advocating the election or defeat of a federal candidate. There are no limits to how much they can raise. These organizations are regulated by the Internal Revenue Service (IRS), but not necessarily the FEC if they do not explicitly advocate for an individual's election or defeat or do not directly subsidize federal elections. Thus this is a major loophole to raising and using soft money. In the 2004 campaign, these entities ran oppositional, and personal, attacks on candidates. Swift Boat Veterans for Truth, Progress for America, MoveON.org, and Voices for Working Families are just a few of the organizations that provided significant media coverage and had a considerable impact on the election. In 2008, these organizations ran advertisements that showed candidates' positions in a very demonstrative and stark manner. For example, John Kerry was portrayed as unpatriotic even though he volunteered and served in Vietnam. George W. Bush was portrayed as supporting child labor because of the large deficits, even though child labor laws were not changed during his term.

Additionally, lobbyists often provide for expenses incurred in "program-related" trips. These payments have caused scandals for national congressional representatives as well as state legislators and governors in the past decade, resulting in calls for and changes to ethics rules so that all persons have access to legislators regardless of socioeconomic means. The same issue has been found at state levels, and recently some officials have been found criminally responsible for taking bribes or inappropriately using their governmental positions to influence policy based on financial donations and arrangements.

Understanding the Legislative Process

An important process to understand is illustrated in *How Our Laws Are Made* (U.S. House of Representatives, 2003; U.S. Senate, 2003), which explains how a bill proceeds through the U.S. Congress. Steps, processes, facilitators, and barriers to enacting legislation at the federal level from introduction of a bill through its enrollment to the president are detailed (Figure 6-1). This illustration also identifies the House and Senate procedures, including leadership roles and responsibilities, committee assignment, readings on the chamber floor, and resolution between the two chambers. Many of the steps and processes, such as the House "hopper" and the system of bells and lights, originated in the late 19th century. The hopper is the box in which representatives initially place a piece of legislation they wish to be brought to the House for action. A system of bells and lights is in place throughout the Capitol building to notify senators and representatives of pending votes and other actions. Also discussed in this document is how to "bury" or "kill" a bill and how the majority party ideas prevail even in the most sacred workings of our democracy. Many state legislations follow similar protocols and procedures. It is incumbent upon nurses to know the major committees and legislators that deal with health and nursing issues in their own state, as well as the major pitfalls or bridges where nurse and health-focused legislation may be delayed or strengthened. The state nursing association can assist with identifying those persons, committees, barriers, and facilitators.

ADMINISTRATION AND COMMITTEES

In addition to the constitutionally mandated process and structure, each Congress or state legislature establishes its own rules for administration and governance that affect how policies are made and which issues are considered. Rules include the number, type, and focus of committees where most of the legislative work takes place. In fact, committee chairpersons, assigned because of seniority, develop the calendar of issues and legislation to be discussed. In the past, and probably continuing into the future, bills that are brought forth for discussion and passage are not necessarily the purview of the particular committee. Rather, these issues may be germane to the constituents of the ranking majority or minority leader, based on the leader's personal beliefs and experience, or related to financial support received from individuals, organizations, and corporations.

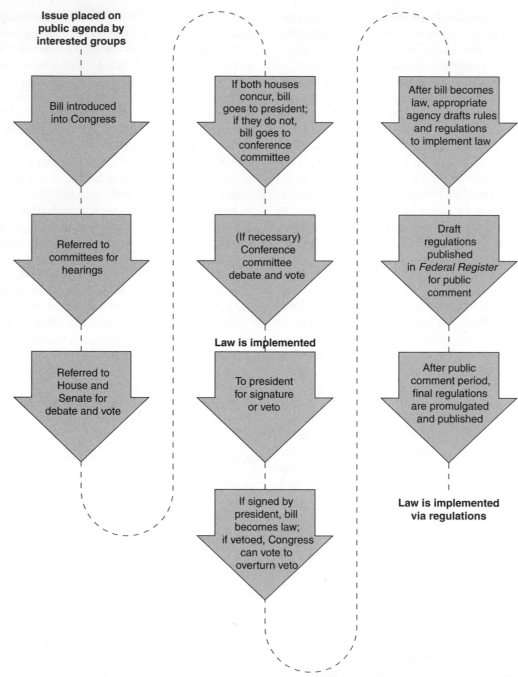

FIGURE 6-1 Formal health care policy process.

Committee structure is also determined for each Congress, with the exception of several mandated committees by U.S. or state constitution. In Congress, committee structure was fairly stable from the 1960s through the early 1990s, years during which the Democrats controlled the House of Representatives and often the Senate. During that time, the Committee on Labor and Human Resources had primary responsibility for health care legislation and issues. With a new Republican majority in the House of Representatives beginning in 1994 and that party's control over the Senate and White House from 2001 to 2008, committee structure was altered and updated. Several committees were terminated, and the names and jurisdictions were changed. A new Health, Education, Labor, and Pensions Committee in the Senate was charged with primary health policy jurisdiction. However, many committees develop health-related bills and send forth authorizations and appropriations for those bills, such as the Senate Agriculture, Nutrition, and Forestry Committee (nutrition bill) and the House International Relations Committee (American Red Cross bill).

CONGRESSIONAL SESSIONS

Each U.S. Congress has two sessions for developing legislation. The 111th Congress began in January 2009 with the first session; the second session began in January 2010. Legislation that has passed both Houses, been resolved in conference committee, been enrolled to the president, and is signed, becomes public law. Laws are signified by the Congress in which they are passed, as well as their chronological order of passage (e.g., PL 110-361: law number 361 passed the 110th Congress). Financial allocations—more precisely, appropriations—are included in bills and usually include funding for 3 to 5 years. However, appropriations depend on the budget bills passed for each calendar year and thus can be revised, reauthorized, or repealed by subsequent congressional action.

CHAMBER RESPONSIBILITIES

A constitutional directive mandates that all budget bills, including an increase in federal income taxes, originate in the U.S. House of Representatives. Thus the Senate cannot initiate an income tax increase, but it can increase spending limits and develop new programs that may result in the need for increased taxes. Either chamber can be the origin of bills that establish or increase funds through other means, such as airport, gasoline, or Medicare fees and taxes. The Ways and Means, Appropriations, and Finance committees have input to the budget and review legislation originating in other committees that require new or continuing appropriations. Any legislation that includes appropriations, whether continuing or new, is required to be submitted by committees and subcommittees to the chamber budget committees for calculation, inclusion in the fiscal year appropriations bills, and estimations of spending in the outlying years. On most occasions the budget committees change or alter the recommended allocations and refer these changes to the committee charged with a specific piece of legislation as well as to the committee of primary responsibility for that specific area (e.g., health care, education, transportation). The Senate has primary responsibility for approval of political appointments, such as judges, ambassadors, the surgeon general, cabinet members, and federal agency directors. In the 1990s the approval hearings were contentiously political and philosophical. Health-related issues such as sexual harassment, sex education, family planning, refugee support, and immigration laws served as litmus tests for appointee approval. Two other health issues, abortion and the death penalty, continue to be major points for discussion that affect health policy and the appointment of judges to state, appellate, and federal courts and the U.S. Supreme Court. More recently, universal health care, terrorism, and environmental issues have resulted in enthusiastic legislative discussions.

STATE ACTIVITIES

Many state legislatures also have two chambers, and leadership is similar to that of the national Congress in that a speaker of the house, a senate majority leader, and party leaders provide day-to-day administration of the legislative body. Chamber and committee leadership is determined by seniority, past party leadership, respective party caucuses, and persons who aspire to the party ideology and philosophy in setting legislative agendas. State legislatures play a large role in the budgetary decisions and health policy and nursing practice, including

Medicaid services, health department auspices, certification of hospitals and nursing homes, and nursing licensure and prescriptive privileges within the state. Many state constitutions require a balanced budget submitted by the governor and approved by the legislature. Thus, even in states, health programs and nursing services can be advanced or be in jeopardy depending on annual budgetary decisions. Several states have instituted lotteries or video gambling to increase revenues directly tied to education or specific health programs. Public health initiatives, such as adolescent tobacco use reduction, drunk driving prevention, and school health programs, may be funded with these nonrecurring funds. Public education may also be supported by this type of fund or by recurring income tax funds. In that case, state-supported community colleges, universities, and public schools (e.g., medical, nursing, pharmacy) can increase enrollment and faculty or offer more online and alternate-schedule courses. Similarly, hospitals and health departments are supported by state and local allocations that affect bed capacity, working environment, salaries, and services provided.

State legislation also may include mandated overtime or nurse staffing levels in health care facilities. Most recently, states have passed bills that do not allow mandatory overtime for nurses. Another route to the same result is for nursing boards or other licensing boards to develop regulations concerning appropriate and safe working hours or limitations on overtime. Approximately one third of states have such statutes. This is where nurses can actively participate in the policy decisions to ensure a quality working situation and maximal patient safety and care. The ANA National Database of Nursing Quality Indicators (NDNQI) and Safe Staffing Saves Lives (SSSL) Initiatives, as well as research by Peter Buerhaus, Linda Aiken, and Susan Letvak and their colleagues, provide a foundation for those efforts.

Budget Process

APPROPRIATION OF FUNDS

Appropriation bills are required to approve funding for running the federal government each fiscal year (October 1 to September 30). Bills, which represent spending by each cabinet department (e.g., Treasury, Labor, Commerce, Health and Human Services, Defense), require congressional approval and presidential signature no later than the beginning of each fiscal year. Near the end of each congressional session, appropriation bills often are combined into one general appropriation bill, which before 1997 was called the *Omnibus Budget Reconciliation Act* (OBRA) and is now known as the *Consolidated Budget Resolution.* In the early 2000s, legislation titles began to be focused on social or financial priorities, such as the Taxpayer Relief Act. Specific bills for the 15 cabinet-level governmental agencies are also titled—for instance, the Homeland Security Act.

Through the president's proposed budget, with input from the Administration's Office on Management and Budget (OMB), this process begins in Congress. After consideration of the proposed budget submitted by the White House, each chamber develops a budget resolution bill by April of each year. Additionally, all legislation under consideration that includes funding recommendations or appropriations is required to be submitted by committees to the Congressional Budget Office (CBO). The CBO reviews and calculates the actual costs to the federal government and considers how a particular appropriation fits into the proposed budget or *reconciliation bill.* One important issue at both state and federal levels is that revenue and expenditure estimates by varying interested parties are calculated with similar factors such as inflation, economic growth, gross domestic product, and consumer price index.

In the late 20th and early 21st centuries, state and federal budgets often were achieved through crisis management. This may have been due to a lack of clarity about legislation, large amounts of legislation to consider and act on, political strife, or budget shortfalls or surpluses. For example, in the late 1990s, disagreements and animosity caused a delay in the mandated federal budget approval in Congress. The lack of approval for a reconciliation or consolidation bill caused the federal government to shut down on more than one occasion. This type of crisis management resulted in special amendments being added to bills at the "eleventh hour" in order to convince certain representatives and senators to agree to vote for the final bill. This deal-making and *"pork barrel"* special interest spending added to what may have been appropriate legislation and allocations in an earlier version of a bill. Many bills were delayed in the early 2000s primarily because of discussions regarding terrorism funding or major disagreements on appropriations. As recently as October 2008, the president signed a continuing resolution (PL. 110-329), which was necessary to keep the government running.

Another type of spending, *emergency spending,* may not be included in the fiscal year reconciliation bill but can be approved through supplemental appropriation bills. For example, after Hurricane Floyd in 1999, Hurricane Ivan in 2004, Hurricane Katrina in 2005, and the terrorist attacks on September 11, 2001, special funds and Federal Emergency Management Agency increases were approved to provide disaster relief. Since 2004, multiple *supplemental bills* have been passed to increase homeland security (Transportation Safety Administration) and defense spending (the war in Iraq) or to deal with other expenses not approved through the traditional congressional budget processes. This is less likely at the state level because of balanced budget statutes.

AUTHORIZATION OF PROGRAMS

Authorization bills/reauthorization (with funding requests) are required to establish or continue programs as well as to fund those mandates. The initial authorization is usually a separate bill named for the issue or program being established—for example, the Older Americans Act, the Ryan White AIDS Act, and the Public Health Service Act. New governmental agencies may be initiated or established, as was the case with the Administration on Aging in 1965 and the Department of Homeland Security (DHS) in 2002. Future authorization and reauthorization bills are required to make changes in governmental agencies, to expand programs, and to continue or alter funding levels. However, some authorization bills that are passed do not contain any funding levels. Rather, these bills are used to establish programs that are to be funded by governmental departments within present allocations or by individual states, or they are *unfunded mandates.* For example, the Brady Bill gun control legislation requires background checks on gun purchasers before a license is issued. This 1993 act was named after James Brady, who was shot during an attempted assassination of President Reagan in 1981. Brady was paralyzed. The federal law contained no continuing funds; thus states must provide funds or be in violation of the law, and as a result often suffer loss of government monies for law enforcement. The No Child Left Behind bill is similar in federal mandate and state funding. Some authorization bills purposely contain no funding recommendations so that members of Congress can support the issue without providing funding. The congressional decision is unfunded (the actual bill has no funding) or underfunded. The regulatory body may not be provided funding to oversee state implementation of the act. Mandating the Culturally and Linguistically Appropriate Services (CLAS) standards is another example where a federal law required states to implement statutes with little or no funding provided.

FISCAL RESPONSIBILITY

Several efforts were made in previous decades to mandate a balanced budget at the federal level. The Gramm-Rudman-Hollings law was passed in 1985 (PL 99-177), but the U.S. Supreme Court subsequently found this law to be unconstitutional. During the 104th Congress, a major effort by the newly Republican-controlled House of Representatives was launched to pass an amendment to the U.S. Constitution to require a balanced federal budget. This attempt failed in Congress; thus citizens did not vote on the constitutional amendment. Congress passed a Balanced Budget Act in 1997, which required a balance of expected revenues and expenditures by the federal government for the 1998 fiscal year. The next year, Congress passed the Taxpayer Relief Act of 1998 as the reconciliation bill that included additional childcare exemptions and capital gains tax reform. In 1999, the reconciliation bill was the Taxpayer Refund and Relief Act. Although it passed both chambers of Congress, President Clinton vetoed the bill. Similar actions occurred with President Bush and the 110th Congress.

Appropriation or budget bills are required for the functioning of the federal government or other legislation, and thus specialized "pet" programs are often attached to the budget bills to get them enacted. For example, several times the Nurse Education Act's appropriation bills were tacked on to the budget to ensure that they were passed during that fiscal year before Congress adjourned. Much of the time, *pork-barrel* amendments are approved to gain the votes of specific members of Congress. Even though the spending will benefit constituencies, the programs often are not federal mandates or related to the responsibilities of the government. Because many of these amendments are added at the eleventh hour and at times in conference committee to resolve the House and Senate differences, the public and some legislators are often not aware of these expenditures until they have been approved. The president does not have *line-item veto authority* and therefore must accept or veto each appropriation bill in its entirety to enact the fiscal year budget. Similar actions occur in state legislatures for appropriation bills for services such as museums, bypass highways, and new post offices.

ECONOMICS

A majority of the budget for the U.S. Department of Health and Human Services (USDHHS) is for *entitlement programs,* which means that only a third or less of the amount appropriated by Congress for this department can be controlled or used in discretionary ways. The NIH, the Centers for Medicare and Medicaid Services (CMS), and the Bureau of Health Professions (BHP) are included in the USDHHS budget. Nursing leaders and others have continually worked to increase these budgets, and these efforts resulted in budget increases during the late 1990s and early 2000s. More recently, those appropriations have been more stagnated. In calendar year 2008, CMS expenditures totaled more than $556.7 billion, with federal Medicaid obligations totaling $267 billion and federal Medicare obligations totaling $283 billion (CMS, 2008). The NIH fiscal year 2008 budget was $27.8 billion, and the National Institute of Nursing Research (NINR) budget was $134.7 million (NIH, 2008). Overall health care spending grew 6.1% from 2006 to 2007, averaging $7421 per person. The health care portion of the gross domestic product (GDP) increased from 16% to 16.2%

(Hartman et al., 2009) This is the slowest growth in 10 years, but hospital care still provided for a third of all expenditures. Various agency heads make budget requests to congressional committees each year through letters, hearings, and routine budgetary processes.

In 1999, a federal surplus of $170 billion resulted from a thriving economy, a leaner governmental structure, and the Balanced Budget Act of 1997. However, Congress has been borrowing from the Social Security Trust Fund since the early 1980s to meet annual operating costs and appropriations across the government. The retirement income and Medicare programs that are funded by current worker payroll taxes do not contain enough money to fund those same workers when they reach 65 years of age. The General Accounting Office (GAO) estimates that the Social Security (SS) Trust Fund will be unable to meet its obligations starting in the year 2040. Debate continues over how a government with a large national debt and a large tax base can best serve its citizens, given the promises made to citizens regarding retirement and health insurance in old age. In 2005, major efforts were proposed to change SS through decreased benefits to younger workers, initiation of private health savings accounts, gradually increasing the salary cap for paying SS taxes, and a means-tested eligibility for full benefits. Some of these passed, but not much change resulted for the long-term commitment of the fund. The financial crisis of 2008 may require the 111th Congress to revise both SS retirement income and Medicare. State legislators also must deal with budget shortfalls and use hiring freezes, layoffs, program cuts, new fees, and increased taxes to meet needs. Local agencies and school boards are often the most successful in dealing with budget shortfalls because they have not had—or have not chosen to use—the ability to borrow funds, incur long-term debt, or move costs from one budget year to another. More detail on the budget and health care costs can be found in Chapter 7.

Health Programs

Two main types of federal health care programs exist, discretionary and entitlement. *Discretionary programs* are subject to annual appropriations by Congress and are considered controllable budgetary items. For this discussion, these programs primarily consist of categorical health services, training, and research programs. Categorical health services are services for somewhat narrowly defined categories of problems, such as programs for communicable diseases and family planning services. An example of a training program is the Nurse Reinvestment Act (PL 107-205), and an example of a research program is the NINR at the National Institutes of Health.

Entitlements are those health care programs in which budgetary expenses are more difficult to control. Citizens who benefit from these programs are "entitled" to the benefits by law because of a specified age, disability, economic status, or prepayment. The federal government is obligated to pay these benefits regardless of the number of enrollees or the costs. The only major avenue to cut costs is by changing either the authorization or eligibility criteria through legislation. Costs cannot be limited by appropriating less money for expenditures. Social Security, veterans' compensation, and pensions are examples of income entitlement programs. Health care entitlement programs are Medicare, Medicaid, and State Children's Health Insurance Programs.

The enactment of the Social Security Act in 1935 marked the first major act of government involvement in health. The act provides federal grants to the states for public health; maternal and child health; services for disabled children; and public assistance for the aged, blind, and families with dependent children. The role of the federal government in the provision of health care was expanded with the 1965 passage of Title XVIII and XIX amendments to the Social Security Act, creating Medicare and Medicaid. These two programs have changed the face of health care and continue to have a large role in the provision of health care services. The addition of disabled persons and those with end-stage renal disease to Medicare in the 1970s increased costs and care. In 1997, Title XXI, the State Children's Health Insurance Program, was added, which dramatically increased the number of children now covered by federal and state legislations and budgets. Much of the discussion in the 105th through the 110th Congresses was related to how to deal with the increasing costs for these entitlement programs as well

as to propose strategies for reforming the programs. The 111th Congress will be faced with more revisions as a result of the significant financial declines in 2008. Medicare and Social Security are major entitlements, but because they affect more than half of Americans, decisions for revision are difficult.

IMPLEMENTATION AND REGULATION

Multiple governmental agencies plan, implement, and evaluate health policy in the United States. The major agencies are headed by political appointment cabinet officials, directors, and administrators but are staffed by career civil servants. For example, the U.S. House of Representatives has 435 elected members, but 10,000 staff members are employed for duties such as cleaning, moving, painting, preparing and serving food, providing mail and phone services, and staffing the infirmary. Congressional legislation and presidential executive orders and mandates can alter workings across staff divisions of the executive, judicial, and legislative branches of government. The last major revisions occurred in 1996 after the Republican Congress and the Democratic vice president requested and mandated streamlining and reorganization of the government. The Balanced Budget Act of 1997 also mandated changes in the administration and implementation of federal programs. Before the 1990s most federal departments or regulatory oversight had changed very little. The Government Performance and Results Act of 1993 was a major effort to enhance accountability of agencies. The Federal Funding Accountability and Transparency Act of 2006, signed by President Bush, was another attempt to clarify governmental action and spending to the public. Several years passed, however, before actual changes occurred. In the 110th Congress, Senator Obama introduced a revision titled the Strengthening Transparency and Accountability in Federal Spending Act of 2008, but the bill died when that congressional session ended.

The USDHHS is charged with protecting and ensuring the health of the nation and is headed by the Secretary of Health. Multiple agencies and divisions are included in the USDHHS, and several assistant secretaries are responsible for administrative aspects. The Surgeon General (SG) is an Assistant Secretary of Health and heads the Office of Public Health and Science (OPHS). An Assistant Secretary for Aging heads the Administration on Aging (AOA) and the Administration for Children and Families (ACF). Other agencies are headed by a commissioner (e.g., FDA) or director (e.g., NIH). Agencies include several sections or divisions. For example, the NIH has 27 institutes or centers, including the NINR, the Eunice Kennedy Shriver National Institute for Child Health and Human Development (NICHD), and the National Institute on Mental Health (NIMH). In Atlanta and other regional offices, the Centers for Disease Control and Prevention (CDC) houses 14 centers, institutes, and offices, including the National Center for Chronic Disease Prevention and Health Promotion (NCCD-PHP), the National Office of Public Health Genomics (NOPHG), the National Center for Health Statistics (NCHS), and the Coordinating Office for Terrorism Preparedness and Emergency Response (COTPER) (CDC, 2009). Most federal government agencies and state agencies have civil rights, legal, public relations, and budget sections staffed by career employees. These agencies have public Internet sites for consumers and professionals to obtain program and contact information. Many political, professional, and health-related agencies and organizations also house websites for rapid and wide public access and dissemination of information.

Each federal agency has specific auspices or sponsorship, although these are not always consistent with the appropriation focus. The Department of Agriculture (DA) directs the commodity distribution program (e.g., nonfat dry milk, cheese products), the national school lunch program, farm programs, and food inspection. CMS directs Medicare, Medicaid, and Children's Health Insurance Programs; the Department of Labor houses the Occupational Safety and Health Administration (OSHA); and the CDC houses the National Institute of Occupational Safety and Health (NIOSH). Most states have similar agencies and auspices to manage public programs. For example, the Tennessee Department of Health (TDH) houses the Tennessee Bureau of TennCare (TBOT) to administer the Medicaid waiver program, and Kansas has a State Secretary for Social and Rehabilitation Services (SRS).

Whereas laws are written in broad language, the *rules and regulations* to implement these laws are very specific and often can be revised without changing the original law. Agencies are charged with implementation, financial oversight, legislative interpretation, and the development of regulations and rules governing their respective programs. Often agencies are required to interpret the purpose and intent of congressional or state legislation to implement such laws. The perceptions, political savvy, and experiences of the agency's director, staff, and proponents have an impact on this interpretation of the issue under consideration. For example, former USDHHS Secretary Tommy Thompson reworded family planning regulations to include abstinence-only programs, President Clinton used presidential directives for regulations to allow stem cell research on embryos not used by couples who went through in vitro fertilization procedures, and President Bush wrote executive orders to allow only currently available stem cell lines to be used rather than new embryonic lines. Interpretations and changes in regulations can be related to the number and types of citizens served in a particular program, the increase or decrease in appropriations, the social or ethical values of directors and department heads, and societal crises.

In some instances, the auspices and appropriations are not consistent. The DA receives appropriations for the elder nutrition programs, but these are administered under the AOA through the state, regional, and local agencies. The Department of Labor (DL) has administrative responsibility for the Senior Community Service Employment Program (SCSEP), which is under the auspices of the AOA. The Bureau of Census (BOC) collects vital data, but the NCHS and the DL analyze those data for developing policy and allocation decisions. Thus some health-related policy legislation and appropriations require extra effort to determine the auspices, regulation, and implementation and whether duplication or omission occurs.

As the health care industry evolves with new emphases, programs, and services, the governmental agencies must develop new strategies for evaluation of their implementation. Evaluation for specific policies and their implementation only recently began at the federal level. This evaluation of process, structure, and outcomes has become an emphasis, especially for the SS, Medicare, and Medicaid programs. Process and structure are often difficult to change in large, bureaucratic organizations of state and federal government. Annual performance plans now required of agencies should assist in more clearly evaluating program effectiveness and efficiency. The recent emphasis on outcomes should lead to changes in process and structure to meet the objectives set forth. Two such health-related efforts are the *Healthy People 2010* and proposed 2020 national objectives and the initiatives to eliminate racial and ethnic disparities at the USDHHS. As these two efforts are revised to reflect new targets and new census health data, they will guide federal, state and local efforts to improve the health of our community through system, policy, and funding decisions. Nursing has a vested interest in those efforts.

Leadership

During the 20th century, several persons and organizations provided leadership to ensure the passage of major health policies and regulation. Surgeon Generals C. Everett Koop, Jocelyn Elders, and David Satcher have supported efforts to deal with chronic diseases, prevent and reduce health risks through education, and target efforts based on *Healthy People* initiatives. Dr. Richard H. Carmona (formerly a nurse), who served as Surgeon General from 2002 to 2006, was a less visible leader partially because of the focus on bioterrorism and the overshadowing of the White House leadership related to stem cell research and abstinence education. There was no Surgeon General from 2006 to 2008, although Steven K. Galson served as Acting Surgeon General for part of that period. David Kessler, Commissioner of the FDA from 1990 to 1997, worked to protect consumers through regulation of nutritional and dietary supplements. He also argued for regulation of tobacco. The Tobacco Master Settlement Agreement was reached in 1998 within the Justice Department between the four largest tobacco companies and 46 state attorneys general, but not under the purview of the FDA. The lawsuit was brought by state departments of justice suing for repayment of public dollars (Medicare and Medicaid) spent on providing health

care to those with tobacco-related illnesses. The $360 billion settlement agreed to by the tobacco industry is to be paid over a 25-year period. Activities associated with the agreement were the termination of soliciting adolescent smokers, bans on tobacco advertisements within specific distances of schools, and further supplementation of education and prevention programs across the country. However, money in most states is not being used for the purposes noted. This is an example of the judicial branch of government playing a role in health policy and planning. Another highly visible leader in health care regulation was Dr. Julie Gerberding, former director of CDC, from 2002 to 2009, whose tenure was marked by multiple national occurrences of food-borne illnesses.

LEGISLATORS

Senators Edward Kennedy (D-Mass.), Barbara Mikulski (D-Md.), Paul Simon (D-Ill.), and Nancy Kassenbaum (R-Kan.) led health-related legislative efforts during the 1980s, 1990s, and early 2000s in the U.S. Senate. In the House of Representatives, efforts were led by Henry Waxman (D-Wisc.), John Lewis, (D-Ga.), Joseph Kennedy (D-Mass.), and Lois Capps (D-Calif.). Legislative efforts during this time were focused on programs for *vulnerable populations* such as children, the elderly, and low-income persons, as well as appropriations for new and continuing programs. During 1999, Senators John Breaux (D-La.) and Bill Frist (R-Tenn.), a heart surgeon, headed the National Bipartisan Commission on the Future of Medicare. Additional health policy efforts in early 2000 were related to managed care (both private and public sector) and consumer rights regarding their health care coverage, use of personal information, the Health Insurance Portability and Accountability Act (HIPAA), and competency of providers. The issues of medical liability and welfare reform were led by Republicans in the House of Representatives and passed in 2003 and 2005. In 2007, Senator Brownback led efforts to develop electronic medical records (EMR) and Senator Akaka worked to block the establishment of electronic records unless privacy could be ensured. In 2008, Medicare, Medicaid, and the Children's Health Insurance Program (CHIP) were a major focus by both parties, with Senators Edward

Kennedy and Hillary Clinton and minority whip James Clyburn in the House leading the efforts. In January 2009, the 111th Congress passed new State Children's Health Insurance Program (SCHIP) legislation that expanded coverage. Also during the 110th Congress, Senators Brownback (R-Kan.), Casey (D-Pa.), Inhofe (R-Okla.), Spector (R-Pa.), and Coleman (R-Minn.), along with Representative Watson (D-Calif.), introduced the compassionate care ACCESS Act to provide for physician and patient FDA options for experimental treatments. Most recently, Senators Mikulski and Collins (R-Me.) and Representative Capps (D-Calif.) are leading supporters of increasing Nursing Workforce Development funds. Representative Lois Capps (a nurse) led the initial Nurse Reinvestment Act effort in 2002 and continues to work with colleagues in both chambers to ensure funding.

NURSES

Many nurses have provided leadership at the national level to contribute to health policy and to ensure that its influence on nursing is positive. Former ANA presidents Virginia Trotter Betts and Beverly Malone were instrumental in setting the original Nursing's Agenda for Health Care Reform (NAHCR). These two nurses also assisted the ANA Council on Practice and various professional practice organizations to promote the passage of third-party reimbursement changes for advanced practice nurses, accreditation of home health agencies, and provision of childhood immunizations. Betts and Malone later were appointed Assistant Secretaries of Health at USDHHS. Debbie Gettis, a registered professional nurse, served as the AIDS advisor to President Clinton. Dorothy Brooten, a nurse researcher, was elected in 1991 to the Institute of Medicine (IOM), which advises Congress on health matters. In 1987 Ada Sue Hinshaw was appointed the first director of the National Center for Nursing Research (NCNR). The present director of NINR, Patricia Grady, is a nurse who has a background in basic sciences, which she has used to develop collaborative agendas with other institutes in the areas of genetics, psychoneuroimmunology, chronic diseases, mental health, and aging. Nancy Bergstrom and Thelma Wells have provided leadership in the development of guidelines for practice for the Agency for Healthcare Research and Quality (AHRQ, formerly the AHCPR), and Nancy Fugate-Woods and Ora Strickland have spearheaded a national focus on women's health. Peter Buerhaus (an economist), Cheryl Jones, and Linda Moody have served as scientists at the national level to develop recommendations and projections for nursing workforce, staffing, and economic needs. Janet Allan, Lucy Marion, and Carol Loveland-Cherry have served on the U.S. Preventive Services Task Force, and Audrey Nelson has led patient safety and quality of care efforts at the Department of Veterans Affairs (DVA).

THINK TANKS, FOUNDATIONS, AND ORGANIZATIONS

Other sources of health policy and planning encompass private or public "think tanks," philanthropic foundations, and policy centers that directly affect nursing. Several large foundations, such as the IOM, the Robert Wood Johnson Foundation (RWJF), and the Pew Charitable Trusts (PCT), play an important role in policy planning and evaluation. The PCT provides grants for health care demonstration and research activities and supports studies of the health care industry. One example is the Pew Health Professions Commission (PHPC), formed to study the future needs of the health care system in the United States. Multiple reports have been issued by this commission (O'Neil, 1993; O'Neil & PHPC, 1998; PHPC, 1995). These reports delineate the nature of health care work, the restructuring of health care professional regulation, the number and types of professionals needed, and the training and education of professionals. Much of the discussion is, by necessity, in the context of an evolving health care system with dynamics not yet known. Although widely heralded, the commission's recommendations are slowly being enacted. The RWJF funds large demonstration projects to address varying health issues and populations. Priorities are reset every few years. In 2010 the RWJF will fund the Initiative on the Future of Nursing, Nurse Faculty Scholars, New Careers in Nursing Scholarship Program, the Interdisciplinary Nursing Quality Research Initiative (INQRI), Disparities Research for Change, and Public Health Law Research.

Nursing

Nursing currently has three main issues. First are the workforce needs; that is, the qualifications and types of roles nurses will be required to fill. The American Association of Colleges of Nursing (AACN) and the PHPC recommends an increase in the number of registered nurses at the baccalaureate level and advanced practice nurses with master's-level preparation (AACN, 2008c). A second issue is that of programs for nurse educators at the doctoral level to prepare nurses for the workforce needs. Although many doctoral programs have opened in the past three decades, the number of doctoral-prepared nurse educators available for appropriate training and education of the projected workforce has not kept pace with market need (AACN, 2000b). This lag can be attributed partly to the large number of nurses retiring in the early 2000s and partly to a lack of incentives to stay in public-sector rather than private-sector positions. A third nursing issue is that of competency-based education and practice, in which nurses demonstrate critical thinking, judgment and decision-making skills, and cultural competence and engage in transdisciplinary practice. Curricular, regulation, and certification changes have been implemented. In the mid-1990s, the National League for Nursing Accreditation Commission (NLNAC) for baccalaureate and master's degree programs placed an increased emphasis on critical thinking and community-based care. The AACN, in 1998 and 2008, put forth revised essentials of baccalaureate and master's degree education, which include health care delivery, ethics, and competency-based education. The Commission on Collegiate Nursing Education (CCNE) and NLNAC (the professional accreditation bodies) required that undergraduate programs target their mission to local and regional health rather than taking a "cookie cutter" approach to curriculum. Master's programs were standardized for clinical and role competence, as well as mastery of the health care delivery system and economic knowledge and skills. This standardization has resulted in an increase in nurses with specialty certification. The American Association of Critical-Care Nurses (AACCN), the Association for Women's Health (AWH), Obstetrical and Neonatal Nursing (ONN), and the Oncology Nursing Society (ONS) offer certification for masters-prepared nurses. The American Nurses Credentialing Center (ANCC) provides both specialty role (e.g., case management, nurse practitioner, clinical specialist) and population (e.g., psychiatric mental health, adult, pediatric) certifications.

Several other organizations have a major impact on health policy and nursing. The IOM, one of the National Academies of Science (NAS), advises Congress on health matters through position papers, expert witnesses, and recommendations for legislative initiation, approval, and funding. The IOM is often involved in discussions of, and decisions for, auspices and allocations for the Division of Nursing and nurse education acts in Congress. In fact, the Higher Education Opportunity Act of 2008 (PL 110-803) requires the USDHHS secretary to negotiate with the IOM to conduct a study on the capacity of nursing schools to meet the needs of the nation.

The American Public Health Association (APHA), the AMA, the ANA, and the American Dental Association (ADA) all provide expert testimony to state and federal agencies and decision-making bodies on topics from product development and liability to school lunch programs, immunizations, disaster relief, and bioterrorism.

Health Policies

Health policies, or decisions regarding the health care system, are developed and implemented through several avenues. Congressional and state legislation; federal, state, and local rules and regulations for agencies; and appropriation decisions are methods to develop health policy. Some health policies are reached only through legislation, whereas others are developed by multiple avenues. All these avenues are affected by public opinion, the economy, societal demographics, professional expertise, technology, and knowledge about health.

HEALTH POLICIES BEFORE 1990

Three of the most influential health policies have been the Social Security Act of 1935 and the amendments that established Medicare and Medicaid in 1965.

Many of our national concerns with health and welfare have been addressed by amendments to these policies. Issues such as abortion, family planning, nutrition, and disability, as well as those related to *vulnerable populations* (the chronically ill, mentally ill, elderly, poor, and minorities), are included as major concerns and foci of programs and payments. These are also the largest programs in terms of population covered and dollars spent. With the aging of the population, technological and pharmaceutical advances, and changes in the racial/ethnic face of society, the original intent and expected costs of these programs have been far exceeded. A major issue today is how to continue these programs as a *safety net* for society. Many bills and acts have been passed that directly and indirectly affect the health of society (Table 6-1). In the 1960s the Hill-Burton Act funded hospital construction. Legislation for payment to nurses was included in the Rural Health Clinics Act of 1977 and extended with OBRA of 1989. In the 1970s and 1980s increased emphasis was placed on disease prevention, risk reduction, and research on the leading causes of death (cardiovascular disease, cancer). OBRA of 1982 established the diagnostic-related groups (DRGs), which resulted in a prospective payment system (PPS) for Medicare hospitalization. Legislation regarding mental health, school lunch programs, disease research, rural manpower, and end-stage renal disease and disability were added

TABLE 6-1	Selected Polices Affecting Nursing and Health Care Before 1990	
Year	**Title**	**Content/Purpose**
1935	Social Security Act (SSA)	Established the Social Security Administration and pension income
1938	Food, Drug, and Cosmetics Act	Provisions of safe and effective drugs through labeling; 1984 amendments applied to generic drugs
1941	Nurse Training Appropriations	Established to assist nursing schools in increasing enrollments and improving programs
1944	Public Health Service Act	Established the U.S. Public Health Service under one statute (Title 42, U.S. Code)
1964	Nurse Training Act	Initial federal act for professional nurse training
1965	Medicare (SSA amendment) Medicaid (SSA amendment)	Established health coverage for the elderly Established health coverage for the indigent
1965	Older Americans Act	Established the Administration on Aging, which provides a broad network of services to elders
1970	Title X Public Health Service Act	Established family planning grant programs aimed at low-income women
1973	Health Maintenance Organization Act	Established alternative to fee-for-service for government-subsidized employers
1982	Omnibus Budget Reconciliation Act (OBRA)	Added the prospective payment system (diagnosis-related groups) to Medicare hospital admission payment
1986	Protection and advocacy of Mental Health Illness Act	Established agencies to investigate and pursue legal action against abuse and neglect of persons with mental illness
1987	Nursing Home Reform Act (OBRA)	Standardized the types of services nursing homes must provide; established standards of quality and patients' rights
1989	Amendments to Nursing Home Reform Act	Allowed nurse practitioner/clinical nurse specialist to certify need for nursing homes
1989	OBRA	Medicaid direct payment for pediatric and family nurse practitioners

to Medicare eligibility. The 1987 OBRA (PL 101-203) changed Medicare payments to hospitals, altered health maintenance organization (HMO) requirements, and authorized nurse practitioners and clinical nurse specialists to certify patient needs for nursing home care.

HEALTH POLICIES 1990 TO 2000

The 1990s have perhaps been the most prolific decade for health policy reform and regulation for specific diseases, conditions, and vulnerable groups (Table 6-2). The Patient Self-Determination Act allowed persons

TABLE 6-2	Selected Polices Affecting Health and Nursing Passed from 1990 to 2000	
Year	**Title**	**Content/Purpose**
1990	Patient Self-Determination Act (PL 101-508)	Required all Medicare/Medicaid-paid health care institutions to provide or ask for advance directives
1990	Occupational Safety and Health Act, amended (PL 101-552)	Describes general working conditions, guidelines for handling blood and body fluids, prevention of infectious disease, and biohazard waste disposal
1990	Trauma Care Systems Planning and Development Act (PL 101-590)	Established guidelines for trauma care services; replaced 1973 Emergency Medical Services Act
1990	Americans with Disabilities Act (PL 101-336)	Prohibits discrimination against persons with disabilities in five specific areas
1992	Breast and Cervical Cancer Mortality Prevention Act (PL 101-354)	Provides grants to states for screening, referrals, educational programs, training, quality assurance programs, and research
1992	Mammography Quality Standards Act (PL 102-539)	Requires certification, accreditation, and inspection of centers, including equipment, technicians, and records
1993	Family and Medical Leave Act (PL 103-3)	Establishes leave (job security) for employees caring for an ill child or family member, experiencing childbirth or adoption, or experiencing own illness
1996	Welfare Reform Act (PL 104-93)	Limits adults to 5 years on welfare; must work within 2 years
1996	Health Insurance Portability and Accountability Act (PL 104-191)	Provides for portability when changing jobs, limits preexisting conditions, requires congressional reports to evaluate the impact
1996	Newborn's and Mother's Health Protection Act (PL 104-326)	Mandates medical decision for minimum 48-hour stay after delivery; *provider* includes midwife and nurse practitioner
1997	Balanced Budget Act (PL 105-33)	Medicare direct payment to advanced practice nurses; Children's Health Insurance program; welfare-to-work
1998	Health Professions Education and Partnership Act (PL 105-392)	Consolidated health professions education and training as well as minority health education and training; nursing education funding
1999	Healthcare Research and Quality Act (PL 106-129)	Changed name of Agency for Health Care Policy and Research (AHCPR) to Agency for Healthcare Research and Quality (AHRQ); mandates and funds quality and outcomes research
2000	Minority Health and Health Disparities Research and Education Act (PL 106-525)	Established the National Center on Minority Health and Health Disparities at NIH

to make decisions regarding their own health care. The Ryan White Act was passed to deal with issues related to HIV and AIDS. New NIH guidelines for inclusion of women and children in research altered past trends, the use of past findings, and subsequent health policies. As the number of homeless persons increased, private and public sectors had difficulty dealing with the costs and spectrum of services, and the McKinney Homelessness Act was passed with both funded and unfunded mandates. The Americans with Disabilities Act has affected health care as well as work and practice environments and the justice system.

Major changes in Medicaid occurred in 1996 with passage of the Personal Responsibility and Work Opportunities Act (Welfare) and Temporary Assistance to Needy Families, which replaced Aid to Families with Dependent Children. The 1997 Balanced Budget Act included SCHIP in the form of block grants to states to provide health care coverage to more low-income children. However, reports indicated that many children remained uncovered, resulting in the subsequent passage of the Children's Health Insurance Program Reauthorization Act (CHIPRA) in 2009.

Policies and new regulations in the 1990s also affected nurses and other health care workers. Parenting and caregiving concerns resulted in the Family and Medical Leave Act. Occupational Safety and Health Administration guidelines were developed regarding work-at-home employees. Reauthorization of programs and allocations for older Americans, children, and indigent care each year also have an impact on nursing and health care. The Health Professions Education Partnerships Act included the Nursing Education and Practice Improvement Act, which established the National Advisory Council on Nurse Education and Practice (NACNEP) workforce needs. A major purpose of the Health Professions Education Partnerships Act was to consolidate health profession education, training, recruitment of minorities, and rural placements. Additionally, Health Care Financing Administration/CMS regulations were revised during the latter part of 1998 and 1999, which changed payment, diagnostic capabilities, and reimbursement for advanced practice nurses as a result of federal legislation. In 2000 the National Center on Minority Health and Health Disparities (NCMHD) was established as part of the NIH.

HEALTH POLICIES 2001 TO PRESENT

Many new policies initiate, establish, or reauthorize nursing and health issues. The Nurse Reinvestment Act, the Medicare Prescription Drug Improvement and Modernization Act, and the Veterans' Health Care Authorization Act (Table 6-3) are such policies. The Medicare Modernization Act is an attempt to provide relief from high-cost prescriptions for the elderly and disabled (CMS, 2005a, 2005b). Drug discount cards were distributed to qualified elderly and disabled persons to be used beginning in January 2006. As of January 2008, 39.6 million Medicare beneficiaries received Part D coverage, with another 6 million eligible (www. cms.hhs.gov/PrescriptionDrugCovGenIn), and more than 90% of persons in Part D had a prescription filled (CMS, 2008, 2009). Consumers and vendors can update or change plans each year. For example, CMS reported that the computation of the drug costs versus administrative fees is changing as a result of the Medicare Improvements for Patients and Providers Act (MIPPA) of 2008. The cost of this law is continually being updated.

Mental health coverage has grown steadily over the past 15 years, culminating in the Paul Wellstone Mental Health and Addiction Equity Act of 2007 (PL 110-343). Politics was a factor even with this legislation, as it was tacked on to the Emergency Economic Stabilization Act of 2008 (which provided for the Troubled Asset Relief Program, or TARP). The growth of genomic medicine and the privacy issues regarding genetic information resulted in the Genetic Information Nondiscrimination Act of 2008 (PL 110-233), which prohibits discrimination or categorization of applicants or employees based on that information and mandates that genetic information be treated as confidential medical information.

MANAGED CARE

The rise in health care costs has contributed to the rise of managed care organizations and more policy focused on health care costs over the past three

TABLE 6-3	Selected Polices Affecting Health and Nursing Passed from 2001 to Present	
Year	**Title**	**Content/Purpose**
2003	Nurse Reinvestment Act (PL 107-205)	Provides funding for nurse recruitment, retention, education, and care for special populations and underserved areas
2003	Medicare Modernization Act (PL 108-173)	Provides prescription drug benefit (Part D); enhances new Medicare Advantage regional health plan choices (Part C)
2004	Asthmatic Schoolchildren's Treatment and Health Management Act (PL 108-377)	Rewards states that require schools to allow students to self-administer medications for asthma or anaphylaxis
2007	Paul Wellstone Mental Health and Addiction Equity Act (PL 110-343)	Requires equity in the provision of mental health and substance-related disorder benefits under group health
2007	Food and Drug Administration Amendments Act (PL 110-85)	Extends the user-fee programs for prescription drugs and medical devices; enhances the postmarket authorities of the FDA with respect to the safety of drugs
2007	Conquer Childhood Cancer Act (PL 110-285)	Amends the Public Health Service Act to advance medical research and treatments into pediatric cancers; ensures patients and families have access to the current treatments and information regarding pediatric cancers
2007	National Breast and Cervical Cancer Early Detection Program Reauthorization Act (PL 110-18)	Established to provide waivers relating to grants for preventive health measures with respect to breast and cervical cancers
2007	Health Centers Renewal Act (PL 110-355)	Established to amend the Public Health Service Act to provide additional authorizations of appropriations for the health centers program under Section 330 of that Act
2007	Older Americans Act Amendments (PL 110-19)	Established to amend the Older Americans Act of 1965 to reinstate certain provisions relating to the nutrition services incentive program
2007	Trauma Care Systems Planning and Development Act (PL 110-23)	Established to amend the Public Health Service Act to add requirements regarding trauma care and for other purposes
2007	Joshua Omvig Veterans Suicide Prevention Act (PL 110-110)	Developed to direct the Secretary of Veterans Affairs to develop and implement a comprehensive program designed to reduce the incidence of suicide among veterans
2007	Head Start Act (PL 110-134)	Established to reauthorize the Head Start Act, to improve program quality, to expand access, and for other purposes
2007	Charlie W. Norwood Living Organ Donation Act (PL 110-144)	Established to amend the National Organ Transplant Act to provide that criminal penalties do not apply to human organ paired donation
2008	Genetic Information Nondiscrimination Act (PL 110-233)	Established to prohibit discrimination of applicants and employees based on genetic information
2009	Children's Health Insurance Program Reauthorization Act (PL 111-3)	Established to amend Social Security Act Title XXI to reauthorize the CHIP program through year 2013 at increased levels

decades. Care provided under costs agreements has become the primary substructure for health care. Capitated costs under Medicare started in 1983 with diagnostic-related groups (DRG). Formal Medicare Choice and Medicare Advantage managed care plans were established through care choice options in the mid- to late 1990s. The number of Americans participating in managed care plans increased steadily during the 1990s and into 2005. In 1998, approximately 80% of Americans with employer-sponsored health insurance had managed care plans. Initial Medicaid managed care plans were established through Health Care Financing Administration (HCFA) waivers to states in the early 1990s. Medicaid managed care covers 25.2 million persons, or 59% of recipients. For Medicare, less than 16% of beneficiaries were enrolled in managed care plans in 2005 (CMS, 2005a). This shows a slower growth of Medicare managed care after the boom from 1993 to 1998, with almost 30% of persons on Medicare+Choice plans (Cowan, Catlin, Smith, & Sensing, 2004). In 2007, a 16% increase in the number of Medicare Advantage beneficiaries were reported, which may partly be due to the Prescription Drug Part D addition by some plans. Medicare Part D enrollment and spending increased for drug costs and administrative fees (CMS, 2009). Similarly, in 2008, almost 30% of Medicare beneficiaries were enrolled in Medicare Advantage programs and overall spending for Medicare has escalated rather than been restrained with Part D (Gold, 2009).

A presidential order required the USDHHS to enact regulations of consumer rights for Medicare and Medicaid beneficiaries with managed care options. However, the bipartisan debate continues over accountability and liability with managed care. State courts, and now the U.S. Supreme Court, are dealing with the issue of whether a patient has the right to sue a managed care organization for services provided or withheld based on economic rationale rather than clinical decision making. Individuals do have the right to notification of denial, changes in benefits, provider network, and network institutions such as hospitals and pharmacies. In addition, some states provide the right to information—written and verbal—concerning the appeal or grievance processes, including a mechanism

for arbitration over disputed denial of care. National- and state-level patient "bills of rights" are required to clarify these issues and ensure equitable care; several states have begun these effort or passed legislation. The Employment Retirement Income Security Act (ERISA) of 1974 and its reauthorizations also ensure certain worker rights regarding health care coverage as part of retirement benefits.

STATE NURSE PRACTICE ACTS

Legislation and related policies that directly affect nurses are addressed in *state practice acts.* The nurse practice acts and corresponding rules and regulations define educational preparation and programs, eligibility for licensure, and the scope of practice. All states require eligible nurses to pass the National Council Licensure Examination (NCLEX) for initial RN (registered nurse) licensure. Candidates for licensure must have graduated from a program approved by the state board of nursing, but the requirements for graduation from a nationally accredited school vary among states. Nursing practice in most states includes research, education, administration, counseling, and clinical practice or direct patient care. The new interstate RN and LPN/VN (licensed practical nurse/vocational nurse) licensure compact was developed through the National Council of State Boards of Nursing (NCSBN) in 1998, and the first states joined in 2000. In 2008 the compact had 23 member states. This compact allows registered nurses to practice in member states without having a separate license; this includes electronic and telehealth practice. A similar compact for advanced practice is in process. These are methods in which a practice act is implemented. Nursing has found that it can often best manage its practice through rules and regulations that require only a state-recognized licensing board or committee to approve changes, rather than a full legislative action. State nurse practice acts are discussed further in Chapter 11.

In addition to state boards of nursing, many national organizations play a role in defining practice. The NCSBN develops the licensure examination for nurses. The ANCC, as well as various national specialty organizations, determines eligibility, educational qualifications, experience, and examinations for national certification required in many states. This is especially true for advanced practice nursing. In some states, an advanced practice nurse can practice without certification but cannot have prescriptive privileges unless national certification is obtained. In other states, certification either is not required or is required for both.

State practice acts are statutes requiring legislative approval for establishment and amendment. In the past, the majority of changes occurred in the legislative arena. More recently, state boards of nursing have developed specific rules and regulations concerning practice that can be changed without legislative activity. This avoids the possibility of undesirable statute revisions that might occur when "opening" the practice act for legislative revision. Additionally, the rules and regulations allow the nursing profession to articulate the practice, roles, and responsibilities of nurses rather than having other entities define nursing. One example is that of anesthesia assistants or unlicensed personnel. For example, there is a national movement to allow anesthesia assistants and other unlicensed personnel to accept responsibilities and use titles traditionally reserved for RNs, LPNs, and certified registered nurse anesthetists (CRNAs).

Nursing and Health Policy

Health policy, regulations, allocations, and care affect nursing and the practice environment and are in turn affected by nursing in several ways. The following sections focus on nursing practice, education, research, and the nursing discipline. The discipline requires professional nurses to conduct scholarly inquiry and participate in social and public policy through multiple avenues.

PRACTICE

Today the health care arena requires nursing administrators and staff to be aware of economic, communication, and ethical issues to a greater extent than previously encountered. This entails knowledge of budgets and health payment, the use of community resources, product evaluation, technology, benchmarking, and outcomes accountability. Consumers are more educated and aware of their health needs and rights in today's world. Although the types of services may be different according to a particular agency, setting, or location, a standard level of competency, transparency, and accountability is required in all practice environments.

One effort to indicate quality and accountability by health care institutions is the magnet hospital program. The ANA, through the ANCC, developed the Magnet Nursing Services Recognition Program (MNSRP) in the late 1990s. This program is a voluntary external professional nurse peer review of the nursing practice and care environment of any hospital that wishes to participate. The review includes examination of the extent to which a hospital meets eight standards of care, which are incorporated within the model of professional practice at each site. The process of applying for magnet status involves both a written application and a site visit by a board of experts. Applicants are required to demonstrate nurse-sensitive quality at the unit or system level and to meet established state, regional, or national benchmarks. Governance, research, patient safety, and feedback processes are all part of magnet criteria. If a facility is designated as a magnet hospital, the effective practice environment and resulting quality of nursing care should be evident (ANCC, 2009; Urlich, Buerhaus, Donelan, & Dittus, 2007).

For individual nurses, standards are provided by professional organizations, including the ANA's *Standards of Clinical Nursing Practice, Scope and Standards of Advanced Practice Registered Nurses,* and the *Scope and Standards of Nursing Administrators,* as well as specialty standards for practice, in response to both societal and professional requests for clarification of nursing. Identification of competencies, such as those for wound and ostomy care, cultural competence, and genetics may be required for nurses across practice settings. Studies examining nurse competence are also needed (Starr & Wallace, 2009). Effectiveness studies that support competent and quality practice also have an impact on legislation. One team found that a intensive case management intervention with low-income women improved substance abuse outcomes (Morgenstern et al., 2006), another nurse reported that school nurse case management improved student outcomes (Bonaiuto, 2007), and Heitkemper and Wolff (2007) addressed challenges in bowel care. To assist in these efforts, Dunston, Boyle, and colleagues at the University of Kansas are leading the effort to develop measures of care through the ANA-supported National Database for Nursing Quality Indicators (NDNQI). These interventions and activities indicate to legislators and the public that nursing contributes to better health outcomes, quality, and cost containment.

Self-development, continuing education, certification, and learning new skill sets (retooling) will be required as the health care delivery system continues to evolve. This learning must be of a transdisciplinary nature, including terminology and new taxonomy languages, client needs, treatment, and evaluation of outcomes, quality, and access. Hospitals and clinics will continue as major settings, but long-term care and alternative care settings and delivery methods that assist clients to achieve health must be initiated and embraced. Case management can assist in meeting the needs of specific populations. Homeless clinics, parish nursing, and collaborative efforts with physician practices and school systems are additional delivery methods that provide community-based care to vulnerable populations.

EDUCATION

Authorization for nursing education originated with the Nurse Training Act of 1964. Between 1965 and 1971, more than $380 million was spent on nursing education for both students and institutions. Doctoral nursing students and nursing doctoral programs received emphasis and support during the mid-1970s, and master's programs received larger allocations for increasing nurses in specific roles in the 1980s and 1990s. However, in the 1990s, with the onset of managed care and increased competition for health care dollars, the nursing education legislation was twice not enacted. Passage of the Health Professions Education Partnership Act in 1998 changed the tradition by which nursing was the only health profession to retain a separate funding law. Congressional funding for nursing education has increased and expanded to include baccalaureate, master's, and doctoral level, but enrollments

have not increased to meet the projected needs in most areas of the country (AACN, 2008a, 2008b, 2008c; U.S. Department of Labor, 2009).

To address the major shortages specific to nursing, the Nurse Reinvestment Act and subsequent legislation have been passed. The focus of these efforts was on funding and implementing strategies for nurse recruitment and nurse retention. Scholarships (Nursing Loan Repayment and Scholarships) are available to those nurses willing to work in health care facilities with a critical nursing shortage. Special grants are provided for schools of nursing to develop and implement programs focused on geriatrics through the Comprehensive Geriatric Education Program (CGEP). Grants and contracts are awarded to schools of nursing that expand their programs by increasing enrollment in 4-year programs, provide internships and residency programs for nursing students, and provide new programs such as distance learning by new technologies. This Nurse Education, Practice, and Retention (NEPR) program fosters the area of practice by providing funding for nurses caring for underserved populations and populations in noninstitutional settings, as well as for nurses interested in developing cultural competencies. Low-interest-rate loans—for instance, through the Nurse Faculty Loan Program (NFLP)—are available to master's and doctoral students who agree to work full-time in a school of nursing or nursing department after graduation. Nursing Workforce Diversity (NWD) grants provide educational funds to persons from disadvantaged backgrounds. The FY 2008 funding was $156 million; the FY 2009 Senate request was $168 million in January 2009. Federal dollars are the largest source of external funding for nursing education, primarily provided through the USDHHS BHP. Most of these federal dollars provide program funding; however, available funding for nursing students themselves is often inadequate (Thaker, Pathman, Mark, & Ricketts, 2008).

The National League for Nursing (NLN) initiated accreditation of nursing programs. Policies relative to accreditation came under scrutiny by the U.S. Department of Education in the 1990s, and the NLNAC was established as a freestanding entity. In 1999, CCNE, which evolved from the AACN, gained recognition from the Department of Education. These accrediting bodies understand the importance of the Pew Commission Report, the Sullivan Commission Report (W. K. Kellogg Foundation, 2004), USDHHS priorities, and congressional requirements and thus encourage schools to initiate new curricula, develop creative teaching methods, stimulate lifelong learning, establish competency-based educational programs, focus on *Healthy People 2010,* address health disparities and diversity issues, and evaluate care delivered at all levels. The AACN "Essentials" for baccalaureate and master's education, the Consensus Model for APRN (Advanced Practice Registered Nurse) Regulation: Licensure, Accreditation, Certification & Education, and the quality indicators for clinical and research doctoral education (www.aacn.nche.edu) are excellent beginning guidelines that will need to be evaluated and revised as the health care industry changes. Clinical doctorate programs, including DNPs (Doctorate of Nursing Practice), are now funded by the Health Resources and Services Administration (HRSA) through the Advanced Education Nursing Program (AENP) grants. In addition, workforce, staffing, and quality of care studies, such as those being conducted by Mark and colleagues (2008), Letvak (2005), Letvak and Buck (2008), Boyle and Miller (2008), Buerhaus (2008), and AHRQ-funded work (Friese, Lake, Aiken, Silber, & Sochalski, 2008; Hanrenhan & Aiken, 2008) are becoming more germane to nurses at the local and state levels as nurses lobby for continued authorization of funding programs and reimbursement and demonstrate quality-of-care benchmarks. Successful efforts to foster collaboration and improve evidence-based practice (de Cordova et al., 2008) and to provide effective education (Bartlett et al., 2008) are needed. These studies and the directions they lead have an impact on the practice environments by identifying appropriate staffing, quality, and effective workforce development.

RESEARCH

The establishment of the NINR at the NIH in 1993 and its reauthorizations have affected nursing research. First established as the National Center for Nursing Research in April 1986, with the purpose of providing a strong scientific base for nursing practice, it became the National Institute of Nursing Research

(NINR) in 2000 and serves as an integral part of the NIH. The NINR National Advisory Council for Nursing Research (NACNR) participates in setting the NIH agenda, budget priorities, and funding recommendations. The NINR has led the NIH efforts to include the elimination of health disparities in their strategic plan. The program areas at the NINR in the 1990s were consistent with the national priorities set by the NIH and *Healthy People 2010.* The priority areas of science identified by the NINR in 2008 were neuroscience, genetics, and symptom management; child and family health and health disparities; immunology, infectious disease, and chronic disorders; and acute and long-term care, end-of-life, and training.

The NINR funds investigators who are not nurses; likewise, nurses receive funding from institutes other than the NINR. An interdisciplinary focus of projects is emphasized across program areas shared with many institutes, including the National Institute on Aging (NIA), the NIMH, the NICHD, the National Center for Minority Health and Health Disparities (NCMHD), and the AHRQ. Agencies such as the NIOSH and CDC have provided funds to support nurse-directed studies on health in agricultural workers (Reed, 2007; Reed & Kidd, 2004). The AHRQ supports evidenced-based practice (EBP) centers (www.ahrq.gov/clinic/epc/epcenters.htm). The Eunice Kennedy Shriver NICHD supports studies related to the Best Pharmaceuticals for Children Act, and the NCMHD funds Centers of Excellence (COE) in Health Disparities. As a final example, the Substance Abuse and Mental Health Services Administration (SAMHSA) has supported demonstration projects to develop tools for Preadmission Screening and Resident Review (PASRR) Screening for Mental Illness in Nursing Facility Applicants and Residents (see www.mentalhealth.samhsa.gov).

Nurses provide leadership in many ways. For example, Dr. Martha Hill, dean of The Johns Hopkins University School of Nursing, co-chaired the committee to develop the IOM's *Unequal Treatment* report, which guides much of the system and disparities interventions. Dr. Hill also leads multidisciplinary and multinational intervention studies to prevent or control hypertension in African Americans and Africans. Dr. Audrey Nelson, as director of the VA Patient Safety Center of Inquiry in Tampa, leads efforts to improve patient safety and quality of care through the Veterans Administration. Dr. Cornelia Beck, Distinguished Professor at University of Arkansas Medical Sciences, provides leadership in the national efforts to alleviate suffering from Alzheimer's disease. In addition, HIV/AIDS work has been led by Dr. William Holzemer at UCSF and by Dr. Nancy McCain at VCU with an emphasis on biobehavioral interventions.

Research directions have been guided by foundations such as the RWJF and the W. K. Kellogg Foundation, which have funded community and rural health initiatives. Findings from nursing investigations and experience have resulted in input to the development of practice guidelines. Nancy Bergstrom and her colleagues' work on decubitus ulcers and Jean Wyman and Thelma Wells' work on incontinence influenced the AHRQ practice guidelines in the 1990s. More recently, nurse researchers have investigated factors related to differing health concerns in U.S. and international populations (Bartlett, Buck, & Shattell, 2008; Hu & Gruber, 2008; Jones, Ivanov, Wallace, & VonCannon, 2006; Moser & Watkins, 2008; Tsai et al., 2008), as well as the effectiveness of interventions for vulnerable populations (Andrews, Felton, Wewers, Waller, & Tingen, 2007; Covelli, 2008; Peden, Rayens, Hall, & Grant, 2005; Peden et al., 2008; Reifsnider & Ritsema, 2008; Tingen et al., 2006). Elaine Larson, Patricia Stone, and colleagues at Columbia Medical Center have built knowledge to prevent infections in hospitals and provided a cost analysis of those interventions.

The NINR, Sigma Theta Tau International (STTI), the four regional nursing research societies (Southern, Midwest, Eastern and Western), specialty organizations, Friends of NINR, and the National Nursing Research Roundtable meet annually to discuss and plan for the direction, implementation, and funding of nursing research. Regional and national conferences and the Council for the Advancement of Nursing Science (CANS) State of the Science Congress highlight nursing research findings that have an impact on health care delivery, costs, access, and outcomes. Congressional members and persons from local, state, and regional political and legislative arenas are invited to attend these meetings to discuss nursing and health care efforts and needs. Additional research activities include the Veterans Administration Nursing Research

Initiative (NRI), the American Nurses Foundation (ANF) awards, and nursing fellowships and grants by the AHRQ, the RWJF, the W. K. Kellogg Foundation, and the Templeton Foundation (TF). Nurses also fill positions as clinical researchers in medical centers across the country and conduct ongoing studies.

OUTCOMES AND QUALITY

Outcomes research is now required to determine the effectiveness and accountability of practice. Much effort is directed to defining what constitutes outcomes and how to measure them. *Outcomes research* is a priority in the area of *health services research.* One policy initiative was the enactment of the Healthcare Research and Quality Act of 1999, which changed the name of the Agency for Health Care Policy and Research (AHCPR) to the Agency for Healthcare Research and Quality (AHRQ). This emphasis provides that research on outcomes and quality will provide a foundation for future policy, regulation, and allocation decisions for health care. National health indicators, *Healthy People 2010* (and the new *Healthy People 2020*), and the USDHHS initiative to eliminate racial and ethnic disparities provide another set of outcomes and measures of quality. Examining system outcomes is one avenue of research. *System outcomes* are those related to direct and indirect material and financial costs, length of stay, manpower, provider qualifications, and provider and payer satisfaction. For example, a hospital-based intervention improved nurse retention and quality of care provided to patients (Meraviglia et al., 2008). Client outcomes such as consumer satisfaction, health status outcomes, adaptation, and function are additional outcomes that require study. Examples are the effective use of emergency department health services studied by Wetta-Hall (2007), a pilot study by Schultz and colleagues (2008) on reducing infant head flattening, and research by Zarate-Abbott and colleagues (2008) on intervention to improve cardiac health in Hispanic women. A final issue to be addressed is how outcomes and quality relate to and affect one another. This will be a specific area for nursing to address in future practice, education, and research efforts. Future nursing efforts will be guided by the ANA's Health System Reform

Agenda (2008) and the new ANA Social Policy Statement (November 2009) that set forth principles for workforce development, quality care, health access, and evolving practice environments.

Nurse Participation in Health Policy

Nurses have increasingly become active participants in the health policy arena as advocates and activists and in writing health policies at the state and federal levels. Nursing has progressed through several stages in its political development and involvement in the policy arena. Nursing is currently at the "leadership" stage, where it is recognized as a political entity with a recognizable agenda that guides health policy. The ANA has been consulted for advice and has offered recommendations on health care reform and on health policies, such as the Women's Health Initiative (WHI). A prime example occurred in September 2008, when Linda J. Stierle, chief executive officer of the ANA, took part in the Kaiser Family Foundation (KFF) interview series *Viewpoints: The Health Care Debate* with various leaders of organizations representing health care providers, insurers, policymakers, employers, labor unions, and consumers. During this series, Stierle shared her views on shortcomings in the nation's health care system and how it could be improved. However, nursing often misses opportunities for input, such as with the Oral Health Initiative, partially because nurses fail to recognize or champion one another as experts.

In 2008, three nurses served as legislators in Congress: Lois Capps (California), Eddie Bernice Johnson (Texas), and Carolyn McCarthy (New York). Representative Capps was instrumental in writing the Nurse Reinvestment Act, which was initially passed in 2002 and provided authority through 2007. The original intent has been accomplished primarily through HRSA funding for graduate programs, nurse scholarships, grants to health care facilities to improve nurse retention and patient safety, faculty loan repayment, and funding for new undergraduate programs. Reauthorization in 2008 was accomplished as part of the Higher Education Act (PL 110-315), which requires awarding of competitive grants to accredited undergraduate RN programs to expand faculty and facilities to accommodate additional students and to fund graduate nursing programs to accommodate advanced practice degrees for RNs and for nurse educator training. Appropriation of adequate funds continues to be a concern.

Nurses have been instrumental in the policy arena, advocating for change in policies that affect nurses. For instance, in Louisiana there was a move to close school-based health centers, and nurses, along with grassroots support, were instrumental through phone calls, faxes, and letters to the governor's office in getting funding to provide for school-based health centers from general fund allocations (Broussard, 2002). In another example, nurses who were members of Virginia's Old Dominion Society of Gastroenterology Nurses and Associates (SGNA) initiated the introduction of legislation to promote insurance payment for colorectal screening. This effort began when a nurse working at a gastroenterology unit in Virginia became concerned about the number of patients that were diagnosed with late-stage colon cancer because they did not get early screening. The President of SGNA contacted Virginia State Senator Emily Couric, sharing the group's concern for the lack of colorectal screening and asking her to write a legislative mandate for insurance coverage of colonoscopies. Through these efforts, Virginia became the first state to pass legislation mandating insurance coverage for colonoscopies to all individuals, including those covered by Medicaid. As of April 2009, the CDC reported that 28 states have enacted legislation mandating insurance coverage for at least one type of colorectal cancer (CRC) screening, and 11 states had introduced legislation that would cover some type of CRC screening (www.cdc.gov/cancer/colorectal/pdf/colorectal_cancer_activities.pdf).

In other areas, nurse practitioners (NPs) have been active in passing state laws dealing with prescription drug rights (Byrne, 2008). Nurse anesthetists have also been active in legislation dealing with their practice. The North Carolina Association of Nurse Anesthetists (NCANA) has been active in fighting to preserve the authority of CRNAs in North Carolina and against legislation that would allow licensing of anesthesiologist assistants (AAs). Julie Ann Lowery, president of the NCANA, has reached out to grassroots groups and North Carolina residents in an effort to get them involved in legislation that would jeopardize CRNAs' practice in North Carolina.

These are only a few examples of nurse activism in the policy arena. As nurses become more informed, passionate, and committed about their leadership role in the policy arena, legislation at the state and federal levels will require input from nurses to advocate for patients, for the public, and for themselves.

Health Care Reform 2010

The historic health care insurance reform law, Patient Protection and Affordable Care Act (PPACA) of 2010 (Public Law 111-148) was signed into law by President Obama on March 23, 2010, and its companion Health Care and Education Affordability Reconciliation Act was signed into law on March 30, 2010. Bills are typed in a particular format that greatly expands the number of pages, and the complexity of the current health care system required the many interconnections be addressed. The federal government website for health care reform (http://www.healthcare.gov/center/authorities/title_v_amendments.pdf) provides an example of how Title V of the PPACA Act was drafted.

The government website (http://healthcare.gov/) provides useful information about specific aspects of the law and includes a section that addresses the law's impact by specific population or issue, including a map that allows the public to see the impact at a specific state level. Table 6-4 provides a summary of the ten titles included in the PPACA Act, including the elements of the companion Reconciliation Act. The Office of Consumer Information and Insurance Oversight (OCIIO) is created within the DHHS to implement many of the provisions of the legislation that address private health insurance. Some provisions will be enacted in 2010, whereas others begin 6 months after enactment. The full act is anticipated to be fully implemented by 2014. Box 6-2 lists the key provisions that will be addressed initially. The OCIIO has published several interim final rules for public comment on www.regulations.gov. As of May 25, 2010, interim final regulations for dependent coverage of children who have not attained age 26, early retiree reinsurance

program, and health care reform insurance web portal requirements are posted for public comment. Request for comments have been posted for medical loss ratio (◉ 2718 of the Public Health Service Act) and premium review process (◉ 2794 of the Public Health Service Act). This allows stakeholders to weigh in on the drafting of interim regulations early in the process.

SUMMARY

As members of the largest group of health professionals and major providers of care, nurses can influence health care policy as individuals and as professionals. Consumers of health care, including nurses, desire affordable, accessible, and high-quality care. Nurses are obligated to ensure that the public has access to quality health care at controlled costs. Identifying and prioritizing client needs with sensitivity to culture and diversity, acquiring and demonstrating a knowledge of treatments and interventions (both nursing and interdisciplinary), maintaining a focus on outcomes (client, system, and provider), and ensuring safe, quality care in multiple environments are basic responsibilities of professional nursing in the 21st century.

Armed with information on how to influence health care policy, nurses serve as advocates for patients and active participants in the formation of effective health care policy. Organizational membership in regional, state, or national organizations and letter writing are two traditional activities for nurses involved in policy making. More focused involvement can be achieved through collective actions as members of PACs and political parties. Social, civic, professional, and lay organizations with interest in specific populations and concerns also provide a mechanism by which nurses can influence legislation and allocation decisions. Another avenue is to run for elected office or sit on boards, committees, councils, or commissions, especially those that make policy and funding decisions that affect health care. Opportunities exist and can be developed to share expertise and communicate nursing needs through consultation to elected officials, health agencies, foundations, educational institutions, and funding agencies.

Policy decisions regarding financial resources influence the type of nursing staff, the number of nurses, the amount and type of management and support services,

TABLE 6-4	Patient Protection and Affordable Care Act (PPACA) of 2010 (Public Law 111-148) and Health Care and Education Reconciliation Act of 2010

ACT SUMMARY WITH DESIGNATION OF NEW AND EXISTING AUTHORITIES

Title I: Quality Affordable Health Care for All Americans	This Act allows individuals, families, and small business owners to make decisions about their health care. Premium costs are reduced for millions of working families and small businesses by providing hundreds of billions of dollars in tax relief—the largest middle class tax cut for health care in history. Out-of-pocket expenses are capped, and preventive care must be fully covered without out-of-pocket expense. For many Americans, their insurance coverage will not change.
	Qualified health plans are more clearly defined, and a health benefit exchange pool will be established for Americans without insurance coverage so they can choose their insurance coverage. The insurance exchange will pool buying power and give Americans choices of private insurance plans that have to compete for their business based on cost and quality. Small business owners will be able to choose insurance coverage through this exchange as well as receive a tax credit to help offset the cost of covering their employees.
	The Act bans insurance companies from denying insurance coverage because of preexisting medical conditions and provides consumers new power to appeal insurance company decisions that deny doctor-ordered treatments covered by insurance.
	The USDHHS Secretary (Secretary) has the authority to implement many of these new provisions to help families and small business owners have the information they need to make the choices that work best for them.
Title II: The Role of Public Programs	The Act extends Medicaid while treating all states equally. It preserves CHIP, the successful children's insurance plan, and simplifies enrollment for individuals and families.
	Community-based care for Americans with disabilities is enhanced, and states will have opportunities to expand home care services to people with long-term care needs.
	The Act gives flexibility to states to adopt innovative strategies to improve care and the coordination of services for Medicare and Medicaid beneficiaries.
	The Secretary has the authority to work with states and other partners to strengthen key public programs.
Title III: Improving the Quality and Efficiency of Health Care	The Act closes the Medicare prescription coverage gap called the *"donut hole."* In addition, the Act provides incentives for doctors, nurses, and hospitals that improve care and reduce errors.
	The Act enhances access to health care services in rural and underserved areas. Funding is provided for school-based and nurse-managed centers to assist in providing this care.
	Another change is the addition of a group of doctors and health care experts, rather than only members of Congress, who identify ideas to improve quality and reduce costs for Medicare beneficiaries.
	The Secretary has the authority to take steps to strengthen the Medicare program and implement reforms to improve the quality and efficiency of health care.
Title IV: Prevention of Chronic Disease and Improving Public Health	The Act directs the creation of a national prevention and health promotion strategy that incorporates the most effective and achievable methods to improve the health status of Americans and reduce the incidence of preventable illness and disability in the United States.
	Included in this title are the availability of science-based nutrition information and waiving co-payments for America's seniors on Medicare for prevention and health screenings.
	The Secretary has the authority to coordinate with other departments, develop and implement a prevention and health promotion strategy, and work to ensure that more Americans have access to critical preventive health services.

Continued

TABLE 6-4	Patient Protection and Affordable Care Act (PPACA) of 2010 (Public Law 111-148) and Health Care and Education Reconciliation Act of 2010—cont'd
Title V: Health Care Workforce	The Act funds scholarships and loan repayment programs to increase the number of primary care physicians, nurses, physician assistants, mental health providers, and dentists in the areas of the country that need them most. In addition, funds are provided to expand, construct, and operate community health centers, with specific funding for nurse-managed health centers.
	Expansions are also noted for the advanced education nursing programs, the Nurse Faculty Loan Program, the Nurse Loan Repayment and Scholarship Program, and the Nursing Student Loan Program.
	The Secretary has the authority to take action to strengthen many existing programs that help support the primary care workforce.
Title VI: Transparency and Program Integrity	The Act includes the Nursing Home Transparency program so that consumers can compare facilities.
	The Act protects whistleblowers, and it requires staffing accountability and disclosure.
	Finally, the Act imposes rigorous disclosure requirements to identify high-risk providers who have defrauded the American taxpayer. It gives states new authority to prevent providers who have been penalized in one state from setting up in another and the flexibility to propose and test tort reforms for improving health care.
	The Secretary has new and improved authority to promote transparency and ensure that every dollar in the Act and in existing programs is spent wisely and well.
Title VII: Improving Access to Innovative Medical Therapies	The Act extends drug discounts to hospitals and communities that serve low-income patients and creates a pathway for the creation of generic versions of biological drugs.
	The Secretary of Health and Human Services has the authority to implement these provisions to help make medications more affordable.
Title VIII: Community Living Assistance Services and Support Act (CLASS)	The Act provides Americans with a new option to finance long-term services and care in the event of a disability.
	It is a self-funded and voluntary long-term care insurance option. Workers will pay premiums to receive a daily cash benefit if they develop a disability. Need will be based on difficulty in performing basic activities such as bathing or dressing. The benefit is flexible—it could be used for a range of community support services, from respite care to home care.
	Safeguards will be put in place to ensure its premiums are enough to cover its costs.
	The Secretary has the authority to establish the CLASS Program.
Title IX: Revenue Provisions	The Act provides new tax credits that will reduce health premium costs for middle class families and allow them exchange pools for insurance purchase. Families making less than $250,000 are the primary targets of these provisions.
	This title will be implemented by the U.S. Department of the Treasury.
Title X:	The Act reauthorizes the Indian Health Care Improvement Act (IHCIA), which provides health care services to American Indians and Alaskan Natives.
	The Secretary, in consultation with the Indian Health Service, has the authority to implement the Indian Health Care Improvement Act.

Modified from Health Reform.GOV at http://www.healthreform.gov/health_reform_and_hhs.html, accessed on May 25, 2010; and Government Printing Office [DOCID: f: publ148.111, Page 124 STAT. 119], accessed July 26, 2010.

BOX 6-2	Key Provisions of PPACA 2010 that Take Effect Immediately or 6 Months after Enactment

1. Small business tax credits
2. No discrimination against children with preexisting conditions
3. Help for uninsured Americans with preexisting conditions until the exchange is available (Interim High-Risk Pool)
4. Guarantees renewable coverage
5. Prohibits discrimination against individual participants and beneficiaries based on health status
6. Begins to close the Medicare Part D Donut Hole for eligible persons
7. Provides free preventive health screenings under Medicare
8. Extends coverage for young people up to their 26th birthday through parent's insurance by certain eligibility
9. Provides reinsurance for early retirees
10. Bans lifetime limits on health insurance coverage
11. Bans restrictive annual limits on insurance coverage
12. Requires free preventive care under new private plans
13. Provides new, independent appeals process
14. Ensures value for premium payments
15. Expands community health centers
16. Increases the number of primary care practitioners
17. Prohibits discrimination based on salary
18. Expands and requires certain health insurance consumer information
19. Monitors insurance companies for fair health insurance premiums

Modified from Health Care.GOV at http://www.healthcare.gov/law/timeline/index.html, accessed on March 3, 2011; and Government Printing Office [DOCID: f: publ148.111, Page 124 STAT. 119], accessed July 26, 2010.

and the extent of educational program and research funding—all of which affect the practice environment and quality of nursing and health care. The settings and payment of care affect access and the spectrum of services available to the most vulnerable populations. Through professional and personal knowledge, expertise, and experience, nurses can take action in research, practice, and education areas. Politics, legislation, and economics provide ample opportunity and challenge for nursing involvement. Taking advantage of these opportunities and meeting the challenge of ensuring access to quality health care for all can be achieved through greater involvement in the health policy arena.

KEY POINTS

- Health policy is influenced by many factors, including politics, economics, demographics, and personal and societal priorities.
- Legislation is a complex process that includes multiple players, takes time, and involves political and special interests at local, state, and federal levels.
- A large portion of the federal budget and expenditures is directed at health programs, specifically Medicare, Medicaid, and Social Security entitlements.
- Federal and state legislation, as well as rules and regulations to implement policies, influence the availability, access, and spectrum of nursing practice and health care.
- New demographics and health needs will require changes in delivery of health care, to whom it is delivered, and the environment and practices of care.
- An outcomes and quality focus is required to ensure quality and useful nursing practice, education, and research.
- Nursing has influenced and has been influenced by policy and allocation decisions.
- Nurses have a responsibility to participate in health policy and planning to ensure quality health care and an effective practice environment.
- Knowledge and involvement are keys to influencing health policy.

CRITICAL THINKING EXERCISES

1. What are the major health care issues in your community, state, and region? What are some solutions to these problems? How might you become involved in implementing these solutions?
2. Discuss how a practice, workplace, education, or research situation in your experience was directly affected by health policy decisions or allocations. What are the options for changing that policy? What are the barriers and facilitators to changing the policy?
3. Discuss how entitlements should be addressed with a health care provider, a health care economist or businessperson, and a client. Develop three strategies and share these with your state or national legislator and your professional organization.

4. Discuss your nursing practice and workplace environment and how these are affected by policy decisions at the local, state, and federal levels.
5. What are your responsibilities to ensure access to quality, timely, appropriate, and cost-effective care?

REFERENCES

American Association of Colleges of Nursing. (2008a, December 3). Enrollment growth in U.S. nursing colleges and universities hits an 8-year low according to new data released by AACN. [Press release]. Retrieved from http://www.aacn.nche.edu/media/NewsReleases/2008/EnrlGrowth.html

American Association of Colleges of Nursing. (2008b, September, last revised). Nursing faculty shortage. [Fact sheet]. Retrieved from www.aacn.nche.edu/Media/factsheets/FacultyShortage.htm

American Association of Colleges of Nursing. (2008c, September last revised). Nursing shortage. [Fact sheet]. Retrieved from http://www.aacn.nche.edu/Media/FactSheets/NursingShortage.htm

American Nurses Credentialing Center. (2009). ANCC magnet recognition program. Retrieved from http://www.nursecredentialing.org/MagnetNewsArchive2008/NewMagnetModel.aspx

Andrews, J. O., Felton, G., Wewers, M. E., Waller, J., & Tingen, M. (2007). The effect of a multi-component smoking cessation intervention in African American women residing in public housing. *Research in Nursing & Health*, *30*(1), 45–60.

Bartlett, R., Bland, A., Rossen, E., Kautz, D., Bwenfield, S., & Carnevale, T. (2008). Evaluation of the outcome-present state test model as a way to teach clinical reasoning. *Journal of Nursing Education*, *47*(8), 337–344.

Bartlett, R., Buck, R., & Shattell, M. M. (2008). Risk and protection for HIV/AIDS in African-American, Hispanic and White adolescents. *Journal of National Black Nurses' Association*, *19*(1), 19–25.

Bonaiuto, M. M. (2007). School nurse case management: Achieving health and educational outcomes. *The Journal of School Nursing*, *23*(4), 202–209.

Boyle, D. K., & Miller., P. A. (2008). Focus on nursing turnover: A system-centered performance measure. *Nursing Management*, *39*(6), 18–20.

Broussard, L. (2002). School-based health centers: Politics and community support. *Policy, Politics, and Nursing Practice*, *3*(3), 235–239.

Buerhaus, P. I. (2008). Current and future state of the US nursing workforce. *Journal of the American Medical Association*, *300*(20), 2422–2424.

Byrne, W. (2008). US nurse practitioner prescribing law: A state-by-state summary. Retrieved January 20, 2009 from http://www.medscape.com/viewarticle/440315

Centers for Disease Control and Prevention. (2009). About CDC. Retrieved January 13, 2009, from http://www.cdc.gov/aboutcdc.htm

Centers for Medicare and Medicaid Services. (2005a). Expenditures for health services and supplies under public programs, by type of expenditure and program. Retrieved January 13, 2009, from http://www.cms.hhs.gov/NationalHealthExpendData

Centers for Medicare and Medicaid Services. (2005b). Medicare Modernization Act. Retrieved January 13, 2009, from http://www.cms.hhs.gov/MMAupdate

Centers for Medicare and Medicaid Services. (2008, October 17). Medicaid spending projected to rise much faster than the economy. [Press release]. Retrieved from http://www.cms.hhs.gov/apps/media/press/release.asp

Centers for Medicare and Medicaid Services. (2009). Medicare releases Part D data for 2006 and 2007. Retrieved February 7, 2009, from http://www.cms.hhs.gov/PrescriptionDrugCovGenIn/Downloads/PartDSymposiumFactSheet_2008.pdf

Covelli, M. M. (2008). Efficacy of a school-based cardiac health promotion intervention program for African-American adolescents. *Applied Nursing Research*, *21*(4), 173–180.

Cowan, C., Catlin, A., Smith, C., & Sensing, A. (2004). National health expenditures, 2002. *Health Care Financing Review*, *25*(4), 143–166.

de Cordova, P. B., Collins, S., Peppard, L., Currie, L. M., Hughes, R., Walsh, M., et al. (2008). Implementing evidence-based nursing with student nurses and clinicians: Uniting the strengths. *Applied Nursing Research*, *21*, 242–245.

Federal Elections Commission. (2000). Campaign finance reports and data. Retrieved January 27, 2009, from http://www.fec.gov

Federal Elections Commission. (2005, March 14). Party financial activity summarized for the 2004 election cycle. Retrieved January 27, 2009, from http://www.fec.gov/press/press2005/20050302party/Party2004final.html

Federal Elections Commission. (2009a). Contribution limits for 2007-08. Retrieved January 27, 2009, from http://www.fec.gov/info/contriblimits0708.pdf

Federal Elections Commission. (2009b). Contributions to all candidates by state. Retrieved January 27, 2009, from http://www.fec.gov/DisclosureSearch/mapApp.do

Friese, C., Lake, E. T., Aiken, L. H., Silber, J., & Sochalski, J. (2008). Hospital nurse practice environments and outcomes for surgical oncology patients. *Health Services Research, 43*(4), 1145–1163.

Gold, M. (2009). Medicare's private plans: A report card on Medicare advantage. *Health Affairs, 28*(1), w41–w54.

Hanrenhan, N. P., & Aiken., L. H. (2008). Psychiatric nurse reports on the quality of psychiatric care in general hospitals. *Quality Management in Health Care, 17*(3), 210–216.

Hartman, M., Martin, A., McDonnell, P., Caitlin, A., & the National Health Expenditure Accounts Team. (2009). National health spending in 2007: Slower drug spending contributes to lowest overall growth since 1998. *Health Affairs, 28*(1), 246–261.

Heitkemper, M., & Wolff, J. (2007). Challenges in chronic constipation management. *Nurse Practitioner, 32*(4), 36–43.

Hu, J., & Gruber, K. J. (2008). Positive and negative affect and health functioning indicators among older adults with chronic illnesses. *Issues in Mental Health Nursing, 29*(8), 895–911.

Jones, E. D., Ivanov, L. L., Wallace, D. C., & VonCannon, L. (2006). Examining the metabolic syndrome in Russia. *International Journal of Nursing Practice, 12*(5), 260–266.

Letvak, S. (2005). Health and safety of older nurses. *Nursing Outlook, 53*(2), 66–72.

Letvak, S., & Buck, R. (2008). Factors influencing work productivity and intent to stay in nursing. *Nursing Economic$, 26*(3), 159–166.

Mark, B. A., Hughes, L. C., Belyea, M., Bacon, C. T., Chang, Y., & Jones, C. A. (2008). Exploring organizational context and structure as predictors of medication errors and patient falls. *Journal of Patient Safety, 4*(2), 66–77.

Meraviglia, M., Grobe, S. J., Tabone, S., Wainwright, M., Shelton, S., Yu, L., et al. (2008). Nurse -friendly hospital project: Enhancing nurse retention and quality of care. *Journal of Nursing Care Quality, 23*(4), 305–313.

Morgenstern, J., Blanchard, K. A., McCrady, B. S., McVeigh, K. H., Morgan, T. J., & Pandina, R. J. (2006). Effectiveness of intensive case management for substance-dependent women receiving temporary assistance for needy families. *American Journal of Public Health, 96*(11), 2016–2023.

Moser, D. K., & Watkins, J. F. (2008). Conceptualizing self-care in heart failure: A life course model of patient characteristics. *Journal of Cardiovascular Nursing, 23*(3), 205–220.

National Institutes of Health. (2008). The NIH almanac-appropriations. Retrieved January 26, 2009, from http://www.nih.gov/about/almanac/appropriations/part2.htm

O'Neil, E. H. (1993). *Health professions education for the future: Schools in service to the nation.* San Francisco: Pew Health Professions Commission.

O'Neil, E. H., & the Pew Health Professions Commission. (1998). *Recreating health professional practice for a new century.* San Francisco: Pew Health Professions Commission.

Peden, A. R., Rayens, M. K., Hall, L. A., & Grant, E. (2005). Testing an intervention to reduce negative thinking, depressive symptoms, and chronic stressors in low-income single mothers. *Journal of Nursing Scholarship, 37*(3), 268–274.

Peden, A. R., Rayens, M. K., Hall, L. A., Hahn, E., Riker, C., Ashford, K., et al. (2008). Nicotine addiction in pregnancy: Preliminary efficacy of a mental health intervention. *Addictive Disorders & Their Treatment, 7*(4), 179–189.

Pew Health Professions Commission. (1995). Critical challenges: Revitalizing the health professions for the 21st century. Retrieved January 27, 2009, from http://future health.ucsf.edu/summaries/challenges.html

Reed, D. B. (2007). Case study: Third degree burn by tincture of iodine. *AAOHN Journal, 55*(10), 393–394.

Reed, D. B., & Kidd, P. S. (2004). Collaboration between nurses and agricultural teachers to prevent adolescent agricultural injuries: The Agricultural Disability Awareness and Risk Education Model. *Public Health Nursing, 21*(4), 323–330.

Reifsnider, E., & Ritsema, M. (2008). Ecological difference in weight, length, and weight for length of Mexican American children in the WIC program. *Journal for Specialists in Pediatric Nursing, 13*(3), 154–167.

Schultz, A. A., Goodwin, P. A., Jesseman, C., Toews, H. G., Lane, M., & Smith, C. (2008). Evaluating effectiveness of gel pillows for reducing bilateral head flattening in preterm infants: A randomized controlled pilot study. *Applied Nursing Research, 21*(4), 191–198.

Starr, S. S., & Wallace, D. C. (2009). Self-reported cultural competence of public health nurses in a southeastern U.S. public health department. *Public Health Nursing, 26*(1), 48–57.

Thaker, S. I., Pathman, D. E., Mark, B. A., & Ricketts, T. C., III. (2008). Service-linked scholarships, loans, and loan repayment programs for nurses in the Southeast. *Journal of Professional Nursing, 24*(2), 122–130.

Tingen, M. S., Waller, J. L., Smith, T. M., Baker, R. R., Reyes, J., & Treiber, F. A. (2006). Tobacco prevention in children and cessation in family members. *Journal of the American Academy of Nurse Practitioners, 18*(4), 169–179.

Tsai, P. F., Beck, C., Richards, K. C., Phillips, L., Roberson, P. K., & Evans, J. (2008). The pain behaviors for osteoarthritis instrument for cognitively impaired elders (PBOICE). *Research in Gerontological Nursing, 1*(2), 116–122.

Ulrich, B. T., Buerhaus, P. I., Donelan, K. N., & Dittus, R. (2007). Magnet status and registered nurse views of the work environment and nursing as a career. *Journal of Nursing Administration, 37*(5), 212–220.

U.S. Department of Labor. (2009). Occupational Outlook Handbook, 2008-09 edition: Registered nurses. Retrieved January 13, 2009, from http://www.bls.gov/oco/ocos083.htm

U.S. House of Representatives. (2003). How our laws are made. Retrieved January 29, 2009, from http://thomas.loc.gov/home/lawsmade.toc.html

U.S. Senate. (2003). How our laws are made. Document 108-93. Retrieved January 17, 2009, from http://www.senate.gov/reference/resources/pdf/howourlawsaremade.pdf

Wetta-Hall, R. (2007). Impact of collaborative community case management program on a low-income uninsured population in Sedgwick County, KS. *Applied Nursing Research, 20*, 188–194.

W. K. Kellogg Foundation. (2004, September). Missing persons: Minorities in the health professions: A report of the Sullivan Commission on diversity in the healthcare workforce. Available at http://www.aacn.nche.edu/Media/pdf/SullivanReport.pdf

Zarate-Abbott, P., Etnyre, A., Gilliland, I., Mahon, M., Allwein, D., Cook, J., et al. (2008). Workplace health promotion: Strategies for low-income Hispanic immigrant women. *AAOHN Journal, 56*(5), 217–222.

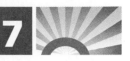

7

Economic Issues in Nursing and Health Care

MATTIA J. GILMARTIN, RN, MBA, PhD

OBJECTIVES

At the completion of this chapter, the reader will be able to:

- Describe how the economic concepts of supply, demand, complements and substitutes, competition, and market failure apply to nursing and health care.
- Define and differentiate methods of cost evaluation.
- Discuss how the cost of care and quality of care are related.
- Compare and contrast the economic foundations of emerging models for health system reform.

PROFILE IN PRACTICE

Elizabeth E. Friberg, DNP, RN
Assistant Professor, University of Virginia School of Nursing, Charlottesville, Virginia

While practicing in direct care for the first 15 years of my career in acute and community-based care, including private practice, I became interested in the production, delivery, and purchasing of health care services and the health care systems that delivered those services. Having a psych-mental health background and a community-based focus, I was interested in the health-seeking behaviors of individuals, groups, organizations, and the larger delivery system, including the relationship of those behaviors to access, cost, and quality. Working with program-level budgets provided an education in the actual cost of producing and delivering health care services. For the next 15 years, my practice was focused at a population level as I moved from community health to managed care and ultimately to the larger health insurance industry. I explored the use of incentives to guide behavior, health benefit design concepts, risk management, role

of prevention, health system fraud and abuse, comparative effectiveness, professional guidelines, and the role of government to protect the public and at times correct behaviors that may negatively affect the public. This focus provided an education on the cost of purchasing health care services—from the varying perspectives of individuals, families, employers, unions, trust funds, and the government. Our system of health care in the United States is extremely complex and inefficient and often fails to produce the outcomes desired by most stakeholders. It tends to satisfy only the few. After 5 years of health care system consulting, I now teach nurses at the undergraduate and graduate level about the complexity and realities of the cost and quality of our health care system.

Nurses need to understand the economic realities of the health care market. Health care professionals need a working knowledge of topics such as delivery models, basic insurance principles, and the fissure between our public health and primary care system. One only needs to listen to recent media dialogue and "town hall meetings" or read op-ed pieces to understand the absolute confusion that exists in the public domain about our current public and private health care system. Nurses have an obligation to know the answers to the following questions: (a) How is the current system designed and how does it operate? (b) What are the drivers of quality health care? (c) What are the market forces that support or impede the delivery of quality health care? (d) What legitimate roles can the government play? and

(e) Where are the opportunities to improve our health care system.

Is health care a legitimate right in our society, and if so, how can we provide it given the limitation of the health care dollar? What models exist that may inform our query and how can we adapt good ideas into a uniquely American approach? As our demographics shift, a solution is imperative because our current path is not sustainable. As nurses, we need to be active and informed participants in the discussion, planning, implementation, and evaluation of a new way forward for ourselves as citizens, for our patients/clients, and for the health and welfare of our nation.

Introduction

Health care professionals historically have been largely unaware of the economic costs and consequences of their clinical decisions. This is due, in part, to the nature of health care financing and the separation of clinical and management functions within health care organizations. However, the spiraling cost of health care as a portion of the nation's overall economy and the inefficient distribution and use of scarce resources within the health care sector (Goodell & Ginsburg, 2008; Institute of Medicine, 1999) underscore the need for health care professionals to understand and incorporate economic principles in their clinical and management decision making.

As the largest professional group in the health care workforce (Hager, Tise, Kuta, Spencer, & Fritz, 2006), nurses are in a unique position to influence the efficient and effective use of scarce health care resources. More broadly, an understanding of economic principles and the tools of economic evaluation enables nurses to demonstrate the contributions of nursing practice that improve resource use in the production of health care services. Nurses involved in clinical practice, administration, education, policy making, and research can use principles of economics to:

- Provide nursing care in the least costly manner
- Protect the scope of nursing practice by demonstrating the quality and value of nursing services in relation to other professionals

- Develop opportunities to expand settings for nursing practice by demonstrating the cost and quality of nursing interventions
- Understand what purchasers and consumers want from nursing and take steps to satisfy these needs and demands
- Promote health system change to expand access, improve the quality, and ensure more equitable distribution of health care resources
- Integrate nursing-specific quality measurement systems and concepts into larger organizational quality improvement initiatives that are largely controlled by nonnurses (Bolton, Donaldson, Rutledge, Bennett, & Brown, 2006; Buerhaus, 1992)

The purpose of this chapter is to introduce the reader to basic economic concepts that affect professional nursing practice and, more broadly, the delivery of health care services. The chapter is organized into three parts. The first part focuses on the economics of nursing with a particular emphasis on the nursing labor market. The next part addresses economic issues for advocacy to improve the quality and effectiveness of patient care and to inform system change. The third part focuses on health care reform, expanding insurance coverage, and consumerism. Common cost evaluation methods useful in demonstrating the economic effects of health care resource allocation decisions and skill development exercises are also presented.

Health Economics

Economics is the study of the distribution of resources across a population. *Health economics* is the study of the production and distribution of health care resources and their impact on a population. Health care resources consist of *medical supplies,* such as pharmaceutical goods, latex gloves, and bed linens; *personnel,* including nurses, physicians, and other allied health professionals; and *capital inputs,* including hospitals and nursing home facilities, diagnostic and therapeutic equipment, and other items used to provide medical care (Santerre & Neun, 2004).

Health care resources are scarce; that is, there is a limit to the quantity that can be produced at a given time, although the demand for these resources can be limitless. Therefore economists are interested in how society makes important decisions regarding the *consumption, production,* and *distribution* of these goods and services within the health care sector and in relation to other societal needs such as education, housing, and defense. As social scientists, health economists seek to answer four basic questions (Santerre & Neun, 2004):

1. What combination of nonmedical and medical goods and services should be produced in a general economy?
2. What particular medical goods and services should be produced in the health economy?
3. What specific health care resources should be used to produce the final medical goods and services?
4. Who should receive the medical goods and services?

Although economic theory is complex, it is guided by a relatively small set of principles and concepts. These concepts are presented in Box 7-1 and provide the foundation for a more detailed explanation of how economic principles underpin current health care issues discussed in this chapter (Henderson, 2008). Typically, economists assume certain conditions to understand human behavior in relation to the production and distribution of resources. Unlike other industries, the health care sector violates a number of assumptions that support general economic theory (Rice, 1998).

UNCERTAINTY

The need for health care services is irregular and cannot be predicted by either consumers or providers (Arrow, 1963). Consumers who demand health care cannot predict when illness or catastrophe will strike, and health care providers cannot forecast the costs of the treatment(s) required. Health care professionals who provide medical interventions also face uncertainty regarding when patients will present themselves for treatment, as well as the extent to which patients will respond to prescribed treatment regimens. The unexpected and often costly nature of illness gives rise to the purchase of insurance as a safeguard against the cost of medical treatment in the event of illness (Folland, Goodman, & Stano, 2007).

INSURANCE AND THIRD-PARTY PAYMENT

Consumers buy insurance to guard against the risk and uncertainty of illness. Insurance introduces an intermediary between the consumer (person requiring medical care) and the providers of care (health care professionals and organizations). Consumers do not pay the full price for their medical care and are separated from making decisions about medical services based on the price of those services. In economic theory, *price* is the key measure used to determine what a consumer is willing to pay for a good or service and enables an organization to gauge its output in relation to consumer desires and buying behaviors. *Insurance* also changes the demand for care, and it potentially changes the incentives for providers to offer certain types of treatments that are reimbursed by insurance (Johnson-Lans, 2006).

PROBLEMS WITH INFORMATION

Economic theory assumes that buyers and sellers have equal information about the cost, price, and quality of goods and services. However, in health care markets, professionals (the sellers) typically have more information about treatment options than do clients (the buyers). In some instances, information is unknown to both the professional and the individual. For

BOX 7-1	Ten Guiding Principles of Economics

1. The principle of scarcity and choice addresses the problem of limited resources and the need to economize. Not enough resources are available to meet all the desires of all the people, making rationing in some form unavoidable. We are forced to make choices among competing objectives—an inescapable result of scarcity.

2. The principle of opportunity costs recognizes that everything and everyone has alternatives. Time and resources used to satisfy one set of desires cannot be used to satisfy another set. The cost of any decision or action is measured in terms of the value placed on the opportunity forgone.

3. Marginal analysis is a way of thinking about the optimal use of resources. Decision makers weigh the trade-offs of a little more of one thing and a little less of another. In this decision-making mode, consideration is given to the benefits and costs of one more unit of a good or service.

4. Self-interest is a primary motivator of economic decision makers. People respond to incentives and practice economizing behavior only when they as individuals can benefit from the behavior. In a just society, the pursuit of self-interest leads each individual to a course of action that promotes the general welfare of everyone in society.

5. Markets and pricing serve as the best way to allocate scarce resources. The market accomplishes this through a system of prices—everything has a price that a consumer is willing to pay for a good or service. Prices decrease if less is desired and increase if more is desired. The price mechanism enables a firm to gauge its output decisions in relation to consumer desires and buying behavior. When supply and demand are in balance, the market is in equilibrium.

6. Supply and demand serve as the foundation for all economic analysis. *Supply* refers to the amount of a good or service available to consumers in the market. *Demand* refers to a consumer's willingness to purchase a particular good or service. Goods and services are allocated among competing uses by striking a balance (equilibrium) between the consumers' willingness to pay and the suppliers' willingness to produce goods and ration those goods by the pricing mechanism.

7. Competition forces those who own resources to use their resources to produce the highest possible satisfaction for society—consumers, producers, and investors. Competition stimulates efficiency in a market environment by rewarding the resource owners who do well in producing a good or service with the best combination of available resources and penalizing those who are inept or inefficient in resource allocation decisions.

8. Efficiency in economics measures how well resources are being used to promote social welfare. Inefficient outcomes waste resources, whereas the efficient use of resources enhances social welfare. Resource allocation is considered efficient when no one can be made better off without making someone else worse off. This equalized allocation state is known as the *Pareto Optimum*.

9. Market failure arises when the free market fails to promote the efficient use of resources by producing either more or less than the optimal level of output.

10. Voluntary exchange in a free market environment promotes economic efficiency and ensures that all mutually beneficial transactions occur. Every transaction will benefit both a consumer and a provider. The market system is grounded in the concept of consumer sovereignty—what is produced is determined by what people want and what they are able to buy. No one individual or group dictates what must be produced or purchased.

Data from Henderson, J. (2009). *Health economics and policy* (with Info Apps 2-Semester printed access card) (4th ed.). © 2009 South-Western, a part of Cengage Learning, Inc.
Reprinted with permission. www.cengage.com/permissions.

example, when a person has cancer that has not yet been detected by regular screenings, a treatment course cannot be formulated because neither party knows that medical services are needed. The lack of symmetrical information is a problem, because it distorts the basic mechanism of consumer sovereignty, in which consumers (clients) dictate what goods and services are produced because they know what they want and what they are willing to pay (Folland, Goodman, & Stano, 2007).

LARGE ROLE OF NONPROFIT FIRMS

Economists assume that organizations seek to maximize profits and that models of firm behavior explain how businesses allocate resources to increase profits. It is important to note that *all* businesses must take in more money than they spend (make a profit or surplus) for continued operations. Many health care providers—including hospitals, nursing homes, and insurance companies—are operated as not-for-profits. Approximately 3000 of the nation's 5700 registered hospitals are organized as privately owned not-for-profit organizations (American Hospital Association, 2008) *Not-for-profit* is simply a tax designation, in which property and earnings are not subject to tax.

RESTRICTIONS ON COMPETITION

Competition is a force that produces the most efficient allocation of resources because owners must use their resources to produce the highest satisfaction for society. Economists assume that markets are perfectly competitive, consisting of numerous buyers and sellers, with no power over price, who have complete information and can enter and exit the market freely by selling similar goods or services. Health care markets violate several of these assumptions. As described previously, health care markets are characterized by asymmetrical information and have weak pricing mechanisms because of third-party payment in the form of insurance. In addition, market entry is blocked by licensure for professional practice, advertising restrictions, and ethical standards that prevent providers from competing with one another. Because health care is considered to be a *public good,* organizations in the sector are subjected to regulation by state and federal government, as well as other outside entities, to ensure the quality of care and distribution of resources across geographic areas (Hoffman, Klees, & Curtis, 2007).

ROLE OF EQUITY AND NEED

Economics is concerned with the distribution of scarce resources so that society receives the highest possible satisfaction from the combination of goods and services produced from these resources. *Distributive justice,* or *equity,* is the extent to which resources are allocated in a fair and equal manner to everyone involved. In pure market economies, the price mechanism is used to strike a balance (equilibrium) between the prices that suppliers charge and the price that purchasers are willing to pay. In pure egalitarian systems, governments ensure that everyone receives an equal distribution of resources (Johnson-Lans, 2006).

The U.S. health care system is a mixed system in which goods and services are distributed both by markets and by government. The mixed system of markets and government is a factor in the inequitable distribution of health care resources, most notably in the lack of universal insurance or universal access to health care services in the United States. Advocates argue that in a just society people ought to get the health care they need, regardless of their ability to pay for these services. We will examine this topic in more detail in the chapter section on health care reform.

GOVERNMENT SUBSIDIES AND PUBLIC PROVISION

The health care sector has more government intervention than other sectors of the national economy because of the uncertainty in the demand for, and provision of, services. In the United States, state and federal governments play major roles as financiers and payers of health care through the Medicare, Medicaid, and State Children's Health Insurance programs. Medicare is the federal insurance program established in 1965 for persons older than 65 years, as well as for selected populations with severe and chronic disabilities. The Medicare program is divided into four parts (Medicare A, B, C, and D) and provides benefits for hospitalization, limited nursing home care, physicians' services, medical supplies, outpatient services, and most recently, prescription drugs. In comparison, Medicaid, also established in 1965, is a joint federal and state-funded insurance program that provides medical and health-related services to America's poorest people. Each state administers its own Medicaid program and sets eligibility requirements for program participation and the type of benefits and services covered. The State Children's Health Insurance Program

(SCHIP) was established in 1997 as part of the Federal Balanced Budget Act to extend health insurance benefits to children of families who do not qualify for the Medicaid program but are unable to buy private health insurance. Together, Medicare, Medicaid, and SCHIP financed $661 billion in health care services in 2005—one third of the country's total health care bill and almost three quarters of all public spending on health care (Hoffman, Klees, & Curtis, 2007).

Economic Concepts Specific to the Nursing Profession

UNDERSTANDING THE SUPPLY AND DEMAND FOR NURSES

In this section we examine the market for nurses to illustrate the concepts of supply and demand. The concepts of complements and substitutes are also presented to examine the use of advanced practice nurses as an alternative to physicians as primary care providers.

Supply refers to the amount of a good or service available to consumers in the market. *Demand* refers to a consumer's willingness to purchase a particular good or service.

Economic theory predicts that as demand increases, so will supply; the pricing mechanism, in the form of wages and other benefits, will create a balance (equilibrium) between firms in need of workers and individuals who are willing to work for the wage offered. When examining the market for labor, economists assume that households have primary and secondary wage earners. Because a very high proportion of nurses are married, they are considered to be part of two-earner families and therefore have more flexibility to respond to employment opportunities as real wages change or in relation to the employment situation of their spouses (Johnson-Lans, 2006).

Nurses' decisions to enter the work force, as well as how many hours they work while employed, are cyclical in nature. In fact, there have been cyclical shortages and surpluses of nurses documented since the 1960s. Current data show that nursing personnel are in high demand as evidenced by an estimated 2.5 million open registered nurse positions across the United States (U.S. Bureau of Labor Statistics, 2007). In addition to the current need for nurses, employment opportunities in the health care sector are expected to grow at a rapid rate, with a 25% projected increase for registered nurses and physician assistants, and a 33% increase in health care support occupations, such as personal and home health care aides (U.S. Bureau of Labor Statistics, 2007). The demand for health care professionals and paraprofessionals is on the rise to care for the nation's 78 million aging baby boomers.

Although employment opportunities in health care are on the rise, the nursing profession is in the midst of a cyclical and worsening shortage that began in 1998, making it the longest in modern history (Buerhaus, Staiger, & Auerbach, 2008; Spetz, 2004). *Shortage* is defined as the excess of the quantity demanded over the quantity supplied at market prices (Folland et al., 2007). The National Sample Survey of Registered Nurses, a comprehensive survey carried out every 4 years to examine trends in the nation's nursing workforce, revealed that the years between 1996 and 2000 marked the slowest growth in the registered nurse population during the 20-year period between 1980 and 2000. On average, the registered nurse population grew only 1.3% each year between 1996 and 2000 compared with average annual increases of 2% to 3% in earlier years. New estimates show that for the period between 2000 and 2004, the number of registered nurses grew by almost 8% to a new high of 2.9 million (Hager et al., 2006). Although progress has been made in expanding the supply of nurses, economists estimate an anticipated shortage of 285,000 registered nurses between 2015 and 2020 (Buerhaus et al., 2008). Box 7-2 and Figure 7-1 illustrate a forecasting model to predict changes in the nursing workforce.

MONOPSONY POWER OF HOSPITALS

In a well-functioning market, a shortage should be resolved by wage increases until a balance is restored (equilibrium) between organizations in need of workers and workers who are willing to participate in the labor force. One argument used to explain the chronic shortage of nurses is the notion that nurses

BOX 7-2	Supply and Demand: Estimating the Nursing Workforce

In the current market environment, the demand for nurses is in flux because of rapid changes in the organization of the health care delivery system. The supply of nurses available to the health care market is affected by five primary components: (1) predictions of the overall growth of the economy; (2) technology, delivery systems, and regulatory factors within the health care system; (3) economic factors influencing resource scarcity; (4) the availability of personnel in the health care sector; and (5) population factors driving the demand for health services. Historically the educational system (responsible for creating the nursing supply) and the health care delivery sector (which creates the demand for nursing services) have acted independently. The uncertainty of the current marketplace and opportunities for new nursing services require the ability to predict accurately the need for appropriate nursing personnel to meet the emerging demand within the changing market environment.

Dumpe, Herman, and Young (1998) present the Forecasting Model of the Nursing Workforce to provide policymakers with information to make accurate decisions regarding the education and employment of nurses. The forecasting model is based on the theory of supply and demand and assumes that the demand for nurses and their services responds in a manner similar to the demand for any other good available in the marketplace. Additionally, the model is based on the assumption that forecasting the demand for nurses is possible. The major economic concepts used in the forecasting model include supply factors, demand factors, the aggregate demand for nurses, the aggregate supply of nurses, contextual factors, market equilibrium, and the nursing workforce.

The monopsony model, which examines how employers set wages and make decisions about hiring workers is used to explain this puzzle and provides a partial explanation as to why the market for registered nurses does not conform to the predictions of supply and demand. More specifically, the monopsony model explains the coexistence of high vacancy rates and lower-than-competitive wages for nurses (Johnson-Lans, 2006).

Although nurses are employed in a number of community settings, hospitals are the main employer of nurses. Approximately 56% of registered nurses are employed in acute care hospital settings (Hager et al., 2006). Therefore most of the information about the market for nursing labor is understood within the context of hospitals. The monopsony model is based on the assumptions that (1) the market has one dominant buyer (employer) or perhaps a few employers in a regional market who control the demand for workers and (2) all persons who do the same work are paid the same wage. Because workers are paid the same wage, if the employer has to offer a higher wage to get additional workers, it must also raise the wages of the workers that it already employs. Eventually, all of the operating budget would go to paying salaries and the hospital would not be able to make a surplus or profit. As discussed previously, organizations need to make a surplus to stay in business.

The hospital using the monopsony model considers the cost of hiring one more nurse in relation to the amount of revenue it will gain from the productivity of that nurse. In effect, the hospital sets nurses' wages so that it maximizes its ability to make a profit. In this situation, the wage level that satisfies the hospital's profit goal is lower than what nurses could be offered if there were more buyers in the market. Because nurses often have choices about participating in the labor force, they may decide that the wage offered by a hospital is too low and decide to forgo working for a particular hospital. Thus the hospital will continue to need nurses and the nurses' wages will be lower than other comparable workers.

In contrast, markets with many hospitals competing for nursing labor conform more closely to the predictions of supply and demand. As noted previously, the presence of multiple competitors (hospitals) in

are underpaid and it is the low wages, relative to other health professionals, as well as other job opportunities outside of nursing and health care, that keep individuals from participating in the workforce as registered nurses. From a purely economic perspective, linking the labor shortage to low wages is curious, in that it violates the basic assumptions of supply and demand.

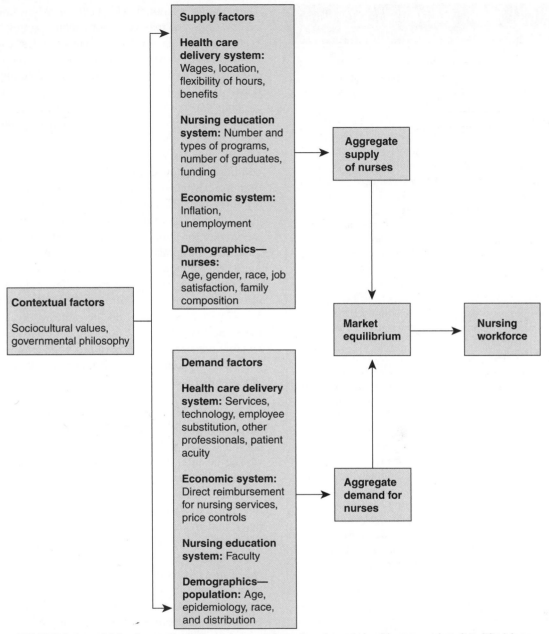

FIGURE 7-1 A model for forecasting the nursing workforce in a dynamic health care market. (Modified from Dumpe, M. L., Herman, J., & Young, S. W. [1998]. Forecasting the nursing workforce in a dynamic health care market. *Nursing Economics, 16*[4], 170. Reprinted with permission of the publisher, Jannetti Publications, Inc., Pitman, NJ.)

one market provides more favorable conditions for workers in terms of the wages employers will offer to satisfy their demand for labor. Under competitive market conditions, when faced with a shortage of nurses, some hospitals will move faster than others and offer a higher wage for nurses. The wage increase brings about two important outcomes that, taken together, help to alleviate the nursing shortage. In the short term, increased wages are incentives for nurses that are currently unemployed to join the workforce.

Additionally, nurses who are currently employed may respond to the higher wages by working overtime hours, taking a second job, or changing from part-time to full-time employment. These responses typically increase the short-term supply of nurses participating in the workforce in RN roles. In the long term, the increased wages offered by hospitals and other organizations influence individuals' decisions to enter the nursing profession and are one mechanism to ensure an adequate supply of nurses (Buerhaus, 2008). Evidence suggests that increases in nurses' wages have reduced the nursing shortage. As of 2004 the average annual earnings for registered nurses were $57,785 (Hager et al., 2006). Buerhaus (2008) reports that between 2002 and 2006 real wages for nurses in the United States increased an average of 6.9%, producing the expected drop in hospital registered nurse vacancy rates from a national average of 13% reported in 2001 to 8.1% by 2006.

Although there have been reports in the popular media about hospitals' somewhat extravagant tactics to attract nurses—for instance, $100,000 annual salaries for experienced nurses and other incentives such as flat-screen TVs, gift certificates, and car leases (Robert Wood Johnson Foundation, 2009)—it is likely that hospitals will begin instituting wage controls in response to the unfolding national recession of 2008-2009, possibly exacerbating the nursing shortage. Wage control, or a freeze on nurses' salaries, is viewed as one way to keep hospital operating costs in check. Historical data on prior nursing shortages suggest that freezing nurses' wages in the face of increasing demand for nursing labor, as characterized by current conditions, will lengthen the duration of a shortage once it begins (Buerhaus, 2008). Given the changing population demographics in combination with the existing labor shortage, widespread use of

wage controls may have destructive consequences for the nursing profession, patients, and hospitals.

It is important to note that nurses' decisions to participate in the workforce are complex and not fully explained by economic theory. Managerial and public policies targeting cost containment, such as efforts to reduce in-patient length of stay (LOS), have had a great impact on the working conditions of nurses and have contributed to the duration of the current shortage (Aiken, 2008). Strong evidence suggests that attributes of the organizational environment, also referred to as the *nursing practice environment,* factor into individual nurses' decisions to stay employed at a particular hospital or to participate in the workforce in the capacity as a registered nurse. Organizational factors such as work load, managers' leadership style, autonomy over nursing practice, promotion opportunities, and work schedules also contribute to nurses' decisions to work (Aiken, 2008; Brewer et al., 2006; Hayes et al., 2006). In their position statement for health system reform, the American Nurses Association advocates for a number of workplace changes to promote the recruitment and retention of nurses and the sustainability of autonomous professional nursing practice (American Nurses Association, 2008).

NURSES AS COMPLEMENTS AND SUBSTITUTES FOR PHYSICIANS

Complements are products or services that are usually consumed jointly, so that an increase in the price of one decreases the demand for both (e.g., intravenous fluids and tubing). If nursing services are complements to physician services, then an increase in the price of physician services will decrease demand for both physician and nursing services.

Substitutes, on the other hand, are goods or services that satisfy the same want or need, so that an increase in the price of one will increase the demand for the other. One example of substitutes in health care occurs when two medications have the same therapeutic effect. Another example is an obstetrician and a nurse midwife. If nursing services are substitutes for physician obstetric services, then an increase in the cost of physician services will increase the demand for nursing midwife services.

In the physician arena an imbalance exists between generalists and specialists, resulting in a shortage of primary care physicians (Hauer et al., 2008; Mitka, 2007). This disparity between consumer demand and physician supply creates favorable opportunities for advanced practice nurses to practice in primary care centers as physician substitutes. Nurses are making arguments for their use as substitutes for more expensive providers of care for services that they have been formally trained to provide. For example, nurse practitioners work as primary care providers in hospital-based outpatient clinics. Similarly, health care delivery organizations, in an effort to reduce input costs, are incorporating the use of unlicensed personnel as substitutes for nurses for those activities that do not require licensure. For example, hospitals and other delivery organizations have changed the nursing staff skill mix to include registered nurses, licensed practical nurses, and nursing assistants. Thus nurses are both substituting for some types of providers and being substituted by other types of providers.

Physicians have traditionally held a monopolistic power as primary care providers because regulations have prevented others from "practicing medicine." As alternative providers of health care services demonstrate their ability to provide comparable services, regulations are being changed to allow these substitutes to enter the market and compete with physicians. Such changes in regulation have come about because consumers have demanded more cost-effective providers while organized physician interests have lost political power (e.g., the journal, *Nurse Practitioner* for an annual legislative review governing advanced nursing practice).

With advanced practice nurses working as physician substitutes, competition between these two providers can occur on the basis of cost effectiveness. Studies have demonstrated that the use of advanced practice nurses as primary care providers can reduce costs of outpatient care, including laboratory costs, per-visit costs, per-episode costs, and long-term management costs (Brown & Grimes, 1993; Fulton & Baldwin, 2004; Schroeder, 1993; U.S. Congress, 1986). Nurse-managed services are typically those services offered by advanced practice nurses (nurse practitioners, clinical nurse specialists, nurse midwives,

and nurse anesthetists) based on the nursing philosophy emphasizing health promotion and preventative care—for example, chronic disease management, case management, or primary care. Research studies have documented that nurse-managed care, when compared with physician-managed care, reduces the frequency of hospitalizations, reduces the acuity of those admitted, reduces lengths of stay, reduces the cost of hospitalization, and results in equivalent ratings for patient satisfaction with service delivery (Brooten, Youngblut, Kutcher, & Bobo, 2004; Mundinger et al., 2000). Given the evidence for the efficacy of nurse-managed services, nurse leaders are developing arguments that move beyond comparing advanced practice nurses as substitutes and complements to physician services and focus on the unique aspects and additional value of advanced practice nurses in achieving optimal patient outcomes (Kleinpell & Gawlinski, 2005; Lin, Gebbie, Fullilove, & Arons, 2004; Mundinger, 2002).

Retail clinics differ from *urgent care clinics* in that they are located within discount stores, grocery stores, or drug stores; are staffed by either nurse practitioners or physician assistants; and offer a limited set of basic medical and preventative services. Retail clinics are an emerging trend whereby advanced practice nurses act as substitutes for physicians to meet consumers' desire for more convenient and lower-cost medical care. Health care services typically offered at retail clinics include preventative care such as immunizations and blood pressure screening, as well as treatment for upper respiratory, sinusitis, ear, or urinary tract infections. Clients mainly pay for retail visits out of pocket, although in recent years many insurance companies, including Medicare and Medicaid, will pay for these visits (Mehrotra, Wang, Lave, Adams, & McGlynn, 2008). There are now more than 700 retail clinics throughout the United States, and their numbers are expected to reach 3000 within 5 years (PricewaterhouseCoopers, 2008).

Retail clinics offer an alternative to urgent care clinics and emergency departments for simple acute problems. Despite the national shortage of primary care physicians, the emergence of these nurse-led clinics has drawn the ire of some medical societies, who question their quality and are asking for increased regulation. For instance, the American Medical Association, the American Academy of Family Physicians, and several state medical societies are recommending certain operating requirements, including limits on the scope of clinical services, the creation of referral systems with physician practices, and the use of electronic patient records (PricewaterhouseCoopers, 2008).

In an early evaluation comparing the client demographics of, and reasons for, visits to retail clinics, primary care physicians, and emergency departments, Mehrotra and colleagues (2008) found that retail clinics show signs of becoming *safety net providers* by offering services to a population that is currently underserved by primary care physicians. Clients seen at retail clinics were more likely to be young adults, between the ages of 18 and 44, who pay out of pocket for their care and are less likely to have an existing relationship with a primary care provider. Approximately 90% of retail clinic visits focus on treating 10 minor acute conditions; these same conditions represent 13% of adult primary care physician visits, 30% of pediatric primary care physician visits, and 12% of emergency department visits. These early data suggest that nurse-led retail clinics serve an important role in expanding access to primary care services and relieve the stress on emergency departments. Whether there will be continued expansion and a widespread shift of uncomplicated acute care services from primary care physicians and emergency departments to retail clinics remains to be seen.

Economic Concepts for Advocacy and Professional Practice

In this section we examine a number of economic concepts and how they affect health care delivery and professional nursing practice. We begin by examining the nature of health insurance markets and the relationship between insurance and access to health care. Next, we discuss relationships among cost, quality, and value and the role of technology as a key driver of health care costs. Finally, we examine the concepts of efficiency and effectiveness and present evaluation tools to assess the distribution and benefits of health care interventions.

PAYING FOR HEALTH CARE: INSURANCE, NATIONAL HEALTH EXPENDITURES, AND ACCESS TO CARE

This section begins with a brief overview of key concepts used to understand how health insurance affects the demand for medical care from the perspectives of consumers and providers. The discussion then turns to comparing the major types of health insurance and concludes by presenting current data on the rising financial burdens faced by U.S. consumers to pay for health care and the problems of the uninsured and underinsured.

Because medical care is costly and it is difficult to predict when one might need medical services, insurance functions as a buffer from the financial risks associated with treating illness or disease. People buy insurance as a way to avoid the *risks* and associated costs of illness and seeking medical treatment. A number of risks are associated with health. There is a risk to one's health or life associated with illness or disease. There is the additional risk that a given treatment course will not cure or alleviate the underlying disease. Also, there may be unavoidable harm from the treatment itself or by the lack of skill or negligence on the part of the provider. There is a risk of incurring the costs that may be substantial to pay for any treatments. Individuals can take certain actions to reduce the risk of illness—getting vaccinations, avoiding dangerous environments, or leading a health lifestyle—but this considerable risk still remains largely uncertain (Johnson-Lans, 2006).

People buy health insurance to avoid the risk of having to pay for expensive medical care. Stated a different way, people are "risk averse" and try to safeguard their wealth or resources by buying insurance as protection from the financial consequences of an unpredictable event. Economists view risk aversion as a characteristic of people's utility functions. Marginal utility is the extra satisfaction, welfare, or well-being (utility) gained from consuming one more unit of a good or service. In the case of insurance, it is believed that people are more likely to buy insurance to cover low-probability events involving large losses than high-probability events that are associated with small losses (Johnson-Lans, 2006).

Although it is difficult to predict when an individual will become sick or need expensive medical care, the risk for large numbers of people (or the expected value of all losses averaged over all people) is quite predictable. Insurance spreads risk across a group of people and involves a series of trades between people. This practice is known as *risk pooling*. Money is shifted between people who are healthy to people who are sick and in need to pay for expensive medical care. Insurance pools potential losses, but it does not eliminate or reduce the losses. That is, insurance companies specialize in *pricing* risks, not in taking risks. Insurance companies sell policies to large groups of people with predictable or average risks. Members pay a premium, which covers all losses across the group of policy holders as well as management fees (Getzen, 2004).

Moral hazard occurs when a person's behavior changes based on his or her insurance coverage. In the event of an illness or other adverse event, the insured person is offered medical care at a reduced price. Moral hazard in health insurance markets occurs to the extent that insurance increases the quantity of medical care used (Chernew, Hirth, Sonnad, Ermann, & Fendrick, 1998; Freeman, Kadiyala, Bell, & Martin, 2008; Jonhson-Lans, 2006; Newhouse, 1992). One way that insurance companies offset the risk of moral hazard is to require cost sharing with consumers. Deductibles and co-payments are two commonly used methods.

Co-payment is a sharing relationship between the consumer and the insurance company, as specified in a given policy. When consumers seek medical care, the insurance company pays for some of the costs and the consumer pays for the remainder (the co-payment). A *deductible* is a fixed amount that the consumer must pay toward a medical bill each year before any insurance payments are made. Deductibles are designed to generate more prudent care decisions on the part of the policy holder because they dissuade consumers from submitting claims to the insurance company for "small" losses or minor services (Getzen, 2004).

Consumers purchase health care depending on their perceptions of the impact of the care on their health (McMenamin, 1990). That is, consumers purchase health care, but their actual desire, with a few exceptions, is health. Thus the demand for health care "is derived from the more basic demand for health" (Feldstein, 1983, p. 81). The decision to purchase health care also depends on the cost of care to the consumer. Total consumer costs of health care include monetary costs (co-payment, deductibles, insurance premiums, out-of-pocket expenses, and lost time from wages and work), as well as nonmonetary costs (e.g., risk, pain, inconvenience).

The demand for health care also depends on the willingness of consumers to purchase services after weighing the expected benefits of the care against the costs of the care. If consumers carry insurance, their direct out-of-pocket expenses for the care will be less than if they are uninsured (Feldstein, 1983). Therefore the insurance status of consumers has an impact on the costs of care (to the consumers) and thus their demand for care.

Despite the fact that consumers make co-payments and pay deductibles, they are generally insulated from the high costs of health care because insurance companies typically pay such a large portion of a bill. This separation of consumers from the price of health care resulting from health insurance coverage (either private or public) has dramatically increased demand for health care services. However, because demand is based on willingness and ability to purchase, demand for health care does not necessarily correlate with the need for health care. Demand for health care services changes over time as societal demographics and morbidity patterns change. For instance, as baby boomers continue to enter middle and old age, their demands for health care will contribute to the already increasing demands of an existing elderly population.

Demand for specific services is also influenced by the recommendations and decisions of health care providers (Feldstein, 1983). Because providers of care possess more knowledge regarding treatment options than consumers do, the practice styles of providers, as well as how much information they share with consumers, can greatly affect the demand and consumption of services (Devers, Brewster, & Casalino, 2003; Rice & Labelle, 1989). Similarly, the risk of litigation by consumers can result in a "defensive" practice style by providers. Fear of litigation can lead to overprescription of (often unnecessary) diagnostic tests or therapeutic interventions and ultimately result in higher health care costs.

The demand for health care services is not directly related to the amount or quality of services purchased as in other industries. This, in conjunction with the high levels of uncertainty and the unequal information among consumers, providers, and payers, leads to a situation called *market failure*. Market failure is characterized by the inability of buyers and sellers to strike a balance in the supply and demand of goods and services and ultimately fail to produce a socially desirable level of output. For example, variation in the quality of care is an example of market failure arising from imperfect consumer information about physician practice patterns. This implies that some patients are getting too much treatment and some too little treatment. In fact, it is well documented that many Americans do not receive care that is based on the best scientific knowledge (Institute of Medicine, 2001). More generally, supply-side drivers leading to market failure include the cost of care for hospital and physician services, access to care because of the prohibitive cost of health insurance, and medical outcomes and population health status in light of invested resources. Demand-side factors of market failure in health care include third-party insurance mechanism, in which the insurance company or government entity under the Medicare and Medicaid programs is the primary purchaser of health care services (Henderson, 2008).

TYPES OF INSURANCE

There are four dominant methods consumers use to pay for their health care in the United States: out-of-pocket payment, private individual insurance, employer-sponsored group insurance, and public or government-sponsored individual or group insurance. Each of these payment modes can be viewed as a historical progression and as a categorization of current health care financing (Bodenheimer & Grumbach, 2005).

Out-of-pocket payment: Out-of-pocket payment for health care services is the simplest form of financing because the consumer directly pays the provider for services. This was the dominant model of paying for health care services in the 19th and early 20th centuries, when the technology and available interventions to cure disease or alleviate the symptoms of illness were relatively weak. However, out-of-pocket payment is a flawed way to pay for health care, especially because health care services have become more complex and increasingly expensive. Individuals cannot save or borrow enough money to pay for health care services.

Private individual insurance: This form of financing adds a third party (the insurance company) to the relationship between the consumer and provider. Payment for health care services is divided into two parts, a premium paid by the individual to the insurance company and a reimbursement payment to the provider from the insurance company. Indemnity insurance adds a third payment transaction: a reimbursement to the individual from the insurance company. Because of the administrative costs in managing these transactions, individual health insurance never became a dominant method of paying for health care (Starr, 1982). Currently, individual policies provide health insurance for only 3% of the U.S. population (DeNavas-Walt, Proctor, & Smith, 2008). Because of the growing burden of uninsurance and underinsurance, individual policies are gaining acceptance as a plausible way to expand insurance benefits, although their use remains limited (Claxton et al., 2007).

Employer-sponsored group insurance came into being during the Great Depression and expanded rapidly after World War II. The American Hospital Association first established the Blue Cross of California in 1939, offering hospital insurance to groups of workers. The first employer-based insurance plans were initiated by physicians and hospitals that were seeking a steady source of income, generous reimbursements, and protection from cost controls (Starr, 1982), all of which had declined during the Great Depression because people were not able to pay for their medical and hospital expenses out of pocket.

With employer-based insurance, the employer pays most of the premium to purchase health insurance on behalf of their employees. Thus in the United States, health insurance became a benefit of employment. The government treats employee health benefits as a tax-deductible business expense for employers. Because each dollar of employer-sponsored health insurance results in a reduction in taxes collected, the federal government is in essence subsidizing employer-sponsored insurance. This subsidy is estimated to be about

$168 billion per year (Employment Benefits Research Institute, 2008). Insurance increased the demand for, and cost of, medical services, which become difficult to control. Moreover, individuals not participating in the labor force, especially the elderly and those with chronic conditions or low incomes, found it increasingly difficult to buy insurance on their own. This lead to the creation of the government-sponsored Medicare and Medicaid programs in the mid-1960s and the more recent State Children's Health Insurance Program in 1997.

Public or government-sponsored insurance: The U.S. government became involved in the financing of health care during the Great Depression. Problems among the elderly and poor in accessing health care services eventually led to the creation of the federally sponsored Medicare and the state-sponsored Medicaid programs. Government health insurance for the poor and elderly adds the taxpayer to the equation as the ultimate payer. Much like private insurance, beneficiaries are required to make a contribution in order to receive benefits. Taxpayers need to contribute a certain amount to social security taxes to be eligible for Medicare.

In comparison, the state-funded Medicaid program is funded by taxpayer contributions, although not all taxpayers are eligible for Medicaid benefits. Because these programs are tax-funded, there is a double subsidy at play for taxpayers. As with private insurance, benefits are shifted from those who are healthy to those who are sick. The government-sponsored programs add an additional distribution of funds between the wealthy and the poor. That is, the healthy middle-income employees generally pay more Social Security taxes than they receive in health services. Unemployed, disabled, and lower-income elderly persons may receive more in health services than they contribute in taxes (Bodenheimer & Grumbach, 2005).

TRENDS IN NATIONAL HEALTH CARE EXPENDITURES AND INSURANCE COVERAGE IN THE UNITED STATES

Individual Americans are spending a greater percentage of their annual income on health services than in the past. Personal health care expenditures are third only to food and housing expenditures in household budgets (Folland et al., 2007). Projections of health care spending are based on data from estimates of per-person income increases, the relative price of medical services, growth in consumers' out-of-pocket share of health care spending, changes in insurance enrollment patterns, and control of public policy initiatives (Smith, Heffler, & Freeland, 1999). Personal health care expenditures grew, per person, from $144 in 1960 to a high of $7421 in 2007. Total personal health care spending is $2.2 trillion, representing 16.2% of the gross domestic product (Smith et al., 1999).

From 2002 to 2004, national health expenditures decelerated rapidly from 9.0% to 6.9% as a result of slowdowns in the net price of private insurance and prescription drug costs, as well as more modest reductions in hospital and public health spending. From 2004 to 2007, national health spending declined from 6.9% to 6.1%, reflecting cost reductions in prescription drugs and hospital spending, the slowest decline since 1998 (Hartman, Martin, McDonnell, Catlin, & National Health Expenditures Accounts Team, 2009). Figure 7-2 demonstrates changes in health care expenditure for selected services for the years 1997 and 2007.

Although national health spending has stabilized in the last 5 years, the overall growth of health spending as a proportion of the GDP has caused an increase in the number of uninsured Americans (people who do not receive health coverage through their employers, do not purchase private insurance out of pocket, and do not qualify for Medicare or Medicaid). It is important to note that the rise in health care costs is related to, but not the same as, rising health insurance premiums. Insurance premiums and health care costs are distinct, yet linked, costs (Ginsburg, 2008). In 2007 the annual employer group premium for a family of four was $12,106, nearly double what it was in 2000 (Kaiser Family Foundation, 2008).

The greatest financial barriers affecting access to health care services are poverty and uninsurance. Race, geographic location, and gender represent the greatest nonfinancial barriers in access to health care services (Rhoades, 2005; Schoen & DesRoches, 2000). The U.S. Census Bureau (DeNavas-Walt et al., 2008) estimates that the number of people without health insurance coverage in the United States declined from

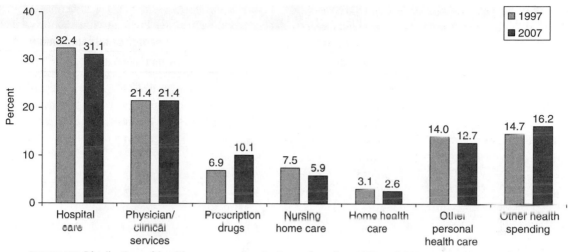

FIGURE 7-2 Distribution of health care spending by type of service, 1997 and 2007. Projections are for services delivered to individuals. Percentages may not total 100% due to rounding. "Other personal health care" includes, for example, dental and other professional health services, durable medical equipment. "Other health spending" includes, for example, administration and net cost of private health insurance, public health activity, research, and structures and equipment. (From "Distribution of National Health Expenditures, by Type of Service, 1997 and 2007," Kaiser Fast Facts, The Henry J. Kaiser Family Foundation, January 2009. This information was reprinted with permission from the Henry J. Kaiser Family Foundation. The Kaiser Family Foundation is a non-profit private operating foundation, based in Menlo Park, California, dedicated to producing and communicating the best possible information, research and analysis on health issues.)

47 million (15.8%) in 2006 to 45.7 million (15.3%) in 2007. The number of people covered by private health insurance (202 million) in 2007 was not statistically different from 2006, while the number of people covered by government health insurance increased to 83.0 million, up from 80.3 million in 2006. For those older than 65 years, 1.1% of the population is uninsured. The widespread coverage of elderly Americans is attributable to the federally subsidized Medicare program.

The majority of uninsured persons come from working families. Nearly 70% of the uninsured have at least one full-time worker in their family and another 12% have only part-time workers. The uninsured are more likely to work either in low-wage blue-collar jobs or for small firms or in service industries. More than half of uninsured workers have no education beyond high school, making it difficult to gain access to jobs that are more likely to provide insurance benefits. Adults between ages 30 and 64 account for nearly 50% of the uninsured. Another 30% of the uninsured are young adults, ages 19 to 29, who are beginning

their careers and have low incomes or are in jobs that are less likely to offer health benefits (Kaiser Commission on Medicaid and the Uninsured, 2008). Hispanics are more likely to be uninsured than non-Hispanic whites or African Americans (Table 7-1). The number of uninsured Hispanics rose to 34.1% or 15.3 million people in 2006 (DeNavas-Walt et al., 2008). Of the 94.7 million women who are 18 to 64 years of age, approximately 18% are uninsured. These women typically do not qualify for Medicaid, do not have access to employer-sponsored plans, or cannot afford individual policies (Kaiser Family Foundation, 2008).

Although progress has been made in extending insurance coverage, underinsurance is a growing trend. People who are underinsured are exposed to greater health care costs as a percentage of their total income. In 2007, an estimated 75 million people, or 42% of the under-65 adult population, were uninsured or underinsured. Of this group, 25 million people were underinsured, a 60% increase since 2003. The rate of increase was steepest among those with income

TABLE 7-1	Health Insurance Coverage, 2007			
	ALL PEOPLE		**PEOPLE OF HISPANIC ORIGIN**	
	No. (in Thousands)	%	No. (in Thousands)	%
Total	299,106	100.0	46,026	100.0
Total covered	253,449	84.7	31,256	67.9
Private	201,991	67.5	20,194	43.9
Employment-based	177,446	59.3	18,551	40.3
Direct purchase	6673	8.9	1804	3.9
Government	83,031	27.8	13,031	28.3
Medicare	41,375	13.8	2887	6.3
Medicaid	39,554	13.2	10,348	22.5
Military	10,995	3.7	801	1.7
Not covered	45,657	15.3	14,770	32.1

Note: The estimates by type of coverage are not mutually exclusive; people can be covered by more than one type of health insurance during the year. Reprinted from DeNavas-Walt, C., Proctor, B. D., & Smith, J. C. (2008). *Income, poverty and health insurance coverage in the United States: 2007. U.S. Census Bureau, current population survey* (pp. 61, 65). 2000-2008 Annual Social and Economic Supplements. Washington DC: U.S. Government Printing Office.

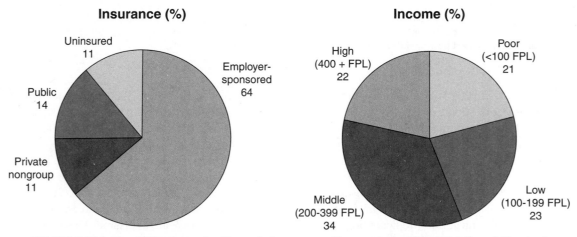

FIGURE 7-3 High financial burden on health care by insurance and income group, 2004. "High financial burden" means that individuals are spending more than 10% of family income on health care. (From "45 Million Nonelderly in Families with High Financial Burden for Health Care, by Insurance and Income Groups, 2004," Kaiser Fast Facts, The Henry J. Kaiser Family Foundation, April 2008. This information was reprinted with permission from the Henry J. Kaiser Family Foundation. The Kaiser Family Foundation is a non-profit private operating foundation, based in Menlo Park, California, dedicated to producing and communicating the best possible information, research and analysis on health issues.)

rates above 200% of the poverty line (Figure 7-3), or those with annual household incomes of $40,000 to $59,999—underinsurance rates among this group nearly tripled between 2003 and 2007 (Schoen, Collins, Kriss, & Doty, 2008). Ziller and colleagues (2006) found that people living in rural areas are more likely to be among the underinsured. One in eight rural residences is underinsured (12%) compared with 10% of people living in rural areas adjacent to urban centers or those living in urban areas (6%). Rural residents are

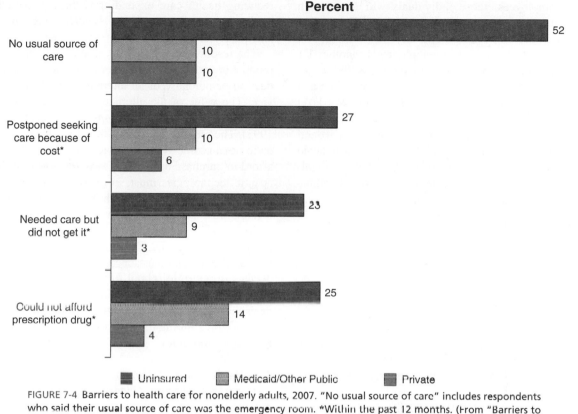

FIGURE 7-4 Barriers to health care for nonelderly adults, 2007. "No usual source of care" includes respondents who said their usual source of care was the emergency room. *Within the past 12 months. (From "Barriers to Health Care Among Nonelderly Adults, by Insurance Status, 2007," Kaiser Fast Facts, The Henry J. Kaiser Family Foundation, October 2008. This information was reprinted with permission from the Henry J. Kaiser Family Foundation. The Kaiser Family Foundation is a non-profit private operating foundation, based in Menlo Park, California, dedicated to producing and communicating the best possible information, research and analysis on health issues.)

more likely to work for themselves or small firms and to have private insurance plans with high premiums and co-payments.

Because of the prohibitive costs of medical care, adequate insurance coverage is a necessary condition to gain access to health care services. The uninsured and underinsured face barriers in obtaining preventative care; they receive a lower standard of care when they do access the system; and they have poorer health outcomes than their insured counterparts (Hadley, 2007). For example, the uninsured or underinsured are more likely to forgo filling prescriptions or to ration their medication, to miss follow-up or routine medical appointments either after a hospitalization episode

or for chronic disease management, and to go without important preventative care procedures such as Pap tests, mammograms, or colonoscopies (Hadley, 2007; Kaiser Family Foundation, 2008a). More alarming, the Institute of Medicine (2004) reports that someone in the United States dies every 24 minutes because they are uninsured and cannot get the medical care they need when they need it. (Figure 7-4 illustrates the effect of being uninsured on nonelderly adults.)

The unfolding economic crisis of 2008 to 2009 will likely reverse the modest gains achieved recently in reducing the rate of uninsured Americans. The number of uninsured or underinsured will surely rise in the face of growing unemployment. As more companies shed employees, these individuals will lose health benefits. According to the Kaiser Family Foundation Commission on Medicaid and the Uninsured (2008), for every 1% increase in unemployment, another 1.1 million people join the ranks of the uninsured. As of January 2009 the U.S. economy was in recession and the unemployment rate increased sharply to a level not seen in decades (Rampell, 2009). In turn, high unemployment rates lead to lower state and federal tax revenues, which are used to finance the Medicaid insurance program and pay hospitals and other organizations for health care services. Those who continue to receive health benefits through their employers will most likely face erosion in the quality of their coverage, as well as higher cost-sharing arrangements as companies seek to minimize their costs (Kaiser Commission on Medicaid and the Uninsured, 2008).

EVALUATING HEALTH SYSTEMS: COST, QUALITY, VALUE, AND TECHNOLOGY

Costs. Costs are resources required by the provider of services to produce health care products and services, as well as the amount a consumer pays to purchase the products and services. The costs to produce health care are the actual costs of inputs incurred for production, whereas the costs to purchase health care services are what the health care economy will bear (i.e., what the consumers and financiers are able and willing to pay). Thus costs depend on supply and demand. Costs may be monetary (pecuniary) or intangible (nonpecuniary). The pecuniary costs of care include salaries of health care providers, insurance premiums, the cost of supplies and equipment used during care, management overhead, pharmaceuticals, transportation, and lost salary of the consumer, as well as construction and maintenance costs and research. Nonpecuniary costs are those associated with the personal loss, pain, suffering, and other consequences associated with the consumption of health care services.

The costs of health care are affected by many factors, including the supply of services, the demand for services, and the use of medical technology. An increase in the input costs of providing a service increases health care expenditures, while the quantity and quality remain constant. Efforts are focused on reducing health care expenditures through reducing the input costs of care without sacrificing the quantity and quality of services.

The resources consumed to produce or purchase a product or service are no longer available for the production or purchase of an alternative product or service. The value of the alternative product or service that is forgone is known as the *opportunity cost* (Pauly, 1993). The opportunity cost is therefore what is given up to obtain some good or service. A hospital that can afford to purchase only one of two diagnostic or therapeutic technologies must, in choosing one, give up known benefits of the other. The value of the forgone benefits (revenue generated, lives saved) is the opportunity cost. The concept of opportunity cost can also be applied to personal economic decision making. In the case of the associate degree–prepared nurse who decides to return to school full time to pursue a baccalaureate degree, the opportunity cost of this career decision includes the lost earnings from not being in the workforce during the time it takes to complete the educational program.

Quality of Care. Nurses play a key role in quality improvement activities. Under managed care, the narrow focus on cost containment has compromised quality improvement activities. Manifest signs of quality of care problems in health care include medical errors, underuse of appropriate medical interventions, lack of integrated services, and poor allocation of resources across different parts of the health care system (Leape, 1994; Wallace, 2004). In their roles as clinicians, managers, researchers, and policymakers, nurses contribute in important ways to advancing the overall quality of health care service. For this discussion, *health care quality* is defined as the degree to which health services for individuals and populations increase the likelihood of desired health outcomes and are consistent with current professional knowledge (Lohr, 1990). From an economic perspective, quality is the value gained from services for the amount of resources used in the production of those services. This section focuses on the contributions of professional nursing practice in quality improvement activities. Background information about systemic and organizational issues related to health care quality and its improvement can be found in the work of Shortell, Bennett, and Byck (1998), as well as the Institute of Medicine's companion reports, *To Err is Human* (1999) and *Crossing the Quality Chasm* (2001).

Clinical nurses: Within organizational settings, clinical nurses play an important role in ensuring the quality of care in three ways. First, clinical nurses act as interpreters among patients, families, physicians, and the system; they bear a responsibility for critical moment-to-moment decision making; and they spend more time than other health care providers in direct contact with patients. Clinical nurses have expertise in evaluating patients' responses to care. This expertise provides a platform to participate in projects that evaluate the costs and outcomes of new or different combinations of clinical interventions.

Second, as consumers of nursing research, clinical nurses play a role in evaluating current practice patterns against best practices and integrating new knowledge into care pathways and unit-based nursing protocols and standards. Finally, as the interface between patients and an organization's care processes, clinical nurses play a role in providing managers with information regarding the extent to which systems and processes enhance or hinder clinical practice.

Nurse managers: Nurse managers and executives play two key roles in quality improvement activities. First, nurse managers, along with their peers, work to create a culture based on principles and practices of quality improvement and clinical excellence. Nurse executives shape the organization's vision and values associated with patient care service. Middle and first-line managers promote behaviors aligned with the organization's vision and values and work to implement the organization's quality improvement goals. Managers remove barriers between departments, lead evaluation activities, and keep the momentum of change going. Second, nurse managers at all levels of an organization develop business cases for investing in technical and structural changes to promote clinical quality. Business cases are detailed arguments advanced by managers to allocate the organization's resources to achieve strategic goals. Senior managers integrate relevant investment proposals originating at the service or nursing unit level into the organization's budget and planning systems. Typical investments to support clinical quality improvement include training and skill development, information systems and electronic patient records, and consultations for data analysis and interpretation.

Nurse researchers: Nurse researchers play a key role in advancing knowledge and sharpening understanding about nursing practice. To this end, nurse researchers have developed conceptual models and documented empirical evidence to articulate nursing's contribution to care quality, patient outcomes, and the costs of service delivery. Nurse researchers have contributed to the field of outcomes research by developing measures of functioning, well-being, and quality of life that are used to assess treatment effectiveness more comprehensively. Additionally, researchers working in the field of nursing administration have led the way in understanding phenomena such as the costs of nursing interventions or the relationships among leadership, staffing, and patient outcomes (Aiken, 2008). Nurses in policymaking roles work at the local, state, and national levels to translate research findings into regulations and laws for nursing and health care delivery.

Nurse educators: Finally, nurse educators promote clinicians' understanding of the economic value of nursing and the profession's key role in providing cost-effective services. Within the higher education arena, nurse educators have developed innovations, such as simulations, to use limited teaching resources in a more creative and economical manner. Further discussion about nursing roles can be found in Chapter 4.

Value. Value is the relationship between quality and cost. In the context of health care markets, *value* is defined as improved health outcomes in relation to the costs of producing services (Ginsberg, 2008). Stated more simply, value is the sum-total of the benefits a provider promises that a consumer will receive in return for purchasing goods or services. In comparison with other industrialized nations, the U.S. health care system suffers from a large value-gap. The United States spends more than any other industrialized country on health care as a percentage of GDP, yet we do not deliver the same levels of quality of care, patient outcomes, improvements in public health, or increases in life expectancy as other nations (Goodell & Ginsburg,

TABLE 7-2	A Comparison of Key Health Care Statistics for the Industrialized Nations, 2009					
	Canada	France	Germany	Japan	United Kingdom	United States
Population (millions)	32,976	61,707	82,257	1277	60,975	301,621
GDP (adjusted for purchasing parity, expressed in millions of U.S. dollars)	$38,500	$32,684	$34,393	$33,603	$35,557	$45,559
Health care spending per capita	$3895	$3601	$3558	$2581	$2992	$7290
Health care spending as percentage of GDP	10.1%	11.0%	10.4%	8.1%	8.4%	16.0%
Life expectancy at birth: females	83.0	84.4	82.7	86.0	81.7	80.7
Life expectancy at birth: males	78.1	77.5	77.4	79.2	77.3	75.4

Reprinted from Organisation for Economic Cooperation and Development. Health at a glance: OECD indicators 2009. Paris: OECD.

2008). Table 7-2 provides a comparison of the health spending patterns of the major industrialized nations (Organisation for Economic Co-Operation and Development, 2009). Although comparisons of U.S. health expenditures with those of other industrialized nations are helpful, they should be interpreted with caution. Henderson (2008) points out that differences in population demographics, per-capita income, disease incidence, and institutional features make direct comparisons difficult.

Rising health care costs and limited health care resources have created a call for documenting the value of professional nursing services. An understanding of the relationship between the quality and the cost of care is paramount because these data inform decisions about the appropriateness and effectiveness of nurses in achieving desired levels of patient care quality (Pappas, 2007; Rutherford, 2008). Under the diagnostic-related group (DRG) prospective payment system used by the Medicare program, hospitals are reimbursed a predetermined amount for services. Hospitals emphasize the daily costs of care, or the ratio of costs to charges for an episode of care, to align the expected reimbursement with profitability. Under this payment system, nursing services become vulnerable to cost-reduction efforts because nursing salaries and benefits make up a large portion of the per-day costs of hospital-based patient care. In an effort to reduce the daily costs of care, many hospitals responded by

reducing nurse staffing levels or substituting registered nurses with unlicensed personnel. Reducing nurse staffing levels emphasizes the cost of nursing without considering how nurses contribute to the quality of patient care (Aiken, 2008).

Nursing research has documented that the quality of patient care is sensitive to the intensity of direct nursing care. More specifically, evidence demonstrates that patients suffer from higher mortality rates and overall failure-to-rescue rates in hospitals where nurses cared for more (rather than less) patients. *Failure to rescue* is the inability of a clinician to save a patient's life when a complication arises. Additionally, higher hours of care from all nursing care providers in conjunction with a higher proportion of registered nurse hours of care are associated with better outcomes for hospitalized patients (Aiken 2008; Pappas, 2007). This research establishes that nurses create value. That is, the costs associated with nursing services bring increased returns to the consumer through nurses' contribution to patient care quality and safety.

Newer approaches to describing the costs related to nursing services consider the process of care and how nursing care offsets the costs related to patient complications (Aiken, 2008; Rutherford, 2008). Methods for describing the costs, quality, and value of nursing services are in the early stages of development and use by nurse managers, researchers, and other leaders to communicate the value of nursing to hospital managers and the public at large. A number of economic evaluation techniques are presented in Box 7-3; these techniques are useful in framing nursing services (as well as other health care services) in terms of their economic value, ultimately supporting increased investments in nursing services and the improved allocation of resources within the health care sector.

Technology. Health care technology has been cited as one of the significant drivers in the escalating costs of service delivery in the United States (Ginsburg, 2008). In its broadest sense, technology is the application of scientific knowledge used to transform inputs into outputs with the goal of improving productivity or economic growth (Henderson, 2008).

The expansion of health insurance since World War II has led to an interdependent relationship between health care technology and insurance and has had a dramatic effect on health care costs (Garber, 1994; Ginsburg, 2008; Weisbrod, 1991). As the financing of services shifted from individuals to insurance companies, individuals became removed from, and insensitive to, the actual costs of health care technologies. Because of the retrospective payment system, in which all services rendered were reimbursed, health care providers (namely physicians and hospitals) had financial incentives to use any and all technologies available regardless of cost. Research and development markets also had the financial incentives of reimbursement to continue to produce new health care technologies at any cost (Iglehart, 2001; Weisbrod, 1991). Consequently, patient and provider demand for greater technology has heightened and become more widespread, as have soaring health care expenditures.

The abundant development and use of technologies have fueled the debate over the appropriateness of many disease-focused clinical interventions in improving health outcomes and overall health status. Because of how health technologies are financed, health care organizations have increased incentives to adopt new technologies, for many of which, the long-term effectiveness or costs are not fully known. Once a new technology is integrated into clinical practice routines, it is very difficult for an organization to disengage from using that technology. Studies suggest that newer technologies tend to complement, rather than replace, older technologies and that hospitals with constrained financial resources are likely to retain ineffective clinical technologies, creating a reverse access problem in which disadvantaged populations have access to ineffective, less effective, or harmful treatments at a higher rate than the population at large (Rye & Kimberly, 2007).

Technology assessment and *outcomes research* are intended to help decision makers deal with the development, acquisition, and use of health care practices and technologies. The goal is to improve patient health, efficiency, and value. Technology assessment, as a form of policy research, evaluates the safety, effectiveness, and costs of technologies to provide the basis for clinical and social policies, including resource allocation. A comprehensive technology assessment encompasses four aspects of the technology: safety, efficacy/effectiveness, costs/benefits, and social impact (Pillar, Jacox, & Redman, 1990).

Health technology assessment (HTA) has grown in popularity and use over the last decade as a tool for evidence based clinical and policy decision making. HTA has evolved from a technique of synthesizing best evidence for policy makers in national governments to disseminating information about the effectiveness of technologies to clinicians and managers to influence the costs, safety, and quality of patient care. Early assessments tended to focus on large, expensive, machine-based technologies, the scope of which has expanded to include "softer" technologies, such as counseling and other process-oriented health care services (Banta, 2003).

Technology assessments are time consuming and costly. Traditional health care markets provide little incentive for investment in the process. During the 1990s technology assessment and the evidence-based practice movement gained importance as tools to inform policy, practice, and health care investment decisions. Nonetheless, these quality improvement methods are not without their limitations. Gilmartin, Melzer, and Donaghy (2004) assessed the extent to which health technology assessments produce recommendations that can and should affect clinical practice. In a sample of 53 therapeutic procedures and pharmacological interventions used in everyday medical practice, such as educational and psychosocial

BOX 7-3	Methods to Evaluate Costs

The two predominant methods of evaluating the economic costs of a service or program are cost-benefit analysis and cost-effectiveness analysis. Other analytic methods used to assess the economic effects of new health care interventions or technologies include cost-minimization analysis, cost-consequence analysis, and cost-utility analysis (Stone, Curran, & Bakken, 2002; Rutherford, 2008).

Cost-Benefit Analysis

Cost-benefit analysis is an analytical technique for evaluating the necessary resources and benefits of producing a particular project, program, or technique. Cost-benefit analysis requires assessment and evaluation of the costs and benefits of a program to determine whether the benefits of a project outweigh its costs. In a cost-benefit analysis all costs and benefits undergo valuation and are stated in monetary terms. This process places a dollar amount on both monetary and nonmonetary costs and benefits so that a comparison can be made between competing projects or programs. In doing so, value or worth is assigned to nonmonetary aspects of the project's costs and benefits.

Cost-benefit analysis is a useful and powerful tool to justify the investment in nurse-managed services to managers responsible for resource allocation decisions. In this era of resource efficiency and service change, a critical skill for nurses across practice settings and role descriptions is the ability not only to speak the language of economics but also to demonstrate the unique value of nursing services in terms of cost, quality, and value. The widespread availability of personal computers and spreadsheet software makes cost-benefit analysis an accessible tool to a broad range of people. The calculations become effortless. Rather, quantification of the tangible and intangible costs is the difficulty of this method.

The comparative nature of cost-benefit analysis is an attractive feature of this analytical technique, but in determining the "worthiness" of a project, it is also a pitfall and a drawback. The major limitation of the application of cost-benefit analysis in health care scenarios is that the valuation of intangible costs such as pain or grief or premature loss of life varies not only from case to case, but also among analysts assigning the values. Specific criteria and arithmetic maneuvers

have been suggested for determining the value of intangible costs and benefits, but these are controversial at best (Klarman, 1982; Pruitt & Jacox, 1991).

Cost-Effectiveness Analysis

Cost-effectiveness analysis is an analytical technique for comparing resource consumption between two or more alternatives that meet a particular objective (e.g., minimum quality of a product or production of a specific patient outcome). Cost-effectiveness analysis measures the costs involved with each alternative and determines the most cost-effective, or least costly, alternative (Kristen, 1983). In a cost-effectiveness analysis, only monetary costs of inputs into each alternative are considered. Because the objective (or outcome) of the alternatives is assumed to be the same, the valuation of benefits is not considered (Folland et al., 1993). Thus cost-effectiveness analysis avoids making valuations while providing empirical evaluation of costs of alternative health care interventions.

Cost-Minimization Analysis

A true cost-minimization analysis (CMA) compares the costs of alternatives. Interventions are assumed to offer equivalent outcomes so that it is possible to determine which intervention is the least costly. In clinical settings this method of analysis is rarely appropriate because different interventions yield different outcomes (Stone et al., 2002).

Cost-Consequence Analysis

In a cost-consequence analysis the consequences and costs of two or more alternatives are measured and evaluated. The cost-consequence analysis method separates the costs and consequences of comparable interventions so that decision makers can form opinions about the relative importance of findings. Brooten and colleagues' (1986) classic work on the early discharge of low-birth-weight infants whose care was managed by advanced practice nurses compared with traditional care is an example of cost-consequence analysis.

Cost-Utility Analysis

Cost-utility analysis is a special type of cost-effectiveness analysis that includes measures for both quantity and quality of life. This analytic method includes an

BOX 7-3	Methods to Evaluate Costs—cont'd

Cost-Utility Analysis, cont'd

individual's preferences, or utilities, for different health outcomes. Preferences are ranked on a scale of 0 to 1, with perfect health represented by 1 and death represented by 0. Preference weights can be calculated for a variety of health states. The preference weights are then multiplied by the amount of time experienced in a health state to determine the number of quality-adjusted health years. Composite outcome analysis such as dollars per quality-adjusted health years is a superior method of assessing the economic effect of clinical interventions because both the quantity and quality of life are determined by using standardized measurements. Thus comparison of people within and across disease states may be possible (Stone et al., 2002).

---

interventions for adolescents with diabetes or laxatives use for the elderly, the clinical effectiveness of 45% of these interventions was assessed as uncertain because of limitations of the primary research base. Additionally, economic analyses of costs and benefits of these clinical technologies went largely unconsidered.

In recent years, the growth of the evidence-based clinical practice and management movements has highlighted the role of the information gained from synthesizing research to improve the quality, safety, and effectiveness of patient care. Many groups have a stake in the outcome of HTAs. These include:

- Policy makers: Broad concern about technology and value for money
- Insurers: Overarching concern for controlling costs of care
- Clinicians: Mostly interested in quality of a technology with a lesser interest in the costs or the equitable distribution of technologies
- Epidemiologists and other researchers: Interested in the poor state of the primary research used in HTAs, with attention to improving research and the dissemination of HTA findings to clinicians and other decision makers
- Industry: Overriding concern for selling products with increasing pressures to demonstrate a given product's efficacy and cost-effectiveness
- The general public: Interested in access to health care that is of acceptable quality (Banta, 2003)

Nursing practice, education, and administration are directly affected by the application of new medical and health care practices and technologies. However, nursing's participation in technology research is small despite its contribution to the implementation and assessment of technology in the clinical setting (Pillar et al., 1990). Nurses directly witness the individual, as well as societal, benefits and burdens that various practices and technologies bring and possess a wealth of clinical knowledge and expertise that could advance technology assessment. Nurses can play an important part in multidisciplinary technology assessment, developing clinical practice guidelines, leading to organizational change initiatives focused on integrating evidence into clinical practice routines, as well as advocating social policy regarding health care technologies. In today's marketplace payers are increasingly willing to pay only for those technologies that are cost effective and medically appropriate. Within this context the nursing profession has an opportunity to develop and demonstrate the effectiveness of nurse-specific interventions and service technologies (Box 7-4).

Health System Reform: Emerging Models and Trends

The final section of this chapter introduces emerging trends shaping patient-provider relationships based on the principles of competition and consumer sovereignty. We also examine proposals for achieving universal health insurance coverage. The economic mechanisms and effects on health care delivery organizations and professional nursing practice are considered. The chapter concludes with a discussion of opportunities for professional nursing to achieve sustainable health system change.

BOX 7-4	How to Read an Economic Analysis Paper

In the contemporary practice environment the allocation of limited resources in the production of health care services is a necessary component of clinical and policy decision making. As this chapter has illustrated, the economic cost of health care service delivery includes many tangible and intangible elements. A key skill for the professional nurse is the ability to analyze critically the quality of a study that reports the economic benefits of an intervention or new service. Greenhalgh (1997) presents the following 10-question checklist that is useful in judging economic analyses of a health care service:

1. Is the economic analysis based on a study that answers a clearly defined clinical question about an economically important issue?
2. From whose viewpoint are the costs and benefits being considered?
3. Have the interventions being compared been shown to be clinically effective?
4. Are the interventions sensible and workable in the setting in which they are likely to be applied?
5. Which method of economic analysis was used, and was it appropriate?
6. How were costs and benefits measured?
7. Were incremental (one unit/one more individual) rather than absolute (overall) benefits considered?
8. Was the "here and now" given precedence over the distant future?
9. Was a sensitivity analysis performed?
10. Were bottom-line aggregate scores overused?

From Greenhalgh, T. (1997). How to read a paper: Papers that tell you what things cost (economic analyses). *British Medical Journal, 315,* 596-599.

ALTERNATIVE MODELS OF ORGANIZING PROVIDER-CONSUMER RELATIONSHIPS

In the last decade, changes in U.S. health systems have been based on principles of market competition. As described in the introductory section of this chapter, competition is a mechanism used to distribute resources in combinations that produce the highest possible satisfaction for society: consumers, producers, and investors. In health care, market approaches focus on improving the efficient allocation of resources to, and within, the sector to minimize the social cost of illness, including its treatment. Efficient resource allocation is achieved when the marginal dollar spent on health care produces the same value to society as the marginal dollar spent on education, defense, personal consumption, and other areas (Enthoven, 1988).

Today, the quality and economic performance of the health care sector remains a concern for citizens, health care professionals, employers, and policy makers. Little change has occurred to improve access to affordable health care to more than 40 million uninsured Americans. Moreover, health care costs continue to rise, and the quality of clinical care has been labeled "a chasm to cross" (Institute of Medicine, 2001). In this context, competition, market mechanisms, and business practices are sometimes cited as the cause of the failing health care system. Economists and organizational theorists have developed a number of arguments for and against the use of market and other institutional forms to govern provider and consumer relationships in health care (Alexander & D'Aunno, 2003; Enthoven, 1988; Gilmartin & Freeman, 2002; Rice, 1998).

From a conceptual perspective, two issues arise from the application of market-based models in health care. First is the appropriate application of economic theory. Rice (1998) argues that economic theory is based on a number of key assumptions that must be satisfied so that the theory can accurately predict the behavior of consumers and providers. As discussed previously, health care markets violate most of these assumptions, thus reducing the predictive power of economic theory. Second, economic theory provides no support for the belief that competition, rather than government regulation and financing, will lead to superior social outcomes. On the basis of these analyses, competition clearly will not solve issues of social welfare, especially access to essential health care services. Ensuring the availability of, and access to, health care services is more likely to be a role played by government policy and regulation.

Nonetheless, as a resource allocation mechanism, particular models of competition can play a role in improving quality and efficiency in the health care system. In health care, competition has come to be associated with profit maximization, cost containment, and limited resources dedicated to patient care. Framed in this manner, competition has been practiced in a winner-takes-all, or zero-sum fashion. Organizational behaviors associated with *zero-sum competition* include (1) cost shifting rather than fundamental cost reduction, (2) pursuit of greater bargaining power between delivery organizations and insurance/managed care companies rather than efforts to provide better care, (3) restriction on choice and access to services instead of making care better and more efficient, and (4) the reliance on the court system to settle disputes among consumers, providers, and payers (Porter & Teisberg, 2004). Zero-sum competition hampers innovation and the adoption of new, more effective technologies, puts health care professionals and clients at odds with one another, and creates a practice environment in which more time is spent taking care of the system than the patient.

A more fruitful model of health care reform is based on *positive-sum competition*. Positive-sum competition recasts the relationships among providers, insurers, consumers and clients, and institutions, with the specific goal of improving the quality and efficiency of health care service. A central goal of positive-sum competition is to create value, which is the economic relationship between cost and quality. Reframing competition in terms of value creation emphasizes the positive aspects of free markets such as invention, innovation, and entrepreneurship. Additionally, in well-functioning free markets consumers and clients play a role in shaping new or better services for themselves and their communities (Gilmartin & Freeman, 2002). Box 7-5 develops possible attributes of a reformed health care system on the basis of principles of positive-sum competition.

Positive-sum competition draws on concepts from economics, systems theory, and ethics to reframe the nature and outcomes of market transactions between buyers and sellers. Positive-sum competition is based on the following four principles:

1. The principle of *stakeholder cooperation.* Value is created because consumers, employers, payers and financers, government, and communities can jointly satisfy their needs. The support of each group is necessary to sustain the activities of the organization. Over the long run, the interests of each group (as opposed to a particular issue) must be satisfied by the organization's activities.

2. The principle of *complexity.* Human beings are complex creatures and act based on many different values. Sometimes human beings act selfishly; sometimes they act for others. Competition works because of the complexity of values and perspectives of individuals and groups. Groups of people (some of whom share like values) will work together to create what they cannot do alone.

3. The principle of *continuous creation.* Managers and leaders cooperate with others to create value. Human creativity is the source of change and progress within well-functioning markets. One creation does not have to destroy another; rather, a continuous cycle of value creation raises the well-being of everyone.

4. The principle of *emergent competition.* Competition arises in a relatively free society so that stakeholders have options. Some forms of cooperation may well satisfy stakeholders' needs better than others, so in a free society stakeholders are free to form many different cooperative schemes (Gilmartin & Freeman, 2002).

Consider the case of the single mother who returns home in the evening to a toddler having an asthma attack. The pediatrician's office is closed, so the mother has two options: she can either visit the local emergency department or the nurse-managed urgent care center at the mall. As an emergency department client she can expect to wait up to 5 hours, fill out a stack of insurance papers, pay a $250 co-payment for the visit, and possibly get a 10-minute consultation with the health care provider. Alternatively, at the nurse-managed clinic, a nurse practitioner is usually available within 15 minutes of arrival, and the consultation usually lasts 30 minutes. In addition to getting the immediate symptoms under control, the nurse practitioner adjusts medication dosages and reviews administration and side effects, teaches symptom management techniques, and makes a referral to a local parent support group. The visit costs $85, and the

BOX 7-5	Zero-Sum and Positive-Sum Competition in Health Care

Features of Zero-Sum Competition

- The wrong level of competition: competition is among health plans, hospitals, and networks
- The wrong objective: cost reduction; participants try to reduce their own costs by transferring them to someone else without reducing total costs
- The wrong forms of competition: competition is to sign up healthy subscribers; methods include discount prices to large payers and groups, consolidating to increase bargaining power, and shifting cost
- The wrong geographic market: competition is local
- The wrong strategies and structure: participants build full-line services, form closed networks, consolidate with others (reducing rivalry), and match their competitors
- The wrong incentives for payers: payers try to attract health subscribers and raise rates for unhealthy subscribers; they restrict treatments and out-of-network services, shift costs to providers and patients, and slow down innovation
- The wrong incentives for providers: providers offer every service but often below prevailing medical standards; they refer patients within the network if at all; spend less time with patients and discharge them quickly; and practice defensive medicine

Features of Positive-Sum Competition

- The right level of competition: competition is to prevent, diagnose, and treat specific diseases or combinations of conditions
- The right objectives: improve value, quality per expended dollars over time
- The right forms of competition: competition is to create value at the level of disease or conditions by developing expertise, reducing errors, increasing efficiency, and improving outcomes
- The right geographic market: competition is at the regional or national level
- The right strategies and structure: participants define their distinctiveness by offering services and products that create unique value; the system has many focused competitors
- The right information: about providers, treatments, and alternatives for specific conditions

- The right incentives for payers: payers help subscribers find the best-value care for specific conditions; they simplify billing and administrative processes and pay bills promptly
- The right incentives for providers: providers succeed by developing areas of excellence and expertise; they measure and enhance quality and efficiency; they eradicate mistakes; they get it right the first time; they meet, exceed, and improve standards

Proposed Changes

No Restrictions to Competition and Choice

- No preapprovals for referrals or treatments
- No network restrictions
- Strict antitrust enforcements against collusion, excessive concentration, and unfair practices
- Meaningful copayments and medical savings accounts with high deductibles, all of which give consumers incentives to seek good value

Accessible Information

- Appropriate information on treatments and alternatives is formally collected and widely disseminated
- Information about providers' experience in treating particular diseases and conditions is made available immediately
- Risk-adjusted outcome data are developed and continually enhanced
- Some information is standardized nationally to enable comparisons

Transparent Pricing

- Providers set a single price for a given treatment or procedure
- Different providers set different prices
- Price estimates are made available in advance to enable comparison

Simplified Billing

- Payer has legal responsibility for medical bills of paid-up subscribers

Nondiscriminatory Insurance

- No re-underwriting
- Assign risk pools for those who need them

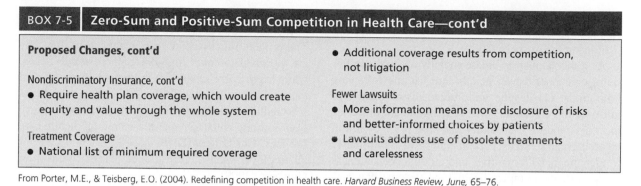

From Porter, M.E., & Teisberg, E.O. (2004). Redefining competition in health care. *Harvard Business Review, June,* 65–76.

registration process is simple. Moreover, a registered nurse from the clinic calls the next morning to see how the mother and her child coped during the night and reinforces information on effective symptom management techniques.

Nurse-led clinics, like the one described in this scenario and the retail clinics profiled earlier, are examples of positive competition based on the principles of stakeholder cooperation and emergent competition. Value is created because services are convenient and affordable and they fill an unmet market need. The nurses involved in these enterprises bring together clients, payers, and the community in a new combination to provide after-hours or expanded-hours primary care and urgent care services that complement overstretched physicians and hospital emergency departments. Additionally, the focus on chronic disease and symptom management distinguishes the nurse-led services from those offered by physicians.

In effect, nurse-led services create a new standard of care that for some clients is superior to that of physician services. This model is not limited to the work of advanced practice nurses. Nurse entrepreneurs, lawyers, and consultants working outside the hospital setting have identified gaps in the market between consumer demand and current provider offerings. Drawing on specialized knowledge, skills, and abilities, these nurses create new services to address an underlying problem associated with health care service.

Finally, magnet hospitals are an example of the power of positive-sum competition in organizational settings. The magnet management and leadership philosophy focuses on developing cultures and systems of clinical excellence. Professionals work in a coordinated yet autonomous manner to deliver patient care services. These organizations emphasize expertise, collegiality, and performance, elements that in turn have a direct effect on the quality of care, patient outcomes, and patient and staff satisfaction ratings (Aiken, 2008; Aiken, Smith, & Lake, 1994; American Nurses Credentialing Center, 2004). In turn, these clinical and service outcomes improve the reputation of the organization among consumers, payers, communities, and potential employees; as a result, all who are associated with the enterprise gain something.

CONSUMERISM

The prolonged U.S. economic prosperity of the 1990s and early 2000s and the Internet revolution are key factors associated with changing consumer expectations for goods and services. Across all sectors of the national economy, citizens expect immediate, low-cost products and services that are tailored to their specific needs. Although many consumers have benefited from more affordable and often expanded health care coverage, restrictions on choice of primary care physicians and access to specialty care, emergency care, and inpatient admissions have led to a retreat from managed care and to a new emphasis on consumers as the central decision makers in U.S. health care (Robinson, 2001). Consumerism in health care can be traced to the women's liberation movement of the 1960s; the new wave of consumerism is squarely based on individual choice and self-responsibility to manage one's own health. The central idea underpinning the consumer movement is that health care belongs in the domain of personal rights and individual decision making (Robinson & Ginsberg, 2009).

As a mechanism to create socially optimal equilibrium, consumer-driven health care has the following limitations: (1) despite widespread dissemination of information, consumers will face significant obstacles in understanding the quality and true price of health insurance and services; (2) consumers vary enormously in their financial, cognitive, and cultural preparedness to navigate the complex health care system—the consumerism model most comfortably fits the educated, assertive, and prosperous and least comfortably fits the impoverished, meek, and poorly educated; (3) consumerism will complicate the pooling of risk between consistently healthy citizens and the chronically ill; (4) consumerism will make transparent and render difficult the redistribution of income from rich to poor that otherwise results from the collective purchasing and administration of health insurance (Robinson, 2001).

Consumerism is a market-based mechanism in which individuals articulate what, when, and how they want health care service delivered. Advocates of consumerism emphasize the potential responses of consumers, employers, insurance companies, delivery organizations, and professionals to create new and better services. The hope is that consumer-driven services will improve many of the problems and limitations that abound in health care. Opponents of consumerism emphasize that consumer choice is not an effective mechanism to allocate health care resources in a manner that will ensure equal access to a basic set of services for all citizens (Coulter, 2000).

In its original conception, the health care consumerism movement focused on the development of convenient, low-cost, high-quality services and client–health care professional relationships based on a partnership model (Herzlinger, 2000; 2007). In this model, health care professionals provide guidance, education, and advice to patients/clients on a plan of care that ultimately is the individual's responsibility to purchase and carry out. The consumerism movement is now entering its second decade and has evolved in ways that diverge from its original intent.

Most of the evolution of health care consumerism has taken place in the form of health insurance benefits, most notably the development of high-deductible health plans (HDHPs) with savings options. These plans function like true insurance in that they are designed to cover high-cost unpredictable needs, while leaving low-cost more predictable types of care to be paid out of pocket. The central idea of these plans is to reduce moral hazard by giving enrollees control over how and when they purchase "minor" health care services. Currently, HDHPs account for only 8% of all employer-sponsored insurance plans (Robinson & Ginsburg, 2009).

It is likely that as consumerism evolves, insurance companies will develop programs seeking to improve the care of enrollees along the spectrum from full health to dire illness. These include preventative and wellness programs for healthy enrollees, service coordination for patients needing acute care, disease management for enrollees with chronic conditions, and intensive case management for enrollees with severe conditions. These services will likely be presented as options rather than mandates, possibly with higher cost-sharing for those who are eligible but choose not to participate (Robinson & Ginsberg, 2009).

In the context of the health consumerism movement, professional nurses occupy a unique position. Nurses advocate personal responsibility and knowledge to achieve an optimal level of health and wellness. In particular, nurses may play a role in promoting more choice for self-management among the seriously ill and vulnerable populations. Nursing's professional value system provides a foundation for important insights to shape new services, organizational strategies, and policies to balance the competing demands of consumerism.

EXPANDING INSURANCE COVERAGE

Observers argue that extending health insurance benefits with the goal of improving access to health care is as much an economic issue as it is a social issue (Lavizzo-Mourey, 2008). Health is an investment that leads to improved national productivity and economic competitiveness. In 2007 alone, the U.S. economy gave up as much as $207 billion in potential output because of the poor health and shorter lifespan of the uninsured (Axeen & Carpenter, 2008). For many observers, expanding health insurance coverage is viewed as the gateway to reforming the U.S. health care system.

Based on the findings of its landmark study on the substantial and compelling effects of being uninsured in the United States, the Institute of Medicine (2004) proposed five principles for expanding insurance coverage and four prototypes to inform public debate on the most effective way to expand health coverage. The five principles are as follows:

- Health insurance should be *universal*—that is, everyone living in the United States should have health insurance.
- Coverage should be *continuous* so as not to disrupt relationships with providers and to ensure timely care for emergencies, as well as chronic conditions.
- Health care coverage should be *affordable for individuals.*
- Health care coverage should be *affordable and sustainable for society.*
- Health insurance should enhance health and well-being by promoting *access* to health care that is *high quality, effective, efficient, safe, timely, patient centered,* and *equitable.*

Using the above five principles, one can then evaluate the costs and benefits of four basic scenarios, or prototypes, currently under public discussion to bring about systems change to achieve universal health coverage:

- *Prototype 1: Major public program expansion and a new tax credit.* The current favorable tax credit for employers would remain. Employers would not be required to offer coverage. Medicare and SCHIP would be combined; Medicare would be expanded to 55-year-olds who pay a premium. A tax credit would be given to moderate-income individuals to purchase private insurance.
- *Prototype 2: Employer mandate, premium subsidy, and individual mandate.* Employers would be required to offer coverage and contribute to their workers' premiums, although a federal premium subsidy would be available to employers of low-wage workers. Medicaid and SCHIP would be merged; Medicare would remain as it

is. Individuals would be required to obtain coverage through work, through enrollment in a public program, or through individual purchase.
- *Prototype 3: Individual mandate and tax credit.* It would be the mandated responsibility of individuals to provide health insurance for themselves and their families through the private market. Each person would be eligible for a tax credit administered by the federal government to offset the cost of purchasing insurance. Medicaid and SCHIP would be eliminated; Medicare would remain as it is.
- *Prototype 4: Single payer.* Everyone would be enrolled in a single, comprehensive benefit package, but persons could purchase supplemental policies for noncovered services. A global budget would help to control aggregate health care spending. Medicaid and SCHIP would be eliminated; those currently eligible for Medicare could be folded into a single-payer model.

OPPORTUNITIES FOR PROFESSIONAL NURSING

In the face of the growing urgency for sustainable national health reform, professional nursing is poised to take a leadership role in defining the attributes of a socially just health care system and bringing about sustainable changes in the organization and delivery of health care services. The American Nurses Association (2008) advocates expanding professional nursing roles and nurse-managed services to address the unmet demand for health care services, working toward universal access to health care services and organizational environments that value nursing's contributions to patient outcomes, care, and safety. Moreover, the profession's clinical expertise for health promotion, disease prevention, and chronic disease management will be integral in addressing the following manifest signs of the ailing U.S. health care system (Lavizzo-Mourey, 2008):

- Tens of millions are uninsured or underinsured.
- Variations in the quality, safety, performance, and treatment are endemic.
- Avoidable medical and hospital errors kill thousands each year.
- Access to care is declining, uneven, and unfair.

- Racial and ethnic disparities in health and health care delivery are pervasive.
- Adult and childhood obesity has become epidemic.
- Prevention is overlooked, and mental health is discounted.
- Public health suffers from years of political neglect.
- Spending trends are unsustainable.
- Resources flood specialty care; resource drought afflicts primary chronic care.
- Demands of profit and process marginalize patients.

One key challenge is nursing's ability to reframe practice into an economic value equation to capture the cost, quality, and service of nursing care within the larger agenda for change (Iowa Intervention Project, 2001; Rutherford, 2008).

SUMMARY

This chapter has provided an overview of the many economic issues that are shaping the national discussion about health care service, its effect on our society, and by extension, its effect on professional nursing practice. Professional nurses must have a basic understanding of economic forces and the ability to apply these principles if they are to participate in shaping a patient-centered, health-focused care delivery system. This chapter serves as a foundation on which to build knowledge and skills to participate in health system reform efforts. Keeping abreast of changes in the dynamic health care economy is one way in which new knowledge shapes the practice environment and professional decision making. Journalistic accounts, professional publications, and Internet resources dedicated to the presentation and discussion of issues in

TABLE 7-3	Web Watch: Keeping Abreast of Economic Issues in Health Care	
Website Description		**Internet Address**
National Institutes of Health		
Provides an overview of programs and activities of the federal government		http://www.nih.gov
National Center for Health Statistics		
The principal health statistics agency in the United States, with the mission to provide accurate, timely, and relevant statistics to inform policy and improve the health of the American people		http://www.cdc.gov/nchs
RAND Corporation		
Not-for-profit institution dedicated to improving public policy through conducts interdisciplinary health sciences research		http://www.rand.org/organization/healthresearch
U.S. Census Bureau		
Provides statistics on population demographics and health insurance		http://www.census.gov status
Nursing World		
The official website of the American Nurses Association; provides access to the online journal *Issues in Nursing*		http://www.nursingworld.org
National Committee for Quality Assurance		
An independent not-for-profit organization that serves as the accrediting agency for the nation's managed care plans		http://www.ncqa.org
Kaiser Family Foundation		
Information and resources about health policy and its communication		http://www.kff.org/
Robert Wood Johnson Foundation		
Information on National health reform initiatives		http://www.rwjf.org/

Modified from Henderson, J. (2009). *Health economics and policy.* (with Info Apps 2-Semester printed access card) (4th ed.). © 2009 South-Western, a part of Cengage Learning, Inc.
Reprinted with permission. www.cengage.com/permissions.

health and nursing economics are widely available (Table 7-3). Professional nurses have the knowledge and expertise to create a socially just health care system. Nursing participation in decision-making activities will occur by placing nursing services within an economic context.

KEY POINTS

- Economics in health care represents the relationships among the supply, demand, and costs of health care.
- The supply of health care refers to the amount of health care facilities, personnel, and financing available to consumers. Supply levels are affected by technological discoveries, costs for services, consumer demands, the level of competition in the marketplace, and the effect of government regulations.
- The demand for health care indicates what health care the consumer is willing to purchase. The demand level revolves around consumer needs and desires, the costs of health care, treatment selections ordered by health care providers, and general societal needs.
- The costs for health care reflect any financial expenditures contributed by providers or consumers to deliver and receive health care, as well as the intangible costs of seeking and receiving care. Factors influencing the cost of health care are numerous, ranging from consumer demands to advancements in medical technology to the status of the nation's economy.
- Economic concepts relevant to nursing practice include opportunity cost, complements and substitutes, and competition. Nurses must be able to incorporate these economic concepts into their management and clinical decision-making processes.
- Cost-containment pressures require that clinicians, managers, and researchers be able to incorporate economic methods such as cost-effectiveness analysis and cost-benefit analysis into practice routines. Such economically and clinically based research can serve as the basis for policy decision making regarding regulatory reform, prioritization, and rationing of health care technologies and services, as well as reimbursement for advanced practice nurses.
- Nurses can bring a unique perspective to the economic analysis of health care that can have an impact on health care delivery systems, health policy, and most important, patient care.

- The rising costs of health care necessitate the provision of more cost-effective ways to provide comparable services. Nurses must continue to demonstrate their accessibility, quality of services, and cost effectiveness to validate existing and expanding roles, to broaden reimbursement policies for services that nurses are trained to render and are capable of providing, and to effectively compete with physicians and other providers of care.

CRITICAL THINKING EXERCISES

1. Discuss the economic concepts of supply, demand, and costs of health care as they relate to your current or future nursing practice.
2. What are the implications of the following issues for the nursing profession?
   a. Access to health care
   b. Cost containment
   c. Quality of care
3. How can nurses in clinical practice become involved in improving the quality and effectiveness of health care services? How can nurses become involved in formulating and evaluating social policies regarding health care?
4. What suggestions do you have for restructuring the health care delivery system to address problems associated with access to care, cost, reimbursement, and quality of care?
5. Using the criteria presented in Box 7-4, critique a paper presenting an economic analysis of a nurse-managed service or intervention.
6. In his 1994 book *Not All of Us Are Saints: A Doctor's Journey With the Poor*, David Hilfiker, MD, tells a story of a homeless man and reveals an extreme example of the economic consequences of health care:

   After breaking his jaw several weeks earlier, Mr. McRae had gone to an emergency room, had his jaw wired shut to heal, and then been discharged back to the streets. Most likely, he had found it impossible to eat and drink enough to keep himself going, and so it was that the police found him severely dehydrated, unconscious, and close to death. [Subsequently,] Mr. McRae had been hospitalized for weeks at a cost of tens of thousands of dollars; attended to by teams of nurses, physicians, and social workers; and fed three carefully prepared meals a day. He was now about to be discharged to the streets, where he would sleep in a shelter, forage for food during the day, and wait in line in the evening in the hope of getting a bed for the night (Hilfiker, 1994, pp. 171-173).

What characteristics of our current health care system contributed to the outcome described by Hilfiker in the above passage? What actions could have been taken, and by whom, to prevent the costly hospitalization? What are some of the broader societal implications of this scenario?

REFERENCES

Aiken, L. H. (2008). Economics of nursing. *Policy, Politics and Nursing Practice, 9*(2), 73–79.

Aiken, L. H., Smith, H., & Lake, E. (1994). Lower Medicare mortality among a set of hospitals known for good nursing care. *Medical Care, 32*(8), 771–787.

Alexander, J. A., & D'Aunno, T. A. (2003). Alternative perspectives on institutional and market forces in the U.S. health care sector. In S. S. Mick (Ed.), *Advances in health care organization theory.* San Francisco: Jossey-Bass.

American Hospital Association. (2008). Fast facts. Retrieved November 20, 2008, from http://www.aha.org/aha/resource-center/Statistics-and-Studies/fast-facts.htmlref

American Nurses Association. (2008). *Health system reform agenda.* American Nurses Association, Silver Springs, MD.

American Nurses Credentialing Center. (2004). *Magnet: Best practices in today's challenging health care environment.* Washington, DC: American Nurses Publishing.

Arrow, K. (1963). Uncertainty and the welfare economics of medical care. *American Economic Review, 53*(5), 851–883.

Axeen, S. & Carpenter, E. (2008). *The cost of doing nothing: Why the cost of failing to fix our health system is greater than the cost of reform.* Retrieved January 10, 2009, from http://www.newamerica.net/files/NAF_CostofDoingNothing.pdf

Banta, D. (2003). The development of health technology assessment. *Health Policy, 63*(1), 121–132.

Bodenheimer, T. S., & Grumbach, K. (2005). *Understanding health policy: A clinical approach* (4th ed.). New York: Lange/McGraw-Hill.

Bolton, L. B., Donaldson, N. E., Rutledge, D. N., Bennett, C., & Brown, D. S. (2007). The impact of nursing interventions: Overview of effective interventions, outcomes, measures and priorities for future research. *Medical Care Research and Review, 64*(Suppl. 2), 123S–143S.

Brewer, C. S., Kovner, C. T., Wu, Y. -W., Greene, W., Liu, Y., & Reimers, C. W. (2006). Factors influencing female registered nurses' work behavior. *Health Services Research, 41*(3, Part 1), 860–866.

Brooten, D., Kumar, S., Brown, L. P., Finkler, S. A., Bakewell-Sachs, S., Gibbons, A., et al. (1986). A randomized clinical trial of early hospital discharge and home follow-up of very-low-birth-weight-infants. *New England Journal of Medicine, 315*(15), 934–939.

Brooten, D., Youngblut, J. M., Kutcher, J., & Bobo, C. (2004). Quality and the nursing workforce: APNs, patient outcomes and health care costs. *Nursing Outlook, 52*(1), 45–52.

Brown, S. A., & Grimes, D. E. (1993). *Nurse practitioners and certified nurse-midwives: A meta-analysis of studies on nurses in primary care roles.* Washington, DC: American Nurses Publishing.

Buerhaus, P. I. (1992). Nursing competition and quality. In M. Johnson, & J. McCloskey (Eds.), *The delivery of quality health care.* St. Louis: Mosby.

Buerhaus, P. I. (2008). The potential imposition of wage controls on nurses: A threat to nurses, patients and hospitals. *Nursing Economics, 26*(4), 276–279.

Buerhaus, P. I., Staiger, D., & Auerbach., D. (2008). *The future of the nursing workforce in the United States: Data, trends and implications.* Boston: Jones and Bartlett.

Chernew, M. E., Hirth, R. A., Sonnad, S. S., Ermann, R., & Fendrick, M. (1998). Managed care, medical technology and health care cost growth: A review of the evidence. *Medical Care Research and Review, 55*(3), 259–288.

Claxton, C., Gabel, J., DiJulio, B., Pickreign, J., Whitmore, H., Finder, B., et al. (2007). Health benefits in 2007: Premium increases fall to an eight-year low, while offer rates and enrollment remain stable. *Health Affairs, 26*(5), 1407–1416.

Coulter, C. H. (2000). The consumer choice model: A humane reconstruction of the U.S. health care system. *The Physician Executive, March-April,* 44–51.

DeNavas-Walt, C., Proctor, B. D., & Smith, J. C. (2008). *Income, poverty, and health insurance coverage in the U.S.: 2007.* Washington, DC: U.S. Census Bureau, U.S. Department of Commerce, Economics and Statistics Administration.

Devers, K. J., Brewster, L. P., & Casalino, L. P. (2003). Changes in hospital competitive strategy: A new medical arms race? Longitudinal changes in communities' health care systems, 1996-2001: Analyses from the Community Tracking Study site visits. *Health Services Research, 38*(1), 447–471.

Dumpe, M. L., Herman, J., & Young, S. W. (1998). Forecasting the nursing workforce in a dynamic health care market. *Nursing Economics, 16*(4), 170–181.

Employment Benefits Research Institute (2008). Fast facts: Tax expenditures and employment benefits. Retrieved November 30, 2008, from http://www.ebri.org/pdf/public ations/facts/0208fact.pdf

Enthoven, A. (1988). Managed competition of alternative delivery systems. *Journal of Health Politics, Policy and Law*, *13*(2), 305–335.

Feldstein, P. J. (1983). *Health care economics* (2nd ed.). New York: Wiley.

Folland, S., Goodman, A. C., & Stano, M. (2007). *The economics of health and health care* (5th ed.). Upper Saddle River, NJ: Pearson, Prentice Hall.

Freeman, J. D., Kidiyala, S., Bell, J. F., & Martin, D. P. (2008). The causal effect of health insurance on utilization and outcomes in adults: A systematic review of U.S. studies. *Medical Care, 46*(10), 1023–1032.

Fulton, J. S., & Baldwin, K. (2004). An annotated bibliography reflecting CNS practice and outcomes. *Clinical Nurse Specialist, 18*(1), 21–39.

Garber, A. M. (1994). Can technology assessment control health spending? *Health Affairs, 13*(3), 115–126.

Getzen, T. E. (2004). *Health economics: Fundamentals and flows of funds* (2nd ed.). New York: Wiley.

Gilmartin, M. J., & Freeman, R. E. (2002). Business ethics and health care: A stakeholder perspective. *Health Care Management Review, 27*(2), 50–65.

Gilmartin, M. J., Melzer, D., & Donaghy, P. (2004). Health technology assessment: More questions than answers for clinical practice? In M. Tavakoli, & H. Davies (Eds.), *Policy, finance and performance*. London: Ashgate.

Ginsburg, P. B. (2008). *High and rising health care costs: Demystifying U.S. health care spending. Research Synthesis Report no. 16*. Princeton, NJ: Robert Wood Johnson Foundation.

Goodell, S., & Ginsburg, P. B. (2008). *High and rising health care costs: Demystifying U.S. health care spending. The Synthesis Project Policy Brief No. 16*. Princeton, NJ: Robert Wood Johnson Foundation.

Greenhalgh, T. (1997). How to read a paper: Papers that tell you what things cost (economic analyses). *British Medical Journal, 315*(7108), 596–599.

Hadley, J. (2007). Insurance coverage, medical care use and short-term health changes following unintentional injury or the onset of a chronic condition. *Journal of the American Medical Association, 297*(10), 1073–1084.

Hager, C., Tise, S., Kuta, L. A., Spencer, W., & Fritz, M. (2006). *The registered nurse population: Findings from the 2004 national survey sample of registered nurses*. Washington, DC: U.S. Department of Health and Human Services, Health Resources and Services Administration, Bureau of Health Professions.

Hartman, M., Martin, A., McDonnell, P., Catlin, A., & the National Health Expenditures Accounts Team. (2009). National health spending in 2007: Slower drug spending contributes to lowest rate of overall growth since 1998. *Health Affairs, 28*(1), 246–261.

Hauer, K. E., Durning, S. J., Kernan, W. N., Fagan, M. J., Mintz, M., O'Sullivan, P. S., et al. (2008). Factors associated with medical students' career choices regarding internal medicine. *Journal of the American Medical Association, 300*(10), 1154–1164.

Hayes, L. J., O'Brien- Pallas, L., Duffield, C., Shaniar, J., Buchan, J., Hughes, F., et al. (2006). Nursing turnover: A literature review. *International Journal of Nursing Studies, 43*(2), 237–263.

Henderson, J. (2008). *Health economics and policy* (4th ed.). Cincinnati, OH: South-Western College Publishing.

Herzlinger, R. (2000). Market-driven, focused health care: The role of managers. *Frontiers of Health Services Management, 16*(3), 3–12.

Herzlinger, R. (2007). *Who killed health care? America's $2 trillion medical problem—and the consumer-driven cure*. New York: McGraw-Hill.

Hilfiker, D. (1994). *Not all of us are saints: A doctor's journey with the poor*. New York: Hill & Wang.

Hoffman, E. D., Klees, B. S., & Curtis, C. A. (2007). *Brief summaries of Medicare and Medicaid*. Washington, DC: Office of the Actuary, Medicare and Medicaid Services, Department of Health and Human Services.

Iglehart, J. K. (2001). America's love affair with medical innovation. *Health Affairs, 20*(5), 6.

Institute of Medicine. (1999). *To err is human: building a safer health system*. Washington, DC: National Academy Press.

Institute of Medicine. (2001). *Crossing the quality chasm: A new health system for the 21st century*. Washington, DC: National Academy Press.

Institute of Medicine. (2004). *Insuring America's health: Principles and recommendations*. National Academy of Sciences. Retrieved December 10, 2008, from http://www.iom.edu/uninsured

Iowa Intervention Project. (2001). Determining costs of nursing interventions: A beginning. *Nursing Economics, 19*(4), 146–160.

Johnson-Lans, S. (2006). *A health economics primer*. New York: Pearson Addison Wesley.

Kaiser Commission on Medicaid and the Uninsured. (2008). *The uninsured and the difference health insurance makes. #1420–10*. Washington, DC: Kaiser Family Foundation.

Kaiser Family Foundation. (2008). *Fact sheet: Women's health insurance coverage. #6000-07.* Menlo Park, CA: Kaiser Family Foundation.

Klarman, H. E. (1982). The road to cost-effectiveness analysis. *The Milbank Memorial Fund Quarterly, 60*(4), 585–603.

Kleinpell, R., & Gawlinski, A. (2005). Assessing outcomes in advanced practice nursing practice: The use of quality indicators and evidence based practice. *AACN Clinical Issues, 16*(1), 43–57.

Kristen, M. M. (1983). Using cost-effectiveness analysis and cost-benefit analysis for health policy making. *Advances in Health Economics and Health Services Research, 4,* 199–224.

Lavizzo-Mourey, R. (2008). *Road to reform: President's message from the 2008 Robert Wood Johnson Foundation Annual Report.* Princeton, NJ: Robert Wood Johnson Foundation.

Leape, L. L. (1994). Error in medicine. *Journal of the American Medical Association, 272*(23), 1851–1857.

Lin, S. X., Gebbie, K. M., Fullilove, R. E., & Arons, R. R. (2004). Do nurse practitioners make a difference in the provision of health counseling in hospital outpatient departments? *American Academy of Nurse Practitioners, 16*(10), 462–466.

Lohr, K. N. (1990). *Medicine: A strategy for quality assurance.* Washington, DC: National Academy Press.

McMenamin, P. (1990). What do economists think people want? *Health Affairs, 9*(4), 112–119.

Mehrotra, A., Wang, M. C., Lave, J. R., Adams, J. L., & McGlynn, E. A. (2008). Retail clinics, primary care physicians, and emergency departments: A comparison of patients' visits. *Health Affairs, 27*(5), 1272–1282.

Mitka, M. (2007). Looming shortage of physicians raises concerns about access to care. *Journal of the American Medical Association, 297*(10), 1045–1046.

Mundinger, M. O. (2002). Perspectives: Through a different looking glass. *Health Affairs, 21*(1), 163–164.

Mundinger, M. O., Kane, R. L., Lenz, E. R., Totten, A. M., Wei-Yann, T., Cleary, P. D., et al. (2000). Primary care outcomes in patients treated by nurse practitioners or physicians. *Journal of the American Medical Association, 283*(1), 59–68.

Newhouse, J. P. (1992). Medical care costs: How much welfare loss?. *Journal of Economic Perspectives, 6*(3), 3–21.

Organisation for Economic Co-Operation and Development. Health at a glance. (2009). *OECD indicators.* Paris: OECD.

Pappas, S. H. (2007). Describing costs related to nursing. *Journal of Nursing Administration, 37*(1), 32–40.

Pauly, M. V. (1993). U.S. health care costs: The untold true story. *Health Affairs, 12*(3), 152–159.

Pillar, B., Jacox, A. K., & Redman, B. K. (1990). Technology, its assessment, and nursing. *Nursing Outlook, 38*(1), 16–19.

Porter, M. E., & Teisberg, E. O. (2004). Redefining competition in health care. *Harvard Business Review,* June, 65–76.

PricewaterhouseCoopers' Health Research Institute. (2008). *Top eight industry issues in 2008.* New York: PricewaterhouseCoopers.

Pruitt, R. H., & Jacox, A. K. (1991). Looking above the bottom line: Decisions using economic evaluation. *Nursing Economics, 9*(2), 87–91.

Rampell, C. (2009). Layoffs spread to more sectors of the economy. *The New York Times,* January 27, 2009, A1 and A 20.

Rhoades, J. A. (2005). *The long-term uninsured in America, 2001 to 2002: Estimates for the U.S. population under age 65.* Rockville, MD: Agency for Health Care Research and Quality. Retrieved January 20, 2007, from http://www.ahrq.gov/about/cfact/cfactbib28.htm#Rhoadespg

Rice, T. H. (1998). *The economics of health reconsidered.* Chicago: Health Administration Press.

Rice, T. H., & Labelle, R. J. (1989). Do physicians induce demand for medical services? *Journal of Health Politics, Policy and Law, 14*(3), 587–600.

Robert Wood Johnson Foundation, Building Human Capital News Digest. (2009). Hospitals offering extravagant incentives to attract nursing talent. Retrieved January 12, 2009, from http://www.rwjf.org/humancapital/digest.jsp?id=9271&;c=EMC-ND137

Robinson, J. C. (2001). The end of managed care. *Journal of the American Medical Association, 285*(20), 2622–2628.

Robinson, J. C., & Ginsberg, P. B. (2009). Consumer driven health care: Promise and performance. *Health Affairs, 28*(2), w272–w281. (Web exclusive). January 27, 2009. Retrieved January 20, 2007, from http://content.health affairs.org/cgi/content/full/28/2/w272

Rutherford, M. A. (2008). The how, what and why of valuation and nursing. *Nursing Economics, 26*(6), 347–383.

Rye, C. B., & Kimberly, J. R. (2007). The adoption of innovations by provider organizations in health care. *Medical Care Research and Review, 64*(3), 235–278.

Santerre, R. E., & Neun, S. P. (2004). *Health economics: theories, insights and industry studies* (3rd ed.). Mason, OH: Thomson, South-Western College Publishing.

Schoen, C., Collins, S. R., Kriss, J. L., & Doty, M. M. (2008). How many are underinsured? Trends among U.S. adults, 2003 and 2007. *Health Affairs, 27*(4), w298–w309. (Web exclusive). Retrieved January 15, 2009, from http://content.healthaffairs.org/cgi/content/full/27/4/w298

Schoen, C., & DesRoches, C. (2000). Role of insurance in promoting access to care. Uninsured and unstably insured: The importance of continuous insurance coverage. *Health Services Research, 35*(1), 187–206.

Schroeder, C. (1993). Nursing response to the crisis of access, cost, and quality in health care. *Advances in Nursing Science, 16*(1), 1–20.

Shortell, S. M., Bennett, C. L., & Byck, G. R. (1998). Assessing the impact of continuous quality improvement in clinical practice: What will it take to accelerate progress? *The Milbank Quarterly, 76*(4), 593–624.

Smith, S., Heffler, S., & Freeland, M. (1999). The next decade of health spending: A new outlook. *Health Affairs, 18*(4), 86–95.

Spetz, J. (2004). Hospital nurse wages and staffing, 1977 to 2002. *Journal of Nursing Administration, 34*(9), 415–422.

Starr, P. (1982). *The social transformation of American medicine.* New York: Basic Books.

Stone, P. W., Curran, C. R., & Bakken, S. (2002). Economic evidence for evidence-based practice. *Image: Journal of Nursing Scholarship, 34*(3), 277–282.

U.S. Bureau of Labor Statistics. (2007). Economic News Release. The 30 occupations with the largest employment growth 2006-2019. Retrieved January 20, 2007, from http://www.bls.gov/news.release/ecopro.t05.htm

U.S. Congress. (1986). *Nurse practitioners, physician assistants, and certified nurse midwives: A policy analysis (Health Technology Case Study 37; Publication No. OTA-HCS-37).* Washington, DC: U.S. Government Printing Office.

Wallace, P. (2004). The health of nations: A survey of health-care finance. *The Economist, July,* 17, 3–18.

Weisbrod, B. A. (1991). The health care quadrilemma: An essay on technological change, insurance, quality of care, and cost containment. *Journal of Economic Literature, 29*(2), 523–552.

Ziller, E. C., Coburn, A. F., & Yousefian, A. E. (2006). Out of pocket health spending and the rural underinsured. *Health Affairs, 25*(6), 1688–1699.

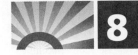

8

Communication Skills and Techniques

KATHARINE C. COOK, PhD, RN, CNE

> We are healed of a suffering only by expressing it to the full.
> Marcel Proust

OBJECTIVES

At the completion of this chapter, the reader will be able to:

- Describe and define the components of effective communication.
- Describe the levels of communication.
- Differentiate between effective and ineffective professional communication.
- Identify the three strategies that enhance interpersonal communication.
- Identify the three types of organizational communication.

PROFILE IN PRACTICE

Barbara Moran, PhD, CNM
Assistant Professor, The Catholic University of America, Washington, D.C.

Nothing is more sacred than the communication between a nurse and a patient. From this interaction, the baseline assessment is laid. Asking sensitive questions is part of taking a complete health history. As nurses we continually learn from our patients how to communicate with them in more effective ways. As a practicing nurse midwife, I became interested in intimate partner violence during pregnancy. I have had opportunity to interview many abused women about their pregnancies and childbirth experiences. These women teach us that better avenues to communicate effectively are always available.

Abuse is a secret that is often kept between a woman and her partner. Breaking that secret by the woman can mean a slap to the face, a hit to the head, or hours of beating. It is incumbent on the nurse to incorporate all his or her communication skills when assessing for abuse.

I want to share with you a lesson learned that represents both intrapersonal and interpersonal communication and the context involved in a communication. Charlotte was a 24-year-old survivor of intimate partner violence. She was pregnant with her second child when I met her. While I was interviewing Charlotte about her pregnancy and birth experience,

I asked if any health care professional had questioned her regarding whether she was in a violent relationship and, if so, whether she had shared her abusive history.

Charlotte's story began when she had her first obstetrical history and physical examination done by a nurse practitioner at a clinic near her home. While doing the exam, the nurse practitioner asked Charlotte if anyone had hurt her at home and whether she felt safe at home. As nurses, we are taught to incorporate sensitive questions regarding abuse within the normal history taking. Although Charlotte was in a very violent relationship, she told the nurse practitioner that she was not in an abusive relationship. This was the first visit Charlotte had had with this practitioner, so she may not have felt comfortable enough to discuss the abuse. However, the reason she did not confide to the nurse practitioner was very revealing. Charlotte's partner was just steps away outside the examination room. Although the questions were asked in a private environment of the examination room, Charlotte was afraid that when the partner was invited back into the room, the nurse practitioner would confront him about what Charlotte had just said and then her partner would know she had told someone about the abuse—which was not in her best interests.

We do not know the skills this particular nurse had in asking about intimate partner violence, but even if the environment had been perfect, the questions sensitively asked, and the body language open and personal, the communication would still have been halted. Charlotte would not have answered the questions with honesty. We learn from Charlotte that we need to be as specific as possible when asking patients about sensitive information. We learn that we need to tell all our patients that what is said between us is confidential and that only with their permission will the information be divulged. Maybe if this nurse practitioner had expressed this to Charlotte, she would have learned about the abuse.

Introduction

Communication is universal yet parochial. All human beings and, as increasing evidence suggests, most living creatures share and try to understand one another's feelings and thoughts, even when not intending to do so. Such is the nature of the world; the deepest interaction is that of communication. Rudyard Kipling likened words to drugs and believed them to be even more potent than pills (1928). Although registered nurses are well trained in the administration of drugs and assessment of drug actions and reactions, most nurses do not understand the powerful actions and potential side effects of communication. Effective communication, like effective drug therapy, requires the five rights: right drug, right route, right dose, right time, and right person. This chapter discusses communication (right drug) in all its universality and in all its peculiarities concerning route, dose, timing, and personal interpretation.

What is communication? Webster's dictionary defines *communication* as "giving or exchanging information signals or messages … by talk, gestures or writing" (Neufeldt & Guralnik, 1997, p. 282). The Latin root is *communicare,* meaning "to share." Thus the key word in the definition is *exchanging,* which implies a giver and a receiver. Communication theory is based on this construct. Many early theories of human communication were built on a linear model, which assumed one person (sender) sent a message to another person (receiver). This conceptualization, however, simplifies a process that is very complex and makes static a process that is dynamic (Kreps & Thornton, 1984).

Contrary to conventional wisdom, communication is complex. The message is created by a process of interacting components: the meanings people actively create, the time and place of the communication, the relationships established between the receiver and sender, the past experiences of both parties, the personalities involved, the purposes of the communication, and the effects of human communication on people and situations. Meanwhile, as all these components dynamically interact, communication is occurring on many levels: intrapersonal communication, which occurs within the individual; interpersonal communication, in which two people interact; small group communication; and organizational communication. Each level builds on another, and successful communication at all levels depends on success at *each* communication level (Kreps & Thornton, 1984).

Intrapersonal Communication

The foundation of the communication pyramid is formed by intrapersonal communication. This level is within the communicator's internal environment, where the critical skills of communication begin. Personal translation processes allow the person to constantly encode or create messages and to decode or interpret messages. During translation, the person creates meanings of the messages given and received from an intensely unique perspective. No word, object, or thing has any inherent meaning. The individual brings to bear influencing factors such as past experiences, personality, and relationships to the interpretation of content (Kreps & Thornton, 1984).

CONTEXT

The biggest influence on interpretation of content is the context in which the message is received. Context is much larger and richer than simply the time and place of communication: "It is more than background; it is the total frame that gives a message its meaning" (Maxwell, 1993, p. 1). Work by language theorists (Clifford & Marcus, 1986; Gergen, 1991; Maxwell, 1993) have led to the belief in a social construction of reality. Instead of one unmitigated universal external reality, what an individual thinks and understands is the result of interaction with others. Each person individually constructs reality; nothing is universal and neutral. All individuals do not necessarily share the same perceptions and conceptual frameworks. One readily given explanation for these phenomena is the traditionally understood differences in culture, but one must be careful not to fall into a static and unchanging viewpoint of culture. Cultural diversity is only a piece of what contributes to multiple understandings of the same word, object, or content. As Maxwell (1993) states, "Postmodern approaches

instead stress how emergent such understandings are as people interact with others, especially in multicultural environments where people have access to interaction with such varied others" (p. 2). Culture and context both help and hinder communication. Language is ambiguous and depends on understanding implicit meanings and nuances of a situation. Returning to the drug metaphor, something as routine as receiving a message that a patient is in pain is ambiguous. Is the patient assigned to you? What kind of pain? Has the patient recently received pain medication? Did something happen that caused the pain? The list of questions is endless and automatic for an experienced nurse. It requires further communication, relying on shared meanings, and incorporating nuances of the situation. Linguists call this experienced communication response *pragmatic competence in communication* (Hearnden, 2008).

SELF-AWARENESS

Given that communication is the underpinning that forms a person's reality, an understanding of the *self*—and how it is influenced by many external factors—is imperative. How does a person come to such an understanding of self?

Johari Window. One helpful framework is the Johari window (Table 8-1), a conceptual framework of the self that is named after its creators, Joseph Luft and Harry Inglam (Luft & Inglam, 1955). The metaphor in this theory is that of a window with four panes—one open, one blind, one hidden, and one unknown. The open pane represents what is personally known and also known to others. When interacting for the first time with a person, the size of this windowpane is small because each person knows little about the other

TABLE 8-1	Johari Window	
	Known to Self	**Unknown to Self**
Known to others	Open area	Blind area
Unknown to others	Hidden area	Unknown area

Based on Luft, J. (1969). *Of human interaction.* Palo Alto, CA: National Press.

person. This window becomes more open as a relationship develops and people self-disclose. The second pane reveals what an outsider knows about another but is unknown to the self; therefore it is called *blind.* This might occur when nonverbal and verbal messages are incongruent and the receiver chooses to believe the nonverbal message, of which the sender may be unaware. The third pane is hidden. This is information that is known to the self but not known to the outsider. The last pane is the unknown, about which neither the person nor others know. This unconscious area can be revealed to one or both as conversation takes place.

The ideal for effective communication is to raise the shade on the open pane of glass so that the self is more transparent to others. However, one should use caution in deciding what information to share with others. In personal relationships it is often not desirable to reveal things that could undo the balance of power in the relationship (e.g., past indiscretions in sexual behavior, mental health problems, life-altering failures). In professional relationships, self-disclosure needs to be in the best interest of the patient. Nurses can encourage reciprocal self-disclosure by revealing the nurse's self as open, honest, and human (Gordon & Edwards, 1995). Storytelling, for instance, is a powerful means of connection, allowing caregiver and patient to understand commonalities and differences (Heilker, 2007).

A good rule of thumb, however, is to withhold any unresolved information. Unresolved information can shift the focus from the patient to the professional and can become an undue burden. This can be especially tempting when interacting with someone who is close to one's own age. Even when teaching adults, the professional must be wary of sharing too much personal information. For example, consider a nurse who shared ongoing personal problems with the orientees she was coaching in a clinical setting. The new nurses tried to understand and be supportive but eventually asked for less self-disclosure from the mentor because it had become a source of worry and distraction.

Values Clarification. Another method for increasing self-awareness is values clarification. Simon, Howe, & Kirschenbaum (1972) set six criteria that must be met for full value development: freedom in choosing, awareness of alternatives, awareness of

BOX 8-1	Values Clarification Exercise

Below is a list of values that people commonly hold. Rank these values in order of the priority each holds for you, with 1 being your top priority and 10 being your last. After completing the list, share your top three values with your peers. Discuss how these priorities affect your interpretations and decisions.

_____ Achievement (sense of accomplishment)
_____ Advancement (promotions)
_____ Adventure (risk taking)
_____ Caring (love, affection)
_____ Economic security
_____ Family
_____ Time freedom
_____ Health
_____ Loyalty
_____ Spirituality

Modified from Simon, S., Howe, L., & Kirschenbaum, H. (1972). *Values clarification: A handbook of practical strategies for teachers and students.* New York: Hart.

consequences for each alternative, happiness with the choice, acting with the choice, and consistently incorporating the choice in one's actions. Values evolve over a lifetime in response to changing circumstances. During values clarification the aim is not to change values but to become aware of what those values are and the priority assigned to each. Only then can the nurse separate his or her values from that of the patient. Box 8-1 provides a list of common values.

Personal values are an important influence on how meaning is assigned to interactions and therefore decisions. The inherent tension between time freedom and economic security is one example. If someone must work to make a living but highly values free time, the person is likely to choose a lower-paying job if it is more flexible than a job with assigned office hours.

Interpersonal Communication

The next level of communication takes place interpersonally between two individuals. Receiver and sender become both intrarelated and interrelated. As one is encoding or creating messages to be sent, the other is already decoding or interpreting the messages being sent. Human beings have an ability to selectively perceive at any given time the information most important to them.

In everyday life, especially in the 21st century, people are barraged by constant external messages. To cope with this noisy environment, three strategies are inherent to the cognitive process. The first, selective attention, is reinforced and made possible by the process of habituation. During selective attention, the most important messages are given more cognitive space than less-important messages. Habituation enhances this adaptation by blocking out extraneous external and internal messages.

Both selective attention and habituation are constantly in a state of flux. What is important to a new nurse in conversation with a patient might be vastly different from the selective attention of an experienced nurse, who might be more attuned to subtle clues about the patient's health status. Both nurses, however, can be influenced by internal messages that interfere with their ability to listen actively. This is especially true in today's health care environment, in which fatigue from 12-hour shifts or too many patients can interfere with communication. To survive in such an environment, habituation allows the nurse to block out fatigue and problems at home to listen to critical messages sent by the patient (Kreps & Thornton, 1984).

One final skill inherent in human beings is the ability for closure. During closure, people make sense out of the messages to which they attended. Educated assumptions are made to fill in the gaps about the message based on the receiver's logic and past experiences. Thus reality is relative and inexorably connected to past experiences (Kreps & Thornton, 1984). The nurse needs to develop particular skills to avoid premature closure, the most important of which is active listening.

ACTIVE LISTENING

Active listening is a learned skill in which the nurse suspends personal beliefs and values, resists categorization, and stays in the present, minimizing the influence of past experiences and self-directed current and future problems. The focus is entirely on the patient. The nurse, however, is not passive but is actively examining the content of the patient's message, sorting the relevant from the irrelevant, and seeking clarification from the sender. Selective attention and habituation undergo change as the nurse identifies themes from the conversation and educated assumptions are voiced for patient validation. Often nurses perceive listening to clients as "doing nothing for them." Active listening properly done, however, provides care and can require as much energy as the nurse expends during physical care of the patient (Pagano & Ragan, 1992; Sheldon, 2004; Williams, 2004).

Silence is an inherent part of active listening. Most nurses are uncomfortable with the use of silence in communication, deeming a pause in conversation as a patient's need for reassurance and a cue for a nurse to "fill in the blanks," often bringing the interaction to premature closure. Silence serves a critical role in communication, allowing both nurse and client to reflect on the interaction and its meaning. Often, letting the patient break the silence is important because it indicates to the sender (patient) that the nurse is willing to listen to the patient's feelings, thoughts, and insights. Occasionally, however, the nurse will need to respond, either by performing a therapeutic technique, moving the conversation in a different direction, or concluding the conversation. The essential interpretation on the part of the nurse is to ascertain carefully whether the silence is uncomfortable for the patient or for the receiver (the nurse); that determination should guide the nurse's actions (Northouse & Northouse, 1998; Sheldon, 2004; Williams, 2004).

THERAPEUTIC RESPONSES

In addition to silence, active listening is enhanced by verbal communication strategies that help the listener accurately receive the sender's intended message. The names of verbal communication strategies vary from author to author. The principal focus should be on the rationale for using any one particular technique and the effectiveness of the response in keeping the receiver selectively attending to the message sent by the receiver and keeping the communication open until closure is truly achieved.

Restatement is a communication approach that has been variously described as repeating verbatim the last few words a patient says or paraphrasing the patient's words. Regardless, the goals of restatement are to let the patient know he or she is being listened to and to encourage the patient to elaborate without asking direct questions. This response technique should be used sparingly because overuse leads to an air of insincerity and could be misconstrued as parroting the patient (Arnold & Boggs, 2003; Sheldon, 2004). Box 8-2 provides an example of restatement.

Reflection is another type of communication nurses can use to let patients know they are attending to their underlying feelings. Often patients will not come out and say how they feel about something, especially to health care providers, where the balance of power is uneven. As nurses, we should actively listen to what patients are communicating, even if the content of the message does not include stated feelings, and then reflect perceptions back to them for validation. Box 8-3 provides an example of reflection.

Clarification is an ongoing strategy to ensure that the message received is the message that was sent. Human beings want to make sense of the world around them and will often move toward premature closure by filling in the gaps by using logic and past experience without checking the accuracy of their assumptions with the sender. This can be one of the most grievous mistakes in therapeutic communication, almost guaranteeing that the patient will feel misunderstood. In a concept analysis of feeling misunderstood, Condon (2008) found that consequences included "termination of activity, such as relationships" (p. 183). Thus the patient will become reluctant to engage. Clarification, therefore, should be used when the patient makes a vague statement or retroactively after the patient finishes a train of thought. Box 8-4 provides an example of clarification.

Minimal cues, leads, and touch are also useful in therapeutic communication. Minimal cues show that the nurse is interested and present for the patient without interrupting the patient's flow of thought. Leaning forward, giving short leads such as "yes," "uh huh," and "go on" convey a clear message that the nurse is actively listening. Touch is a basic sense and need that all human beings share. Intentionally touching the patient lightly on the arm or shoulder sends a message of comfort that is more powerful and deep than many words (Arnold & Boggs, 2003). The nurse should carefully discern when the patient would accept touch in the context of cultural influences and past experiences.

Summarization helps both the patient and the nurse integrate the meaning of the interaction by relating

---

BOX 8-2 | **Restatement**

Patient: I don't know when to schedule my surgery. The surgeon has offered me Monday or Tuesday.
Nurse 1: Monday or Tuesday …?
Nurse 2: You are unsure of which day would be best to schedule surgery.
Note that in both responses, the nurse is offering the patient an opportunity to discuss why deciding when to schedule surgery is difficult.

BOX 8-3 | **Reflection**

Patient: I don't want to take this treatment anymore. It just makes me sicker than when I came in to the hospital. How is this helping me?
Nurse: You are afraid that the treatment we are giving you will not make you well.
Note that the nurse identified an underlying fear the patient has about the effectiveness of the treatment.

BOX 8-4 | **Clarification**

Patient: I cannot stand that other nurse. She comes in and only looks at the IV pump and then quickly leaves the room.
Nurse 1: Tell me more about what happened with the nurse this morning.
Nurse 2: You said earlier in the conversation that you were having trouble with one nurse. Can you give me an example?
Note that Nurse 1 immediately follows up to help the patient clarify what he perceives in the nurse's actions. Nurse 2 reminds the patient of an earlier remark and asks the patient to elaborate. In both cases, the nurses are asking for specifics to help both them and their client be clear about the situation.

ideas and feelings expressed during the conversation in a short synopsis for review by both of the participants. The nurse is responsible for critically thinking about the material and offering a brief summation. In turn, the patient's responsibility is to add to the nurse's observations or correct them. With summarization both nurse and client can move on to a different topic or terminate the interaction.

Questioning is a strategy that every nurse uses on a daily basis to obtain information about the client. Questions can be closed or open ended. Contrary to the belief that all close-ended questions must be answered with a yes or no response, the basic premise of a close-ended question is to compel a direct response from the patient. Examples include asking the patient's age, as well as inquiries that require the patient to answer yes or no. Open-ended questions, on the other hand, allow patients to respond in any direction they wish and give the nurse new information about their concerns and goals. Patients are given a general invitation to respond to when, where, and how they sought help in the health care system. Asking "why" is not a helpful strategy because it puts the patient on the defensive by asking reasons for behavior that even the patient might not understand (Arnold & Boggs, 2003; Williams, 2004).

Many nursing students, especially experienced RNs, get caught up in the minutiae and appear stilted and uncomfortable when trying to implement these communication strategies. The best approach is to be oneself and put specific, concrete strategies into a larger picture. There is tension among nursing professionals about the use of strategies, which some believe to be a task-based approach. The crux of intentional dialogue is to focus on creating ease in the relationship; to set aside "self-focus to be truly present and gather another's story about a health challenge" (Smith & Liehr, 2008, p. 176). A more comprehensive framework helps the nurse to draw together the whole and incorporates four of the rights mentioned at the beginning of the chapter: the right route, right dose, right time, and the right person.

DETERMINING THE RIGHT ROUTE

There is more to communication than talking and listening. A powerful alternative route to understanding the client is the use and interpretation of nonverbal behavior. The nurse gives and receives nonverbal cues that greatly influence the interaction. Important nonverbal behaviors include facial expression, eye contact, hand and arm gestures, posture, and use of personal space. Facial expressions are informative in terms of their congruence with the subject matter under discussion. If the patient is recalling a frightening event, is his expression serious and reflective of his feelings? A broad smile or laugh would indicate an inconsistency between the spoken and nonspoken message that needs to be explored. One approach to this situation is to confront the patient directly with the incongruence by stating, "You are telling me about a very frightening experience, yet you are laughing about it."

The meaning of eye contact varies from person to person and from culture to culture. Looking someone in the eye can convey many things: a sense of respect and trustworthiness, a confidence in oneself, a personal interest in the speaker, and conversely, hostility or insult. Culture is the main influencing factor regarding the interpretation of eye contact. For example, Asians and Pacific Islanders understand a downward glance as a sign of respect, whereas Americans might interpret looking away as disinterest or boredom (Sheldon, 2004).

Arm and hand gestures inform the nurse during the interaction. Open gestures indicate a willingness to share and be open, whereas folded arms convey unwillingness to talk or vulnerability and a need for self-protection (Sheldon, 2004). Posture also reveals underlying feelings. Leaning forward conveys a sense of interest and active listening, whereas a rigid posture could imply, "I don't want to talk to you." In addition, the use of personal space is telling. Although different cultures use personal space in varying ways, Americans generally understand this distance to be 18 inches to 4 feet. These boundaries, which help people maintain a sense of identity and assert safety and control in a vulnerable situation, must be observed (Northouse & Northouse, 1998; Sheldon, 2004).

An appropriate setting, the use of understandable language, boundaries set with a clear contract, and the establishment of confidentiality are also routes to effective therapeutic communication. Although difficult in today's health care environment, a quiet, private setting to talk with a patient is fundamental, as is the use of language that the patient understands. A noisy public setting will cause distractions and fear of being overheard, and professional jargon confuses the patient, who will rarely ask for clarification. A clear contract gives the patient insight into the purpose of the interaction, how long the professional relationship is expected to last, and what the patient can expect of the health care provider. Confidentiality is an expectation that should be overtly stated; under Health Insurance Portability and Accountability Act (HIPAA) regulations, this should be given to the patient in writing.

THE RIGHT DOSE

Although the nurse cannot precisely measure the dose of communication as is possible with drug therapy, several guidelines can help determine the intensity, the depth, and the content of a therapeutic interaction. Simply put, the client is the one person who directs the dose of the intervention. Mirroring the client depth or lack thereof during the interaction is important. If the client is exploring deeper feelings, then the nurse must go there with him or her. However, when the patient gives a superficial response, responding with intensity is contraindicated. In addition, verbal responses need to match the patient's words without embellishment or minimization. Before the nurse can make assumptions, enough data must be available to warrant an interpretation (Arnold & Boggs, 2003).

The use of humor, reframing, presentation of reality, metaphors, and the sharing of personal information all must be given in the right dose. Humor is effective when purposely inserted into the conversation for a specific purpose. It can help reduce an overly intensive situation and allow the patient to appreciate the absurdities of life and humanity. Occasional use is more therapeutic than constant humor, which can minimize the seriousness of the patient's concerns. Another strategy, reframing, helps the patient see the larger reality and put things into perspective. One clue that reframing may be helpful is when the patient uses black-and-white phrases such as "always" or "never." Rarely in life, if at all, do such absolutes exist. Having the patient reexamine statements helps ameliorate

feelings and opens the opportunity for a patient to move on. The use of metaphors can be overdone but is sometimes crucial to aid in the patient's understanding. Consider how this chapter uses a metaphor that equates the effective use of therapeutic communication with the correct method of drug administration in terms of how essential each task is to the patient's health. Finally, the right dose of personal information must be determined when interacting with a patient. A general guideline is to share only those issues that are fully resolved and pertinent to the conversation at hand to help the patient better understand himself or herself (Arnold & Boggs, 2003).

THE RIGHT TIME

Timing is of the utmost importance when deciding how to respond in a therapeutic interaction. The first consideration is the stage of the relationship. Therapeutic relationships typically have four sequential phases: preorientation, orientation, working, and termination (Peplau, 1952). Preorientation takes place before the nurse even meets the client. During this phase the nurse reflects on professional roles and responsibilities, sets broad goals for the interaction, gets an overview of the patient's status, anticipates obstacles or difficulties, and thinks about the physical environment to maximize privacy and comfort.

The second stage, orientation, is when the therapeutic relationship begins. The main objective during this phase is to establish trust. The nurse is unfamiliar to the patient, who might be in new surroundings as well. To lay the groundwork for trust, the nurse needs to give the client basic information about himself or herself and explain why the nurse is there. The focus is the immediate problem that brought the patient to the health care system; deep exploration is avoided. Honesty and commitment are essential. If a nurse cannot keep an appointment, the patient deserves an explanation. Content is kept fairly superficial as the nurse bonds with the patient over everyday life interests; the nurse listens to the patient's story. Even seasoned registered nurses often ask how to begin a therapeutic conversation with a client they might be treating over a number of months. A helpful rule is to start a social conversation, perhaps asking about family pictures that may be on display or about something of interest to the client based on environmental clues (Smith & Liehr, 2008; Williams, 2004).

The third stage is when the work of the therapeutic relationship begins, thus the name *working phase*. During this phase, rapport has been established and the interaction becomes more focused and intense for both the nurse and the patient. The nurse uses active listening and indirect verbal responses as the client reveals health care concerns. Because part of the relationship is more interactive, the importance of mirroring the client cannot be stressed enough. The nurse follows the client's lead, pursuing in-depth those issues that the client indicates a readiness to explore (Smith & Liehr, 2008). During RN to BSN gerontology courses, where students refine therapeutic communication, older adults will often tell students things they have never discussed with anyone.

The termination phase actually begins at the start of the relationship. During preorientation the nurse reflects on feelings about past experiences with endings. During orientation the nurse needs to be clear about the length of the contract, and the topic of termination needs to be revisited by the nurse and client during the working phase, when both parties have an opportunity to discuss what this ending might mean to them. Despite preparation, the client and even the nurse might resist termination. Behaviors that indicate resistance might be cancellation of appointments, anger, or an expressed disinterest in talking about important issues or termination itself. The responsibility of the registered nurse student is to accept these feelings nonjudgmentally and help the client understand their meaning. If client issues need further intervention, the nurse should help connect the client to other resources.

Registered nurse students often become uncomfortable with the notion of leaving the client at a potentially important juncture in their work together and feel that they have "used" the client to further their own education at the client's expense. Students could be correct in that assumption if adequate preparation for termination has been ignored during the other phases of the relationship. Most often, however, this anxiety is part of student-centered issues around past losses that the student is reluctant to face.

THE RIGHT PERSON

The patient determines the right person to whom to entrust their deepest thoughts and concerns. The nurse can only prepare intrapersonally (see beginning of chapter) and offer a safe and therapeutic environment for interpersonal interaction. If the patient is not ready or chooses someone else to confide in, the nurse should follow the patient's wishes and avoid taking the patient's decision personally.

Organizational Communication

An organization is by definition an interdependent entity whose members strive toward a common purpose of accomplishing stated goals: "Organizational communication refers to human communication between organization members (as well as between organization members and related others) during the performance of organizational tasks and the accomplishment of organizational goals" (Kreps & Thornton, 1984, p. 155). This discussion focuses on the basic understanding of the dynamics of organizational communication and group process.

Systems theory is a helpful way to understand the complexity of organizations. This theory posits that systems have both environmental inputs and outputs, which are vastly different by virtue of the synergy or added energy that occurs from the interactions among system parts. Therefore the product of the system is uniquely different from the mere summation of its parts or, as is often noted, the whole is greater than the sum of its parts. Think of the organization (hospital or health care system) as the system whose input (various patient and community health needs) is processed by the many levels of health team members, allowing its output to be flexible in providing health care services for many client groups (Kreps & Thornton, 1984). Figure 8-1 illustrates some of the influencing factors (throughput) on the product (output) of a health care organization. These influencing factors include upward, downward, and vertical or horizontal communication within the organization itself and the group

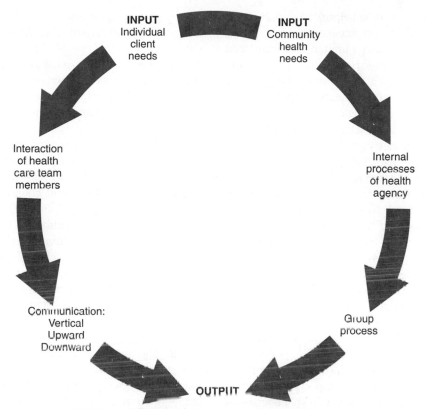

FIGURE 8-1 Influencing factors of a health care organization.

process of its team members. Systems theory is also discussed in Chapter 5.

TYPES OF ORGANIZATIONAL COMMUNICATION

Three types of formal organizational communication exist: upward, downward, and vertical. These formal networks follow the chain of command. Upward communication from subordinates to superiors usually takes on the form of reports. Downward communications from administration to workers on lower levels often are commands about decisions to be implemented, rules, and regulations.

Vertical communication, on the other hand, can be part of a formal or informal network. Formal ways of communicating horizontally are work groups and vertical connections among departments. Informal networks are formed by employees and are not controlled by management. These "grapevines" are faster

than formal channels and are busy when employees feel insecure, are threatened, or are faced with organizational change. These communications are approximately 75% accurate and are the main source of practical job information (Baskin, 1984).

A key to successful outputs in a health care organization is professional-to-professional communication. Given the complexity of patient care problems, collaboration and cooperation are essential to deliver quality health care services. The nurse is often the coordinator of care and, as such, takes the lead in communication. This communication can be adversely influenced by three factors: role stress, lack of interprofessional understanding, and autonomy struggles (Northouse & Northouse, 1998).

Role stress is familiar to registered nurse and baccalaureate-degree students when roles are complicated by the addition of academic demands in already overscheduled lives. To better understand role stress, looking at two components is helpful: role conflict and role overload. Role conflict occurs when competing demands vie for attention in a limited time frame and the nurse is faced with choices that affect patient care. One example is the decrease in hospital days and the need to hurriedly discharge patients to open beds for other admissions. The new patient needs the hospital care, but the patient being discharged also needs teaching and planning for care outside the health care setting. Role overload is also common in today's settings, where the nursing shortage requires regular overtime and the responsibilities of the nurse increase as staffing decreases (Northouse & Northouse, 1998). Chapter 4 explores these aspects of "role" in more detail. Additionally, the impacts of professional-to-professional communication are addressed in Chapter 20.

Lack of interprofessional understanding is cited as a significant impediment to communication. In a study by Laschinger and Weston (1995), groups of nursing and medical students were asked to describe their perceptions of one another's role. Not surprisingly, each group misunderstood the other group's expertise. The consequences of these misperceptions were profound and produced an inverse relationship in collaboration. The greater the gap in interprofessional understanding, the more negative the participants were toward shared decision making.

Autonomy struggles between health care professionals also disrupt professional-to-professional communication. Historically, the nurse has been seen as the handmaiden of the physician. This perception is rapidly changing as physicians and nurses must work together in critical care settings, emergency departments, community-based practices, and long-term care of an increasingly aging population to achieve quality patient outcomes (Northouse & Northouse, 1998).

GROUP PROCESS

Contrary to the popular notion of group inefficiency and ineffectiveness, groups tend to formulate effective solutions by building on one another's ideas, bringing different perspectives to the problem at hand, and increasing commitment to a decision formed by consensus. To lead and participate in productive work groups, the nurse needs to understand group processes and behaviors.

Two important dynamics are the life cycle of groups and group functions (Arnold & Boggs, 2003).

Group Phases. The typical group phases are forming, storming, norming, performing, and adjourning. When the group first forms, anxiety by group members is focused on acceptance. During this forming phase, group members are polite as they establish commonalities around goal setting, group identification, explicit norms of behavior, and methods of communication. As group comfort increases, members begin to challenge one another about boundaries, methods of goal achievement, group format, and discussion topics. This storming phase, although essential to deeper levels of group understanding, can be uncomfortable and thus sometimes not acknowledged. During this phase, group members must acknowledge the tension and work toward developing group norms so that the group can progress to the next phase of group development (Arnold & Boggs, 2003).

During the next phase, norming, communication is more spontaneous and personal. Consensus is reached about group behavior that will increase the likelihood of the group achieving its goal. Members are more comfortable with divergent opinions but are able to agree on the best way to proceed. Consensus does not mean that all members must wholeheartedly agree on all the particulars, but rather each member supports group decisions enough to prevent conscious or unconscious undermining of their implementation. Group cohesiveness increases, and the members move on to the performing phase. An *esprit de corps* facilitates the accomplishment of group goals and group members feel a sense of both intellectual and emotional fulfillment. With the group's purpose realized, the group is no longer needed and the adjourning phase occurs. During this termination, members share feelings about group members and personal contributions to the group's work. Closing comments can help reframe previous interactions, blend emotional and cognitive experiences, and "summarize the group experience" (Arnold & Boggs, 2003, p. 320).

Group Functions. More than a half-century ago, Bennis and Shepard (1956) separated group participant roles into three distinct functions: maintenance, task, and self-serving. Maintenance role functions help increase group satisfaction, whereas task role functions move the group toward goal accomplishment. Self-serving role functions serve individual needs that are unrelated to the group's purpose and thus interfere with group work toward a common mission (Arnold & Boggs, 2003; Northouse & Northouse, 1998).

Tables 8-2 to 8-4 give examples of task, maintenance, and self-serving behaviors. These behaviors occur in all groups. Therefore vital tasks include

TABLE 8-2	Task Behaviors in Groups	
Task Behaviors	**Definition**	**Example**
Initiator/contributor	Suggests new ideas	"Have you thought of ...?"
Information seeker	Asks for clarification or information	"Do you mean ...?"
Opinion seeker	Clarifies values	"What do you think ...?"
Information giver	Offer facts or personal experiences	"I read in this research article ... "
Opinion giver	States personal beliefs	"I think we should ... "
Elaborator	Expands on ideas	"We could also ... "
Coordinator	Pulls ideas together	"Sally suggested ... and Tim's idea is similar ... "
Orientor	Defines present position or raises questions about direction of group	"Where are we as a group on this?"
Evaluator-critic	Explores practicality and logic of discussion	"Given _____, will this idea work?"
Energizer	Urges group toward action	"Have we had enough discussion to move toward a decision?"
Procedural technician	Carries out routine tasks	Sets up chairs in a circle before meeting
Recorder	Writes down proceedings	E-mails group members a summary after each meeting

Modified from Northouse, L. L., & Northouse, P. G. (1998). *Health communication: Strategies for professionals.* Stamford, CT: Appleton & Lange.

TABLE 8-3	Maintenance Behaviors in Groups	
Maintenance Behaviors	**Definition**	**Example**
Encourager	Praises and accepts others' contributions	"I really think that is a useful idea."
Harmonizer	Acts as a go-between	"I think you two are really saying the same thing."
Compromiser	Modifies position	"I see that some of the things I value are included so I can agree to ..."
Gatekeeper	Regulates flow of group discussion	"We have 15 minutes left to discuss ..."
Standard setter	Points out group goal	"I think we are getting off track ..."
Group observer	Offers comments on group process	"Everyone seems to be much more comfortable offering different opinions on ..."
Follower	Goes along with group	"If everyone else thinks ..."

Modified from Northouse, L. L., & Northouse, P. G. (1998). *Health communication: Strategies for professionals.* Stamford, CT: Appleton & Lange.

TABLE 8-4	Self-Serving Behaviors in Groups	
Self-Serving Behaviors	**Definition**	**Example**
Aggressor	Verbally attacks others	"I think that idea is silly."
Blocker	Consistently disagrees with group ideas	"This situation is not going to change."
Recognition seeker	Calls attention to self	"I thought of that idea last night."
Self-confessor	Expresses unrelated personal feelings	"I felt awkward in that situation … "
Playboy/playgirl	Plays around and not involved	"Did you see on television last night …?"
Dominator	Interrupts other group members	"Before you finish, let me … "
Help seeker	Tries to elicit sympathy	"I just can't get this task done because … "
Special interest pleader	Champions positions of particular groups	"I know the union would … "

Modified from Northouse, L. L., & Northouse, P. G. (1998). *Health communication: Strategies for professionals.* Stamford, CT: Appleton & Lange.

understanding, observing, and for task and maintenance behaviors, putting into practice group communication strategies that help move the group toward task accomplishment.

SUMMARY

Effective communication can be analyzed using the processes developed for medication giving. Communication is dynamic and includes intrapersonal, interpersonal, and organizational communication. By using values clarification and other techniques, nurses can strive to improve their professional communication skills.

KEY POINTS

- Effective communication is conceptually similar to medication administration; it includes the right route, right dose, right time, and right person.
- Communication is the giving or exchanging of information signals or messages through gestures, writing, and talk.
- Communication occurs dynamically at many levels, including intrapersonal, interpersonal, small group, and organizational.
- Johari's window is a conceptual framework of the self expressed through a four-pane window metaphor. This framework is helpful in identifying boundaries for self-disclosure, depending on the intended form of communication.

- In professional relationships, self-disclosure is based on what is in the best interest of the patient.
- Values clarification is a method of developing self-awareness. Values clarification assists the nurses in separating their values from those of the patient.
- Strategies that enhance the cognitive processes involved in interpersonal communication include selective attention, habituation, and active listening.
- Nonverbal communication cues greatly influence interactions.
- Therapeutic communication is an important and effective intervention that is essential to a patient's health.
- The dynamics and complexity of organizational communication are best understood by using systems theory. Systems theory proposes that the environmental inputs and outputs of a system are greater than the sum of its parts because of the synergy of the interactions among its parts.
- A lack of interprofessional understanding among nursing and medical students of different disciplines has an inverse relationship on their ability to collaborate.

CRITICAL THINKING EXERCISES

1. Complete the value clarification exercise in Box 8-1 and discuss the results with your peers. Consider how your values could affect your ability to therapeutically communicate with patients.
2. Practice active listening by asking a peer to talk about her or his day. Lead with a broad statement such as "Tell me about your day." At various intervals use different responses to encourage the speaker to continue and to

feel understood. Pay particular attention to reflecting feelings and content, restatement, and clarification. Have the speaker and a third person comment on your use of communication responses.

3. Reflect on your clinical/work experiences at various organizations and identify differences in upward, downward, and vertical communication patterns. Consider how the difference in organizational communication patterns affected the unit work environment (e.g., mentorship, staff morale, orientation processes).

4. Using Table 8-2, identify your role in group interactions. Obtain feedback from peers regarding their perceptions of your group communications and compare the feedback to your self-evaluation.

5. Visit http://empathy.colstate.edu/Exercises/sugar_test. htm to read about the Sugar Test by Thomas Endres (1998). Demonstrate the two sugar exercises and lead a class/group discussion on systems theory and the interdependence of group members.

REFERENCES

Arnold, A., & Boggs, K. U. (2003). *Interpersonal relationships: Professional communication skills for nurses* (4th ed.). Philadelphia: Saunders.

Baskin, O. W. (1984). *Interpersonal communication in organizations.* Glenview, IL: Scott Foresman.

Bennis, W., & Shepard, H. (1956). A theory of group development. *Human Relations, 9,* 415–437.

Clifford, J., & Marcus, G. (Eds.) (1986). *Writing culture: The poetic and politics of ethnography.* Berkley, CA: University of California Press.

Condon, B. B. (2008). Feeling misunderstood: A concept analysis. *Nursing Forum, 43*(4), 177–191.

Endres, T. G. (1998). The sugar test: Demonstrating interdependence. Presented as part of the GIFTS program, NCA Convention, November 1998, New York, NY. Retrieved August 30, 2009, from http://empathy.colstate.edu/Exercises/sugar_test.htm

Gergen, K. (1991). *The saturated self.* New York: Basic Books.

Gordon, T., & Edwards, W. S. (1995). *Making the patient your partner: Communication skills for doctors and other health care professionals.* Westport, CT: Auburn House.

Hearnden, M. (2008). Coping with differences in culture and communication in healthcare. *Nursing Standard, 23*(11), 49–59.

Heilker, D. (2007). Story sharing: Restoring the reciprocity of caring in long-term care. *Journal of Psychosocial Nursing and Mental Health Services, 45*(7), 20–24.

Kipling, R. (1928). *A book of words: Selections from speeches and addresses delivered between 1906 and 1927.* Manchester, NH: Ayer.

Kreps, G. L., & Thornton, B. C. (1984). *Health communication: Theory and practice.* New York: Longman.

Laschinger, H. K., & Weston, W. (1995). Role perceptions of freshman and senior nursing and medical students and attitudes toward collaborative decision making. *Journal of Professional Nursing, 11*(2), 119–128.

Luft, J., & Ingham, H. (1955). *The Johari window: A graphic model of interpersonal awareness.* Proceedings of the Western Training Laboratory in group development. Los Angeles: UCLA.

Maxwell, M. (1993). The authenticity of ethnographic research. *Journal of Childhood Communication Disorders, 13,* 1–12.

Neufeldt, V., & Guralnik, D. B. (Eds.) (1997). *Webster's new world college dictionary.* New York: Macmillan.

Northouse, L. L., & Northouse, P. G. (1998). *Health communication: Strategies for professionals.* Stamford, CT: Appleton & Lange.

Pagano, M. P., & Ragan, S. L. (1992). *Communication skills for nurses.* London: Sage Publications.

Peplau, H. E. (1952). *Interpersonal relations in nursing.* New York: Putnam.

Sheldon, L. S. (2004). *Communication for nurses.* Thorofare, NJ: Slack.

Simon, S., Howe, L., & Kirschenbaum, H. (1972). *Values clarification: A handbook of practical strategies for teachers and students.* New York: Hart.

Smith, M. J., & Liehr, P. (2008). Theory guided translation: Emphasizing the human connection. *Archives of Psychiatric Nursing, 22*(3), 175–176.

Williams, C. (2004). *Therapeutic communication in nursing.* Thorofare, NJ: Slack.

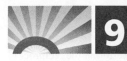

9

Critical Thinking, Clinical Judgment, and the Nursing Process

BRENDA MORRIS, EdD, RN, CNE

The author acknowledges the important foundational work for this chapter developed by Dr. C. Fay Raines in the previous edition of this book.

OBJECTIVES

At the completion of this chapter, the reader will be able to:

● Define critical thinking.
● Describe the components and characteristics of critical thinking.
● Understand the relationship of critical thinking to clinical judgment and the nursing process.
● Describe the steps of the nursing process and the relationships among those steps.
● Discuss nursing activities associated with each step of the nursing process.
● Evaluate the utility of the nursing process as a systematic framework for the delivery of nursing care.
● Apply critical thinking in nursing practice situations.

PROFILE IN PRACTICE

Elizabeth R. Lenz, PhD, RN, FAAN
Dean and Professor, College of Nursing, The Ohio State University, Columbus, Ohio

Critical thinking: it's recognizable when someone does it well and certainly evident when it is not happening. During the past 20 years we have talked increasingly about critical thinking in nursing, but that wasn't always the case. In the early 1960s, when I was entering the profession, serious efforts to change the "handmaiden" image of nursing were only just beginning. Clearly, if one's role is defined as handmaiden, rather than as colleague or independent decision maker,

critical thinking is not deemed particularly important or even desirable. Rather, blind, noncritical obedience is the order of the day. Fortunately, as nursing has become more truly professional and nurses have functioned with increasing autonomy in increasingly complex situations, critical thinking has become a most important and valued competency.

What elements converge to produce a good critical thinker? It seems to me that there are several requisites, not the least of which is intelligence. However, even though intelligence is a necessary condition, critical thinking is not guaranteed to occur without training and a nourishing environment as well. We assume that critical thinking is something that can be learned; hence we address it at all levels of nursing curricula.

Based on my experience, I believe that two essential types of learning provide the basis for critical thinking. The first is substantive. It is impossible to think truly critically about something you do not understand or about which you possess only partial information. Mastery of the theory and research findings that relate to the problem or issue to be addressed is critical, but this is not something that nurses always take time to achieve. Unfortunately, we have been less successful than other professions (namely, medicine) in socializing our practitioners to value learning as a career-long pursuit; yet pursuit of the most state-of-the-science information is an essential ingredient of critical thinking.

The second type of learning involves the process of critical thinking itself. The skills of raising questions, using logic, and comprehensively considering alternative perspectives, explanations, and courses of action can often best be learned experientially within a structure that encourages and, in fact, mandates that kind of thoughtful consideration. The model that comes to mind is the daily medical rounds in which physicians-in-training are challenged to present cases and to lay out their diagnostic reasoning clearly for others to critique. Equally valid as an environment for cultivating critical thinking is that found in many of the social sciences and humanities, where freewheeling debate and open challenge of ideas are encouraged. At first frightened by that kind of candor during my doctoral studies in sociology, I later came to value greatly the critical input of my peers. More of that kind of willingness to challenge one another's assumptions and ideas within an atmosphere of mutual respect would benefit our profession.

For me, the groundwork for critical thinking was laid early in my education. Fortunately, the faculty responsible for the BSN program I attended were forward-thinking and highly committed to the emerging definition of nursing as a true profession, with the requisite obligation to base action on scientific knowledge and clear and logical thinking. Without labeling the goal as such, we were consistently encouraged, groomed, and enabled to be critical thinkers. We were continually challenged by being asked to provide rationales for our decisions, to make explicit all of the alternative approaches and explanations we had considered and rejected, and to explain why. Not inconsequentially, the school was in a small liberal arts institution, where we were exposed on a daily basis to a wide range of points of view and disciplinary perspectives and assumptions. If anything, the nursing students were the "oddballs" whose pragmatism and goal-directedness seemed strange to the arts, sciences, and music majors. I wrestled more than once with how in the world assignments such as dissecting the symbolism in *Moby Dick* might be relevant to my career in nursing, but I now appreciate the mind-expanding contribution that such activities made to my ability to think critically.

The base hopefully having been laid during one's professional education, critical thinking depends not only on training but also on an environment or context that enables, encourages, and rewards it. Regretfully, today's employment picture in nursing is typically one with precious little time for contemplation. Downsizing, high proportions of nonprofessional personnel, high levels of acuity, and high productivity requirements may discourage critical thinking. That means every effort must be made to counter the tendency to let critical thinking slide and, instead, to encourage, nurture, and reward it, even if that means bucking the tide and incurring some additional short-term costs.

The "community of scholars" type of environment to which top educational institutions aspire should, by definition, be conducive to critical thinking. Nevertheless, even in those settings, time and energy to engage in deliberation, to exchange ideas, and to critique those ideas openly are scarce, and the kind of culture that encourages such scholarly dialogue is relatively rare. When it is in place, it is wonderful. One of my most exciting opportunities to engage in intense and prolonged critical thinking occurred when a group of four colleagues and I were "freed up" from many of our routine responsibilities to plan a doctoral program "from scratch." In weekly full-day sessions we argued, debated, challenged, cajoled, compromised, and created.

We drew on what we knew substantively about nursing, science, philosophy, and the disciplines of our respective doctoral degrees (none of which were in nursing). It was hard work, but invigorating. The ground rules were that no idea was to be belittled or rejected out of hand; all perspectives were heard and considered. We were given time to think with minimal interruption and maximal flexibility; accordingly, the end product was excellent and the process truly energizing. Such time away from the routine is rarely available in today's environment, but the model is certainly not without merit. Essential are a culture and leadership that permit and encourage critique without recrimination.

In clinical settings, time to engage in deliberative critical thinking is even more difficult to attain. Rather, critical thinking seems to be expected to occur routinely without much cultivation. Benner's model of progression from novice to expert suggests that excellent clinical experience fosters critical thinking that eventually becomes almost automatic and intuitive. However, I assert that the level of critical thinking displayed by clinical experts needs to be developed deliberately and strategically. The clinical environment in which I have seen critical thinking encouraged most effectively was one in which the expectations were explicit, critical thinking was measured routinely in the practice context, relevant learning and growth opportunities were provided, and critical thinking was taken into account in performance evaluation. In other words, the nursing leadership in that academic medical center truly valued critical thinking and was willing to assign it priority.

Nursing has reached the point in its evolution in which a consistent and continuous pattern of critical thinking by its practitioners is a mandate—a *sine qua non*. The assurance that critical thinking will be truly woven into the fabric of our profession will depend on our ability to recruit and retain intelligent, interested, and committed nurses; to provide challenging educational opportunities that develop the requisite competencies; and to provide and sustain the kinds of environments in which critical thinking is valued and demanded.

Introduction

The ability to process information from multiple sources and make decisions is a fundamental ability of professional nursing practice. Dramatic changes in the health care system and the practice of nursing have occurred during the past decade as a result of an aging population, cost containment efforts, technological advances, increased complexity of clients' health care needs, decreased average hospital length of stay, and a shift from acute care to community-based care. All of these changes have emphasized the need for professional nurses to think critically in order to provide safe and effective client care to diverse populations. To function effectively in complex, rapidly changing health care environments, nurses must use higher-order thinking skills and apply content knowledge to clinical practice. The critical thinking process provides nurses with the ability to use purposeful thinking and reflective reasoning to examine ideas, assumptions, principles, conclusions, beliefs, and actions in the context of professional nursing practice (Brunt, 2005). Professional nurses must think critically to process complex data from multiple sources and make intelligent decisions in planning, managing, delivering, and evaluating the health care of their clients. Nurses also use their critical thinking skills to reduce health care errors and improve client safety (Fero, Witsberger, Wesmiller, Zullo, & Hoffman, 2008). To become a critical thinker, a nurse must understand the concept of critical thinking; possess or acquire the essential knowledge, skills, and attributes required to think critically; and deliberately apply critical thinking principles in making clinical judgments. This chapter covers both classical and current sources to examine critical thinking, clinical judgment, and the nursing process.

Defining Critical Thinking

Critical thinking, as a concept, has been examined and presented from a variety of perspectives. An early definition, proposed by Watson and Glaser (1964), described critical thinking as the combination of abilities needed to define a problem, recognize stated and unstated assumptions, formulate and select hypotheses, draw conclusions, and judge the validity of inferences. A less prescriptive definition was offered by Ennis (1989), who characterized critical thinking as "reasonable reflective thinking focused on deciding what to believe or do" (p. 4). Paul (1992) stated that critical thinking is a process of disciplined, self-directed rational thinking that "certifies what we know and makes clear wherein we are ignorant" (p. 47). Alfaro-LeFevre (2006) presented critical thinking for nursing as informed, purposeful, and outcome-focused thinking that requires the ability to identify problems, issues, and risks and make judgments based on evidence. Bandman and Bandman (1995) describe critical thinking for nursing as "the rational examination of ideas, inferences, assumptions, principles, arguments, conclusions, issues, statements, beliefs, and actions" (p. 7) and include the following functions:

- Discriminating among use and misuse of language
- Analyzing the meaning of terms
- Formulating nursing problems
- Analyzing arguments and issues into premises and conclusions
- Examining nursing assumptions
- Reporting data and clues accurately
- Making and checking inferences based on data
- Formulating and clarifying beliefs
- Verifying, corroborating, and justifying claims, beliefs, conclusions, decisions, and actions
- Giving relevant reasons for beliefs and conclusions
- Formulating and clarifying value judgments
- Seeking reasons, criteria, and principles that justify value judgments
- Evaluating the soundness of conclusions

Conclusions are drawn as a result of this reasoning process. In nursing practice, the desired outcome of this reasoning is effective action.

Conflicting viewpoints exist regarding whether critical thinking is subject specific or generalizable (U.S. Department of Education, 1995). Most authors agree that the critical thinking processes are not discipline specific but, rather, are generalizable (Ennis, 1987; Facione, 1990; Paul, 1992; Watson & Glaser, 1964). The same critical thinking skills of interpretation, analysis, inference, and evaluation are applied in different subjects. However, the difference lies in how the critical thinking processes are applied to

specific disciplines. For example, professional nurses apply critical thinking skills to client care situations in order to make sound clinical judgments, whereas engineers apply critical thinking skills to business or industrial situations in order to make sound decisions. Meyers (1991) and McPeck (1990) believe that mastery of basic terms, concepts, and methodologies must occur before critical thinking skills can be developed. Ennis (1987) agrees that some familiarity with subject matter is necessary for the development of critical thinking; however, some principles of critical thinking bridge many disciplines and can transfer to new situations.

An attempt to define critical thinking by consensus was begun in the late 1980s, and the results became known as the Delphi Report. The Delphi research project used an expert panel of theoreticians representing several disciplines from the United States and Canada to develop a conceptualization of critical thinking from a broad perspective (Facione, 1990). The resulting work described critical thinking in terms of cognitive skills and affective dispositions. The outcome was a definition of critical thinking as the process of purposeful, self-regulatory judgments: an interactive, reflective reasoning process (Facione & Facione, 1996). A critical thinker gives reasoned consideration to evidence, context, theories, methods, and criteria to form a purposeful judgment. At the same time, the critical thinker monitors, corrects, and improves the judgment. The Delphi project produced the following consensus definition from its panel of experts:

We understand critical thinking (CT) to be purposeful, self-regulatory, judgment which results in interpretation, analysis, evaluation, and inference, as well as explanation of evidential, conceptual, methodological, criteriological, or contextual considerations upon which that judgment is based. … CT is essential as a tool of inquiry. As such, CT is a liberating force in education and a powerful resource in one's personal and civic life. (American Philosophical Association, 1990)

The Delphi participants identified core critical thinking skills as interpretation, analysis, inference, evaluation, and explanation. These critical thinking cognitive skills and subskills are listed in Box 9-1.

BOX 9-1	Critical Thinking Cognitive Skills and Subskills

Interpretation	**Inference**
Categorization	Querying evidence
Decoding sentences	Conjecturing alternatives
Clarifying meaning	Drawing conclusions
Analysis	**Explanation**
Examining ideas	Stating results
Identifying arguments	Justifying procedures
Analyzing arguments	Presenting arguments
Evaluation	**Self-regulation**
Assessing claims	Self-examination
Assessing arguments	Self-correction

Critical Thinking in Nursing

Scheffer and Rubenfeld (2000) replicated the Delphi study with a panel of 55 nurse educators to obtain a consensus definition of critical thinking for nursing. That study resulted in the identification of 17 dimensions of critical thinking and agreement on the definition of critical thinking for nursing as:

> … an essential component of professional accountability and quality nursing care. Critical thinkers in nursing exhibit these habits of the mind: confidence, contextual perspective, creativity, flexibility, inquisitiveness, intellectual integrity, intuition, open-mindedness, perseverance, and reflection. Critical thinkers in nursing practice the cognitive skills of analyzing, applying standards, discriminating, information seeking, logical reasoning, predicting and transforming knowledge. (p. 7)

Although many areas overlap with the American Philosophical Association's (1990) Delphi Report definition of critical thinking, some important differences also exist. According to Allen, Rubenfeld, and Scheffer (2004), the dimensions of creativity, intuition, and transforming knowledge that are so crucial to effective clinical practice were not included in the Delphi Report definition. These dimensions emerged in the consensus definition of critical thinking for nursing.

SUMMARY OF DEFINITIONS OF CRITICAL THINKING

Although a universally accepted definition of critical thinking has not emerged, agreement exists that it is a complex process. The variety of definitions helps provide insight into the myriad dimensions of critical thinking. Commonalities in definitions include an emphasis on knowledge, cognitive skills, beliefs, actions, problem identification, and consideration of alternative views and possibilities (Daly, 1998). The definitions presented earlier are summarized for comparison in Table 9-1, and characteristics of critical thinking are listed in Box 9-2.

The activities involved in the process of critical thinking include appraisal, problem solving, creativity, and decision making. The interrelationships among these concepts are illustrated in Figure 9-1. These activities are embedded in the critical thinking process in both nursing education and nursing practice.

CRITICAL THINKING AND THE NURSING PROCESS

In nursing, critical thinking has often been portrayed as a rational, linear process that is synonymous with clinical judgment, problem solving, and the nursing process (Ford & Profetto-McGrath, 1994; Huckabay, 2009; Jones & Brown, 1993; Kintgen-Andrews, 1991; Wilkinson, 1996). However, some critics believe that the problem-solving emphasis of the nursing process constrains critical thinking because it does not incorporate the creativity and open-mindedness components of critical thinking (Conger & Mezza, 1996; Duchscher, 1999; Jones & Brown, 1993; Miller & Malcolm, 1990).

Although critical thinking skills are important components of the nursing process and problem solving, these are *not* synonymous terms. The nursing process serves as a tool for applying critical thinking to nursing practice. The nurse uses critical thinking throughout the nursing process, by sorting and categorizing data; identifying patterns in the data; drawing inferences; developing hypotheses that are stated in the form of outcomes; testing these hypotheses as care is delivered; and making criterion-based judgments

TABLE 9-1	Definitions of Critical Thinking
Author(s)	**Definition**
Watson and Glaser (1964)	Combination of abilities needed to define problems, recognize assumptions, formulate and select hypotheses, draw conclusions, and judge validity of inferences
Ennis (1989)	Reasonable reflective thinking focused on deciding what to believe or do
Paul (1992)	Process of self-disciplined, self-directed, rational thinking that verifies what we know and clarifies what we do not know
The Delphi Report (American Philosophical Association, 1990); Facione, Facione, and Sanchez (1994)	Purposeful, self-regulatory judgments resulting in interpretation, analysis, inference, evaluation, and explanation
Bandman and Bandman (1995)	Rational examination of ideas, inferences, assumptions, principles, arguments, conclusions, issues, statements, beliefs, and actions
Alfaro-LeFevre (2006)	Informed, purposeful, and outcome-focused thinking that uses evidence to make clinical judgments

BOX 9-2	Characteristics of Critical Thinking

Involves conceptualization
Is rational and reasonable
Is reflective
Is partially attitudinal
Is autonomous
Includes creativity
Is fair
Focuses on what to believe and do

From Wilkinson, J. M. (2001). *Nursing process: A critical thinking approach* (2nd ed.). Upper Saddle River, NJ: Prentice-Hall.

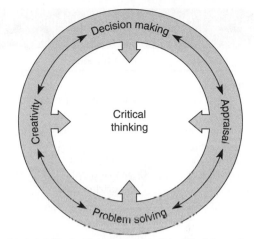

FIGURE 9-1 Critical thinking model. (Modified from Strader, M. K., & Decker, P. J. [1995]. *Role transition to patient care management.* Upper Saddle River, NJ: Prentice-Hall.)

of effectiveness. Therefore critical thinking can distinguish between fact and fiction, providing a rational basis for clinical judgments and the delivery of nursing care. Although an argument can be made that the nursing process constrains critical thinking because of its structured format, general agreement exists that critical thinking skills and subskills are evident throughout the nursing process (Alfaro-LeFevre, 2006). Although the components of the nursing process are described as separate and distinct steps, they become an integrated way of thinking as nurses gain more clinical experience. An overview of critical thinking throughout the nursing process is presented in Table 9-2. A thorough understanding of the nursing process reveals that critical thinking is indeed an integral part of its most effective use.

The Nursing Process

The nursing process is a systematic, problem-solving approach used extensively in the United States and Canada for the delivery of nursing care. The nursing process was first described in the literature in 1955 by Lydia Hall. Her approach was built around three interrelated spheres of nursing activity: care, core, and cure. The focus in the *care sphere* is the body, including

TABLE 9-2	Overview of Critical Thinking Throughout the Nursing Process
Nursing Process	**Critical Thinking**
Assessment	Observing
	Distinguishing relevant from irrelevant data
	Distinguishing important from unimportant data
	Validating data
	Organizing data
	Categorizing data
Analysis/diagnosis	Finding patterns and relationships
	Making inferences
	Stating the problem
	Suspending judgment
Planning	Generalizing
	Transferring knowledge from one situation to another
	Developing evaluative criteria
	Hypothesizing
Implementation	Applying knowledge
	Testing hypotheses
Evaluation	Deciding whether hypotheses are correct
	Making criterion-based evaluations and judgments

Modified from Wilkinson, J. M. (2001). *Nursing process: A critical thinking approach* (2nd ed.). Upper Saddle River, NJ: Prentice-Hall.

assessment and evaluation of the client's ability to perform basic functions and activities of daily living. The focal point in the *core sphere* was on the therapeutic use of self in providing nursing care, whereas nursing activities related to the *cure sphere* centered on the administration of treatments and therapies, as well as supporting the patient and family during the treatment process.

Subsequently, many others have described a "nursing process," but the model that has withstood the test of time is that developed by Yura and Walsh (1988). They proposed a four-step nursing process model that consisted of assessing, planning, implementing, and evaluating. The current model closely resembles the Yura and Walsh model, but with the addition of a

diagnostic component. The five-step nursing process consists of the following elements:

- *Assessment*—gathering and validating client health data, strengths, risks, and concerns
- *Analysis/diagnosis*—processing client data and identifying appropriate nursing diagnoses
- *Planning*—designing strategies to solve identified problems and build on client strengths
- *Implementation*—delivering and documenting the planned care
- *Evaluation*—determining the effectiveness of the care delivered

The American Nurses Association (ANA), in its publication *Nursing: Scope and Standards of Practice* (2004), parallels the steps of the nursing process and supports its use. Outcome identification, which follows the nursing diagnosis phase and precedes the planning phase, is identified as a separate step in the ANA model.

The nursing process is sometimes depicted as a systematic, linear model proceeding from assessment through diagnosis, planning, implementation, and evaluation. It is more appropriately conceptualized as a continuous and interactive model (Figure 9-2), thereby providing a flexible and dynamic approach to client care. This model can accommodate changes in the client's health status or failure to achieve expected outcomes through a feedback mechanism. The interactive nature of the model with its feedback mechanism permits the nurse to reenter the nursing process at the appropriate stage to collect additional data, restructure nursing diagnoses, design a new plan, or change implementation strategies. This model is consistent with the concept of critical thinking as a continuous reflective process. Further examination of the elements of the nursing process reveals the multiple activities embedded in each step.

ASSESSMENT

In the assessment phase, the nurse deliberately and systematically collects data to determine the client's health, functional status, strengths, and risk factors (Carpenito, 2008). Data collection centers on the use of multiple sources and types of data, a variety of data collection techniques, and the use of reliable and valid

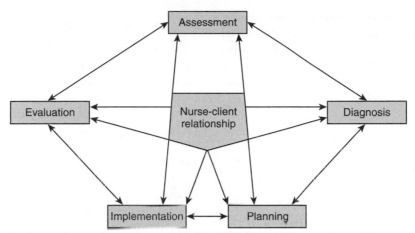

FIGURE 9-2 The interactive nursing process model. (Modified from Christensen, P. J., & Kenney J. W. [1995]. *Nursing process: Application of conceptual models* [4th ed.], St. Louis: Mosby.)

measurement instruments. All these elements are critical to building a comprehensive database.

Sources of Data. The primary source of data is the client, whether the client is defined as the individual, the family, or the community. Secondary sources of data include written records, other health care providers, and significant others (e.g., family members, friends). To strengthen the overall assessment and validate client data, it is important to use primary and secondary data sources.

Data Collection Techniques. Assessment techniques include measurement, observation, and interview. Measurement is used to determine the dimensions of a given indicator (e.g., blood pressure) or to ascertain characteristics such as quantity, size, or frequency. Measurement may require the use of specialized equipment (e.g., stethoscope, thermometer) or specialized assessment tools (e.g., pain scale, depression scale) to assess functional, behavioral, social, or cognitive domains. Data collection by observation requires the use of the senses, including visual observation and tactile (palpation) and auditory techniques (auscultation). Observation provides a variety and depth of data that may be difficult to obtain by other methods. A structured or unstructured interview may be used to obtain information such as a health history and demographic data. A structured interview is commonly used in emergency situations when the nurse needs to gather specific infor

mation. An unstructured interview is commonly used in situations in which the nurse wishes to elicit information from the client's perspective or gain insight to the client's understanding of a problem. The unstructured interview allows the nurse to use active listening skills while building rapport with the client through the use of an open-ended interview format. These communication techniques are discussed in chapter 8.

Types of Data. To complete a comprehensive assessment, objective and subjective data are obtained. Objective data are factual data, usually obtained through observation or measurement. An example of objective data occurs when the nurse uses an otoscope to assess the client's tympanic membrane and observes that it is reddened and inflamed. Subjective data are based on the client's perception of the health problem. An example of subjective data occurs when the client states that he is having pain in his right ear. It is important to collect both objective and subjective data to complete a comprehensive assessment. Care should be taken to record data factually and to avoid personal or biased interpretations.

Data Collection Instruments. The use of selected data collection measures and instruments can assist the nurse in compiling a comprehensive database and organizing data into meaningful patterns. Assessment usually begins by taking a nursing history and conducting a physical examination. Many clinical areas have developed nursing history and physical forms specific to the type of agency and the clients served. Regardless of the format, the nursing database should include the following categories of information (Edelman & Mandle, 1994):

- Demographic data
- Current and past medical problems
- Family medical history
- Surgical and (if appropriate) obstetrical history
- Childhood illnesses
- Allergies
- Current medications
- Psychological status
- Social history
- Environmental background
- Physical assessment

The amount of detail may vary; for example, a history obtained in an emergency department may be different from one taken in an extended care facility. The focus of the assessment and history may also vary on the basis of the type of client served. For example, on an oncology unit emphasis may be placed on assessment of pain, social support networks, and coping skills, whereas in a prenatal clinic the focus would be on assessment of fetal growth, knowledge of nutrition, and the need for community resources such as childbirth education classes. Beyond the areas of particular concern, however, all dimensions of the client, including physiological, psychological, sociocultural, developmental, and spiritual aspects, should be assessed (Carpenito, 2005).

To ensure appropriate identification of client health problems, it is important to perform a comprehensive assessment. The nurse may also use the assessment phase as a time to establish the nurse-client and nurse-family relationships and begin the discharge planning process. Completion of a comprehensive assessment lays the foundation for making effective clinical judgments and implementing appropriate nursing care to meet the client's identified health needs. To accurately assess a client, the nurse must apply the critical thinking skills of observing, distinguishing relevant from irrelevant data, validating the accuracy and completeness of the data, and organizing the data to provide the basis for subsequent analysis and diagnosis.

ANALYSIS/NURSING DIAGNOSES

Analysis involves processing the data by organizing, categorizing, and synthesizing the information. The nurse uses critical thinking skills to make inferences in the data from which conclusions can be drawn. Analysis gives meaning to the data as client strengths, problems, and risks are identified. Client data may be compared against known norms, such as the stages of growth and development or disease-specific behaviors or expectations. Gaps or incongruities in the data are identified, and patterns of behavior are ascertained. Analysis occurs while the nurse is actively listening and questioning the client, and later, when the nurse processes the information to formulate a plan of care. Analysis is an ongoing process that is initiated when new information is obtained or changes in the client's health status occur. The end result of data analysis is the formation of a *nursing diagnosis.*

As noted in Carpenito (2008), the North American Nursing Diagnosis Association (NANDA) defines nursing diagnosis as a "clinical judgment about individual, family or community responses to actual or potential health problems/life processes. The nursing diagnosis provides the basis for selection of nursing interventions to achieve outcomes for which the nurse is accountable" (Carpenito, 2008, p. 10). Diagnosis involves drawing conclusions through the use of critical thinking skills from identified patterns in the data and includes the elements of deliberation, inference, interpretation, and choice (Wilkinson, 1996). The nurse uses inductive and deductive reasoning to determine an appropriate nursing diagnosis. *Inductive reasoning* is used to draw broad or generalized conclusions from specific data (Bandman & Bandman, 1995). A nurse uses inductive reasoning when making the observation that clients who underwent bowel resection surgery experience intense postoperative pain. From this observation, the nurse concludes that all clients who undergo bowel resection surgery will probably experience pain postoperatively and therefore will have the nursing diagnosis of acute pain. *Deductive reasoning* is used to draw specific conclusions from generalized data or facts. If the nurse accepts the premise that pain in the left arm and jaw is a cardinal sign of a myocardial infarction, then when a client presents to the emergency department complaining of left arm and jaw pain, the nurse uses deductive reasoning to suspect that the client is having a myocardial infarction until it can be proved otherwise. Diagnosis entails back-and-forth movement between these two modes of reasoning.

Nursing diagnoses reflect actual or potential health problems that can be treated within the scope of nursing practice (Carpenito, 2008). A nursing diagnostic statement differs from a medical diagnosis in both content and context. The medical diagnosis describes a pathological condition or symptom that requires treatment aimed at curing the disease or alleviating the symptom. The nursing diagnosis, on the other hand, describes the human response to the illness or life event.

It is important for the nurse to accurately identify the client's nursing diagnoses and to validate these nursing diagnoses with the client. If the nursing diagnoses are not validated with the client before nursing interventions are implemented, the nursing care plan may be ineffective and may not meet the client's health care needs. The client's nursing diagnosis guides the planning, implementation, and evaluation phases of nursing care.

PLANNING

During the planning phase of the nursing process, the nurse collaborates with the client to establish the priority nursing diagnosis or diagnoses, determine client outcomes, and identify nursing interventions to assist the client toward optimal achievement of outcomes (Carpenito, 2008). It is important to involve the client, family, and significant others in the planning process, when appropriate, to gain their support for implementing the plan of care.

Prioritizing nursing diagnoses consists of ranking them according to importance. In general, the highest-priority nursing diagnoses address basic survival needs, life-threatening client problems, and safety. Additional considerations in setting priorities are the need for early resolution of health problems that have the potential to impair functioning or normal growth and development; the client's individual needs, values, and overall health status; and constraints of time and resources. Ideally, the client and nurse mutually determine the priority nursing diagnoses; however, this is not always possible

Once priorities are established, desired outcomes are identified. *Outcomes* are client centered, specific, realistic, and measurable, and they include a time frame. Outcomes are written to reflect attainment of an optimal level of health, alleviation or minimization of a health problem, or modifications of lifestyle. It is recommended to begin the outcome statement with the phrase "The client will …" This helps the nurse to write the outcome from the client's perspective rather than the nurse's perspective. It is helpful to use the following format when writing an outcome statement: "The client will *(insert action verb and behavioral criterion)* by *(insert time frame).*" An example of a well-written outcome is as follows: "The client will ambulate 50 feet with the assistance of a walker by the first postoperative day." In this example, the phrase "ambulate 50 feet with the assistance of a walker" includes the action verb and behavioral criterion; the phrase "by the first postoperative day" describes the time frame. In clinical situations a specific date and time (e.g., 9 AM on 10/10/2009) may be used. See Table 9-3 for another example of a well-written client outcome.

Each outcome must be accompanied by one or more *nursing interventions* aimed at helping the client achieve the outcome. Bulechek and McCloskey (1987) define a nursing intervention as "an autonomous action based on scientific rationale that is executed to benefit the client in a predicted way related to the nursing diagnosis and stated goals" (p. 37). Therefore nursing interventions are what nurses do with and for the client to treat a specific nursing diagnosis or client health problem (Bulechek & McCloskey, 1987). Nursing interventions may be performed by the nurse or delegated to assistive personnel as appropriate. It is

TABLE 9-3	**Example of a Measurable Behavioral Outcome**
Outcome	**Characteristic**
The client will walk	Performance
One half the length of the hall	Criterion
Unassisted	Condition
On the second postoperative day	Condition

important to select nursing interventions that are specific to the nursing diagnosis, acceptable to the client, feasible to implement, realistic, and supported with scientific rationale or evidence.

Nursing diagnoses, client outcomes, and nursing interventions are incorporated into a nursing care plan. The *nursing care plan* is used as a communication tool between nurses and other health professionals and serves as a guide for nursing care. It is more common for clinical agencies to use standardized care plans or care maps created by clinical experts. Standardized care plans or care maps contain common nursing diagnoses, client outcomes, and nursing interventions for clients experiencing common medical and surgical illnesses. Nurses customize the standardized care plans or care maps to meet the specific needs of their client.

IMPLEMENTATION

During the implementation phase, the nurse executes the previously identified plan of care by using intellectual, interpersonal, and technical skills to provide care that is client focused and outcome oriented and meets the needs of the client. Common nursing interventions initiated during the implementation phase include performing assessments to monitor client health status; providing or assisting the client with personal care; assisting the client to perform activities of daily living; administering medications or other prescribed treatments; teaching the client; or consulting with other health care professionals. During implementation, the nurse uses critical thinking skills to apply knowledge to client care situations, reflect upon implementation of the plan of care by assessing for changes in the client's condition, evaluating the effectiveness of the nursing interventions, and making changes to the plan of care based on this assessment.

The final step in the implementation phase is careful documentation. The system of documentation may be agency specific, but the content should reflect the client's concerns and the nursing process. It is important to include the following information in the record:

- A description of the nursing intervention that was performed
- The client's response to the intervention

- Any new data that may have emerged
- Progress (or lack of it) toward achievement of client care outcomes

Documentation should also include a description of any planned interventions that did not occur and the reasons why they were not implemented. It is very important to ensure that all information is documented correctly; therefore it is recommended that nurses review their documentation for errors prior to finalization.

EVALUATION

Evaluation is an ongoing activity that occurs at each stage of the nursing process. The overall purpose of the evaluation phase of the nursing process is to determine whether the client met the identified outcomes. The nurse evaluates the attainment of outcomes by comparing the predicted outcome with the client's actual progress toward meeting the outcome.

Evaluation occurs within each step of the nursing process. During the assessment phase, evaluation focuses on the appropriateness and completeness of data collection. During the analysis and diagnosis phase, evaluation centers on whether the data are appropriately clustered; whether the nursing diagnoses reflect the data and the client's health concerns; and whether the nursing diagnoses are clear, concise, and relevant. During the planning process, evaluation activities are directed toward determining the appropriateness of the outcomes, nursing diagnosis priorities, and selected nursing interventions. During the implementation stage, evaluation focuses on the relevance and effectiveness of specific nursing interventions. The nurse and client continue to evaluate these components until the client's health concerns are resolved, the outcomes are achieved, or the episode of care ends.

Another way to focus evaluation activities is to judge the appropriateness, effectiveness, and efficiency of the plan of care and its implementation. The ideal plan of care is relevant to the client's health concerns and focuses on mutually desirable outcomes; is effective in achieving desired outcomes within the specified time frame; and is efficient in maximizing the use of client, provider, and agency resources.

Guidelines for Evaluation. As previously mentioned, evaluation includes comparing actual outcomes against predicted outcomes and evaluating the nursing care plan. If the outcomes are not met, the nurse and client must determine the reason. The following questions may be asked:

- Were the assessment data appropriate and complete?
- Were the data interpreted correctly?
- Were nursing diagnoses appropriate?
- Were outcomes realistic, attainable, and measurable?
- Was the nursing care plan directed toward resolution of nursing diagnoses?
- Was the implementation of the plan individualized in accordance with the client's strengths and limitations?
- Were both the nurse and the client working toward the same outcomes?

Based on the answers to these questions, the nurse will modify the plan of care.

Nursing Judgment Model

Clinical judgment, which makes use of reflective thinking, is strongly rooted in the critical thinking process (Duchscher, 1999). Kataoka-Yahiro and Saylor (1994) describe a model for nursing judgment and assert that the critical thinking process is "reflective and reasonable thinking about nursing problems without a single solution and is focused on deciding what to believe and do" (p. 352). This model identifies the outcome of critical thinking as discipline-specific clinical judgments.

THE CRITICAL THINKING MODEL FOR CLINICAL JUDGMENT

The critical thinking model for clinical judgment presents five components of critical thinking: specific knowledge, experience, competencies, attitudes, and standards of care.

Knowledge. Domain-specific knowledge is essential to successful clinical reasoning because knowledge provides the data for critical thinking processes.

For example, one cannot identify appropriate actions for unexpected clinical symptoms without understanding the physiology involved. This example highlights the fact that for critical thinking to be productive, nurses must have a sound knowledge base.

Experience. The lack of practical experience and opportunity to make decisions can limit the development of critical thinking. Understanding complex situations comes through experience in analyzing similar and contrasting situations. The importance of experiential knowledge as a nurse moves from novice to expert clinician has been emphasized by Benner (1984).

Competencies. The nursing judgment model features cognitive rather than psychomotor competencies. *Cognitive competencies* are of three types: general critical thinking competencies, specific critical thinking competencies in clinical situations, and specific critical thinking competencies in nursing. General critical thinking competencies are common to other disciplines and nonclinical situations and therefore are not unique to nursing. Examples include the scientific process, hypothesis generation, problem solving, and decision making. Specific critical thinking competencies in clinical situations are used by nurses and other health care providers and include diagnostic reasoning, clinical inferences, and clinical decision making.

Attitudes. *Attitudes* are "traits of the mind" and are central aspects of a critical thinker (Paul, 1992). According to Paul, critical thinking is impossible if one does not persevere at reasoning, does not fairly weigh evidence for an opposing viewpoint, or does not value curiosity or discipline. The cultivation of independence, confidence, and responsibility is essential, as is acknowledgment of the limits of one's personal knowledge or viewpoint. Thus the critical thinking model for nursing judgment includes attitudes of confidence, independence, fairness, responsibility, risk taking, discipline, perseverance, creativity, curiosity, integrity, and humility.

Standards. Both intellectual and professional standards are important to the nursing judgment model. Critical thinking must meet the universal intellectual

PERFECTION............VS..............IMPERFECTION
OF THOUGHT

Clear...........................vs...............Unclear

Precise.......................vs...............Imprecise

Specific.......................vs...............Vague

Accurate.....................vs...............Inaccurate

Relevant......................vs...............Irrelevant

Plausible......................vs...............Implausible

Consistent...................vs...............Inconsistent

Logical........................vs...............Illogical

Deep...........................vs...............Superficial

Broad..........................vs...............Narrow

Complete....................vs...............Incomplete

Significant...................vs...............Trivial

Adequate for purpose...vs...............Inadequate

Fair.............................vs...............Biased or one-sided

FIGURE 9-3 Intellectual standards for thinking. (From Paul, R. [1992]. *Critical thinking: What every person needs to know to survive in a rapidly changing world.* Santa Rosa, CA: Foundation for Critical Thinking.)

standards identified by Paul (1992) and presented in Figure 9-3. Critical thinking also must be consistent with standards of professional nursing (e.g., the ANA's *Code for Nurses* and *Standards of Professional Nursing Practice*). That is, nurses engage in critical thinking for the good of individuals or groups rather than to cause harm or to undermine a situation. Professional standards include criteria for ethical nursing judgment, evaluation, and professional responsibility.

LEVELS OF CRITICAL THINKING

In addition to the five components of critical thinking, three levels of thinking are included in the Kataoka-Yahiro and Saylor model (1994). These levels are basic, complex, and commitment.

At the *basic* level, nurses view answers as dichotomous and assume that authorities have a correct answer for every problem. They also acknowledge and accept the fact that a diversity of opinions and values exists among authorities. Although the goal is to move to higher levels of thinking, movement can be restricted by lack of knowledge and experience, as well as by inadequate competencies, inappropriate attitudes, and nonutilization of standards.

At the *complex* level, the nurse continues to recognize diversity in outlooks and perceptions and also has the ability to detach, analyze, and examine alternatives systematically. At this level the best answer to a problem might be "it depends." Alternatively, perhaps conflicting solutions are recognized. An example of complex thinking is deciding to deviate from standard protocols or roles in a specific complex client situation.

At the *commitment* level, the nurse anticipates the necessity of making a personal choice after the relative merits of alternatives have been examined. The nurse chooses an action or belief on the basis of alternatives identified at the previous level. If the chosen action is unsuccessful, alternative solutions are considered and used.

The three levels of thinking can be illustrated in a practice situation in which a nurse receives a physician's medication order. Notice in the following examples how nurses functioning at different levels of thinking handle the same situation in different ways:

Basic: "Since Dr. Jones wrote it, it must be correct. However, last week we had a client with the same problem, and Dr. Smith ordered a different medication. There must be two ways to treat this problem."

Complex: "I wonder why we are treating identical clients in two different ways. I am going to explore this issue in more detail."

Commitment: "I have examined all the information I can find, and I think Dr. Jones made a mistake in the order. I am going to call and confer with her."

The requirement for critical thinking in nursing judgment is based on the complexity of sound clinical reasoning that is "characterized by analysis, reasoning, inference, interpretation, knowledge, and open-mindedness … and requires knowledge of the area about which one is thinking" (Turner, 2005, p. 276). Effective nursing care demands that the nurse avoid simplistic generalizations about procedures and routines in favor of rational individualized clinical judgment based on critical thinking. As Alfaro-LeFevre (1999) states, "Being able to make effective clinical judgments comes from a marriage of theoretical and experiential knowledge" (p. 83). This statement may explain in part why only 35% of new registered nurse graduates meet entry-level expectations for clinical judgment (del Bueno, 2005).

Characteristics of Critical Thinkers

Eight interdependent traits of mind are essential to becoming a critical thinker (Paul & Elder 1999):

- *Intellectual humility*—an awareness of the limits of one's knowledge and sensitivity to the possibility of self-deception
- *Intellectual courage*—a willingness to listen and examine all ideas, including those that trigger a negative reaction
- *Intellectual empathy*—imagining oneself in the place of others to better understand them; allows reasoning from the viewpoint of others
- *Intellectual integrity*—the application of rigorous and consistent standards of evidence and the admission of errors when they occur
- *Intellectual perseverance*—willingness to seek intellectual insights continually over a period of time and in the face of difficulties
- *Faith in reason*—confidence in one's own ability to think rationally
- *Intellectual sense of justice*—holding to intellectual standards without seeking one's own advantage
- *Intellectual autonomy*—having rational control of one's beliefs, values, and inferences

Individuals who are critical thinkers have specific sets of characteristics. According to Alfaro-LeFevre (1999), active thinkers ask themselves such questions as: *"Am I seeing things correctly?" "What does this really mean?" "Do I know why this is?" "How can I be*

more sure?" Other characteristics identified by Alfaro-LeFevre include the following:

- Knowledgeable about biases and beliefs
- Confident, patient, and willing to persevere
- Good communication skills and the realization that mutual exchange is essential to understanding the facts and finding the best solutions
- Open-minded, willing to listen to other perspectives and to withhold judgments until all evidence is weighed
- Humble, realizing that no one has all the answers
- Proactive, anticipating problems and acting before they occur
- Organized and systematic in the approach to problem solving and decision making
- An active thinker with a questioning attitude
- Flexible, changing approaches as needed
- Cognizant of rules of logic, recognizing the role of intuition but seeking evidence and weighing risks and benefits before acting
- Realistic, acknowledging that the best answers do not mean perfect answers
- Creative and committed to excellence, looking for ways to improve oneself and the way things get done

The Delphi Report description of an ideal critical thinker also describes the attributes of a nurse with ideal clinical judgment:

> The ideal critical thinker is habitually inquisitive, well-informed, trustful of reason, open-minded, flexible, fair-minded in evaluation, honest in facing personal biases, prudent in making judgments, willing to reconsider, clear about issues, orderly in complex matters, diligent in seeking relevant information, reasonable in the selection of criteria, focused in inquiry, and persistent in seeking results which are as precise as the subject and the circumstances of inquiry permit. (American Philosophical Association, 1990, p. 3)

Disposition Toward Critical Thinking

Becoming a critical thinker involves more than developing a set of skills. It involves nurturing the disposition toward critical thinking to ensure the use of critical thinking skills outside a structured setting, such as a classroom. Seven aspects of critical thinking disposition, based on the findings from the Delphi Report, are incorporated into the California Critical Thinking Disposition Inventory (CCTDI) (Facione, Sanchez, Facione, & Gainen, 1995). The following dispositional subscales, designed to be discipline neutral, have relevance for nursing practice:

- *Inquisitiveness* is intellectual curiosity and desire for learning even when application for the knowledge is not readily apparent. For nurses, a deficit here might signal a limited potential for developing expert knowledge and clinical practice ability. Nurses who routinely ask, "I wonder why ..." in the absence of a specific problem display inquisitiveness.
- *Systematicity* is the tendency toward organized, orderly, focused, and diligent inquiry. Questions such as "In what order did the client's symptoms occur?" and "Is there more information we should consider?" are examples of systematic inquiry. Organized approaches are essential for competent clinical practice.
- *Analyticity* is applying reasoning and the use of evidence to resolve problems, anticipating difficulties, and remaining alert to the need to intervene. An analytical nurse connects clinical observations with the theoretical knowledge base to anticipate clinical events.
- *Truth seeking* is eagerness to seek the best knowledge in a given context, courage in asking questions, and objectivity and honesty, even if findings do not support self-interests or preconceived notions. Truth seeking leads to continual reevaluation of new information. In nursing practice, the rationale for doing things a certain way is often described as "we have always done it that way." This response is contrary to truth-seeking behavior. Not being disposed to truth seeking can lead to nursing practice that is based on habit rather than on tested theory and may therefore hamper the development of more effective practice.
- *Open-mindedness* is tolerance of divergent views and sensitivity to one's own biases. This disposition is central to the goal of culturally competent

care. Absence of open-mindedness might preclude provision of effective nursing care to populations that are different from that of the nurse.
- *Self-confidence* is trust in one's own reasoning processes. It permits trust in one's judgment and promotes leadership of others in resolving problems. The nurse who makes excellent assessments of client care situations but who is reluctant to bring these observations forward in interdisciplinary situations, especially if they differ from those made by the physician, shows a lack of self-confidence. Self-confidence to present the results of one's thinking is important in improving client care.
- *Maturity* is the disposition to be judicious in one's decision making. The critically thinking mature person approaches problems, inquiry, and decision making with the understanding that some problems are ill structured; some situations have more than one plausible option; and many judgments must be made based on standards, contexts, and evidence for which the outcome is uncertain. This trait has important implications for ethical decision making in nursing.

Strategies to Build Critical Thinking Skills

Critical thinking is enhanced in environments that are caring, nonthreatening, flexible, and respectful of diverse points of view. Nurses who are familiar with the nursing process, the scientific method, and research methods already know much about critical thinking because they are based on some of the same principles.

Strategies to enhance critical thinking include the following (Alfaro-LeFevre, 1999):

- Evaluates and corrects one's own thinking—Is aware of strengths, capabilities, limitations, and predispositions.
- Anticipates questions others might ask—This helps identify a wider scope of questions that need to be answered to obtain relevant information. For example, ask "What will the client's family want to know?"

- Maintains a questioning attitude—Asks questions that seek further information and clarification.
- Develops good habits of inquiry—These are habits that aid in the search for truth, such as keeping an open mind, clarifying information, and taking enough time.
- Maintains a sense of inquisitiveness—Uses phrases such as "I need to find out" rather than "I don't know" or "I'm not sure."
- Turns errors into learning opportunities.

Persistent use of these strategies develops the skills and nurtures the disposition for critical thinking. Becoming a critical thinker is a lifelong process; everyone can improve by working at it.

CURRICULUM INNOVATIONS FOR TEACHING CRITICAL THINKING

With a focus on critical thinking, nursing education is shifting from a purely problem-solving approach to one in which critical reflection mediates the relationship between knowledge and action. The ever-expanding rate of change in health care requires that students learn more, evaluate new knowledge, and monitor their own practices in light of the changes. In addition, the emphasis on critical thinking in education has been formalized in outcome measures for regional and specialized accreditation criteria. Although the need to develop critical thinking skills within educational programs is generally accepted, agreement on the methods of teaching these skills is lacking. Reviews of research in the literature reveal mixed findings, with no consistent evidence that nursing education contributes to an increase in critical thinking abilities in nursing students (Adams, 1999).

Incorporating and measuring critical thinking outcomes is a complex task leading to a variety of teaching methods. Keeping journals and using them to create action plans, using Socratic questioning, analyzing case studies from clinical practice, developing innovative clinical experiences, and modeling reflective problem solving are among the methods suggested for teaching critical thinking to students at all levels (Baker, 1996; Brock & Butts, 1998; Callister,

1996; Colucciello, 1999; Daley, Shaw, Balistrieri, Glasenapp, & Piacentine, 1999; Feingold & Perlich, 1999; Kelly, 1997; Mastrian & McGonigle, 1999; Paul & Heaslip, 1995; Perciful & Nester, 1996; Rossignol, 1997; Schumacher & Severson, 1996; Sedlak & Doheny, 1998; Wade, 1999). One carefully constructed framework for teaching and evaluating critical thinking was developed at the Indiana University School of Nursing (Dexter et al., 1997). Competencies were based on cognitive skills derived from the Delphi Report's definition of critical thinking. These cognitive skills of interpretation, analysis, evaluation, inference, explanation, and self-regulation were operationalized and leveled for associate degree, baccalaureate, master's, and doctoral programs. Suggestions for faculty use in evaluating critical thinking accompany these definitions. Such frameworks provide useful guidance for teaching and measuring what is often seen as an elusive concept. The University of Wyoming School of Nursing incorporated the analysis of newspaper articles in a course on professional issues (Beeken, Dale, Enos, & Yarbrough, 1997). Other strategies for teaching critical thinking skills include process-focused group discussion (Bell, Heye, Campion, & Hendricks, 2002), critical thinking vignettes (Eerden, 2001), and computer-assisted instruction (Saucier, Stevens, & Williams, 2000). At the University of Alabama College of Nursing at Huntsville, registered nurse students present paradigm cases of a clinical situation when refining their critical thinking abilities.

The goal of these strategies is to help students think critically and reflectively. The effective strategies support and encourage students in seeing new possibilities by going beneath the surface of a situation to examine underlying assumptions that constrain discourse and autonomous action. Critical reflection requires a disposition to listen; a tolerance for diversity, disagreement, and uncertainty; and an openness to new ideas. It includes critical examination of one's own practices. This self-examination enables an understanding of the personal perceptions and assumptions of a situation that guide one's practice. It also requires understanding a situation and the way the system works to maintain the status quo. This action involves risk taking, challenges the status quo, and requires a more active learning environment.

Research and Measurement Issues Associated with Critical Thinking

Challenges in measuring the concept of critical thinking include lack of a clear definition of the concept, as well as problems associated with instruments that measure critical thinking (Adams, 1999; Brunt, 2005; Rane-Szostack & Robertson, 1996). Few fully tested measures of critical thinking skills exist, and research with subjects other than students is quite limited.

CRITICAL THINKING MEASURES

The most commonly used measures of critical thinking include Watson-Glaser Critical Thinking Appraisal (WGCTA), Cornell Critical Thinking Test (CCTT), California Critical Thinking Skills Test (CCTST), and California Critical Thinking Dispositions Inventory (CCTDI). All of these instruments measure generalized concepts of critical thinking and are not discipline or subject specific.

Historically, one of the most widely used measures of critical thinking skills is the Watson-Glaser Critical Thinking Appraisal (WGCTA). This test is composed of a series of objective items designed to measure five aspects of critical thinking: inference, recognition of assumptions, deduction, interpretation, and evaluation of arguments. Scores on the five subtests are equally weighted to derive a total score.

The Cornell Critical Thinking Test (CCTT) is a multiple-choice test. It assesses deductive reasoning, identification of faulty reasoning, judgment of reliability of statements, evaluation of evidence, choice of useful hypothesis-testing predictions, and determination of assumptions.

The California Critical Thinking Skills Test (CCTST) is a 34-item multiple-choice test, based on the Delphi Report's consensus definition of critical thinking. It provides an overall critical thinking score, and subscale scores on analysis, evaluation, inference, deductive reasoning, and inductive reasoning. The CCTST companion instrument, the California Critical Thinking Dispositions Inventory (CCTDI), is designed to measure dispositions toward critical thinking.

Research

Much of the research on critical thinking in nursing has been done with students rather than with practicing nurses. Brunt (2005) conducted an integrated review of 18 studies from 1992 to 2003 to analyze critical thinking in nursing. The findings from this study reveal inconsistent results in the relationships among critical thinking abilities, clinical judgment (clinical decision making), and nursing education. These inconsistent findings may be related to wide variations in the definitions and descriptions of critical thinking, as well as variation in the instruments used to measure critical thinking, leading to difficulties in comparing and contrasting results of research studies.

In an integrative review of 20 studies from 1977 to 1995, Adams (1999) found varied and contradictory results about the relationship between critical thinking abilities and skills and nursing education. Some explanations for the inconsistency might be the design of the study (e.g., lack of randomization), an imprecise definition of critical thinking, lack of instruments to measure critical thinking in nursing (as opposed to general critical thinking abilities), and the failure to determine whether teaching methods facilitated critical thinking.

The results of longitudinal studies that address the relationship between nursing education and critical thinking are mixed. Using the CCTDI, Stewart and Dempsey (2005) found no significant differences in students who were tested in their sophomore year and their final senior semester. Several studies that used the WGCTA also found no significant difference in critical thinking between entry to and exit from upper-division nursing study (Bauwens & Gerhard, 1987; Maynard, 1996; Vaughan-Wrobel, O'Sullivan, & Smith, 1997). Sullivan (1987) also used the WGCTA and found no significant differences between entry and exit among registered nurse students in a baccalaureate program. Similarly, Kintgen-Andrews (1988) found no significant gain over an academic year among practical nursing students, pre-health science freshmen, associate degree nursing students, and generic baccalaureate sophomore students. On the other hand, Frye, Alfred, and Campbell (1999); McCarthy, Schuster, Zehr, and

McDougal (1999); and Miller (1992) reported a positive relationship between education and critical thinking, with both associate degree and baccalaureate students scoring significantly higher as they moved through their programs.

Cross-sectional studies also report mixed findings. Baccalaureate senior students scored higher on critical thinking than did second-year associate degree students (Frederickson & Mayer, 1977). Baccalaureate seniors also scored higher on the WGCTA than did associate degree and diploma nursing students (Brooks & Shepherd, 1992; Scoloveno, 1981). However, no significant differences were found between graduate and undergraduate students on the WGCTA (Matthews & Gaul, 1979).

Research relative to critical thinking in clinical practice is sparse. A study of critical thinking ability of practicing nurses was conducted by Pardue (1987). Baccalaureate- and master's-prepared nurses scored higher on the WGCTA than did those with diplomas or associate degrees, but no significant differences were found in self-reported difficulty in making decisions. Maynard (1996) explored the relationship between critical thinking and level of competence as defined by Benner's (1984) stages of skill acquisition and reported that the experiential component appears to have an influence on critical thinking development. May, Edell, Butell, Doughty, and Langford (1999) also postulate that critical thinking might emerge as a factor associated with clinical competence as nurses become more experienced clinicians. Howenstein, Bilodeau, Brogna, and Good (1996) studied 160 nurses practicing in two urban hospitals and found that age and years of experience were negatively correlated with critical thinking ability. Beeken (1997) interviewed and tested 100 staff nurses to determine the relationship between critical thinking and self-concept. Comparison among nurses with varying levels of education showed higher levels of critical thinking ability in baccalaureate-prepared nurses.

None of these studies are definitive in their findings. The mixed findings might be attributed to the fact that critical thinking is a complex process that is very difficult to measure, or to other factors in the research design such as the interval between the pretest and posttest. Brunt (2005) recommends that educators and researchers develop a clear definition of critical thinking and use a consistent operational definition in research so that findings can be compared across studies.

Application of Critical Thinking in a Clinical Situation

All disciplines have a logic and nursing is no exception ... Nursing content is infused through, with, and continually shaped by nursing goals, nursing questions and problems, nursing ideas and concepts, nursing principles and theories, nursing evidence, data and reasons, nursing interpretations and claims, nursing inferences and lines of formulated thought, nursing implications and consequences, and a nursing point of view. (Paul & Heaslip, 1995, p. 47)

Nursing information and data are transformed into knowledge, which then becomes the basis of sound and critically monitored nursing practice. The following example uses the elements of reasoning (Paul, 1993), which work together to create a critical thinking environment.

SITUATION

Representatives of various agencies have come together to discuss the adequacy of health services for the elderly in their community. A registered nurse is selected as the leader of the group. Because the group is a loosely constructed one representing many different constituencies, the leader recognizes the potential for the lack of focus and the possibility of producing a product that does not meet the stated purpose or needs of the community. The nurse decides to use the elements of critical thinking consciously in leading the group through its task.

Identify the Purpose. At the beginning of the first meeting, the leader states that the group's purpose is to analyze the adequacy of community health services for the elderly. During the course of subsequent meetings, the leader reiterates the purpose to keep the group focused. The major purpose often has to be distinguished from related purposes, such as expanding services for the elderly or assessing all health services in the community. Frequent reminders help achieve the purpose and focus thought and action.

Clearly and Succinctly State the Question Being Asked, the Problem Being Solved, or the Issue Under Discussion. In this situation the major question is, "Are there adequate health services for the elderly of the community?" This question can be further broken down into subquestions related to the type of services available, access to those services, the amount of use of the services, and unmet health needs of the elderly in the community. The questions should relate to the overall purpose and be answerable and relevant.

Recognize That All Reasoning Is Done from Some Point of View. Because the group itself represents different constituencies, multiple points of view are expected to surface. In guiding the group, the challenge to the leader is to become aware of his or her own point of view and that of others, be fair in having all relevant points of view expressed, and allow evaluation of all perspectives while keeping the discussion focused on the purpose and relevant questions.

Understand That All Reasoning Is Based on Assumptions. Because assumptions are often deeply embedded in reasoning, identifying them is sometimes difficult. However, not doing so places serious constraints on critical thinking and may distort the outcome. For example, the leader hears statements from one member of the group that health services for children are a greater problem than for the elderly. Another group member comments that because of their previous contributions to the community, health services for the elderly should have the highest priority and no amount of service is adequate. The challenge to the nurse leader is to help the group to identify assumptions that influence the group's work, check the validity of the assumptions, and reexamine the questions being asked in light of the assumptions.

Clarify Concepts and Ideas Necessary to Explore the Issue. The group should first define what is meant by "adequacy" and what is meant by

"health services." These terms may have a wide range of meanings depending on the points of view and assumptions of the group members. Clarifying these ideas may lead to further discussion and explication of assumptions stated earlier.

Examine the Empirical Data. At this point the group examines the available data. Examples of information that might be useful include the number and types of health services available in the community, whether elderly people are able to get access to those services, and the existence of health needs for which no services are provided. The challenge to the leader is to ensure that the data presented are complete and relevant to the question, disregard information that is not relevant to the current issue, and state the evidence clearly and fairly.

Draw Inferences from the Data. The leader must be sure that a link exists between the data and inferences, that it is reasonable given the data, and that any links are consistent. In this situation, the group determined that institutional services were adequate for those elderly who could get to them. However, the lack of transportation services prevented many of the elderly from getting to the settings where services were delivered. The group also determined that a lack of primary care and nutritional services existed in the community.

Develop Implications and Consequences. At this stage the group must examine the conclusion of their reasoning and project the implications and consequences of that reasoning. Precise consequences for addressing or not addressing the issues must include both positive and negative consequences.

SUMMARY

Today's health care environment requires nurses to solve complex problems, explore unique client situations, and evaluate the effectiveness of a wide range of interventions. Critical thinking is an integral part of effective nursing action. It is a complex process through which nurses can explore practice situations and search for effective outcomes. The conscious application of critical thinking principles can result in effective decision making and ultimately enhance the quality of care.

KEY POINTS

- Critical thinking is an evolving concept that is not easily defined.
- Critical thinking skills are important components of the nursing process and problem solving, but *critical thinking, nursing process,* and *problem solving* are not synonymous terms.
- Clinical judgments are outcomes of critical thinking in nursing.
- Appraisal, problem solving, creativity, and decision making are interrelated concepts in critical thinking.
- Nurses with expert clinical judgment display characteristics of high-level critical thinking.
- Critical thinking skills are used throughout the nursing process.
- To think critically, nurses must be able to see connections; use logic; differentiate fact, inference, and assumptions; evaluate arguments; consider many sides of an issue; be creative; and believe in their ability to think and reason.
- Becoming a critical thinker involves acquiring a set of skills and developing a disposition toward critical thinking.
- Becoming a critical thinker is a lifelong process.
- More work needs to be done to enhance and examine critical thinking embedded in nursing practice. Two areas needing particular attention are the development and refinement of instruments to measure critical thinking in practice and further exploration of the relationship between clinical judgment and critical thinking.

CRITICAL THINKING EXERCISES

1. Differentiate critical thinking, problem solving, and decision making.
2. Think about a recent patient care situation you experienced. What questions would your colleagues likely ask you if you presented this situation to them?
3. Mr. Jones, age 82 years, is admitted to your hospital unit. In conducting his initial assessment, you notice that Mr. Jones is somewhat confused. His admitting notes indicate that he takes digoxin and Lasix. Describe the process that you will use to determine whether Mr. Jones is experiencing side effects from his medication. Focus on the questions you will ask yourself or others, not on the side effects themselves.
4. Evaluate the nursing assessment instrument used in your current area of practice in terms of its adequacy for your clinical setting, usefulness in other clinical settings, and comprehensiveness. What additional data would be useful, and how might you collect this information?
5. Describe the best and worst decision making you have seen by a nurse in a client care situation. Compare these two situations in terms of the thought process used, the underlying assumptions of the nurse, the accuracy of available information, the interpretation of information, and the soundness of the decision reached.

WEBSITE RESOURCES

Alamo Colleges, Strategies for Success: Critical thinking: http://www.accd.edu/sac/history/keller/ACCDitg/SSCT.htm

Foundation for Critical Thinking: http://www.critical thinking.org

How the Language Really Works: The Fundamentals of Critical Reading and Effective Writing: http://www.criticalthinking.com

Insight Assessment—Measuring Critical Thinking Worldwide: http://www.insightassessment.com/articles.html

Institute for Critical Thinking, Montclair State University: http://www.chss.montclair.edu/ict/homepage.html

National Center for Teaching Thinking: http://www.nctt.net

REFERENCES

Adams, B. L. (1999). Nursing education for critical thinking: An integrative review. *Journal of Nursing Education, 38,* 111–119.

Alfaro-LeFevre, R. (1999). *Critical thinking in nursing: A practical approach* (2nd ed.). Philadelphia: Saunders.

Alfaro-LeFevre, R. (2006). *Applying the nursing process: A tool for critical thinking* (6th ed.). Philadelphia: Lippincott, Williams & Wilkins.

Allen, R. D., Rubenfeld, M. G., & Scheffer, B. K. (2004). Reliability of assessment of critical thinking. *Journal of Professional Nursing, 20*(1), 15–22.

American Nurses Association (2004). *Nursing: Scope and standards of practice.* Washington, DC: Author.

American Philosophical Association (1990). *Critical thinking: A statement of expert consensus for purposes of educational assessment and instruction. The Delphi Report: Research findings and recommendations prepared for the Committee of Pre-college Philosophy.* Newark, DE: Author.

Baker, C. R. (1996). Reflective learning: A teaching strategy for critical thinking. *Journal of Nursing Education, 35,* 19–22.

Bandman, E. L., & Bandman, B. (1995). *Critical thinking in nursing* (2nd ed.). Norwalk, CT: Appleton & Lange.

Bauwens, E. E., & Gerhard, G. G. (1987). The use of the Watson-Glaser Critical Thinking Appraisal to predict success in a baccalaureate nursing program. *Journal of Nursing Education, 26*, 278–281.

Beeken, J. E. (1997). The relationship between critical thinking and self-concept in staff nurses and the influence of these characteristics on nursing practice. *Journal of Nursing Staff Development, 13*, 272–278.

Beeken, J. E., Dale, M. L., Enos, M. F., & Yarbrough, S. (1997). Teaching critical thinking skills to undergraduate nursing students. *Nurse Educator, 22*(3), 37–39.

Bell, M. L., Heye, M. L., Campion, L., & Hendricks, P. B. (2002). Evaluation of a process-focused learning strategy to promote critical thinking. *Journal of Nursing Education, 41*, 175–179.

Benner, P. (1984). *From novice to expert: Excellence and power in clinical nursing practice.* Menlo Park, CA: Addison-Wesley.

Brock, A., & Butts, J. B. (1998). On target: A model to teach baccalaureate nursing students to apply critical thinking. *Nursing Forum, 33*(3), 5–10.

Brooks, K., & Shepherd, J. (1992). Professionalism versus general critical thinking abilities of senior nursing students in four types of nursing curricula. *Journal of Professional Nursing, 8*, 87–95.

Brunt, B. A. (2005). Critical thinking in nursing: An integrated review. *Journal of Continuing Education in Nursing, 36*(2), 60–67.

Bulechek, G. M., & McCloskey, J. D. (1987). Nursing interventions: What they are and how to choose them. *Holistic Nursing Practice, 3*(3), 38.

Callister, L. C. (1996). Maternal interviews: A teaching strategy fostering critical thinking. *Journal of Nursing Education, 35*, 29–30.

Carpenito, L. (2005). *Nursing diagnosis: Application to clinical practice* (11th ed.). Philadelphia: Lippincott, Williams & Wilkins.

Carpenito, L. (2008). *Nursing diagnosis: Application to clinical practice* (12th ed.). Philadelphia: Lippincott, Williams & Wilkins.

Christensen, P. J., & Kenney, J. W. (1995). *Nursing process: Application of conceptual models* (4th ed.). St. Louis: Mosby.

Colucciello, M. L. (1999). Relationships between critical thinking dispositions and learning styles. *Journal of Professional Nursing, 15*, 294–301.

Conger, M. M., & Mezza, I. (1996). Fostering critical thinking in nursing students in the clinical setting. *Nurse Educator, 21*, 11–15.

Daley, B. J., Shaw, C. R., Balistrieri, T., Glasenapp, K., & Piacentine, L. (1999). Concept maps: A strategy to teach and evaluate critical thinking. *Journal of Nursing Education, 38*, 42–47.

Daly, W. M. (1998). Critical thinking as an outcome of nursing education. What is it? Why is it important to nursing practice? *Journal of Advanced Nursing, 28*, 323–331.

del Bueno, D. (2005). A crisis in critical thinking. *Nursing Education Perspectives, 26*(5), 278–282.

Dexter, P., Applegate, M., Backer, J., Claytor, K., Keffer, J., Norton, B., & Ross, B. (1997). A proposed framework for teaching and evaluating critical thinking in nursing. *Journal of Professional Nursing, 13*, 160–167.

Duchscher, J. E.B. (1999). Catching the wave: Understanding the concept of critical thinking. *Journal of Advanced Nursing, 29*, 577–583.

Edelman, C. L., & Mandle, C. L. (1994). *Health promotion throughout the lifespan.* St. Louis: Mosby.

Eerden, K. V. (2001). Using critical thinking vignettes to evaluate students' learning. *Nursing and Health Care Perspectives, 22*, 231–234.

Ennis, R. H. (1987). Critical thinking and the curriculum. In M. Heiman, & J. Slomianko (Eds.), *Thinking skills instruction: Concepts and techniques.* Washington, DC: National Education Association.

Ennis, R. H. (1989). Critical thinking and subject specificity: Clarification and needed research. *Educational Researcher, 18*, 4–10.

Facione, P. A. (1990). Critical thinking: A statement of expert consensus for purposes of educational assessment and instruction (executive summary). In *The Delphi Report* (pp. 1–19). Millbrae, CA: California Academic Press.

Facione, N. C., & Facione, P. A. (1996). Externalizing the critical thinking in knowledge development and clinical judgment. *Nursing Outlook, 44*, 129–136.

Facione, N. C., Facione, P. A., & Sanchez, C. A. (1994). Critical thinking disposition as a measure of competent clinical judgment: The development of the California Critical Thinking Disposition Inventory. *Journal of Nursing Education, 33*, 345–350.

Facione, P. A., Sanchez, C. A., Facione, N. C., & Gainen, J. (1995). The disposition toward critical thinking. *The Journal of General Education, 44*(1), 1–25.

Fero, L. J., Witsberger, C. M., Wesmiller, S. W., Zullo, T., & Hoffman, L. A. (2008). Critical thinking ability of new graduate and experienced nurses. *Journal of Advanced Nursing, 65*(1), 139–148.

Feingold, C., & Perlich, L. J. (1999). Teaching critical thinking through health-promotion contract. *Nurse Educator, 24*(4), 42–44.

Ford, J. S., & Profetto-McGrath, J. (1994). A model for critical thinking within the context of curriculum as praxis. *Journal of Nursing Education, 33,* 341–344.

Frederickson, K., & Mayer, G. G. (1977). Problem solving skills: What effect does education have? *American Journal of Nursing, 77,* 1167–1169.

Frye, B., Alfred, N., & Campbell, N. (1999). Use of the Watson-Glaser Critical Thinking Appraisal with BSN students. *Nursing and Health Care Perspectives, 20,* 253–255.

Hall, L. (1955). Quality of nursing care. In *Public health news .* New Jersey State Department of Health.

Howenstein, M. A., Bilodeau, K., Brogna, M. J., & Good, G. (1996). Factors associated with critical thinking among nurses. *Journal of Continuing Education in Nursing, 27*(3), 100–103.

Huckabay, L. A. (2009). Clinical reasoned judgment and the nursing process. *Nursing Forum, 44*(2), 72–78.

Jones, S. A., & Brown, L. N. (1993). Alternative views on defining critical thinking through the nursing process. *Holistic Nurse Practitioner, 7,* 71–76.

Kataoka-Yahiro, M., & Saylor, C. (1994). A critical thinking model for nursing judgment. *Journal of Nursing Education, 33,* 351–356.

Kelly, E. (1997). Development of strategies to identify the learning needs of baccalaureate students. *Journal of Nursing Education, 36,* 156–162.

Kintgen-Andrews, J. (1988). Development of critical thinking: Career ladder PN and AD nursing students, pre-health science freshmen, generic baccalaureate sophomore nursing students. Resources in Education, 24(1), (ERIC Document Reproduction Service No. 297 153).

Kintgen-Andrews, J. (1991). Critical thinking and nursing education: Perplexities and insights. *Journal of Nursing Education, 30,* 152–157.

Mastrian, K. G., & McGonigle, D. (1999). Using technology assignments to promote critical thinking. *Nurse Educator, 24,* 45–47.

Matthews, C. A., & Gaul, A. L. (1979). Nursing diagnosis from the perspective of concept attainment and critical thinking. *Advances in Nursing Science, 2*(11), 17–26.

May, B. A., Edell, V., Butell, S., Doughty, J., & Langford, C. (1999). Critical thinking and clinical competence: A study of their relationship in BSN seniors. *Journal of Nursing Education, 38,* 100–110.

Maynard, C. A. (1996). Relationship of critical thinking ability to professional nursing competence. *Journal of Nursing Education, 35,* 12–18.

McCarthy, P., Schuster, P., Zehr, P., & McDougal, D. (1999). Research briefs: Evaluation of critical thinking in a baccalaureate program. Are there differences between sophomore and senior students. *Journal of Nursing Education, 38,* 142–144.

McPeck, J. E. (1990). *Teaching critical thinking.* New York: Routledge.

Meyers, C. (1991). *Teaching students to think critically.* San Francisco: Jossey-Bass.

Miller, M., & Malcolm, N. (1990). Critical thinking in the nursing curriculum. *Nursing and Health Care, 11*(2), 67–73.

Miller, M. A. (1992). Outcomes evaluation: Measuring critical thinking. *Journal of Advanced Nursing, 17,* 1401–1407.

Pardue, S. F. (1987). Decision-making skills and critical thinking ability among associate degree, diploma, baccalaureate, and master's prepared nurses. *Journal of Nursing Education, 26,* 354–361.

Paul, R. (1992). *Critical thinking: What every person needs to survive in a rapidly changing world.* Santa Rosa, CA: Foundation for Critical Thinking.

Paul, R. (1993). The art of redesigning instruction. In J. Willsen, & A. J.A. Binker (Eds.), *Critical thinking: How to prepare students for a rapidly changing world* (pp. 319). Santa Rosa, CA: Foundation for Critical Thinking.

Paul, R., & Elder, L. (1999). *The miniature guide to critical thinking concepts and tools.* Dillon Beach, CA: Foundation for Critical Thinking.

Paul, R., & Heaslip, P. (1995). Critical thinking and intuitive nursing practice. *Journal of Advanced Nursing, 22,* 40–47.

Perciful, E. G., & Nester, P. A. (1996). The effect of an innovative clinical teaching method on nursing students' knowledge and critical thinking skills. *Journal of Nursing Education, 35*(1), 23–28.

Rane-Szostack, D., & Robertson, J. F. (1996). Issues in measuring critical thinking: Meeting the challenge. *Journal of Nursing Education, 35*(1), 5–11.

Rossignol, M. (1997). Relationship between selected discourse strategies and student critical thinking: The clinical post-conference. *Journal of Nursing Education, 36,* 467–475.

Saucier, B. L., Stevens, K. R., & Williams, G. B. (2000). Critical thinking outcomes of computer-assisted instruction versus written nursing process. *Nursing and Health Care Perspectives, 21,* 240–246.

Scheffer, B., & Rubenfeld, G. (2000). A consensus statement on critical thinking in nursing. *Journal of Nursing Education, 39,* 352–359.

Schumacher, J., & Severson, A. (1996). Building bridges for future practice: An innovative approach to foster critical thinking. *Journal of Nursing Education, 35,* 31–33.

Scoloveno, M. (1981). Problem solving ability of senior nursing students in three program types. *Dissertation Abstracts International, 41,* 1396B.

Sedlak, C. A., & Doheny, M. O. (1998). Peer review through clinical rounds: A collaborative critical thinking strategy. *Nurse Educator, 23*(5), 42–45.

Stewart, S., & Dempsey, L. F. (2005). A longitudinal study of baccalaureate nursing students' critical thinking disposition. *Journal of Nursing Education, 44*(2), 81–84.

Sullivan, E. J. (1987). Critical thinking, creativity, clinical performance, and achievement in RN students. *Nurse Educator, 12*(2), 12–16.

Turner, P. (2005). Critical thinking in nursing education and practice as defined in the literature. *Nursing Education Perspectives, 26*(5), 272–277.

U.S. Department of Education (1995). *National assessment of college student learning: Identifying college graduates' essential skills in writing, speech and listening, and critical thinking.* Washington, DC: U.S. Government Printing Office.

Vaughan-Wrobel, B. C., O'Sullivan, P., & Smith, L. (1997). Evaluating critical thinking skills of baccalaureate nursing students. *Journal of Nursing Education, 36,* 485–488.

Wade, G. H. (1999). Using the case method to develop critical thinking skills for the care of high-risk families. *Journal of Family Nursing, 5*(1), 92–109.

Watson, G., & Glaser, E. M. (1964). *Critical thinking appraisal.* Orlando, FL: Harcourt Brace Jovanovich.

Wilkinson, J. M. (1996). *Nursing process: A critical thinking approach* (2nd ed.). Menlo Park, CA: Addison-Wesley Nursing.

Yura, H., & Walsh, M. B. (1988). *The nursing process: Assessing, planning, implementing, evaluating* (5th ed.). Norwalk, CT: Appleton & Lange.

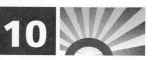

10

Challenges in Teaching and Learning

TAMI H. WYATT, PhD, RN, CNE

The author acknowledges the important foundational work for this chapter developed by Dr. Joan Creasia in the previous edition of this book.

OBJECTIVES

At the completion of this chapter, the reader will be able to:

- Compare and contrast major teaching-learning theories
- Discuss the principles and practices of effective teaching-learning experiences.
- Discuss the role of technology in teaching and learning.
- Design teaching-learning experiences for both individuals and groups.

PROFILE IN PRACTICE

Patricia Biller Krauskopf, PhD, RN, FNP-BC
Associate Professor, Family Nurse Practitioner Coordinator Shenandoah University, Winchester, Virginia

Cutting-edge technology is essential in health care delivery, and consequently, nursing education must keep up the pace. In busy outpatient practices, where the primary care goal is improved clinical outcomes and streamlined visits, innovations that enhance clinical decision making and fast-track care provision are essential and welcomed. As a family nurse practitioner with over 20 years in clinical practice, I recognize the need for technology that supports practice. Early on, I was enamored with personal digital assistants (PDAs) and felt certain they would be a valuable resource for health care practitioners' clinical practice. However, evidence to support how PDAs improve accuracy and efficiency of practice was absent.

My earliest research, "Accuracy and Efficiency as Outcomes of Clinical Scenarios by Novice Nurse Practitioners Using Personal Digital Assistants," found significant outcomes that helped to validate the use of PDAs in clinical practice. The purpose of this study was to determine whether using PDAs, as compared with textbooks, for the evaluation of clinical scenarios increased accuracy and efficiency of clinical decisions made by novice nurse practitioners. The sample consisted of 40 subjects, and the study examined novice nurse practitioners' efficiency when making decisions regarding laboratory values, diagnosis, and treatment. This study demonstrated that in all of these areas, the PDA users were more efficient in determining an answer to a clinical question and with a level of accuracy that was at least equal to the textbook users. I routinely use a PDA with drug database applications, medical calculators, and other time-saving resources to quickly locate information during patient visits in the clinical setting.

As a faculty member engaged in the teaching of nurse practitioner students, I am an advocate for the use of technology, not only in clinical practice but also in the classroom and via the Internet to aid student learning. Web-enhanced courses through the use of courseware management systems, such as BlackBoard Learning System, allow students access to all course syllabi, information, class materials, and each other through forums, emails, and chats. This is a valuable component when completing course assignments or preparing for classroom discussions. Another way to enhance classroom teaching is through the use of iPod technology to review podcasts of course lectures and presentations.

More recently, my students and I were involved in a research study with the University of Tennessee at Knoxville, evaluating the effectiveness of mobile e-learning among NP students within a multisite environment. All students used PDAs with Skype to communicate with their counterparts in all universities to complete specific assignments. Skype, a free voice-over-Internet protocol application, was found to be useful as a communication tool when costly or inaccessible alternative methods were not available. For example, Skype would be valuable to support global learning and support cost-effective communication between international students.

I fully expect that as technology evolves, it will continue to be at the cutting edge of practice and education. In the future we will be using applications that presently we can only imagine. Keeping up with these advancements is the challenge we all undertake.

Introduction

It can be said that those who practice nursing are not only nurses, but also teachers and students. Nurses engage in teaching and learning while studying to become nurses, in their everyday practice, and as they further their professional development. Clearly, readers of this text are experiencing some form of teaching and learning either through formal (course-required readings) or informal (professional development) methods of learning. Furthermore, readers either have already taught patients and colleagues or they will in the very near future. Most readers have encountered patient-teaching situations similar to the following:

- A 16-year-old female inquires about the "morning-after pill" after reporting she might be pregnant because she has felt nauseous every morning for 2 weeks.
- A 50-year-old wife accompanies her husband to the doctor. She states, "He won't take aspirin for his heart because it upsets his stomach, and he thinks it will make him bleed internally. Is this true?"

- The mother of a 2-year-old boy recently diagnosed with insulin-dependent juvenile diabetes states, "There is no way I will be able to give him shots. I faint at the site of blood."
- A 54-year-old man newly diagnosed with hyperlipidemia states, "I don't know how this happened; no one in my family has high cholesterol."

Few nurses have had formal preparation or coursework in teaching and learning, but recognition of the importance of this knowledge for nurses is growing. Nursing programs are integrating teaching and learning content into their curricula, which might very well be the reason you are reading this chapter. Whether you are a hospital nurse, an educator, an administrator, or a student, it is necessary to have basic knowledge of the teaching-learning process and the ways that technology influences teaching, learning, and information seeking. This chapter reviews the more commonly used learning theories in health education, discusses the ways technology influences teaching and learning practices, and presents effective teaching-learning practices with relevant supporting research, including similarities and differences between individual and group teaching-learning experiences.

Teaching and Learning Theories

Most commonly and simply stated, *teaching* is defined as the act or process of imparting knowledge (Merriam-Webster, 2009). This definition implies that those who teach present information and those who learn passively accept the knowledge. However, *learning* represents a change in meaning for the learner that is based on previous meaningful experiences. More than 200 teaching and learning theories exist, and numerous Internet sites provide information about these theories (e.g., http://tip.psychology.org). Although it is unrealistic to review all of the theories in this chapter, this section will compare and contrast several viewpoints and reflect on the comparisons by presenting learning principles and teaching

applications for each of the following theory viewpoints: behaviorism, cognitivism, change, and humanism. This chapter will reference the classical works of theorists to allow the reader the opportunity to explore teaching and learning principles in more depth.

BEHAVIORIST THEORIES

Teaching based on a behaviorist model, known as *behaviorism* or *instructivism,* presents objectives and content in a stepwise progression from basic to complex information with minimal learner engagement in the experience. Many of the assumptions of behaviorist models are built on the classic work of Thorndike (1913), Pavlov (1927), Skinner (1953), and Wolpe and Lazarus (1966), as well as some of Bruner's earliest writings (1966). Table 10-1 summarizes certain learning principles and teaching applications relative to the ideas of behaviorist learning and cognition theorists such as Piaget, Vygotsky, Bruner, and Dewey (Russell, 2002).

TABLE 10-1	Learning Principles and Teaching Applications Relative to Behaviorist Theory
MAJOR THEORIES AND THEORISTS Connectionism—Thorndike (1913) Stimulus-response—Pavlov (1927) Operant conditioning—Skinner (1953) Stimulus substitution—Wolpe & Lazarus (1966) Modeling—Bruner (1966)	
Learning Principle	**Teaching Application**
Human beings learn through trial and error.	Provide opportunity for problem solving.
Learning develops over time.	Provide adequate practice time; plan retesting or repeat demonstrations both immediately and at later intervals.
Given a stimulus, the learner responds.	Plan teaching strategies to trigger desired response; avoid unnecessary information that may detract from desired response.
Positive and negative feedback influence learning; positive feedback is remembered longer.	Reward learner for all correct behavior; praising positive behavior is better than punishing mistakes.
Learning is strengthened each time a positive response is received or a negative consequence is avoided.	Continue praise and positive reinforcement throughout the teaching transaction.
Learning occurs through linking behavior with an associated response.	Proceed from simple to complex; provide information to show that learning is occurring.
Learning remains until other learning interferes with original learned response.	Assess prior experience with subject; some "unlearning" may be needed before new learning can take place.

COGNITIVE THEORIES

As more scientists focused on teaching and learning, behaviorist theories and their assumptions evolved from teacher focused to learner focused. Theorists such as Piaget (1954), Lewin (1951), Gagne (1974), Bloom (1956), and Johnson, Johnson, and Stanne (2000) examined cognition and the ways that learners process information. By the mid-20th century, a new method of teaching and learning, known as *constructivism,* appeared in the literature (Bruner, 1966). This method of teaching and learning proposes that learners construct new ideas based on previous knowledge and experiences. Today, many cognitive and behavioral psychologists support this view, which asserts that learners engage or become active in the learning process instead of passively receiving information. In this view, learners actively seek information, problem-solve, collaborate with others, and apply information to realistic problems. Most cognitive and learning experts believe that active learning is superior to passive learning. A summary of cognitive theory and applications is presented in Table 10-2 .

CHANGE THEORIES

The more common teaching-learning methods used by nurses while teaching patients require strategies that empower the patient to exercise healthy behaviors that do not conflict with the patient's value system. The themes of patient empowerment and patient value systems are based on change models and concepts such as Rosenstock's health belief model (1974), Bandura's concept of self-efficacy (1977), Rotter's locus of control (1990), Festinger's cognitive dissonance theory (1957), and stages of readiness described by Prochaska and DiClemente, (1982). A summary of learning principles and teaching applications based on change theories are presented in Table 10-3 .

HUMANISTIC THEORIES

In humanistic theory, learning is self-motivated, self-directed, and self-evaluated. The teacher provides information and support to help learners increase their cognitive and affective functioning. Humanistic theories are the oldest classic theories and include

TABLE 10-2	Learning Principles and Teaching Applications Relative to Cognitive Theory
MAJOR THEORIES AND THEORISTS	
Cognitive discovery—Piaget (1954)	
Field theory—Lewin (1951)	
Information processing theory—Gagne (1974)	
Hierarchal structure—Bloom (1956)	
Cooperative learning theory—Johnson, Johnson, & Stanne (2000)	
Learning Principle	**Teaching Application**
Learning is based on a change in perception.	All learning cannot be readily observed; information must be internalized.
Perceptions are influenced by the senses.	Use multisensory teaching strategies; adjust environment to minimize distractions.
Perception depends on learning and is influenced by both internal and external variables.	Assess attitude toward learning, past experiences with similar situations, culture, maturity, developmental level, and physical ability before designing teaching plan.
Personal characteristics have an impact on how a cue is perceived.	Identify learning style and target it in the teaching process; develop a flexible approach.
Perceptions are selectively chosen to be focused on by the individual.	Focus learner on what is to be learned; provide support and guidance.

TABLE 10-3	Learning Principles and Teaching Applications Relative to Change Theory

MAJOR THEORIES AND THEORISTS
Health belief model—Rosenstock (1974)
Social cognitive theory—Bandura (1977)
Locus of control models—Rotter (1990)
Cognitive dissonance theory—Festinger (1957)
Transtheoretical model of behavior change—Prochaska & DiClemente (1982)

Learning Principle	Teaching Application
Learning occurs with motivation.	Provide incentives.
Motivation may be internal or external.	Set goals and expectations that match motivators.
Learning occurs with improved self-efficacy.	Use repetition, reward, reinforcement.
Learning occurs if relevant to learner needs.	Assist learners in identifying their own risks.

TABLE 10-4	Learning Principles and Teaching Applications Relative to Humanistic Theories

MAJOR THEORIES AND THEORISTS
Self-directed learning—Rogers (1969)
Hierarchy of needs—Maslow (1970)
Perceptual-existential theory—Combs (1965)
Values clarification—Dewey (1938)
Reality theory—Glasser (1965)
Andragogy—Knowles (1980)

Learning Principle	Teaching Application
Learning is self-initiated.	Promote self-directed learning.
Learning is an active participant in teaching-learning transaction.	Serve as a facilitator, mentor, and resource for learner to encourage active learning.
Learning should promote development of insight, judgment, values, and self-concept.	Avoid imposing own values and views on learner; support development of learner's self-concept.
Learning proceeds best if it is relevant to learner.	Expose learner to new, necessary information; pose relevant questions to encourage learner to seek answers.

andragogy or adult-centered learning (Knowles, 1984), hierarchy of needs (Maslow, 1970), self-directed learning (Rogers, 1969), reality theory of self-awareness learning (Glasser, 1965), perceptual-existential theory or self-determined learning (Combs, 1965), and values clarification learning (Dewey, 1938).

Teachers who use humanistic theories will encourage learners to set their own goals and work toward them. For example, a nurse might ask a client with diabetes, "When do you think you'll be ready to give your own insulin injection? What activities or steps would help you get ready to do this?" Table 10-4 summarizes teaching applications and learning principles relative to humanistic theories.

Chances are that as a nurse, you have or will use a combination of the above theories in teaching and learning, depending on the type of instruction, the learner, and the desired outcome. Regardless of the theoretical approach of the teaching-learning process, all effective instruction is based on fundamental principles that include matching the instruction with the type of learning that is required and developing a sense of mutuality and trust between teacher and learner.

Teaching and Learning Principles

Teaching and learning can be formal or informal in nature. Formal teaching-learning is planned instruction with objectives or goals that match the intended learned skills or concepts with the most effective method of delivery. According to the classic cone of learning theory by Edgar Dale (1969), learners remember:

- 10% of what they read
- 20% of what they hear
- 30% of what they see
- 50% of what they see and hear
- 60% of what they write
- 70% of what they discuss
- 80% of what they experience
- 95% of what they teach

Although reading and listening to information may be the most ineffective method of learning, it is often the most appropriate method, especially if the information or content is abstract in nature and requires few or no motor skills. On the other hand, content that requires motor skills are best learned by actively engaging in the learning such as experiential learning, simulations, or role play (Dale, 1969). Regardless of the level of learning required, the more an individual engages in the content, the more likely the person is to learn the material. Learners, whether they are patients, family care givers, or colleagues, learn best by teaching the information to someone else. Table 10-5 provides examples of types and levels of learning and matching strategies based on Dale's cone of experience theory.

Informal ways of learning are also effective. Informal learning results from interactions with others through networking, coaching, and mentoring. Learning that occurs in groups or from interactions with others, known as *collaborative* or *cooperative learning,* engages the learner in the information (Johnson et al., 2000; Walker & Elberson, 2005). Furthermore, learners who participate in their own learning are able to attach purposeful meaning to the content based on previous experiences. Perhaps this is one reason why the most successful learning often takes place in groups, such as weight loss groups, grief support groups, and parenting groups, where individuals help one another and the teacher is seen more as a guide or a facilitator.

Self-directed learning may also be another form of informal learning. Incidental learning consists of learning from mistakes, assumptions, beliefs, attributions, and internalized meanings and is often a byproduct of another activity. With more and more learners turning to the Internet for information or to complete formal online coursework, emphasis on ways to enhance self-directed learning has increased. Although self-directed learning may be incidental, it can also be purposeful when combined with tutorials, access to resources, and guided lessons.

TRANSFER OF KNOWLEDGE

The key to successful learning is determining how important the information is to the learner's ability to function effectively in his or her daily life and world. The more the learning environment resembles the actual environment, the more likely learning will be applied (Knowles, 1980). Learning transfer can be enhanced by focusing on behavior rather than

TABLE 10-5	Teaching and Learning Based on Dale's Cone of Experience Theory (1969)	
Information/Skill	**Level of Learning**	**Teaching-Learning Strategy**
Insulin injections	Concrete motor skill	Simulation, demonstration
Heart-healthy diet	Cognitive skill	Audiovisual or media, pictures, or audio only
Medical vocabulary terms	Abstract information	Text, reference materials

knowledge, setting realistic expectations, and establishing rewards. Behavior, however, is not changed by knowledge alone. To influence behavior, a learner must not only have knowledge of the desired behavior but also believe that he or she is able to perform or adopt the new information (self-efficacy) and must value or desire (attitude) the behavior (Bandura, 1977). Factors that inhibit transfer of learning include, but are not limited to, readiness to learn, anxiety level, environmental factors, stress levels, complexity of the content or tasks, ability to learn, and emotional readiness (Bastable, 2006).

MUTUALITY AND TRUST

The most successful teaching-learning experiences involve a process in which an interpersonal relationship of shared mutuality and trust is established between the teacher and the learner. This relationship might be instructor to student nurse, nurse to nurse, or nurse to patient. In such a relationship, the teacher is viewed as the knowledge and information expert, and the learner is seen not only as the individual in need of information and support, but also as the expert on how the information is best suited to his or her life. The emphasis is on the learner actively engaging, discovering, and taking responsibility for new ways of acting and problem solving. Mutuality and trust is prevalent in nurse and patient relationships because the nurse is often considered the expert on health matters and the patient is the information seeker.

Characteristics of Effective Teachers

Most of us teach the way we were taught, imitating the behaviors of the best teachers we have known and minimizing behaviors of those teachers we did not like. To be an effective teacher, however, requires that we develop a sound educational theory and research base, learn the specifics of the teacher-learner roles, find new ways of interrelating, and continually explore new teaching methods that we might use in our various roles (as a nurse, teacher, or peer). In addition, we must be able to critique our own performance and be willing to accept constructive criticism from others.

Many lessons can be learned from classroom teachers, but sometimes learning that occurs in a classroom involves nothing more than obtaining information on a topic. Nurses engaged in patient education often require more advanced teaching skills because patients may need not only to gain information but also to change their health behaviors. Sometimes nurses practice paternalism—that is, they overextend their power of authority over the patient. This method is ineffective; instead, nurses should practice a shared decision-making model with patients.

Regardless of the type of learning required, all teaching should be tailored to be appropriate to the learner's age, culture, and native language. This is a challenge for nurses who must teach complex medical processes to the lay public; however, numerous websites provide information and learning materials for various populations. For example, EthnoMed (http://ethnomed.org/ethnomed) is a site dedicated to providing material and information for culturally diverse populations. In addition, the National Network of Libraries of Medicine (http://nnlm.gov/outreach/consumer/multi.html) houses patient information in more than 12 different languages. With all educational material, but especially web-based information, nurses must ensure accuracy and reliability of the information obtained.

Characteristics of Effective Learners

The process of learning often requires engaging in a relationship with a teacher, a nurse, or another person with knowledge. At other times, learners must manage their own learning (self-directed learning), which requires self-discipline in completing assignments. Either way, learners must be motivated or accountable for retrieving or receiving information to gain the desired or required knowledge.

Learners are motivated for different reasons. For some, knowledge is necessary to remain healthy, whereas other learners may seek knowledge for professional opportunities or for enjoyment. The motivation for learning can be powerful and should be harnessed to enhance learning. For example, a man who needs to learn how to use an inhaler is generally quite motivated because without it, he has trouble breathing. On the other hand, some learners are less interested in learning if they perceive that gaining knowledge or changing behavior is less important than some other factor. For example, a 46-year-old woman has learned that as a result of being overweight, along with other factors, she has developed hypertension. As part of her treatment regimen, she has been prescribed hypertensive medications and instructed to lose 20 pounds. Unless she perceives that her weight is a true cause of the hypertension, she is not likely to change her eating and exercise behaviors—especially if she experiences positive results with the hypertensive medication alone.

Learners must understand their own motivating factors for seeking knowledge and use those factors to enhance learning. Furthermore, learners are most effective when they understand their own ways of learning, what works best, and how they might engage in activities to promote the best learning outcomes.

LEARNING STYLES AND PREFERENCES

All individuals have experienced some form of teaching and learning; therefore, it is likely that most learners can identify their own best method for learning. Each learner has a unique way of processing information, and the various delivery methods can either enhance or distract from the learning that takes place. For this reason, teachers must be aware of the learning styles of learners so that appropriate strategies can be used to promote learning. The classifications of learning styles are dependent on the type of learning inventory that one completes and the source that is used to determine the learning style. Many scientists have examined learning styles, which has lead to numerous classifications of learning styles. Nonetheless, three domains of learning have come to be considered essential: visual, auditory, and tactile/kinesthetic. These three domains may be combined and then aligned with styles of learning based on individual preferences. You can determine your own learning style by taking a free online learning style survey (http://metamath.com/lsweb/dvclearn.htm).

Learning strategies for individual styles are also provided on this website.

Working with individuals with various learning styles or assuming responsibility for your own learning will lead to more successful outcomes if you consider the following basic principles in relation to learning styles (Bastable, 2006):

1. Knowledge of the style of the teacher and the style of the recipient offers clues about the way one learns, and learning activities can be adjusted accordingly.
2. Nurses functioning in the role of teacher should refrain from teaching exclusively by their own learning style. A full range of techniques are often necessary to deliver content, even when teaching to individuals with similar learning styles.
3. Teachers should help learners (even patients) to identify their own style of learning so that the best learning approach can be identified.
4. All learners should have the opportunity to learn through techniques that are best suited to their learning style. For example, individuals who are visual learners prefer videos, movies, or simulations.
5. All learners should be encouraged to explore their various learning preferences to seek out strategies that are most conducive to their learning.
6. Those functioning as teachers must have a "toolbox" full of resources, strategies, and techniques rather than relying on one source for delivering content. Often, learners will need remediation or review, which requires several different sources.

TECHNOLOGY INFLUENCES ON TEACHING AND LEARNING

Learners, whether students enrolled in formal coursework or everyday information seekers (e.g., health consumers), have access to information that until about 15 years ago was available only to a select few. With the advent of the World Wide Web, finding information is no longer the problem. Instead, paring down volumes of information and ensuring that the information is accurate and reliable is the challenge. Before the Internet, information was available through print, video, or word of mouth. Obtaining accurate information involved in-depth research, numerous phone calls, or interviews with reliable sources. In essence, experts served as the clearinghouses of information. If, for example, a patient needed information about his or her newly diagnosed disease, the physician or nurse gave information verbally, by phone, or by printed brochures available only at a health care facility. Internet-empowered information seekers are leading a revolution of informed consumers, including health care consumers. Armed with unprecedented access to health-related information via the Internet, today's health care consumer is demanding more involvement in his or her own care, as well as access to more choices about how health care is organized, delivered, and reimbursed. This development alone influences the teaching-learning methods that nurses must adopt while accessing information and teaching patients or other nurses (see Chapter 13).

INTERNET-SUPPORTED TEACHING AND LEARNING

Access to information via the Internet has become one of the most significant defining characteristics of the present *Information Age,* in which computers network with one another. In 2008, 73% of the 303,824,646 people in the United States accessed the Internet. That was an astounding 131% increase in Internet usage since 2000 (Internet & World Stats, 2009). Of those accessing the Internet, 8 in 10 users searched online for information on health topics including diet, fitness, drugs, health insurance, and experimental treatments (Fox, 2005). This increase in Internet use is due, in part, to more readily available access to computers and the Internet, the ever-increasing amount of information that can be obtained quickly, and the development of more online multimedia technologies. Teaching styles that use a variety of methods and audiovisual devices (e.g., information presented on the Internet) can enhance learning and attend to a variety of learning styles.

Because individuals rely on the Internet for information ranging from personal health to financial investments, it is crucial for learners to evaluate these resources. Currently, standards do not exist to ensure accuracy of online information. Essentially, anyone can publish anything on the Internet. Unlike traditional print resources, web resources rarely use editors or content experts. Multiple tools and criteria are available for evaluating websites, but there are key elements to guide learners in evaluating information on the Internet (Box 10-1).

Health on the Net (HON) is a foundation that guides Internet users to reliable and trustworthy

BOX 10-1	Evaluating Information on the Internet

Credibility
- Is it current? Or updated?
- Is there an editorial process?

Content
- Is it accurate?
- Is it complete?
- Is it error free?
- Is it a reliable source?
- Look for a header or footer showing affiliation.
- Look at the domain or site sponsor located after the "dot" in the address. For example: .edu = education, .gov = government, .org = organization, .com = commercial, .mil = military
- Look for a disclaimer.
- Does the author of the website have the education, expertise, or experience to be a trustworthy source?

Disclosure
- What is the purpose of the site?

Links
- Are they appropriate to the content being described?

Design
- Is it readable and appealing?
- Is it easy to navigate, and does it have a search function?

Interactivity
- Is there a mechanism for feedback?
- Are there listservs?
- Is there a contact source?

Caveats
- Are there advertisements?

sources of health information. HON is considered the gold standard for evaluating health-related web-based information. A website that displays the official HON seal has applied for and met HON criteria. HON has also developed a toolbar that automatically verifies the accreditation status of health-related websites (this toolbar can be downloaded at www.hon.ch).

By far, most individuals use the Internet as a self-directed learning tool to access information; however, the Internet is capable of supporting other teaching-learning methods. For example, the Internet connects networked computers so that the scope of learning extends beyond the physical walls of a learning institution or facility. Web conferencing, for example, connects individuals who are not physically located in the same place. This method of connecting individuals in real time by videostreaming is known as *synchronous learning*. Alternatively, *asynchronous learning* allows individuals to share information or ideas in delayed time. Examples of asynchronous learning are email correspondence, electronic bulletin boards, listservs, blogs, or information posted on websites. Both forms of learning have advantages and disadvantages. Overall, asynchronous learning does not promote live discussion, but it may be advantageous to learners who need additional time for processing information. It may also improve writing skills because all responses are text-based. Of course, it has been well documented that the greatest advantage of asynchronous learning is the scheduling flexibility for learners (Billings & Halstead, 2009). Because this form of learning does not take place in real time, a learner can choose to engage in the learning at a time that is convenient and fits his or her busy schedule.

Synchronous learning, on the other hand, engages the learner in the teaching-learning process at the same moment with the teacher and/or other learners. This method promotes collaborative or cooperative learning because information is processed with a group of learners. This real-time dialogue may be necessary for some learners or for comprehension of some forms of information. However, synchronous learning requires the use of robust and advanced technology by both the teacher and the learner. At a minimum, the learner and teacher must have broad bandwidth Internet access to support videos, audio, videostreaming, chat rooms, webcasts, or other synchronous methods.

INSTRUCTIONAL TECHNOLOGIES

The Internet has dramatically changed the ways information is obtained, but technology itself also influences teaching and learning. To offer effective teaching, whether with patients, colleagues, or children, nurses need to seek technology-rich and interactive learning environments that engage the learner. In fact, the generation of children and young adults who have been exposed to technology their entire lives—known as "Generation Y" (Internet generation)—learn best in environments that are rich in multimedia, moving and navigating freely through their experience (Mayer, 2001). The Pre-Y generation, those who remember a world without personal computers (PCs), typically process information in a sequential order similar to a book, but engage in the learning more readily when the information is interactive or presented in multiple mediums (multimedia). Technologies that support multimedia have changed how learners access information and how they interact with information, other learners, and the teacher. For example, collaborative learning (learning in teams, pairs, or small groups) to problem-solve (situated learning) is no longer limited to individuals who are physically located in the same room. With networked notebooks/laptops, handheld technology such as tablet PCs and personal digital assistants (PDA), or with a PC, groups can connect from around the world to learn and problem-solve together. The EDUCAUSE Center for Applied Research (ECAR) is investigating the ways that mobile technologies, such as handheld technology, enhance learners' educational experiences. Overall, the research suggests that mobile technology shows promise as a teaching-learning tool and will likely penetrate most formal education settings in the future (Wentzel, Lammeren, Molendijk, Bruin, & Wagtendonk, 2005).

Most recently, the Internet supports collaborative teaching-learning groups through IP telephony or voice-over-IP (VoIP). This technology allows individuals to talk to one another online. This method of collaboration is cost effective because there are several free applications to support VoIP and there are no additional costs to establish the voice connection (Federal Communication Commission, 2009). Clearly, the advantage of VoIP is to connect learners who, before networking capabilities, would have been difficult (if not impossible) to connect without extensive time commitments, travel, and expenses. Each member of the learning group brings unique experiences and perspectives to the situated learning environment, which promotes constructivist approaches to learning. Of course, there are associated disadvantages, including the technical support needed to connect learners via networked computers, the learning curve associated with using collaborative technologies, and the change in the way learners must communicate so that the technology does not interfere with their learning (pauses, delays in audio transmission, frequent disconnections).

Other more extensive web tools, known as Web 2.0 tools, are available for students and teachers. With technology advancements and more users of the Internet, some fascinating tools have emerged, many of which were never intended to be learning tools. Social networking, or tools designed to connect people, have evolved and become mainstream for Generation Y learners. These tools serve not only to connect individuals but also to share information and promote collaboration. For example, Facebook connects friends, friends of friends, and those with common interests. The tool supports photo and video sharing, live chat sessions, links, and notes. Other similar social networking and collaborative tools allow people or learners to share documents, files, and contact information and to set up live meetings using chat features or video applications. Nurses and other professionals may use these applications to connect with like-minded individuals or those with similar expertise. One such tool, LinkedIn, allows professionals to connect and share friends, resources, and contact information. Moodle, a free open-source collaborative tool, also supports networking but is slightly different because it is not secure and available to the public, which means that only individuals who are invited to the site may participate in networking. This application is most commonly used to support classrooms because it can be a secure site and it organizes and manages content.

Blogs and services such as Twitter also connect people with common interests; both allow document and image sharing, posting, and journaling. A blog or a "tweet" can be used to update learners about ongoing activities and store information for easy retrieval. These tools are often used to supplement professional conferences for those persons unable to attend but interested in learning more about the conference presentations and proceedings.

Social bookmarking is another type of Web 2.0 tool that allows individuals with similar interests to share their bookmarks, or favorite websites. Because the Internet lacks a clear organized structure, it is often difficult to find information or to retrace previous search steps. Bookmark sharing increases one's capacity to locate specific information. Bookmarks are shared when individuals post their bookmarks to a public server, rather than on their personal Internet browser. Individuals who subscribe to the same social bookmarking service then have access to one another's bookmarks. Many bookmarking services, some free, are available: SocialMarking (http://socialmar king.com), AddThis (http://addthis.com), and Delicious (http://delicious.com).

Video, film, audio equipment, software applications, interactive whiteboards, projection systems, and PCs are other forms of technology frequently used by teachers and learners to promote learning. Each technology is best suited for a particular form of learning and should be matched to the type of expected learning. In many cases, multiple forms of technology (multimedia) are used to support teaching and learning and are effective when matched with the appropriate level of learning. Caution, however, should be used when selecting the delivery method for instruction because selecting the wrong medium can distract the learner, making the instruction ineffective. This will be discussed in the next section.

Designing Teaching-Learning Plans

The effectiveness of a teaching-learning plan is limited to the teacher's knowledge and skill on the topic to be taught, as well as the teacher's knowledge about learning, teaching, and evaluation. Nurses, therefore, must have knowledge about teaching and learning. Developing a teaching-learning plan is similar to the nursing process and includes assessing the learner, developing learner objectives, selecting teaching-learning strategies, implementing the teaching plan, and evaluating outcomes.

ASSESSING THE LEARNER

There are some key elements that should be explored when assessing the learning needs of learners. These include (1) knowledge level, (2) developmental characteristics (e.g., age, reading ability), (3) preferred learning style, (4) motivation or readiness to learn, (5) anxiety level, (6) health values, and (7) health status. Many of these factors have already been discussed in this chapter. It is, however, necessary to gather information about these factors through questioning or interviewing. Susan Bastable, a well-known patient education expert, suggests that interviewing (or any form of communication with a patient) can be enhanced by beginning with short phrases (2006). This technique can apply to any type of learner, whether a patient, a student, or a peer. These short phrases are ice-breaker questions such as, "How was the traffic coming in today?" This strategy not only helps to develop rapport with the patient but also allows the nurse to assess the general well-being of the patient, such as discomfort or irritability. During the initial stages of the interviewing, teachers (nurses) should give patients a sense of what is about to occur, thereby developing trust and setting the stage for the educational experience. This map of what is to occur may be an outline of the material or simply a spoken phrase informing the patient of the information that will be reviewed.

ASSESSING SPECIAL GROUPS

Learners who are from an unfamiliar culture or who are challenged in some way often have complex and unique learning needs. Assessing the special characteristics of these learners will aid in identifying learning needs and choosing teaching strategies that are appropriate and effective.

Cultural Considerations. Nurses who are teaching to diverse populations must be sensitive to cultural traditions, taboos, and values that facilitate or interfere with the teaching-learning process. For example, in the Asian population it is important to "save face," and these learners may not indicate a lack of understanding or may be uncomfortable answering questions, especially those concerning bodily and sexual functioning. Because Africans respect authority figures, they may be reluctant to ask questions if the questions seem to challenge the teacher.

When a learner from an unfamiliar culture is being assessed, a systematic appraisal of his or her beliefs and values is essential. If the learner is a patient, then the nurse must gather information about the patient's cultural preferences and health care practices. Barriers to communication and preferred methods of learning must also be identified, because both may be culturally based. Several free web-based programs are available to assist in translating documents into different languages (e.g., http://babelfish.com). Such tools are useful as a beginning step in translating teaching materials. However, all documents translated in this manner should be checked by a native speaker to ensure cultural congruency.

Challenged Populations. It is critical for the teacher to carefully assess the learner's reading level and ability to understand the written word when printed materials are used for teaching. This assessment must respect the learner's dignity, because many people are embarrassed by their reading difficulties. For instance, a statement about forgetting one's reading glasses may indicate illiteracy. In this case, nurses should offer to read the content to the learner and attempt to find materials that illustrate the information. When developing or selecting reading materials, the nurse must ensure that the reading level is appropriate for the target audience. The reading level of printed materials can be determined by most word processing programs. Websites that evaluate readability and grade level of content are also available (http://juicystudio.com). As a general rule of thumb, experts recommend that all materials prepared for adults be written at a sixth-grade level (Badarudeen & Sabharwal, 2008).

Individuals who are visually or hearing impaired may require adapted educational materials. Reading materials in large print or audiotapes can be used with visually impaired learners, and sign language or closed-captioned videos can be used with those who are hearing impaired. Advances in technology offer many opportunities for visually impaired learners. Adaptive reading devices can translate websites so that the information these learners receive is as similar as possible to that accessed by learners who are not visually impaired. For those with language barriers, an interpreter may be needed. Individuals who have impaired mobility may require adaptations in the teaching plan to accommodate their level of functioning.

DEVELOPING LEARNER OBJECTIVES

It is sometimes difficult for new teachers to develop concise and measurable learner objectives. The purpose of learner objectives are (1) to communicate what the leaner is to know and do, (2) to guide the selection and use of teaching materials, and (3) to evaluate whether the learner actually learned what the teacher tried to teach. For example, "Today we will watch a video of patients giving themselves insulin injections (media), tomorrow we will practice preparing an insulin injection together (demonstration and return demonstration), and the next day you will have the opportunity to give your own insulin injection (evaluation)."

Bloom divided learning objectives into two categories: cognitive (Bloom, 1956) and affective (Krathwohl, Bloom, & Masia, 1964). Cognitive objectives are concerned with the learner's mastery of different levels of cognition along a continuum from simple to complex: (1) knowledge, (2) comprehension, (3) application, (4) analysis, (5) synthesis, and (6) evaluation. Below are examples of cognitive objectives:

- Lists correct signs and symptoms of health problem (knowledge)
- Describes relationship between exercise and weight loss (comprehension)
- Schedules 30 minutes of exercise three times weekly (application)
- Calculates amount of hidden fat in restaurant offerings before ordering (analysis)
- Prepares and cooks meals for self and family with more low-fat choices (synthesis)

- Revises exercise and dietary choices as needed (evaluation)

Affective objectives describe changes in the learner's interests, attitudes, appreciations, values, and emotional sets or biases. Levels of affective objectives include (1) receiving, (2) responding, (3) valuing, (4) organizing a value system, and (5) characterizing a value complex. Below are examples of affective objectives:

- Accepts that present weight is unhealthy (receiving)
- Shows willingness to comply with health belief of increased exercise to decrease weight (responding)
- Desires to attain optimal weight (valuing)
- Forms judgment about the responsibility of the individual for maintaining optimal weight (conceptualization of a value)
- Revises health beliefs about weight, diet, and exercise as new information becomes available (value complex)

Much more has been written about cognitive objectives than about affective objectives in the general educational and nursing literature. This may be due, in part, to the complexities of influencing affective domains of knowing. Present changes in society, the global economy, and health care would seem to indicate the need to pay as much, if not more, attention to the affective domain of learning.

The psychomotor domain of learning requires learners to perform motor skills, which is accomplished through practice to master the skills with precision, accuracy, and complete execution of the task. Psychomotor skills are most commonly associated with lab or clinical learning. Psychomotor skills are best learned by observing the skills of a more experienced person, imitating the behaviors in a controlled environment through practice, and adapting the skills to other situations.

The following are examples of psychomotor objectives:

- Demonstrates proper techniques for specified physical activity (demonstration)
- Illustrates documentation of physical activity in log sheet (application)
- Prepares a meal following the recommended healthy eating guidelines (synthesis)

SELECTING TEACHING-LEARNING STRATEGIES

Primary steps in effective teaching and learning are setting the climate and selecting appropriate strategies. Some obvious ways to facilitate a climate conducive to learning include attention to room size, temperature, noise level, seating arrangements, and availability of supplies. The degree of formality that sets the tone of the teaching-learning experience is also important. For example, teaching about dietary and activity recommendations to patients recovering from stroke may involve a more formal presentation. In contrast, a class for new parents on how to bathe a baby may be more informal and relaxed.

Cognitive capacity, psychosocial development, and physical maturation and abilities of the learner are important considerations when one is choosing a teaching strategy (Billings & Halstead, 2009). Selection of appropriate strategies is also influenced by cultural and environmental factors.

Questioning Techniques. Teacher questioning that enhances critical thinking has a positive impact on meeting learner needs. Two aspects of the teacher's questioning technique are important: phrasing the questions and probing the responses. Clearly phrased questions are stated simply, using words that are easily understood; they focus on the content and emphasize specific thinking skills. For example, "When you had your last asthma attack, were you near someone who was smoking?" or "How do you plan to increase your physical activity without jeopardizing your cardiac status?"

After a learner has responded, the teacher should follow up with probing questions to clarify exactly what the patient means (e.g., seeking a more exact description of pain intensity). Probing strategies include asking questions that increase awareness of potential motivations, refocusing the conversation when it begins to wander from the topic at hand, and inquiring about emotional reactions to the situation.

Lecture. In many situations a lecture format of teaching is used; this format is most appropriate when the learner needs basic knowledge on a topic before more advanced forms of learning can occur (Billings & Halstead, 2009). The lecture may be supplemented by written materials or more interactive learning techniques (Novotny & Griffin, 2006). For example, an experienced nurse who is mentoring a new RN might inquire (use questioning techniques) about the mentee's knowledge about blood gas analysis. If the new RN has minimal knowledge about blood gas analysis and interpretation, it will be necessary to review the basic information about oxygen and carbon dioxide before practicing blood gas analysis and interpretation. This teaching would most likely be presented in a lecture format because the information is fundamental to understanding how to analyze blood gas results. The learning could be enhanced for a tactile, or hands-on, learner if the lesson also included a demonstration of collecting a blood sample along with a return demonstration.

Demonstration. Frequently a learning situation involves a demonstration in which a teacher shows an individual or group how to perform a particular task. To facilitate a demonstration, prepare the materials before the audience gathers and analyze the steps ahead of time. Additional tips include:

1. Start the session on time.
2. Arrange the groups around you so that all can see.
3. Explain ahead of time what will happen and what to expect.
4. Demonstrate slowly and deliberately.
5. Explain each step.
6. Allow time for questions after each step.
7. Use humor to keep people alert.
8. End with a final summary and more questions.
9. Have the learners return the demonstration.

Group Discussions. A group discussion is a purposeful conversation and deliberation on a topic of mutual interest conducted under the guidance of the leader. Discussion enables participants to express opinions and to learn about topics of mutual interest. This technique provides maximum opportunity for the acceptance of personal responsibility for learning and sharing experiences and opinions with others. Focus groups are types of group discussions that are often used in research and to obtain information from the patient-consumer point of view.

Role-Playing and Case Studies. Case studies, or fictitious data regarding a situation, often guide role-playing activities. This technique requires that selected members of a learning group spontaneously act out specific roles. Role-playing is used to bring participants into the closer experience of feeling and reacting to a problem. It promotes understanding of one's own and others' feelings and viewpoints. Types of role-playing include the following:

1. Drama: Helps participants gain insight into other people or situations (plot, characters, and scenes are developed previously).
2. Exercise: Larger, more complex, and prolonged version of role-playing in which groups are interacting.
3. Psychodrama: Directed primarily at the therapeutic treatment of individuals.
4. Simulation games: Learners act out their understanding and insight in handling "live" problems or "critical incidents" using gaming techniques.

Choice of media can also enhance teaching and learning and may help determine the strategy selected for learning. Questions to ask in choosing and using media, as well as their individual differences and special considerations, are summarized in Table 10-6.

Evaluating the Teaching-Learning Experience

Evaluation consists of determining the worth of something. This process includes obtaining information for use in judging the worth of a program, product, procedure, or objective, or the potential utility of alternative approaches designed to attain specified objectives. In planning, designing, implementing, and validating teaching-learning experiences, knowledge of the theories and methods of evaluation is extremely important.

Three evaluation methods can be used concurrently in teaching and learning: formative, summative, and peer evaluation. *Formative evaluation* takes place while the teaching-learning experience is in progress. Its purpose is to identify needed changes in material, content, or teaching style in order to better meet overall program learning objectives (Billings & Halstead,

2009). *Summative evaluation* occurs near the end of a teaching-learning episode and may focus on learner satisfaction, the level of learner performance, the incidence of occurrences related to the subject area (e.g., fewer episodes of hyperglycemia secondary to testing blood glucose levels more frequently), improved self-care skills documented through a home visit, or satisfaction with a lifestyle change (e.g., change in diet or exercise documented through a follow-up phone call). Information from summative evaluations is used to judge the value of the present teaching-learning experience as compared with alternative methods of experiences.

Although learners are certainly important evaluators of teacher effectiveness, teachers should also be evaluated by peers, particularly if they are novices and are expected to grow and develop. *Peer evaluation* conducted by a colleague or an outside observer offers a different perspective on the effectiveness of the entire teaching-learning episode. An evaluation of this type requires an experienced teacher who can evaluate against more sophisticated criteria, such as selection and organization of content, utilization of the literature, evidence of learning needs assessment, ability to ask or answer difficult questions, and quality of teaching style.

Despite efforts to plan effective teaching and learning, learners may not learn or gain the desired outcome. According to Bastable (2006), barriers to learning may include any of the following: (1) lack of time to learn, (2) stress related to the need for learning or the circumstance that requires learning, (3) negative influences from the teaching-learning experience, (4) personal characteristics of the learner, (5) inappropriate level or amount of required learning, (6) lack of support, (7) denial that learning needs exist, and (8) the inconvenience and complexity of the information to be learned. In cases where barriers exist, it is helpful to identify the factors that impede learning and determine what methods of teaching will improve learning based on the barriers. This may require repeated efforts with a variety of methods. Engaging other family members, support individuals, or caretakers in the teaching-learning experience is appropriate and may be absolutely necessary in some cases.

TABLE 10-6	Choosing and Using Teaching-Learning Materials	
Media	**Advantages**	**Considerations**
Audiotapes	Useful for individuals and groups; involves auditory sense Economical, easy to prepare Can be used independently	Assess hearing with individuals, room size with groups
Books/pamphlets/printed materials	Useful for individuals; involves visual sense Easy to use Allows learner to self-pace Easy to reference	Assess reading ability and level of material Cost; must obtain permission to copy Texts go out of date rapidly
Computer applications	Allows self-pacing, multisensory involvement Sequential programs; can be used by all learner levels	Requires added time to learn computer use Expensive equipment Professional programming required
Internet websites	Appeals to visual and auditory learners if sites use multimedia to present material Interactive, multisensory Hyperlinks to additional resources Can support video, sounds, images, animation, and text	Limited to only users with Internet access Computer monitors not designed for paragraph reading; therefore limits information to list format Requires more development time
Films	Suitable for groups; involves sight, hearing Can stimulate emotions, build attitudes May be available from a public library Useful for compression of time and space	Does not permit self-pacing Difficult to produce Expensive to buy; allow time for order Requires special equipment
Flipcharts/chalkboards	Suitable for groups; involves sight Allows step-by-step sequence of material Inexpensive	Bulky to transport Teacher's back to audience while writing Not reusable
Models/real objects	Useful for individuals/small groups Multisensory involvement Permits demonstration and practice	May not be easy to obtain Can be costly Models often easily damaged
Posters/overheads	Useful for individuals/small groups; involves sight Easy to produce, inexpensive May be reused, easy to store	Requires viewing space and/or equipment Avoid crowding; consider color, size, and space For best appearance, have professionally developed
Slides/electronic slides	Suitable for large groups Inexpensive, easy to produce and duplicate Easy to add or subtract material	Requires expensive equipment to develop and to project slides once developed

☀ Future Trends in Teaching and Learning

Technology is changing the way we teach and learn. Future teaching-learning experiences will focus on information management, problem solving, decision making rather than memorization, and collaboration with teachers and learners through global access. Nurses and patients have access to devices that fit in the palms of their hands. These devices are not only promoting quick and easy access to information but also influencing the way health is managed. For example, applications are available on handheld devices (or PDAs) that allow patients with asthma or diabetes to store daily health logs and send the information via the Internet to their health care providers. These logs can also be accessed online on any computer for those who do not own handheld technology. Such technology allows teachers and students to connect with one another for sharing information, teaching, and learning; therefore teaching methods in the future will center on more experiential learning, such as interactive online simulations. Technologies that are currently available via handheld devices are also available through cellular phones that connect to the Internet using VoIP. This technology has endless potential because cellular phone technology is the fastest-growing market in the world.

At present, some teaching and learning occurs in virtual environments, whereby users become characters (known as *avatars*) acting in simulated settings such as emergency departments or operating rooms to learn skills and techniques. The most common virtual environment used in education is Second Life (learn more by visiting http://secondlife.com/whatis).

SUMMARY

This ongoing explosion of knowledge and emergence of major scientific developments means that nurses must become continuous lifelong learners who recognize the importance of how to think critically, how to accept the need to relearn, and how to deal with change. Teaching and learning remain essential aspects of the professional nurse's role. To effectively implement the teaching or learning role, the nurse must possess or acquire a thorough understanding of the teaching-learning process.

Furthermore, nurses must take into account variations in a learner's health status, risk factors, cultural considerations, and myriad other factors to develop effective teaching-learning experiences. The need to adapt teaching and learning to new practice environments and the ever-changing health values of the nation will continue to challenge the nursing profession.

KEY POINTS

- Behaviorist theories are based on the premise that learning occurs through a stimulus-response sequence, followed by consistent feedback.
- Cognitive theories propose that learning is related to an internal change in perception that is influenced by both internal and external variables.
- Change theories are based on strategies that empower patients to exercise healthy behaviors or health-managing behaviors that are not in conflict with the patient's value system.
- Humanistic theories state that learning is self-initiated and should promote the development of insight, judgment, values, and self-concept.
- Learners have different preferred styles of learning (ways in which they perform best). Awareness of the various learning styles influences the choice of teaching-learning strategies and can enhance learning.
- The Internet is dramatically changing the teaching-learning process because teachers and learners now have access to information that, just decades ago, was available only to a select few.
- Advancing technology is changing the way teachers deliver information and the way individuals learn information.
- The teaching-learning process parallels the steps of the nursing process—assessment, planning, implementation, and evaluation.
- Assessment of the learner is multifaceted and includes demographic, psychosocial, cultural, physical, behavioral, and cognitive factors.
- Planning the teaching-learning experience focuses on developing learner objectives and selecting appropriate teaching-learning strategies.
- For successful implementation of the teaching plan, the environment must be conducive to learning.
- Evaluation of the teaching-learning experience includes the level of achievement of learner objectives and the effectiveness of the teacher.
- Among the future trends in teaching and learning are a reliance on information management, the development of critical thinking and problem-solving skills, and a focus on experiential learning for the continuous lifelong learner.

CRITICAL THINKING EXERCISES

1. Evaluate the effectiveness of the teaching-learning process in your own area of clinical practice. What are the typical activities of the teacher and the expected outcomes of the learner? What evaluation methods are used to determine whether learning objectives are achieved? What changes would you make in the teaching-learning process to improve its effectiveness?

2. Select a learning theory and disease of your choice (e.g., behavioral theory and diabetes). Develop learning objectives in the cognitive and affective domains. What teaching strategies would be effective in achieving those objectives with an adolescent client and an older adult?

3. Select a disease in a specific population (e.g., asthma in children) and search the Internet for resources. Evaluate two websites based on evaluation criteria. Do the sites meet HON criteria? Explain.

4. Select a disease in a specific population (e.g., diabetes in adults) and search the Internet for tools that help patients manage their condition (e.g., health logs, daily journals). How can these tools be used?

5. Analyze teaching materials (e.g., care plans, pamphlets, audiovisuals) in use at your clinical facility for evidence of educational, gender, or cultural bias. Select two of these and describe the changes needed to make them culturally acceptable.

REFERENCES

Badarudeen, S., & Sabharwal., S. (2008). Readability of patient education materials from the American Academy of Orthopaedic Surgeons and Pediatric Orthopaedic Society of North American websites. *The Journal of Bone and Joint Surgery, 90*, 199–204.

Bandura, A. (1977). Self-efficacy: Toward a unifying theory of behavioral change. *Psychology Review, 84*, 191–215.

Bastable, S. B. (2006). *Essentials of patient education.* Sudbury, MA: Jones and Bartlett.

Billings, D. M., & Halstead, J. A. (2009). *Teaching in nursing: A guide for faculty* (3rd ed.). St. Louis: Saunders.

Bloom, B. (1956). Taxonomy of educational objectives: Handbook I. *Cognitive domain.* New York: Davis McKay.

Bruner, J. (1966). *Toward a theory of instruction.* Cambridge, MA: Harvard University.

Combs, A. (1965). *The professional education of teachers.* Boston: Allyn & Bacon.

Dale, E. (1969). *Audiovisual methods in teaching* (3rd ed.). New York: Holt-Dryden.

Dewey, J. (1938). *Experience and education.* New York: Macmillan.

Federal Communication Commission (2009). Voice over internet protocol. Retrieved March 28, 2009, from http://www.fcc.gov/voip

Festinger, L. (1957). *A theory of cognitive dissonance* (1st ed.). Stanford, CA: Stanford University Press.

Fox, S. (2005). Health information online. Pew Internet & American Life Project. Retrieved May 18, 2005, from http://www.pewinternet.org

Gagne, R. (1974). *Essentials of learning for instruction.* Hinsdale IL: Dryden.

Glasser, W. (1965). *Reality therapy.* New York: Harper & Row.

Internet and World Stats Internet usage statistics: The big picture. Retrieved March 26, 2009, from http://www.internetworldstats.com/stats.htm

Johnson, D. W., Johnson, R. T., & Stanne, M. B. (2000). Cooperative learning methods: A meta-analysis. Retrieved April 18, 2005, from http://www.co-operation.org/pages/cl-methods.html

Knowles, M. (1980). *The modern practice of adult education: From pedagogy to andragogy.* Chicago: IL: Follett.

Knowles, M. (1984). *The adult learner: A neglected species* (3rd ed.). Houston: Gulf.

Krathwohl, D. R., Bloom, B. S., & Masia, B. B. (1964). *Taxonomy of educational objectives: Handbook II. Affective domain.* New York, NY: David McKay.

Lewin, K. (1951). *Field theory in social science.* New York: Harper & Row.

Maslow, A. (1970). *Motivation and personality.* New York: Harper & Row.

Mayer, R. E. (2001). *Multimedia learning.* New York: Cambridge University Press.

Novotny, J. M., & Griffin, M. T. (2006). *A nuts and bolts approach to teaching nursing* (3rd ed.). New York: Springer.

Pavlov, I. (1927). *Conditioned reflexes.* (G.V. Anrep, Trans.). London: Oxford University Press.

Piaget, J. (1954). *The language and thought of the child* (3rd ed.). London: Routledge & Kegan Paul.

Prochaska, J. O., & DiClemente, C. C. (1982). Transtheoretical therapy toward a more integrative model of change. *Psychotherapy: Theory, Research, and Practice, 19*(3), 276–287.

Rogers, C. (1969). *Freedom to learn.* Columbus, OH: Merrill.

Rosenstock, I. (1974). Historical origins of the health belief model. *Health Education Monographs 2*(4), 324–473.

Rotter, J. B. (1990). Internal versus external control of reinforcement: A case history of a variable. *American Psychologist, 45*(4), 489–493.

Russell, G. (2002). Constructivist vs. behaviorist: A search for the "ideal learning environment." Retrieved May 10, 2005, from http://www.uca.edu/divisions/academic/coe/students/GR/portfolio1/Constructivist%20VS%20Behaviorist.htm

Skinner, B. (1953). *Science and human behavior.* New York: Macmillan.

teaching (2009). In Merriam-Webster Online Dictionary. Retrieved March 19, 2009, from http://www.merriam-webster.com/dictionary/teach

Thorndike, E. (1913). *The psychology of learning.* New York: Teachers College Press.

Walker, P. H., & Elberson, K. L. (2005). Collaboration leadership in a global technological environment. *Online Journal of Issues in Nursing.* Retrieved June 10, 2010 from http://www.nursingworld.org/MainMenuCategories/ANAMarketplace/ANAPeriodicals/OJIN/TableofContents/Volume102005/No1Jan05/tpc26_516012.aspx

Wentzel, P., Lammeren, R. V., Molendijk, M., Bruin, S. D., & Wagtendonk, A. (2005). *Using mobile technology to enhance students' educational experiences.* Boulder, CO: Educause.

Wolpe, J., & Lazarus, A. (1966). *Behavior theory techniques: A guide to the treatment of neurosis.* Oxford: Pergamon Press.

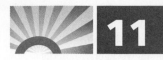

11

Legal Aspects of Nursing Practice

NAYNA C. PHILIPSEN, PhD, JD, RN, CFE, FACCE
PATRICIA MCMULLEN, PhD, JD, CNS, CRNP

OBJECTIVES

At the completion of this chapter, the reader will be able to:

- Describe the constitutional and administrative law principles foundational to nursing practice.
- Analyze contract law and its effect on the nurse's employment relationships.
- Differentiate torts of relevance to nursing practice.
- Discuss strategies the nurse can use to reduce legal exposure.

 PROFILE IN PRACTICE

Elizabeth Frey, JD, RN
Dugan, Babij & Tolley, LLC, Baltimore, MD

As a nurse attorney in Baltimore, Maryland, I handle medical malpractice cases on behalf of the plaintiff (the patient or injured party). I thoroughly enjoy handling these cases for three primary reasons.

First, my goals as a practicing nurse were and are the same as my present goals. They are to be a patient advocate and to improve the quality of patient care. I believe that I am able to reach these goals as a lawyer practicing in the area of plaintiff medical malpractice.

Second, I believe that the patient who has been injured as the result of medical negligence is the underdog, if you will, and I prefer to represent those who are less fortunate. The patient generally does not have the same level of resources that physicians, hospitals, and insurance companies have, such as money, influence, and advanced education. Other factors that place the plaintiff at a comparative disadvantage in these cases include tort reform and the difficulty and cost involved

in finding a qualified physician who is willing to review records and be an expert witness (which usually means testifying against a fellow physician). And, of course, the plaintiff has the burden of proof.

Third, I believe plaintiff medical malpractice is one of the best areas of law in which to utilize a nursing background. Most of my time is spent investigating cases before the filing of a lawsuit and then, after the suit is filed, performing discovery, in which a nursing background is invaluable. As with any case, you must know and understand the facts and applicable law. To obtain the facts in a medical malpractice case, it is necessary to acquire the client's medical records, review them, and know and understand the client's condition, as well as the care and treatment that he or she received. When the client contacts you because of an unfavorable outcome, you need to determine whether that negative outcome is a risk or consequence that occurred in the absence of negligence or whether it was the result of medical negligence. To do this, you must research the medical literature and determine what kind of medical experts are needed to render the necessary opinions. Then you must contact and retain the required experts. Where I have found my nursing background most helpful is in discussing cases with expert witnesses and in deposing physicians and other health care providers. You must have a strong knowledge and understanding of medicine to handle such cases, and my nursing background has been invaluable in this regard. In fact, almost every medical malpractice law firm (plaintiff and defense) that I am familiar with has at least one nurse attorney on staff.

Introduction

Nurses practice within a framework of legal principles on a daily basis. Legal concepts, expectations, and consequences surround all health care professionals in the United States. An informed and safe nurse must be aware of the effect these legal aspects have on nursing practice to reduce exposure to adverse legal consequences.

Law is the sum total of human-made rules designed to help people maintain order in their society and settle their problems in a nondestructive manner. *Statutory law* is established through the legislative process and expands each time Congress or state legislatures pass new legislation. *Common law* is established by previous court decisions and expands each time a judge makes a legal ruling in a case.

The function of law is to create and interpret relationships. *Public law* defines and interprets relationships between individuals and the government. The major categories of public law are constitutional law, administrative law, and criminal law. *Private law* defines and interprets the relationship between individuals. Private law includes contract law and tort law.

These areas of law have an effect on the practice of nursing. Constitutional law defines the clients' and nurses' constitutional rights and remedies. Administrative law includes the licensing and regulation of nursing practice, as well as areas such as collective bargaining. Criminal law usually involves the nurse as a witness. However, it can also involve the nurse as a defendant who is accused of a criminal offense. Contract law identifies the common types of employer-employee relationships and determines the risks and protections inherent in each type of relationship. Tort law is concerned with the reparation of wrongs or injuries inflicted by one person on another. It defines the legal liability for the practice of nursing and identifies the elements essential for each tort. This chapter describes the interaction between law and nursing in three major areas: administrative law, employment law, and civil (or tort) law.

Administrative Law in Nursing

All states have a "police power" to enact legislation to protect the health, safety, and welfare of their citizens. The power of the state to license nurses and other health care professionals originates in the U.S. Constitution (*Dent v. West Virginia*, 1889). The 10th Amendment allows the states to enact legislation that is not preempted or prohibited by federal law. Each state constitution has a health and welfare clause empowering it to pass such legislation.

Boards of Nursing (boards) are state agencies legislatively created by the state nurse practice acts (NPAs). Like other government agencies, the boards develop regulations that give the public "notice" of how laws passed by the legislature will be implemented in their agency. The boards also enforce their regulations.

Nurses are licensed under state NPAs. The NPAs establish entry requirements into the profession, set definitions of nursing practice, and establish guidelines for professional discipline when a nurse fails to obey state laws or becomes incompetent. For most nurses, licensing will be their only direct contact with the board. However, many will find themselves tangentially involved with the board through some level of conflict about the definition of nursing. Fewer nurses will have direct contact with the board's disciplinary unit.

LICENSURE

Licensure is an exercise of the state's police power that the state legislature uses to protect the health, safety, and welfare of its citizens. Through state licensure statutes, the state controls entry into the profession, the discipline of licensees who fail to comply with minimal standards, and the nursing activities of unlicensed practitioners ("nurse imposters"). Boards are composed largely of the professionals that they regulate. Nurses themselves, typically with some consumer representation and input, implement the standards because their specialized knowledge best qualifies them to evaluate and oversee nursing practice.

All the states, the District of Columbia, and the U.S. territories have laws and regulations controlling nursing licensure and practice. National guidelines serve as useful references for nurses in proposing and implementing state laws. The American Nurses Association, the American Association of Colleges of Nursing, the National Organization of Nurse Practitioner Faculties, and other professional groups develop definitions and standards of nursing education, practice, and ethics that are often incorporated into state NPAs. These NPAs are implemented through a state agency called the *health professions board, nursing board,* or a similar title. Rules and regulations promulgated by the board give meaning to the NPA.

The most visible function of NPAs is the control over entry of new members into the nursing profession. Nursing and other professions have been scrutinized for entry requirements that may contain bias, discriminate against minorities, or discourage diversity. Entry requirements typically include completion of an approved nursing education program, satisfactory performance on a standardized licensure examination, competency in spoken English, and strong moral character. Laws regulating nursing practice vary from state to state, with each state placing its individual requirements on the profession. All state NPAs, however, intend to ensure the health and safety of the patients receiving care by nurses. Licensing is supposed to

protect the public from incompetence and abuse. Does a blanket license, covering practice over a broad range of specialties, accomplish that purpose? Do recredentialing tests scrutinize actual competence? Other licensure questions facing the nursing profession include the following: Is licensure too restrictive in its limits on entry into the profession? Do the tests and criteria used actually identify the individuals who are safe and competent nurses, or do they shut out good nurses who are different from a homogenized stereotype? Do licensure requirements protect the public, or do they protect nursing professionals by eliminating competition? Should a national licensure for nurses be established so that nurses could easily practice across state boundaries?

Although a national nursing license is not currently available, an interstate mutual recognition model of nurse licensure, also known as the *Nurse Multi-State Licensure Compact* (or "the Compact"), was approved by the National Council of State Boards of Nursing (NCSBN) in 1998. To participate in the Compact, each state legislature must enact the model Compact. The first state to pass the Compact into law was Maryland in 1999. As of 2009, 23 states had passed the nurse licensure Compact (NCSBN, 2009). The Compact allows a nurse who holds a license in the state of legal residency (the state used as residence on the federal tax return) to practice in other states that have enacted the Compact. The Compact for nursing works like the compact law of a century earlier, which enabled states to recognize automobile licenses so that drivers could cross state lines (Philipsen & Haynes, 2007). The nursing licensure compact is the result of technological advances, including the Internet and the increasing ease of transportation and communication in health care. The goal of the Compact is to ensure public protection and enhance access to safe and competent nursing care for patients who are across state lines from their nurse. These patients may be receiving services through telenursing, by a traveling nurse, or by a nurse who regularly drives across a state line to get to work. Nurses must have licenses in all of the non-Compact states where they practice. Because the nurse who is practicing on a Compact license is subject to each state's laws, the Compact nurse must be familiar with and comply with the NPA for each state in which he or she works.

Because state laws governing advanced practice registered nurses (APRNs) vary more significantly than those governing entry into nursing, a model setting standards for multistate certification took longer to develop. In September 2008 the NCSBN endorsed a new Consensus Model for APRN Regulation: Licensure, Accreditation, Certification, and Education. However, until states pass model legislation agreeing to recognize one another's advanced practice regulations, APRNs must continue to obtain APRN certification (a procedure that is in addition to, and separate from, RN licensure) in each state where they are practicing.

CONTROL OVER PRACTICE

The power to control entry into the profession and the power to take disciplinary action on the license of practitioners were developed to assure the public of safe, qualified practitioners. An indirect result of those powers is that the boards have some ability to exert control on the nursing market. Licensure grants a privileged place in the occupational hierarchy, but it is a position challenged both by the public and by other professionals who fear the surrender of power. Nurses also control the quality and standards of nursing care in the state through the disciplinary process of nurses in the NPAs. Thus, as in many other professions, NPAs leave public consumers of nursing care dependent to a large degree on members of the profession to control access to nursing services and to maintain the quality of nursing care. The result is that nurses have the duty to advocate for patients, at the bedside and before the licensing board, for high-quality care from competent licensed practitioners. The ability of nurses to meet this great responsibility is sometimes challenged by members of the public who fear competing professional incentives. Some have also argued that this is too much power to give any profession because professionals may be reluctant to discipline their own colleagues.

This power is also challenged by other professionals, from physicians to wound care specialists and lay midwives, who are afraid that nursing's scope of practice will compete with their own professional and financial incentives. NPAs permit nurses to function

under a broad definition of nursing while restricting the practice of nonnursing personnel who might otherwise deliver many services provided by nurses.

Enforcement of the prohibition against the unauthorized practice of nursing is exemplified by the practice of lay midwifery. Some states define midwifery as an advanced practice area within nursing and prohibit the practice of midwifery by nonnurses. Practicing lay midwives are not registered by the board of nursing and may be served with cease-and-desist orders. Boards may also request criminal charges for misrepresentation against lay midwives with the local office of the state's attorney (*People of the State of Illinois v. Jlhan,* 1989). Some boards have administrative fining powers for unlicensed practitioners, which they can impose on lay midwives. These powers are invoked regardless of client satisfaction and often in spite of public protest. Boards argue that a threat to the public safety and welfare is inherent whenever unlicensed practice occurs, regardless of the specific situation. Similar policies and procedures have prevented nursing from taking over functions that have been absorbed into medical specialties. The jurisdiction of the nursing board may overlap with other professions that perform some of the same functions as nursing. For example, the expanded role of the nurse has resulted in clashes with physicians at the regulatory level (*Sermchief v Gonzalez,* 1983). While nursing boards have moved to limit the practice of unlicensed lay midwives, medical boards and organizations have moved to limit the practice of several types of advanced practice nurses.

The above arguments illustrate the restrictive nature of licensing by limiting entry and practice. Is licensing too restrictive, or is licensing too permissive by granting "blanket" licenses? Does licensure today permit nurses to practice beyond their actual competence? No individual nurse can competently perform all the services that nurses are licensed to deliver. Although most nurses practice only in a limited field (e.g., surgery, obstetrics, oncology), a nursing license permits a nurse to practice in all areas of nursing. In addition, after initial licensure, many states require little or no demonstration of continuing competency to practice. However, initial credentials do not guarantee competency in the indefinite future. For this reason, some states and health care agencies are requiring mandatory continuing education or advanced certification as an indicator of ongoing competency (Philipsen, Lamm, & Reier, 2007).

DELEGATION IN NURSING PRACTICE

Most state NPAs authorize registered nurses to delegate, or assign, certain nursing care tasks to a non-nurse, although the nursing process itself cannot be delegated. Some nurses, knowing that they are accountable for the care that they delegate to their nursing assistants and other nursing extenders, are fearful of delegation. However, nurses who delegate reasonably and responsibly do not need to fear the task of delegating. Safe delegation requires that the nurse understand the requirements for delegation, such as assessing the task, selecting a nursing assistant/delegatee who is both competent and allowed by law to perform the task, explaining the importance of the task, and evaluating and giving feedback after the delegated task is complete. The 2006 Joint Statement on Delegation by the NCSBN and the ANA is (NCSBN and ANA, 2006) available online (www.ncsbn.org/Joint_statement.pdf).

DISCIPLINARY AND ADMINISTRATIVE PROCEDURES

A board of nursing usually has both regulatory and adjudicatory power. The regulatory power authorizes the board to develop rules and regulations for nursing licensure, nursing education, and nursing practice. The adjudicatory power authorizes the board to investigate, hear, and decide the outcomes of complaints that involve violations of the act and of the rules and regulations promulgated by the board. As mandated by the NPA, the board must ensure that a licensed nurse continues to practice within the standard of care, behaves professionally and ethically, and obeys all relevant state laws. The NPA contains or incorporates a number of grounds to achieve this. The disciplinary action is on the license of the nurse, and that license may be suspended or revoked by the board.

It is important to understand that the responsibility of state boards is to protect the current and future safety of the public. Their delegated powers are to protect the public from unfit nurses, not to punish bad nurses. Boards can only limit or deny a nursing license. They cannot incarcerate a nurse, and they cannot require a nurse to compensate a patient for damages, financial or otherwise. Most board actions cannot be used in a lawsuit against a nurse. If an injured patient does seek monetary damages, he or she must file a civil lawsuit against the nurse. If an individual thinks a nurse has acted criminally, that person must contact the office of the state attorney.

A professional license is property protected by the U.S. Constitution. This means that it cannot be limited or taken away without due process. Each state has an Administrative Procedure Act that guides the procedures within state agencies to guarantee this due process right. Each state agency has its own regulations that describe how the agency implements the law. These regulations can vary greatly from state to state and even among professional boards within a state. A board of nursing in one state may hear all arguments concerning nursing issues. The board in a neighboring state may delegate this action to an administrative law judge or a hearing officer. Within a state, a board of nursing may hear its own cases, whereas another professional board in the same state may have its cases heard by an outside hearing officer.

Due process requires the right to be heard, and it requires notice. A licensed nurse has a duty to be aware of the state's NPA. The NPA is considered notice to nurses in that state about the grounds for which they may lose their license to practice. Further notice comes when a nurse receives a charging document. This paper advises the nurse that the board has probable cause to believe that the nurse is violating the NPA. It has to be specific enough to give the nurse notice about what any defense could be and about the time and place of the hearing.

Due process further requires that a nurse be afforded the right to appeal any decision made by the board that seems improper. This appeal is usually to the state civil courts. Appeal is typically limited to procedural issues, such as whether the board had a right to hear the case or whether the board gave the nurse proper due process rights.

Although all NPAs have commonalities, each state has its own unique legislation. The nurse who moves from one state to another or practices in multiple states through the Compact should obtain a copy of each state's NPA. The differences in state NPAs can be significant. For example, one state may impose no legal duty on a nurse to report the incompetence of a physician. In the next state, the nurse may find that failure to report such a physician can result in the loss of the nurse's license. The nurse needs to be familiar with the requirements of the local NPA for licensure, the boundaries and definitions of practice, the areas for discipline on practice, and the procedures in place to protect the nurse in case the board challenges the license.

THE AMERICANS WITH DISABILITIES ACT

In 1990, the federal government enacted the Americans with Disabilities Act (ADA). The ADA (U.S. Department of Justice, 1990) prohibits discrimination based on disability in employment. It also prohibits disability-related discrimination by state and local governments, by private companies, and by commercial facilities. This is a federal law and, like the constitutional right to due process, it applies to all state boards. Updated information about ADA requirements can be found online (www.ada.gov). The entire text of the ADA is also available online (www.ada.gov/pubs/ada.htm).

Formerly, the boards could interact with disabled nurses without regard or accommodation for their disability. Now disabled nurses, such as those with a drug dependence who are compliant with treatment, those with a physical impairment, and those with a mental illness, are granted special confidentiality, as long as it is consistent with patient safety. This is intended to encourage nurses to seek treatment and self-report, to report other nurses who need treatment, and to ensure that the disabled are not the object of discrimination. Some boards have responded to this mandate by creating their own internal resources to comply with the ADA, such as a rehabilitation committee. Others have made arrangements with external groups, such as rehabilitation services that are provided privately or by a professional organization. A nurse in treatment for a protected disability does not have a public record connected with that disability.

The ADA also requires the professional boards to make any special arrangements to facilitate access to practice by nurses. Examples are special communication services for the sensory impaired and reasonable accommodations at the entrance to the site for licensure examinations or disciplinary hearings.

Nursing and Employment Law

Most nurses work as employees rather than as employers or independent contractors. Nurse employees deal daily with the tension of being professionally independent and responsible for their actions in practice, while simultaneously being constrained by the standards and requirements of their employer. At some time, every nurse will be faced with making a decision about accepting a work assignment. Similarly, the nurse is likely to be faced with decisions about delegation of nursing functions to unlicensed assistive personnel. How can nurses' voices be heard and valued in creating work environments that promote the delivery of high-quality care? What avenues of redress do nurses have if they experience employee/management problems, such as hospital downsizing or cross-training of nonprofessionals to carry out nursing functions under their supervision? How can nurses tell whether they are employees or part of management for bargaining purposes?

CONTRACT LAW

Nurses who are employed work under some form of contract. A contract is a promissory agreement between two or more parties that creates (or modifies or destroys) a legal relationship (Schwartz, Kelly, & Partlett, 2005). A contract can be in writing, or it can be in spoken language with specific terms, in which case it is called an *express contract.* A contract can also be based solely on the conduct of the parties. These contracts are referred to as *implied contracts.*

An enforceable contract must first be for the performance of legal goods or services. A nurse cannot contract to practice medicine. Second, the parties must have legal capability to make the contract. For example, they must all have the mental ability to understand their actions and must be old enough to make a legal agreement. Third, all parties at the time of the contract must agree to do something, and they must agree on what that something is. Finally, there must be "consideration" (i.e., some kind of trade in which each party gets something from the contract). In a typical nurse employment situation, the employer receives nursing services, and the employee receives financial reimbursement.

All states have a "statute of frauds" that limits the enforcement of some contracts that are not written. These vary and are usually not significant to a nurse employee situation. However, a nurse who wants to prove the specific terms of a contract will obviously have difficulty with an oral contract.

Of more significance is the state "parole evidence rule." This rule provides that if oral agreements are made that differ from the written contract, the courts will not allow them to add to or change the written contract. Overcoming a written contract can be difficult for nurses, although it can be done—for example, by showing fraud or duress by the employer. When a nurse agrees to an employment position, he or she should be familiar with the employment contract, should obtain it in writing, and should not rely on oral agreements that are not part of that written contract. What about the role of the contract when the nurse is being terminated from employment or wants to leave that employment? A contract can be legally terminated when it has been completely performed, its terms have been met, both parties agree to a change, it becomes impossible (e.g., through the death of a party or the destruction of the subject matter), or both parties agree to annul the contract. A contract can also be terminated by a breach, which means that one of the parties fails to meet the terms of the agreement. When that happens, the other party can sue in civil court for any damages. For instance, an employee could sue for lost wages, and an employer could sue for lost profits. The Fair Labor Standards Act (FLSA) sets standards for overtime pay, minimum wage, family and medical leave, child labor, and workers' compensation. The U.S. Department of Labor provides a detailed description of the provisions of the

FLSA online (www.dol.gov/compliance/laws/comp-flsa.htm). A nurse employee in a private setting could also file a grievance with the National Labor Relations Board (NLRB). Of utmost importance for nurses to understand is that most employment contracts are not individual contracts but are "at will." The following section clarifies this concept.

EMPLOYMENT AT WILL

Employment at will means that the employee has the right to quit employment at any time for any reason, or "at will." The employer has the parallel right to terminate the employee at any time for any reason, also at will. The law of employment at will considers the employee and employer to have equal power, an assumption that nurse employees know does not reflect employee-employer realities. For this reason, it is a harsh legal doctrine. An example is an employee who is terminated for reasons that are against the public good, such as for joining a union or serving on a jury. Courts have found ways to restrict this doctrine, but they are limited to public policy, implied contract, and good faith. Employees terminated against an implied contract are those who can show that this contract included hospital procedural manuals and personnel handbooks, employer's conduct or policy, or (rarely) oral promises. An informed nurse employee must be familiar with such manuals and handbooks, document any oral promises, and get them in writing as soon as possible. What else can nurses do to enhance their protection as employees?

LABOR LAW

Collective bargaining by nurses is a relatively recent activity. In 1974, Congress extended coverage of the National Labor Relations Act (NLRA) to apply to workers in certain health care organizations. By the early 1990s, approximately 20% of nurses employed in hospital settings were represented by unions (McMullen & Philipsen, 1994). This means that they had formed a collective bargaining unit and could bargain with the employer as a group, in good faith, to make an agreement regarding similar interests in wages, hours, and working conditions. Collective bargaining agreements contain grievance procedures guaranteed to all employees. Furthermore, they usually contain a clause protecting the nurse employee from discharge except for "good cause." Nurses who work in a unionized facility cannot bargain individually with the employer. The employer must bargain with the union, which must represent all employees, whether or not they join the union (McMullen & Philipsen, 1994). Nurse employees can enforce employment agreements under the NLRA, enacted on July 5, 1935 (29 U.S.C. 141-178). The provisions of the NLRA are enforced through the National Labor Relations Board (NLRB) and various federal courts. The NLRB is a federal agency charged with implementing the NLRA, in much the same way that the nursing board implements the NPA. Because the NLRA is federal law, its protections apply in all states.

Only nurses who are employees can participate in collective bargaining with the union. The NLRA also has a special provision allowing "professionals" to bargain collectively. In the past, many nurses who supervised health care workers, such as nursing assistants, were able to participate in collective bargaining under the professional exemption. Some nurse supervisors, however, were, and still are, excluded from collective bargaining participation and protection. In May 1994, the Supreme Court narrowed the NLRA coverage of professional nurses. In a split decision, the court found that nurses who supervised others in a nursing home were part of management because such activities were "in the interest of the employer" (*NLRB v. Health Care and Retirement Corporation of America,* 1994). Of note, subsequent NLRB cases have determined that many types of nurses do not fall into the supervisory category and are eligible to participate in collective bargaining. In the case of *Providence Alaska Medical Center v. Alaska Nurses' Association and the American Nurses Association* (1996), affirmed on appeal to the federal court, the NLRB determined that charge nurses, neurological outpatient rehabilitation nurses, and on-call home health leaders were not supervisors under Section 2 (11) of the NLRA because they did not exercise "independent judgment in directing employees" and were therefore able to engage in collective bargaining. In *NLRB v. Kentucky River Community* (2001) the Supreme Court concluded that charge

nurses are supervisors, and not employees, under the NLRA. As a result, every nurse has to ask whether supervision of other employees might be interpreted as "management," thereby depriving the nurse of the right to bargain collectively and its protections.

COMPLIANCE PROGRAMS

Nurses are often employees of health care organizations, which have to comply with multiple state and federal laws and programs. A compliance office is responsible for developing and implementing related policies and procedures. The purpose of the compliance program is to promote conformity to legal requirements within the institution by identifying potential concerns and correcting and preventing the recurrence of any identified problems. Compliance programs should include a confidential disclosure program, such as a toll-free telephone line, that allows employees to report suspected violations of federal or state health care program requirements or of the company's policies and procedures to the compliance officer. Nurses should be able to make these reports anonymously and be protected from retaliation or any other adverse action for making a report in good faith. Nurses should become familiar with their employer's written standards of conduct and compliance program. Nurse employees typically receive annual training that covers health care compliance policies, procedures, and related legal requirements.

GOVERNMENT EMPLOYEES

The NLRA applies only to privately employed nurses. Federal employees, such as nurses who work for the Veterans Administration, are covered under the Civil Service Reform Act of 1978. The employment rights of state employees are governed by each state's public employee statutes.

Tort Law in Nursing

Another area of the legal system of particular importance to nurses is that of tort law. Torts are private or civil wrongs, in contrast to crimes, which are wrongs committed against the state (McHale, Tingle, & Peysner, 1998; Scott, 1998). The plaintiff, or person filing the lawsuit, files a tort action to recover damages for personal injury or property damage occurring from negligent conduct or unintentional misconduct (Schwartz et al., 2005). Unintentional torts are those in which persons incur harm or injury as a consequence of an unintended, wrongful act by another person. Negligence and the related legal concept of malpractice are examples of unintentional torts (Sharpe, 1999). Several types of torts are often encountered in legal actions against nurses. These include negligence, assault, battery, false imprisonment, lack of informed consent, and breach of confidentiality. A brief discussion of each of these types of torts follows. Case examples of various torts are included in Box 11-1.

NEGLIGENCE AND MALPRACTICE

Negligence occurs when a person fails to act in a reasonable manner under a given set of circumstances (Schwartz et al., 2005). For example, if a person drinks excessively at a party, drives down the highway, and injures another motorist, the injured motorist could file a tort suit for negligence. Driving a car under the influence of alcohol or drugs is not typically considered reasonable conduct. Consequently, in addition to possible criminal action by the state where the accident happened, a negligence lawsuit would probably also result.

Unreasonable conduct by a nurse or other professional is a specific type of negligence, one referred to as *malpractice*. The nurse has the legal duty to provide the patient with a reasonable standard of care. This is usually described as "what the reasonably prudent nurse would do under the same or similar circumstances." In malpractice cases, the issue is whether the conduct of the nurse is below the standard established by law for the protection of others or whether the care given by the nurse involves an unreasonable risk for causing damage to another (McHale et al., 1998; Sharpe, 1999). The courts, based on long-established legal precedent, usually place the responsibility of establishing that the nurse acted wrongly on the injured patient. The nurse is initially assumed to be innocent of the malpractice charge. Consequently, the plaintiff patient has the responsibility of proving

BOX 11-1	Examples of Cases Involving Nurses

Mississippi Bd. of Nursing v. Hanson, 703 So. 2d 239 (1997). The state board of nursing had substantial evidence supporting its decision to revoke the nursing license of a nurse holding a naked infant around its neck with one hand, carrying babies by their armpits, and flipping levers on incubators to stimulate babies.

Karney v. Arnott-Ogden Memorial Hospital, 251 A.D.2d 780, 674 N.Y.S.2d 449, 1998 N.Y. Slip Op. 05900 (N.Y.A.D. 3 Dept. June 11, 1998). Patient was admitted to labor and delivery for evaluation of possible preterm labor. Initial testing excluded preterm labor. However, over time, patient reported worsening contractions. For several hours, nurse failed to notify the physician of the patient's continuing complaints. Patient delivered a preterm infant with initial low Apgar scores. Jury awarded family $13.7 million. This award was appealed.

Kovacs v. Kawakami, 1:93cv02576 (D.C. Dist Ct. Dec 16, 1993). Physician refused to see deaf patient at the time of a scheduled appointment unless she brought a qualified interpreter. Patient filed suit against physician under the Americans with Disabilities Act.

Nowak v. High, 209 Ga.App. 536, 433 S.E.2d 602 (Ga.App. June 8, 1993), certiorari denied (Oct 12, 1993). Nurse permitted to testify as an expert regarding whether a physician negligently administered intramuscular Phenergan to a patient.

Harris County Hosp. Dist. v. Estrada, 872 S.W. 2d 759 (1993). A nonphysician nurse who was familiar with the medical standard of care was qualified by experience to testify as a medical expert in a medical malpractice action.

that the nurse's conduct was unreasonable. In some cases, the nurse will be able to resolve the patient's charges out of court through an alternative dispute resolution strategy (Philipsen, 2008). To successfully negotiate a settlement or defend in court, the nurse will be responding to a patient complainant/plaintiff who must provide evidence related to four elements:

1. Duty. A duty is a legal obligation toward the patient (Scott, 1998). A nurse's signature in the patient's medical record may be enough to prove

that the nurse had a duty to the patient. For purposes of establishing the element of duty in a malpractice case against a nurse, the question is, "Did the nurse have a legal obligation toward this patient?"

2. Breach of duty. This element of negligence and malpractice considers whether the nurse's conduct violated the duty to the patient (McHale et al., 1998). To determine whether a breach of duty occurred, the plaintiff must show that the nurse's conduct did not comply with reasonable *standards of care* rendered by an average, like-specialty provider under similar circumstances (Schwartz et al., 2005). A number of methods are used to determine whether the nurse's care was reasonable. Expert witness testimony, nursing texts, professional journals, standards developed by professional organizations, institutional procedures and protocols, and equipment guidelines developed by manufacturers can all be used to decide whether the nurse's care complied with reasonable care (Aiken & Catalano, 1994; McHale et al., 1998; Schwartz et al., 2005; Sharpe, 1999). Use of careful documentation techniques, such as those specified in the documentation guidelines, will help the nurse to establish that the care delivered was reasonable (Box 11-2).

A defendant's breach of duty, or failure to comply with the standard of care, is usually proven in court by the oral testimony of another health care provider. A nurse can testify to the standard of care and whether a defendant nurse has breached the standard of care if the nurse testifies within his or her knowledge, skill, experience, and training (*Crocker v. Paulyne's Nursing Home,* 2002).

Generally, courts will only allow testimony of breach of the standard of care by a professional holding the same licensure as the defendant. In *Mills v. Moriarty* (2003), New York's Supreme Court held that a nurse practitioner could not testify that a physician breached the standard of care in ordering the drug Haldol for the plaintiff. As basis for dismissing the plaintiff's action, the appellate court held that the nurse practitioner

"lacked the qualifications to render a medical opinion as to whether the [doctor and hospital] had deviated from the standard."

3. Causation. This element addresses two issues: whether the nurse's action or inaction caused the patient's injury and whether the patient's injury was foreseeable (Aiken & Catalano, 1994; Schwartz et al., 2005). To determine whether the nurse's actions or inaction caused the injury to the patient, lawyers frequently use the "but for" test (Schwartz et al., 2005), which asks, "But for the acts or inaction of the nurse, would the injury to the patient still have occurred?" The second part of the causation element looks at whether the nurse could have reasonably anticipated that his or her conduct might lead to patient harm (Aiken & Catalano, 1994; Sharpe, 1999).

4. Damages. For a patient to recover damages from a nurse in a malpractice suit, he or she must have suffered some type of damage (i.e., injury, harm). For example, if the nurse gave the patient the wrong medication but the patient did not experience any adverse effects, the damage element would be missing and the malpractice suit would be unsuccessful.

If sufficient evidence is established concerning all four of these elements and the defendant nurse does not provide an adequate defense, the plaintiff patient can recover damages for pecuniary (monetary) and nonpecuniary (pain and suffering) injuries (Scott, 1998). The defendant nurse usually tries to ward off an adverse verdict by producing evidence that the nursing care was reasonable, that the patient's conduct contributed to the injury, that the time for filing the lawsuit (statute of limitations) has expired, or that he or she is immune from the lawsuit (Schwartz et al., 2005). If, however, a defendant nurse is called to give testimony in a legal action, the strategies for giving oral testimony presented in Box 11-3 could prove useful.

ASSAULT AND BATTERY

The common law has long recognized the right to be free from offensive touching or even the threat of offensive touching. An assault is a deliberate act in which

BOX 11-2	Charting Basics

Documentation is always vital for nurses. Knowledge of a few basic rules can help nurses protect themselves in the event of a lawsuit. These rules can also help communicate the quality of nursing care that is delivered. Helpful tips include the following:

- Never alter or falsify a record. You will lose all your credibility if it is discovered that you altered or falsified a record.
- If you make a written error, draw one line through it and explain why (e.g., wrong chart). Never use correction fluid or a sticker over an error. You want others to clearly see what you have changed so that you maintain your credibility and your client goals.
- Know and adhere to your agency's policies and guidelines. Policies and guidelines help convey what the expectations are in your facility. They are frequently evaluated in lawsuits to determine whether what the nurse did or did not do complies with reasonable standards of care. Consequently, the policies and guidelines need to delineate what the reasonable expectations are. But they should not be so stringent that they cannot reasonably be accomplished.
- Document in clear and chronological order. If you need to go back, chart a "late note." If a lengthy delay in charting occurs, explain why. Keeping orderly records is important. Remember always to date and time all notations. Nurses often leave blank spaces in the chart so that others can come back and make additions. However, blank spaces leave room for a sanitized record. Avoid gaps in charting. No one expects you to prolong a code to make a timely nursing entry. If you code a patient at 0900 and your adrenaline finally becomes manageable at 1100, make a late entry note. This will make sense to attorneys, judges, and other health team members.

- Record accurate and complete information. If an abnormality occurs, chart your appropriate actions. Complete information is data that another member of the health care team would need to care for that particular patient reasonably. If you fill your charting with irrelevant details, other providers will have a hard time locating the important facts. Part of your nursing role is to separate the critical information from the filler.
- If you identify a patient abnormality, chart your appropriate nursing actions. Remember to record the physician's response to your concerns. An unsatisfactory response (or no response) from a physician warrants a call to your nursing superior.
- State objective, factual information. Avoid conclusive statements such as "well," "good," "fine," and "normal."
- Sign your legal name and title. Always make your charting legible. A plaintiff's attorney can use illegible charting to his or her advantage.
- Keep records in a safe and confidential manner. Institutions and professionals are charged with the responsibility of maintaining a patient's privacy.
- Unusual circumstances warrant an incident report, but do not refer to the incident report in your notes. Incident reports are designed to improve the quality of care rendered in an institution. They are not designed to communicate the needs of a particular patient. Generally, incident reports are not discoverable during a lawsuit. Courts want to promote quality care in institutions. However, if you refer to the incident report in your patient's chart, a little-known legal doctrine, incorporation by reference, may be applied. Under this doctrine, the incident report becomes part of the patient's record and not just the institution's quality assurance program and is consequently discoverable.

Modified from McMullen, P., & Philipsen, N. (1993a). Charting basics 101. *Nursing Connections, 6*(3), 62–64.

one person threatens to harm another person without his or her consent and has the ability to carry out the threat (Schwartz et al., 2005). A battery is a nonconsensual touching, even if the touching may be of benefit to the patient (Schwartz et al., 2005). For example, a lawsuit for assault could result when a nurse threatens to medicate a competent person against his or her will. Battery would occur when the nurse actually administers the medication to the unwilling patient.

In some circumstances, such as restraint situations, the law allows providers to touch patients without their consent. However, special circumstances and

BOX 11-3	Giving Oral Testimony

- Bring your own attorney with you to review any records, for depositions or trials, to answer interrogatories, or for other legal requests if you are a party to a lawsuit.
- Never go to a deposition or a trial after working an off-shift, when you may be mentally exhausted.
- Thoroughly prepare for your testimony.
- Bring a recent, thoroughly updated copy of your resume or curriculum vitae with you to the deposition or trial.
- During your testimony, always tell the truth.
- Dress professionally for your trial or deposition.
- If you are asked a question that is lengthy or convoluted, ask that it be restated and then rephrase it in your own words.
- Do not testify regarding the medical standard of care.
- If you become fatigued during your testimony, ask for a brief break.
- Try to remain calm throughout the testimony.
- If asked whether a source is "authoritative" or a "classic," almost always answer "no."
- Maintain eye contact during testimony.
- Do not waive your signature.

Modified from McMullen, P., & Pepper, I. (1992). Surviving the legal hot seat. *Nursing Connections, 5*(2), 33–36.

procedural safeguards must be adhered to in order to excuse the battery. Initially, courts will look at whether the battery was needed to protect the patient, health care team members, or the property of others (e.g., a patient threatens to set a fire in an emergency department). Next, courts will examine whether restraining the patient was the least intrusive method to control the patient. For example, could the patient have been placed in a quiet room rather than being placed in a restraint? Finally, courts typically inquire whether the health care team regularly reassessed the need to continue using the restraint. If the health care team can demonstrate that it has complied with these requirements and with institutional procedure, nonconsensual touching will be excused. Consequently, nurses need to be sure that they provide detailed documentation to indicate that (1) the patient was a threat to self, others, or the property of others; (2) the restraint was the

least intrusive means to control the patient; (3) regular reassessment of the need to continue the restraint occurred; and (4) the restraint was discontinued as soon as possible. Many hospitals and clinical facilities have specific procedures and protocols dealing with the application of restraints. Every nurse needs to be familiar with applicable agency policies.

INFORMED CONSENT

Informed consent lawsuits focus on whether the patient was given enough information before a treatment to make an informed, intelligent decision, including the decision to refuse treatment. The legal mandate for informed consent in the United States is unambiguous and overwhelming. It is based on the 14th Amendment constitutional right to privacy and self-determination and the liberty interest, on the 1st Amendment constitutional Free Exercise Clause, and on state and federal legislation, as well as on common law. Informed consent requires that the patient receive adequate information concerning the nature of the proposed treatment and its purposes, the material risks and benefits of the proposed treatment and of doing nothing (based on best evidence and including discomfort), and the choice to refuse or accept. In other words, did the patient get enough information so that he or she was the ultimate decision maker regarding whether to pursue or abandon the proposed treatment?

Courts have made strong statements supporting informed consent. The right to informed consent was articulated in a landmark 1914 New York Court of Appeals case in which the court stated that, "Every human being of adult years and sound mind has a right to determine what shall be done with his own body" *(Schloendorff v. Society of New York Hospital)*. In 1997 a Massachusetts court stated, "Basic to the informed consent doctrine is that a physician has a legal, ethical and moral duty to respect patient autonomy" *(Feeley v. Baer, 1997)*. Consent may be express or implied. Express consent is given in spoken or written direct words. Implied consent is consent inferred from the patient's conduct. Even if the patient does not sign a consent form expressly consenting to a proposed treatment or procedure, courts sometimes find that the patient gave implied consent to the treatment or procedure by coming to the health care facility and submitting to the treatment or procedure. For example, coming to an emergency department implies that the patient is seeking emergency treatment. An early case found that holding out an arm to receive a vaccination implies consent to the vaccination (*O'Brien v. Cunard S.S. Co.*, 1891). In most circumstances, express written consent is the standard.

The patient may accept or refuse any treatment, even lifesaving procedures. Nearly all states today treat the failure to provide the necessary information so that a patient can make an informed decision regarding the risks and benefits of care as negligence under the informed consent doctrine. In other states the plaintiff files a battery action alleging that the failure to give adequate treatment information constituted nonconsensual touching. The right to informed consent and informed refusal was affirmed at the federal level by the Patient Self-Determination Act of 1991.

Recognized exceptions exist to the doctrine of informed consent. If a patient was admitted to an emergency department with a severe, hemorrhaging abdominal injury that required the immediate removal of his spleen, this would be within the *emergency exception* to the mandate to provide the usual explanation of the splenectomy procedure and obtain informed decisions about care from the patient. Some courts have allowed a provider to avoid full disclosure to a patient if disclosure of information might lead to further harm to the patient. This exception is known as *therapeutic privilege*. For example, if the provider thought a psychiatric patient's knowledge of terminal cancer would lead the patient to commit suicide, the provider might exert therapeutic privilege and not reveal the cancer to the patient.

Regardless of the situation, the caregiver does not have authority to stand in the place of the patient to provide informed consent for the treatment that he or she is providing (Philipsen, 2000). Consent must be obtained from the patient or the patient's legal representative. In any exception, the practitioner must seek the best possible substitute for informed consent by the patient. In emergencies, implied consent permits the caregiver to save a life but does not waive the patient's right to informed consent as expeditiously as practical. Patients who are unconscious, incompetent,

or minors are unable to provide their own informed consent. The caregiver must locate the person with (1) the patient's power of attorney for health care, (2) the next-of-kin designated by state law, or (3) the court-appointed guardian who has the power to make decisions for the patient, in that order. Parents are generally responsible for making the health care decisions for their minor children, unless the parents are not acting in the child's best interest. The caregiver must inform the patient, the patient's guardian, or the patient's *surrogate for health care decisions* of the patient's care options and must obtain consent for treatment. A true exception is court-ordered care; for example, drug treatment or psychiatric care ordered during sentencing by a criminal court. When in doubt, the nurse should consult with the facility's attorney.

Typically, responsibility for the consent procedure rests in the hands of the practitioner who will be performing the treatment, frequently a physician, and the nurse serves as a witness. When the nurse signs the witness portion of the consent form, he or she is attesting that the signature on the consent form is the patient's. If the nurse witnesses the physician giving the pertinent information regarding the treatment or procedure, the nurse may want to write "consent procedure witnessed" below his or her signature. If a lawsuit later develops concerning whether the provider gave the patient information concerning the procedure or treatment, the "consent procedure witnessed" statement can furnish powerful evidence that the patient did receive adequate information. Today's advanced practice nurses often perform procedures and treatments that require consent, such as suturing, obstetrical care, and administration of medications. In these circumstances, the APRN is the practitioner who must ensure that the patient has enough information to make an informed decision regarding a proposed treatment.

FALSE IMPRISONMENT

False imprisonment occurs when a person is unlawfully confined within a fixed area. The confined person must be aware of the confinement or harmed as a result of the confinement. To prevail in a false imprisonment action, the patient must prove that he or she was physically restrained or restrained by threat or intimidation and that he or she did not consent to the restraint (Schwartz et al., 2005). False imprisonment suits may involve situations in which a patient was kept in a mental health facility against his or her will and without a judicial order, or a restraint device was applied to a patient against his or her will.

The laws on false imprisonment vary from state to state. Most states allow some degree of patient confinement if the patient poses a serious threat of harm to self, others, or the property of others. In deciding whether a valid confinement occurred, judges and juries often look at the reasonableness of the decision to confine the patient, how long the patient was confined, whether the need for the confinement was regularly reassessed, and whether the least restrictive methods for detention of the patient were used.

BREACH OF CONFIDENTIALITY

Confidentiality is the duty of health care providers to protect the secrecy of a patient's information, no matter how it is obtained (McMullen & Philipsen, 1993b). Until recently, patients had few legal remedies when the privacy of their medical records was breached. Today, state and federal laws provide patients with legal remedies to compensate them for confidentiality breaches.

One such law is the Health Insurance Portability and Accountability Act (HIPAA), which was enacted by Congress in 1996 (PL 104-191; 42 U.S.C. §§1320d et seq.), along with the regulations issued under HIPAA governing the privacy of personal health information (the Privacy Rule, at 45 C.F.R. §§160 and 164) and the security of such information (the Security Rule at C.F.R. 164.302 et seq.), which set a minimum standard governing uses and disclosure of this information. This legislation also protects individuals from losing their health insurance when leaving or changing jobs (portability), and it increases the government's authority over health care fraud and abuse (accountability). HIPAA established that although the health care practitioner who created a health record owns that record, the information that it contains belongs to the patient. The HIPAA Privacy Rule prohibits the release of identifiable personal health information in any form without the patient's permission. Penalties for failure

to comply with the Privacy Rule involve a substantial fine and/or prison term for those who use individual health information for commercial or personal gain or to inflict harm. The Security Rule provides two standards to ensure the authenticity of electronic patient records: The Integrity Standard and the Person or Entity Authentication Standard (45 C.F.R. §§164.31). As the electronic medical record becomes commonplace and new patient privacy issues surface, nurses should expect that additional regulations will be promulgated under HIPAA.

Several cases demonstrate why valid concerns exist about medical record confidentiality. In *Doe v. Roe* (1993), a flight attendant asked her treating physician not to reveal her HIV status to her insurer or her employer. The physician verbally promised not to reveal her HIV status. Several months later, the flight attendant found that her entire chart, complete with HIV information, had been forwarded to her employer. The attendant recovered damages against the physician for breach of confidentiality and for breaching his expressed oral promise not to disclose her HIV status. Breach of confidentiality lawsuits have also resulted when psychiatric, drug, and alcohol treatment information was released.

A strict level of confidentiality typically exists for patients receiving drug or alcohol abuse treatment. Providers are usually prohibited from even disclosing information on whether a certain person is a patient. In addition, the state where a nurse is practicing may have laws that identify who has authority to control access to medical records of patients who are incapacitated, incompetent, minors, or deceased. Information concerning special situations is available through the office of the state's attorney general and through the employer's legal counsel.

DISASTER NURSING

Nurses who respond to disaster are typically volunteer nurses, working either through a recognized nonprofit organization such as the American Red Cross or through a government agency. As long as the volunteer nurse acts in good faith and within the scope of practice of nursing, he or she is protected from tort actions. Special provisions in most nurse practice acts permit practice across state borders for emergencies. The Good Samaritan Acts, which were designed to encourage individuals to volunteer to help in emergencies, also protect volunteer nurses. In addition, special tort laws protect nurses who may be working as disaster volunteers under the coordination of a state or federal government agency, in the same way that employees of that agency are protected.

Criminalization of Unintentional Error

In rare cases, officials of the local criminal courts have charged health care providers criminally for patient deaths that resulted from unintentional error. This is an extreme example of a common response to error: to punish the individual who made the error. Errors are seldom due to one individual failure, and that reaction is unlikely to make the system safer. In addition, one element of a crime is that it must include the *intent to do wrong*. Carelessness is not a crime, unless the individual was so reckless as to show intentional disregard for others, as in the case of drunk driving or waving a loaded handgun. All nurses make mistakes, but mistakes do not create criminal intent, regardless of patient outcome. Criminalization of health care providers in the past decade has been initiated by complaints related to medication errors, patient abandonment, and disaster care.

When bad outcomes in health care are criminalized, they are likely to receive public attention. In 1998 workers at the Faith Clinic in Libya were sentenced to death when the government blamed them for spreading AIDS to the children they were treating for AIDS. They were freed after negotiations with the European Union in 2007 (Garrett, 2006; U.S. Department of State, 2008). In 1996 three nurses at Centura St. Anthony Hospital North outside Denver, Colorado, were charged with administering the wrong dose of a medication to an infant, who died. Two of the nurses pled guilty in a plea bargain, but the nurse who refused to plead guilty was acquitted by a jury (Plum, 1997). In December 2008 in San Luis Obispo, California, Dr. Hootan C. Roozrokh was acquitted after being charged criminally with speeding the death of an organ donor (Superior Court of California County of San Luis Obispo, 2008). Perhaps the case with the greatest amount of publicity in recent times involved the Hurricane Katrina tragedy. With no food, water, oxygen, or basic medical supplies, in sweltering heat, and with outside help late in arriving, nurses and doctors at Memorial Medical Center in New Orleans, themselves victims of the disaster, were unable to save all of their patients. The Louisiana attorney general charged one physician and two nurses with euthanasia (*Louisiana v. Anna M. Pou, Lori L. Budo, and Cheri A. Landry*, 2006; Night, 2007). Eventually, charges were dropped against the nurses in return for their testimony, and in July 2007 a grand jury refused to indict the physician. In another high-profile case, nurses recruited to the United States from the Philippines were charged in New York's Suffolk County Court with abandoning their patients when they resigned from their job because of abuse by their recruiter. Details are available online from the Philippine Nurses Association of New York (www.pnanewyork.org/articles/sentosa.html).

These cases discourage the recruitment of nurses and other caregivers, discourage the reporting of errors, discourage participation in lifesaving organ donation, and discourage caregivers from volunteering in disaster. In response, authoritative bodies have begun to emphasize the need to stop blaming the individual for bad outcomes in health care systems. The Joint Commission (TJC) sets standards for health care organizations and issues accreditation to institutions that meet those standards. In 2006 TJC stated that solutions must make health care systems safer and prevent mistakes from reaching patients instead of focusing on individuals. The Institute of Medicine, in their 2004 report, *To Err Is Human: Building a Safer Health System*, stated, "The focus must shift from blaming individuals for past errors to a focus on preventing future errors by designing safety into the system ... when an error occurs, blaming an individual does little to make the system safer and prevent someone else from committing the same error. Health care is a decade or more behind other high-risk industries in its attention to ensuring basic safety" (p. 5). The Committee for Disaster Medicine Reform (www.cdmr.org) is an organization that was formed in response to the criminal charges following Hurricane Katrina. It promotes legislation and takes other measures to protect health care professionals from "unwarranted criminal allegations and wrongly placed lawsuits" (www.cdmr.org/intro.html). Nurses and other health care professionals must work together to enforce a policy against the criminalization of error. Belonging to an authoritative professional organization, such as the ANA, is one act that every nurse can take to effectively advocate for nursing and for patients.

SUMMARY

A basic understanding of the impact of legal principles on nursing practice is essential to safe and effective performance as a nurse. An understanding of the role of the state board of nursing in the control and regulation of nursing practice is also important. A thorough knowledge of employment rights and responsibilities when nurses enter into employment contracts can make nurses better negotiators. Knowledge of tort law is crucial to understand the duties and liabilities in our system and to serve as both a professional and patient care advocate.

KEY POINTS

- The power of the state to license nurses is derived from the U.S. Constitution.
- Licensing of health professionals is intended to protect the health, safety, and welfare of the public.
- Nurse practice acts (NPAs) define the practice of nursing, identify the scope of nursing practice, set the requirements for licensure, and provide guidelines for licensure disciplinary action.
- A nurse who is charged with a violation of a state's NPA has a right to due process in the investigation and hearing of the charge.
- The Americans with Disabilities Act grants special confidentiality to nurses who are in treatment for protected disabilities.
- Nurses work under a contract, which is an express or implied agreement with an employer that creates a legal relationship.
- A collective bargaining agreement establishes a contractual relationship between the union and the employer.
- Torts are private civil wrongs against individuals, in contrast to crimes, which are wrongs against the state.
- Negligence occurs when a person fails to act in a reasonable manner.

- Malpractice occurs when the conduct of a nurse or other professional practices below the established standard.
- Assault is a threat to touch or harm another person.
- Battery is nonconsensual touching, even if the touching is beneficial to the patient.
- The principle of informed consent requires that the patient be given enough information before treatment to make an informed, intelligent decision about whether to pursue or abandon treatment.
- False imprisonment occurs when a person is unlawfully confined within a fixed area.
- Information about a patient belongs to the patient; the health care provider is duty bound to keep information about a patient confidential and generally cannot share it unless the patient gives permission.
- Disaster nurses who act in good faith and within their scope of practice are protected from tort claims.
- The criminalization of nursing errors is rare and a violation of public policy.
- One way that nurses can advocate for changes in health care policy or law is to join an authoritative professional organization such as the American Nurses Association.

CRITICAL THINKING EXERCISES

1. Review your state NPA and delineate the definition and scope of nursing practice. Evaluate its relevance for today's health care environment.
2. Discuss the administrative and disciplinary functions of state boards of nursing.
3. How does the right of due process protect the nurse? How does it protect the public?
4. What must a plaintiff prove to recover damages in the following situation?
   An IV was left in place for 5 days, although the hospital policy specified 2 days. As a result, the patient sustained a thrombosis and inflammation at the site.
5. Discuss the concepts of employment law as they relate to your employment situation.
6. Apply knowledge of tort law to formulate risk reduction strategies that could protect the nurse against legal action.

WEBSITE RESOURCES

National Institutes of Health, Institute of Medicine. To err is human: Building a safer health system: www.nap.edu/books/0309068371/html. This report by the Institute of Medicine estimates that as many as 98,000 people in the United States die each year as a result of medical errors. The report examined primarily hospital-based errors. Common errors and suggested solutions are addressed.

National Labor Relations Board: www.nlrb.gov. Facts about the NLRB, labor law, weekly summaries, press releases, rules and regulations, and decisions are all available on this free government website. Information is available in Spanish and English.

Nurses Service Organization: http://www.nso.com. This free website provides the Risk Advisor Newsletter, a nursing malpractice case of the month, and valuable information on malpractice/liability questions. Malpractice insurance information is also available.

U.S. Department of Justice. Americans with Disabilities Act: http://www.usdoj.gov/crt/ada/adahoml.htm. The ADA website gives valuable information on the history of the ADA, provisions of the Act, enforcement considerations, settlement information, technical assistance, new or proposed regulations, and ADA mediation information.

VersusLaw: www.versuslaw.com. VersusLaw is a legal search engine. Cases from all states and the federal government are available. There is a modest fee to use the site.

REFERENCES

Aiken, T. D., & Catalano, J. T. (1994). *Legal, ethical and political issues in nursing*. Philadelphia: Davis.

Committee for Disaster Medicine Reform. Retrieved March 8, 2010, from http://www.cdmr.org/intro.html

Crocker v. Paulyne's Nursing Home, 95 S.W. 3d 416 (Texas, 2002).

Dent v. West Virginia, 129 U.S. 114, 9 S. Ct. 231, 32 L. Ed. 623 (1889).

Doe v. Roe, No. 0369 N.Y. App. Div., 4th Jud. Dept. (May 28, 1993).

Feeley v. Baer, 424 Mass. 875, 876, 679 NE2d 180, 181 (1997).

Garrett, L. A. (2006). Six imprisoned health care workers in Libya are pawns in a far larger strategic game, with enormous repercussions. Council on Foreign Relations. Retrieved March 16, 2009, from http://www.cfr.org/publication/11821/six_imprisoned_health_care_workers_in_libya_are_pawns_in_a_far_larger_strategic_game_with_enormous_repercussions.html?breadcrumb=%2Fregion%2F146%2Flibya

Institute of Medicine (2004). *To err is human: Building a safer health system*. Washington, DC: Institute of Medicine.

McHale, J., Tingle, J., & Peysner, J. (1998). *Law and nursing*. Woburn, MA: Butterworth-Heinemann Medical.

McMullen, P., & Pepper, J. (1992). Surviving the legal hot seat. *Nursing Connections*, *5*(2), 33–36.

McMullen, P., & Philipsen, N. (1993a). Charting basics 101. *Nursing Connections*, *6*(3), 62–64.

McMullen, P., & Philipsen, N. (1993b). Medical records: Promoting patient confidentiality. *Nursing Connections*, *6*(4), 48–50.

McMullen, P., & Philipsen, N. D. C. (1994). The end of collective bargaining for nurses? *NLRB v. Health Care and Retirement Corp. Nursing Policy Forum*, *1*(1), 34–39.

Mills v. Moriarty, 302 A.D 2d 436, 754 N.Y.S.2d 901; N.Y. App. Div. LEXIS 1312, (2003).

National Council of State Boards of Nursing and American Nurses Association (2006). Joint Statement on Delegation. Retrieved January 28, 2009, from https://www.ncsbn.org/Joint_statement.pdf

National Council of State Boards of Nursing and American Nurses Association (2008). Consensus model for APRN regulation: Licensure, certification, education & regulation. Retrieved March 12, 2009, from https://www.ncsbn.org/7_23_08_Consensue_APRN_Final.pdf

National Council of State Boards of Nursing (2009). Nurse licensure compact. Retrieved January 19, 2009, from https://www.ncsbn.org/1100.htm

Night, S. S. (2007). Hurricane force winds destroy more than physical structures. University of Hawaii. Retrieved March 15, 2009, from http://www.law.uh.edu/healthlaw/perspectives/2007/(SN)%20Pou%20New%20Orleans.pdf

NLRB v. Health Care and Retirement Corporation of America, 511 U.S. 571, 114 S. Ct. 1778, 128 L.Ed. 586, 62 U.S.L.W. 4371, 146 L.R.R.M. (B.N.A.) 31, 18 Lab. Cas. 11,090 (May 3, 1994).

NLRB v. Kentucky River Community, 121 S.Ct. 1861 (2001).

O'Brien v. Cunard S.S. Co., 28 N.E. 266 (Mass. 1891).

People of the State of Illinois v. Jihan, 537 N.E.2d 751m 127 Ill.2d 379, 130 Ill. Dec. 422 (1989).

Philipsen, N. (2000). In the patient's best interest: Informed consent or protection from the truth? *The Journal of Perinatal Education*, *9*(3), 243.

Philipsen, N. (2008). Resolving conflict: A primer for nurse practitioners on alternatives to litigation. *The Journal for Nurse Practitioners*, *4*(10), 766–772.

Philipsen, N., & Haynes, D. (2007). The multistate licensure compact: Making nurses mobile. *The Journal for Nurse Practitioners, 3(1),* 36-40. Retrieved January 19, 2009, from http://www.medscape.com/viewarticle/551037

Philipsen, N., Lamm, N., & Reier, S. (2007). Continuing competency for nursing licensure. *The Journal for Nurse Practitioners, 3*(1), 41–45.

Plum, S. D. (1997). Nurses indicted: Three nurses may face prison in a case that bodes ill for the profession. *Business Network*. Retrieved March 1, 2009, from http://findarticles.com/p/articles/mi_qa3689/is_199707/ai_n8766289

Providence Alaska Medical Center v. Alaska Nurses' Association and the American Nurses Association, 121 F.3d 548(1997), 320 NLRB No. 49 (Jan. 3, 1996).

Schloendorff v. Society of New York Hospital, 211 N.Y. 125, 105 N.E. 92 (1914).

Sermchief v. Gonzalez, 660 S.W.2d 683 Mo. (1983).

Schwartz, V E., Kelly, K., & Partlett, D. F. (2005). *Prosser, Wade, Schwartz, Kelly and Partlett's cases and materials on torts* (11th ed.). St. Paul, MN: Thomson West/Foundation Press.

Scott, R. W. (1998). *Health care malpractice: A primer on legal issues for professions.* New York: McGraw-Hill.

Sharpe, C. C. (1999). *Nursing malpractice.* Westport, CT: Auburn House/Greenwood.

State of Louisiana v. Anna M. Pou, Lori L Budo, and Cheri A. Landry. (2006). Retrieved March 1, 2009, from http://news.findlaw.com/nytimes/docs/katrina/lapoui706wrnt.html

Superior Court of California County of San Luis Obispo (2008). *The People of the State of California v. Hootan Roozrokh, Defendant.* Case No. F405885. Ruling After Preliminary Hearing. Retrieved February 1, 2009, from http://media.sanluisobispo.com/smedia/2008/03/19/17/8-19_rrozrokh_ruling.source. prod_affiliate.76.pdf

U.S. Department of Justice (1990). Americans with Disabilities Act of 1990 (ADA). Retrieved January 19, 2009, from http://www.ada.gov/pubs/ada.htm

U.S. Department of State (2008). Country reports on human rights practices. Retrieved March 1, 2009, from http://www.state.gov/g/drl/rls/hrrpt/2007/100601.htm

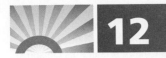

12

Ethical Dimensions of Nursing and Health Care

HEATHER VALLENT, RN, MS
PAMELA J. GRACE, PhD, APRN

OBJECTIVES

At the completion of this chapter, the reader will be able to:

● Describe the foundations of ethical nursing practice.
● Identify the ethical content of everyday practice situations.
● Analyze difficult practice and health care problems using a moral reasoning framework.
● Use appropriate strategies and resources to address practice problems.
● Delineate the scope of nursing's responsibilities for ethical care environments.

 PROFILE IN PRACTICE

Heather Vallent, RN, MS
Clinical Assistant Professor, Boston College, Chestnut Hill, Massachusetts

My interest in ethics started as an undergraduate nursing student when I double-majored in philosophy. At the time, it seemed foolish—What was a nursing student doing studying philosophy? The joke was that as a student, I just spent more time asking "Why?" about everything. The necessity of understanding ethics became much more obvious to me in my first year working as a registered nurse.

As a new graduate, I was grappling with many tasks and technical issues. One of the hardest things for me to learn was how to deal with the unpredictable, especially death and dying. Unfortunately, that first year, I had many experiences with dying patients. Dealing with

death and dying has never become an "easy issue," but it was especially difficult as a brand-new nurse. Such questions as "Did I do right by my patient or their family?" or "How could this have been done better for all?" kept me perplexed for a long time. Once I was able to identify where my angst was coming from, I began to organize my thoughts, but I still needed an outlet to process them. My philosophy background helped me do this. I knew that I wanted to do "good" for my patients, but it took some time to fully understand that doing "good" does not always yield good results.

In my first year, I also saw first-hand what was meant by a scarcity of resources and the effect this has on the patient, the patient's family, and also the nurse. The desire to do good was further complicated by the fact that I could not always be perfect and that doing good for one patient sometimes seemed to mean not doing as good for another. For example, a very sick patient on my general medical floor may have been too sick to be on that floor and ideally would have had an ICU bed; yet there were no patients in the ICU well enough to leave the unit and relinquish their bed to my sick patient. So, if my patient could not be moved to the ICU, where there was a better chance of "fixing" the patient, the problem then became doing the best job I could to help this patient, even though this was not the best-case scenario. Understanding the idea of scarcity of resources can often mean that doing justice is compromised. It definitely takes time to realize that "best" cannot always be achieved if there is a desire to do "good" for all. Over time, my understanding of ethics

helped me to realize this and gave me the tools to move forward as an advocate for change.

After a few years of working as a staff nurse at Massachusetts General Hospital (MGH) in Boston, I decided to pursue my MS degree at Boston College. During graduate school, I took an advanced ethics course, where I was given more knowledge and resources to continue my interest in ethics and begin my journey toward becoming a nursing ethics expert. One of my CNS clinical practica was with a very knowledgeable nurse ethicist at MGH, Ellen Robinson, RN, PhD. Learning from Dr. Robinson was truly an enlightening experience. The majority of our consults were spent resolving conflicts around end-of-life care. Since then, I have also become a member of MGH's Optimum Care Committee (OCC). This committee provides consultation for difficult patient cases and ethical dilemmas. Being surrounded by such great ethical minds inspires me to continue asking myself, "What is the ethical good for each—and for all—of my patients?"

Introduction

So what does it mean to be an ethical person? More specifically, what does it mean to be an ethical *nurse*? As alluded to in the Profile in Practice, there is no prescription or formula to memorize in order to be an ethical nurse; rather, it is a process. This process will take time and an understanding of ethics to proceed. Studying philosophy (ethics is a form of philosophy) is unlike studying any other discipline in that, at the end of the day, there still may be no answer to your question. However, you will better understand all the implications of the question and have a framework to help you proceed with a plan of action.

Overview of Ethics

Ethics is a form of philosophy that has many implications for everyday use, especially when exploring very complex issues. It is derived from the Greek word *ethos,* which is roughly interpreted as "character." The term *ethics* can be used and interpreted in many

different ways. In a broad sense, ethics is an attempt to establish a foundation (or a philosophical inquiry) for what determines good conduct in human behavior. When it is used to describe an action, it denotes the ability to know what is right and wrong—and then to act on the right. Ambiguity exists not only in the *practice* of ethics, but in the word itself.

When discussing the conduct of a whole group, the term *ethics* is used; however, when referring to an individual, it has become common practice to use the term *morals. Ethics* is synonymous with *moral philosophy*; they are simply derived from two different languages (*ethics* from Greek; *morals* from Latin). Essentially, morals become your personal ethics.

Many famous philosophers (e.g., Plato, Aristotle, Immanuel Kant, David Hume, Thomas Hobbes, John Stuart Mill, Friedrich Nietzsche) have debated what constitutes a moral action and a moral person. From these debates, many "guidelines" have been developed to evaluate a person's or a group's ability to act on a moral philosophy. Subsequently, many professions, including nursing, have developed their own "code of ethics" to determine whether a member of the profession demonstrates moral reasoning.

☀ Foundations of Ethical Nursing Practice

MORAL PHILOSOPHY

Moral philosophy is the pursuit of understanding human values (*doing* ethics). So what are values? Values are a way to qualify an action. Morally good choices must be supported by good reasons and must take into consideration other individuals, with impartiality (Rachels, 2007). Many philosophers have dedicated their life to defining the complexities of moral theory. Some variations include deontology, the concept that we should act according to a perceived duty, and utilitarianism, the idea that we ought to maximize the greatest good for the greatest number. Such theories arose out of the needs and struggles of particular eras and as such are useful to varying degrees in general life. It is beyond the scope of this chapter to discuss the complexities of such theories.

The various moral theories do provide some structure and perspective regarding the underlying concern; however, they are complicated and all are to some degree flawed or have been criticized as such. For this reason, in health care settings, we do not rely on any one moral theory to give us answers to a problem. As Grace (2009) states, "We must understand the limits of the theory and what its flaws are, rather than uncritically relying on theories to answer difficult issues in health care" (p. 13).

Moral philosophy can be utilized as a framework or thought process from which to decide which actions are appropriate. For example, imagine a nurse named Molly, who has made a mistake that has not caused harm to a patient but could have. Should Molly report this error to the patient and/or the physician? The debate that is going on in Molly's head (Should she report her error or ignore it? What are the consequences either way?) is Molly doing moral philosophy. From her thought process, Molly will pursue an action; this is Molly doing applied ethics.

APPLIED ETHICS

Applied ethics is the application of the thoughts determined by moral reasoning. It is not enough to know what is good and what is the right thing to do; the ethical person needs to be able to act on his or her thoughts. This is often not an easy thing to accomplish. There are many people in this world, all of whom have a position on what they consider the right thing to do. One individual's version can easily conflict with another's: "Similarly, there is no reason to think that if there is moral truth everyone must know it" (Rachels, 2007, p. 11). Furthermore, what about the possibility that not all people are even *capable* of moral reasoning?

A more complex task is establishing the right conduct for a group of people engaged in the same work—individuals who should have the same goals in mind. This is especially true of groups who provide an important societal service. The group needs to come to consensus on what they consider ethical actions. In order to remain as part of the group, each individual is responsible for good actions as conceptualized by the thought process of the whole. Such a group distinguishes themselves by their idea of applied ethics, thus forming a branch of applied ethics. Individual branches are termed *professional ethics*.

PROFESSIONAL ETHICS

To be considered a true profession, nursing must have a code of ethics from which to practice. A professional code acts as a guide to what the profession considers professional conduct and the scope of its practice.

It may seem obvious at this point that different professions are going to follow different codes of conduct based on the goals and duties of their particular professions. For comparison, let us explore the difference between business ethics and nursing ethics: it would likely not be ethical for a businessman to ask a client to undress for the purpose of clarifying his or her needs; however, it could be very normal for a nurse to ask a patient to undress (while maintaining the patient's dignity) in order to gain data to clarify his or her needs. A different profession, a different setting, and a different relationship exist between the businessman and client and the nurse and the patient. It is this difference that greatly determines what constitutes an ethical action. Whether an action is considered ethical or nonethical is partially dependent on the goal of the profession.

NURSING ETHICS

To explore nursing ethics more specifically and to distinguish nursing ethics from health care ethics or medical ethics, we need to understand the professional goals of nursing and how these relate to promoting individual and societal good. According to Nightingale, nursing "ought to signify the proper use of fresh water, light, warmth ... all at the least expense of vital power to the patient" (1969, p. 8). The means to this goal is complex; a nurse utilizes his or her own knowledge base, experience, personal limitations, a general understanding of ethics, and many other attributes to promote the good for the patient. Furthermore, "it is the discipline's explicit aim of contributing both to the health of individuals and the overall health of society that makes nursing itself a moral endeavor" (Grace, 2009, pp. 52-53).

We can think of nursing ethics in two different ways—a form of study that looks at nurses' responsibilities or nurses' actual practice of doing good (Grace, 2009). In Fry (2002), the main concerns for nursing ethics are the ability to describe the characteristics of the "good" nurse and to identify nurses' ethical practices. From this we can deduce that the idea of the ethical nurse is one who can or does recognize a potential problem that must be differentiated as morally right or morally wrong. This struggle between right and wrong is often convoluted by the fact that rarely is one option completely right and another completely wrong; instead, we experience the inevitable gray area. For example, Mike, who lives with his family in a small but well-populated town, has tuberculosis, a highly contagious respiratory disease. Within the town, there is only one small hospital. Unfortunately, all of the hospital beds are currently occupied with very sick townspeople. Should Mike be admitted to the hospital, where he could be isolated to prevent him from spreading TB to his family, but thereby causing one of the very sick townspeople to be discharged prematurely from the hospital? Or should Mike stay

at home with his family without precautions, thus exposing his family members to serious illness, but not displacing any current patients in the hospital? What would a "good" nurse do in this situation? Does a straightforward answer to this question even exist? To further expand on this thought, consider that the patient may not represent one individual, but rather a family or even a whole community or society at large. In moral reasoning, when neither option is ideal, the resulting gray area is called a *dilemma*.

Abma and colleagues (2008) have reviewed multiple approaches to defining the characteristics of the "good" nurse or "good" care. From their research they have summarized that the concept of the "good nurse" is an outcome of a nurse's reflective inner dialogue with other nurses and health care members, as well as with patients (i.e., "thinking through" a hypothetical conversation between oneself and others). They found that nurses, by engaging in these dialogues, "develop richer understandings of their practice" (Abma et al., 2008, p. 790). They postulate that if nurses are allowed the time for this reflective inner dialogue, then the attributes of a "good nurse" will develop over time, growing with each experience encountered and improving practice. Embodying these characteristics, a morally good nurse would be able to identify a problem, to articulate why it is a problem, to determine how a nurse would be affected by this problem, and to determine how the patient would be affected by this problem. Presumably, this would be followed by good action.

For the good nurse to be able to identify all of these issues, a framework or a body of knowledge is required that can help the nurse decipher and process the problem. A nurse's knowledge base is broad and draws on theories and evidence from a multitude of disciplines. This knowledge is filtered through the nursing perspective as developed over time by nursing's scholars and clinicians. Nursing's perspective is that human beings are unique, complex, and contextual. This perspective plus the goals of the profession related to facilitating health and relieving suffering provide a framework that allows us to appraise nursing actions. Nursing actions, then, are ethical if they use knowledge and skills to provide good nursing care. This precedent then essentially becomes a moral responsibility for the nurse to expand upon nursing's goals of practice not only in individual situations but also in the interest of good practice as a whole (Grace, 2009). That is, good (ethical) nursing actions include addressing the source of obstacles to good practice that may arise from any levels of the health care system.

Nursing Ethics History. Historically, nursing ethics was more concerned with the nurse's personal behavior or virtues instead of his or her professional behavior (Fowler, 1997). An ethical nurse was one who was obedient and followed orders (Fry, 2002). According to Fowler (1997), in the late 1960s, nursing ethics evolved, along with general changes in society, to a more duty-based ethics, in which nurses were held accountable for their actions. However, Fowler argued that nursing ethics should be a combination of virtue-based and duty-based ethics; that is, nurses should be concerned not only with their actions, but also with the environment in which they practice.

With this new sense of accountability, nursing needed guidelines from which to demonstrate ethical care. This concept of needing a code upon which to base nursing actions started in Detroit, Michigan, in 1893 with Lystra Gretter, who wrote the Nightingale Pledge. In 1896, a group of nurses formed an organization that later came to be known as the American Nurses Association (ANA). The group began the process of developing a code of ethics for nursing at that time, although the ANA did not formally accept a code until 1950. Since then, there have been several published revisions; the latest, *Code of Ethics for Nurse with Interpretive Statements*, was released in 2001 (Box 12-1).

The International Council of Nurses (ICN), a federation of national nurses' associations serving nurses in more than 128 countries, also published a code of ethics in 1953, with its most recent revision appearing in 2006 (ICN, 2006). Any code of ethics is established to protect the population it serves and to uphold the goals of the profession. Although many health care professions have similar goals, the perspective on how these goals can be met and the context in which the individual professions practice lead to profession-specific codes of ethics.

BOX 12-1	ANA's Code of Ethics for Nurses, 2001

1. The nurse, in all professional relationships, practices with compassion and respect for the inherent dignity, worth, and uniqueness of every individual, unrestricted by considerations of social or economic status, personal attributes, or the nature of health problems.
2. The nurse's primary commitment is to the person, whether an individual, family, group, or community.
3. The nurse promotes, advocates for, and strives to protect the health, safety, and rights of the patient.
4. The nurse is responsible and accountable for individual nursing practice and determines the appropriate delegation of tasks consistent with the nurse's obligation to provide optimum patient care.
5. The nurse owes the same duties to self as to others, including the responsibility to preserve integrity and safety, to maintain competence, and to continue personal and professional growth.
6. The nurse participates in establishing, maintaining, and improving health care environments and conditions of employment conducive to the provision of quality health care and consistent with the values of the profession through individual and collective action.
7. The nurse participates in the advancement of the profession through contributions to practice, education, administration, and knowledge development.
8. The nurse collaborates with other health professionals and the public in promoting community, national, and international efforts to meet health needs.
9. The profession of nursing, as represented by associations and their members, is responsible for articulating nursing values, for maintaining the integrity of the profession and its practice, and for shaping social policy.

Reprinted with permission of American Nurses Association, *Code of Ethics for Nurses with Interpretive Statements*, © 2001 Nursesbooks.org, Silver Spring, MD.

Nursing Ethics Professional Values. The nursing profession has identified with the practice of ethics for years. As Fowler (1997) stated, ethics "has been the very foundation of nursing practice since the inception of modern nursing in the United States in the late 1870s" (p. 17). Implicit in the idea of having a Code of Ethics (2001) is the understanding that all actions of the individual nurse reflect on the actions of the nursing profession as a whole; therefore all actions should be congruent within the context of the Code. If any action by the nurse does not allow for the goals of the Code (Principle 1), then it is nursing's obligation to fix this (Principle 10). It is in the best interest of nursing students to familiarize themselves with the Code and to reflect on its statements throughout their years of practice.

Appropriate to ask at this time is, "Who determines what constitutes a good action? And what if I do not agree?" We are all born into different cultures and are subject to different social standards, not to mention different religious perspectives. So how can we be expected to all agree on the concept of "a nurse's good action"?

Research on Nursing Ethics. Nursing has conducted its own research on its practice conduct. As society has changed over time, so has the nursing profession. With the advent of increasing responsibility and technological growth, the nursing profession's ethical inquiry has evolved. The scope of knowledge developed from research on nursing ethics continues to shape the trajectory of our profession's future.

Before discussing nursing's research on ethics, it is necessary to review the historical aspects of the ethics surrounding research on human subjects. It is important to understand that all research is subject to ethical scrutiny. For a brief history of research ethics and human subject protection, refer to Box 12-2. Only by reviewing this history can one comprehend the growth that has occurred in this field.

The concept of ethics in research has evolved over time with the change in nursing's responsibilities, as discussed in the history of nursing ethics. In the early 1900s, the aim of studying nursing ethics was to gain clarity on nurses' behavior and conduct in caring for the sick (Fry, 2002). After World War II,

more nurses attended college and became more independent and accountable for their own clinical judgment (Grace, 2009). By the 1990s the topics explored by nurses had increased; however, Tschudin (2006), who served as editor of *Nursing Ethics* since its inception in 1994 until 2008, undertook a content review of the articles published over the first 10 years. She noted that initially the articles were "timid" and not particularly in-depth, but rather focused more on facts or legal issues without taking a stance on the issue. However, by 2003, many articles emphasized care and virtue ethics influenced by an intuitive response and with an affirmation of their beliefs. Some similarities throughout the 10 years of publication included the analysis of end-of-life care, nursing education, morality, moral decision making, and carrying out research (Tschudin, 2006). Contemporary nursing ethics analyzes nursing's ability to meet the profession's established goals. More emphasis is placed on virtue ethics and the intuitive process, rather than conduct and laws: "Nursing ethics remains a subject that will change and grow with what is given and taken, tried and not tried, and used or not used" (Tschudin, 2006, p. 74).

Ethical Nursing Practice

From our previous discussion, we can now say that ethical nursing practice is in fact the same thing as *good* nursing practice. A nurse is practicing well when that nurse uses knowledge, experience, skills, and an understanding of the patient as a unique individual in order to facilitate that patient's well-being. That is, the nurse uses these characteristics to meet nursing goals. However, in today's health care settings and environments of care, nurses may not always be able to carry out those actions that will best meet their patients' needs. They are often faced with barriers to giving the care that they believe is important and necessary. Additionally, nurses may sometimes be confronted with situations in which it is not obvious what is actually in the best interests of patients and their families. Under such circumstances, there are further questions about how to proceed and what are likely to be the best or most effective actions. This next section provides foundations and resources for nurses as they try to give

BOX 12-2	Overview of Research History in Relation to Ethics

When discussing ethics in relation to research, it is important to mention a few very important historical cases that have shaped biomedical ethics of today. The Nuremberg Code was enacted in 1949, after reviewing the experiments taken place in Nazi Germany. This Code stated that the protection of the research subject is always more important than any potential benefit to society and most important, the voluntary participation of the research subject should be sought. The World Medical Association (WMA) developed the Helsinki Declaration in 1964 as a follow-up to the Nuremburg Code. It was realized that ensuring voluntary participation, as required by the Nuremburg Code, meant that research could not be carried out on children or the cognitively incapacitated; yet research with the potential to benefit these groups is important. Concepts that the WMA considered in more detail included therapeutic versus nontherapeutic experiments, consenting minors, and consent by proxy (substitute).

Even with the advent of the Helsinki Declaration, many unethical research studies continued. In the 1960s the Willowbrook Hepatitis Studies intentionally injected hepatitis into "mentally retarded" children who resided at Willowbrook School. The Stanford Prison Experiment by Zimbardo in 1971 explored the psychological effect that imprisonment would have on college students. In 1972, the media publicized the unethical practices of the Tuskegee Syphilis Study, in particular the lack of informed consent and the lack of full disclosure of

information. From all of these horrific "studies" came the development of the National Research Act of 1974 (Grace, 2009).

The National Commission for the Protection of Human Subjects of Biomedical and Behavioral Research was created as a result of the National Research Act. This commission published the Belmont Report in 1979. The Belmont Report provided a framework for the establishment of three ethical principles—respect for persons, beneficence, and justice. By identifying these principles, the Belmont Report also established boundaries between the practice of research and the practice of medicine, determined the criteria for risk versus benefits to the subjects, developed guidelines for the selection of participants, and defined the concept of informed consent (National Institutes of Health, Office of Human Subjects Research, 1979). Another important outcome of the Belmont Report was the origin of independent review committees, also known as *institutional review boards* (IRBs). IRBs ensure the ethical conduct of the research for any institution that is funded by the U.S. government (Grace, 2009).

From this brief review of historical events, it is clear why research on humans has significant implications for ethics and how promoting human good can be lost in the actual science. Utilizing the knowledge gained from unfortunate, sometimes devastating, historical choices, ethical practices related to research has taken on a new meaning.

good care to patients in difficult situations. Responsibilities exist at two levels. The first and priority level is to meet the immediate needs of patients and families. The second level of responsibility is to address the unit, institution, or public policies that are unjust or do not serve patients and/or the public well.

PERCEIVING ETHICAL CONTENT

Studies have shown that nurses sometimes do not understand that ethics is infused throughout all of their professional activities. For example, from an extensive survey (N = 2090) of nurses in the New England region who were asked about ethical issues encountered in practice, a small but significant proportion

responded that they either never encountered ethical issues in the course of their work or that they rarely did (Grace, Fry, & Schultz, 2003). Additionally, in a research study that the authors of this chapter conducted related to understanding what experienced nurses see as essential characteristics of good nurses, some interesting themes are emerging as data are analyzed. This qualitative phenomenological study provides some tentative support for the idea that good nurses take all of their nursing role–related activities to be ethical in nature. Nurses who were not deemed "good nurses" by the respondents tended to focus on completing the day's tasks in a timely manner rather than being responsible for their patients' individual needs. Developing a nurse-patient relationship, when this is possible, tends to weaken the task-orientation of nurses and strengthens the focus on providing good care. This focus on the interests of the particular individual and his or her unique needs has long been considered part of the nurse's caring function.

The nurse-patient relationship, like the physician-patient relationship, has been described as *fiduciary* in nature (Grace, 1998, 2009; Spenceley, Reutter, & Allen, 2006; Zaner, 1991). What this means is that the person who presents to us in need of health care is vulnerable as a result of their needs. They are relying on us to work toward meeting their needs and are counting on us not to be distracted by other issues. They are hoping, if not expecting, that their interest remains our most important concern. This places a heavy burden on nurses who often practice within institutions and settings that limit their actions. Many nurses see this as too much to ask. Any number of things might influence their ability to do best for a given patient. Consider a few examples: staffing is poor, and the nurse is forced to juggle the care needs of several very critical patients; the institution is trying to cut costs and does not have the best drug or the most effective monitoring equipment for the patient; changes in health care system financing lead to shorter lengths of stay (LOS), and patients are often released home before they are ready; a frail, elderly patient is sent home with no capable adult available to provide the needed care.

In addition to institutional constraints on good care, the nurse may be experiencing difficulties in his or her personal life, may be emotionally or physically exhausted, or may be suffering from residual "moral distress." First described by Jameton (1984) and later studied by other scholars (Corley, 2002; Corley, Minnick, Elswick, & Jacobs, 2005; Eizenberg, Desivilya, & Hirschfeld, 2009; Mohr & Mahon, 1996), moral distress is a feeling of unease that accompanies the inability to do what one knows to be right. Left unaddressed, moral distress can have long-lasting effects on people and has been shown to cause nurses to leave nursing. Nurses who remain may distance themselves from and cease to engage with patients. Both of these actions, leaving nursing and failing to interact with patients, are thought to be defense mechanisms that nurses have used to cope with moral distress. Here are some common examples of situations that can lead to a nurse's distress: the seemingly uncaring attitudes of one's colleagues, physicians who do not listen to a nurse's account of what the patient wants, families who disagree about what treatments a patient should have, and so on.

Although nurses sometimes feel powerless to do the right thing under difficult conditions, there are appropriate and effective paths of recourse. Learning how to evaluate complex issues and analyze aspects of difficult cases with personal reflection and dialoguing with others (Abma et al., 2008) is one way to come to terms with and diffuse moral distress. Taking action to remedy a problem is a further way to disperse residual feelings of moral distress. However, before appropriate action can be identified and taken, we must understand our professional obligations as nurses.

The ANA's Code of Ethics for Nurses (2001) has clearly articulated the professional obligations for nurses in the United States. These obligations are all rooted in the goals that nursing as a profession has determined over time by nursing scholars and practicing nurses. The goals are concisely articulated in the ANA's Social Policy Statement (2003):

> Nursing is the protection, promotion, and optimization of abilities, prevention of illness and injury, alleviation of suffering through the diagnosis and treatment of human response, and advocacy in the care of individuals, families, communities and populations. (p. 6)

Understanding disciplinary goals and our responsibilities to further them is a first step in responding appropriately to the needs of our patients. The second step is to use our knowledge, experience, and skills (clinical judgment) to grasp the unique needs of the particular patient. The third step is to give them the care required or access the appropriate resources so that their needs can be met. Implicit in this process is the idea that we understand the limits of our own knowledge and skills and consult with others as necessary.

But what is the extent of our responsibility when obstacles to good care are present or when it is unclear what is the right action in a complex case? At that point, we need to use the tools of ethical decision making to gain clarity about the issues and, in doing so, try to uncover and propose appropriate courses of action, all the while utilizing appropriate resources.

Decision-Making Tools. What is a decision-making tool? It is a helpful framework or structure for working through a difficult problem. Figure 12-1 is a schematic approach to visualize the many elements that are involved in moral decision making. There are many decision-making frameworks available in both nursing and ethics textbooks. The one used in this chapter is synthesized by one of the authors (Grace) from her clinical and educational experiences and the extant literature, and it is presented later in the chapter.

Although they are called *frameworks,* decision making tools do not always proceed in a direct line but rather pose questions to be answered, forcing us to ask more questions and to seek out more information. They will cause us to weave back and forth through the information until we have exposed as many aspects of the issue as possible. Such frameworks help us see the hidden aspects of a case or problem. They do not necessarily give us the "right" answer. There are sometimes no clearly right answers. The reason for this is that we are dealing with human beings and cannot absolutely predict the outcome. We can, however, often be reasonably sure we are on the right track. This is what decision-making tools do for us: they help us deliberate about the issue so that we can gain confidence about available courses of action. They keep us focused on the main goal of action. For the most part, in practice this will be an individual human being, although the needs of family members may also be important considerations. In working through a situation, it is often helpful to involve others. These different perspectives can shed light on hidden aspects and illuminate solutions not previously considered.

Using an ethical decision-making tool does require a basic understanding of the language of health care ethics. Grasping the meaning of generally accepted ethical principles helps with decision making in two ways: it helps us isolate problematic issues and it helps us articulate these issues in language that is understood by other professionals. This next section explores the origins and meaning of ethical principles and uses clinical examples to illustrate their meaning. The practice of analyzing complex cases using decision-making tools is common in health care ethics committees and in education settings. The purposes of case analyses are clarity, direction, and learning from experience. The goals are to determine the best (beneficent) actions and to minimize harm (nonmaleficence). The main focus is the good of a particular human being; a secondary focus is the good of other human beings who may be affected by decisions made. As a professional nurse who has knowledge of ethical decision making, you will be equipped to start your own ethics discussion group on your unit and to serve as a resource for other nurses.

What Are Ethical Principles? Ethical principles are "rules, standards, or guidelines for action that are derived from theoretical propositions ... about what is good for humans" (Grace, 2009, p. 17). More simply put, they are statements that capture what humans have over time come to believe is important in ensuring a reasonably good life for individuals living within mutually beneficial societies. Societies are, of course, made up of individuals who work together to meet collective needs. No one person is capable of solely providing for his or her own needs. Ethical principles have

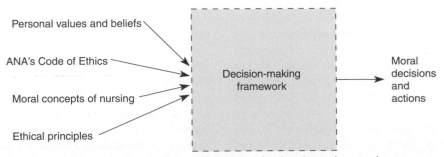

FIGURE 12-1 Essentials of moral decisions and actions in nursing practice.

their roots in different philosophical points of view, but historically they have come to be seen as useful for "imposing order on a situation, highlighting important considerations in problem-solving complex issues" (Grace, 2009, p.17) and holding people accountable for their treatment of others. They are reflective of cultural, religious, and social values, and thus different cultures may stress certain principles over others.

Ethical principles themselves, many of which derive from moral theory, have proven useful in providing clarity and in bringing out underlying assumptions that are being made in a situation. For example, in the Western world, autonomy is often viewed as the most important principle, whereas in other cultures social harmony may be seen as more important than an individual's right to make his or her own decisions. This next section discusses the four principles (beneficence, nonmaleficence, justice, and autonomy) that Beauchamp and Childress (2008) highlighted, as well as some other concepts that have been seen as important in enabling good nursing practice.

Ethical principles serve as a "beginning or starting point for reasoning" (Thompson, Melia, & Boyd, 2000, p. 13). They are not absolutes. That is, no one principle will lead to the right action in every circumstance, because they are derived from a variety of ethical theories and perspectives over time. Consequently, principles that have proven helpful to ethical reasoning in health care settings can conflict with each other. It is important to keep this in mind because we may have to choose which principle to favor in a given situation. This decision most often will depend on the particular situation and the goals for the main focus of the decision making—most often an individual patient.

Ethical principles, however, are helpful in providing clarity about the salient issues to consider in a problematic situation. They trigger more questions and permit the revelation of underlying assumptions. Thus ethical principles are the most helpful in the analysis phase of the problem-solving process. They help determine the most critical issues, such as what is at stake and for whom. Beauchamp & Childress (2008) have stated that ethical principles are action guides to moral decision making and are an important element in the formation of moral judgments in professional practice. For nurses, our overriding action guide is the

"good" of the patient in front of us. This idea is captured by the principle of beneficence.

Beneficence. Beneficence is the obligation to provide a good. When nurses enter the profession and start to practice, they are essentially promising that they can provide a good. If there were no benefit that nurses could bring to patients, there would be no need for nurses. In broader terms, *beneficence* means that not only are we as nurses obliged to provide a good, but we are charged with avoiding harm as a byproduct of our good actions. In health care ethics language, acting on this principle means helping others to gain what is of benefit to them. However, in order to do this, we must understand what *benefit* means in terms of others' (patients') desires and needs. The obligations of beneficence, then, are stronger for the nurse when acting as a nurse than when acting as a citizen in everyday life. This is because the purposes and goals of nursing are explicitly to provide for the patient's good. The ANA's Social Policy Statement affirms nursing's commitment to provide "safe, effective, quality care" (ANA, 2003, p. 1). The goals of nursing are generally understood to be "the prevention of illness, the alleviation of suffering, and the protection, promotion, and restoration of health" (ANA, 2001, p. 5). All of these services are "goods" because they address critical human needs; thus the goals of nursing are beneficent goals.

Applying the principle of beneficence in nursing practice, though, may not be as simple as it sounds. For example, is the nurse obliged to consider all the ways in which the patient might be benefited? What should the nurse do if obstacles exist to giving good care that are beyond his or her immediate control? A second problem in applying this principle is deciding whether the obligation to provide benefit is stronger than the obligation to avoid harm. Some ethicists claim that the duty to avoid harm—also known as the ethical principle of *nonmaleficence*—is a stronger obligation (at least in contemporary health care relationships) than the obligation to benefit (Beauchamp & Childress, 2008). This opinion has risen, in part, because we now have powerful biological and technological advances that can be used to treat or save critically ill patients, but these tools can also have extreme side effects.

Nonmaleficence must be balanced by the provision of benefit, and acceptable ranges of both benefits and risks of harm need to be established. For example, getting a patient out of bed after surgery is likely to cause pain despite premedication with an analgesic. Nevertheless, mobilization is still encouraged because we know that in the long run more good than harm is likely to be achieved. Another example is the availability of tests that can highlight a person's genetic susceptibility to develop a disease such as cancer. Although genetic testing can provide positive benefits (e.g., relieving a person's anxiety if the test gives a negative result or facilitating early intervention if the test yields a positive result), such testing can also cause extreme anxiety, depression, and guilt. Nurses need to anticipate these concerns when asked for advice or when counseling patients.

A third problem in applying the principle of beneficence in nursing practice concerns the limits of providing benefit to patients. At what point do benefits to other parties (one's own family, the employing institution, co-workers) take priority over the benefits to the patient? Is the nurse obliged to provide benefits broadly or simply to the specific patient? Nurses need to be clear about the boundaries of their obligation to provide benefits and avoid harm in patient care. More examples of this follow later in this chapter.

Justice. Another consideration in ethical decision making is how benefits and burdens should be distributed among patient populations (Fry & Veatch, 2006). Nurses generally care for several patients during any given shift. A decision may have to be made about what is a just or fair allocation of resources among patients under the nurse's care. Should the priority be based on the greatest need, the sickest patient, or the patient most likely to recover? In addition, nurses are also often faced with the end results of unjust social arrangements. In the United States, we see quite often very sick patients who do not have easy access to, or cannot afford, preventive health care or health-promoting care. This puts these patients at a disadvantage in many ways and causes harm in the sense that they do not seek care early in their illness. Consequently, these patients' illnesses may likely become more severe and result in irreversible damage.

The principle of justice is likely to lead nursing to work towards change. Both the ANA's Code of Ethics (2001) and the ANA's Social Policy Statement (2003) highlight the nurse's responsibility to join with others and address inequities at the institutional and societal level. In *A Theory of Justice,* Rawls (1971) hypothesizes that those who are the *least* advantaged in terms of possessing material goods and/or personal abilities should receive the *most* benefit from social structures that serve the public. When this does not happen, Rawls argues, nurses and other health care providers who see first-hand the results of these inequities have a responsibility to act to change the situation. A further discussion of health care disparities occurs in Chapters 14 and 19.

Currently, health care arrangements in the United States cannot be described as just, because many individuals are uninsured and have inadequate access to health care. The U.S. Census Bureau, in 2007, estimated that more than 45 million Americans were without health insurance (DeNavas-Walt, Proctor, & Smith, 2008). Nurses are among those who are the most likely to see the effects of poor health monitoring and maintenance on the severity of their patients' illnesses. Nurses thus have responsibilities for social and political activism related to ensuring just health care. Provision 8 of the ANA's Code of Ethics for Nurses (2001) delineates nursing's responsibilities to be collectively active in promoting societal health (see Box 12-1). Socioeconomic factors and roles of the professional nurse are also addressed in Chapters 7 and 4, respectively.

Autonomy. The idea that individuals have the right, and should have the freedom, to decide for themselves which actions are acceptable is captured in the principle of autonomy. This principle has ancient origins but was emphasized by Immanuel Kant (1724 to 1804). Kant noted, as described by Grace (2004), that "the human capacity for reason gives each person dignity and requires that they be permitted to decide for themselves what actions are morally correct" (p. 33). This is another way of saying that because human beings have the capability to reason and might be expected to know themselves and their beliefs, values, and desires better than others, they have the right to make their own decisions. John Stuart Mill (1806 to 1873), another moral philosopher who was almost certainly influenced by Kant's writing, noted that indeed we are only justified in interfering with a person's freedom of action if the possibility exists that the person might injure or obstruct someone else.

In health care practice, although we acknowledge the ideal that people ought to be able to make their own decisions, we also recognize that people are only autonomous in varying degrees. Autonomy is a "more or less" idea. Patients cannot make choices about their care entirely free from internal and external constraints. *Internal* constraints on patient autonomy include mental ability, level of consciousness, age, and disease states. For example, someone who is in a great deal of pain, who is distressed, who is hypoxic, or who is fearful of authority figures is not necessarily able to make an informed autonomous choice. *External* constraints on patient autonomy include the hospital environment, nursing resources, information for making informed choices, and financial resources. Autonomy, viewed as the right to self-determination, underlies the idea of informed consent to treatment (Grace & McLaughlin, 2005). Responsibilities of nurses related to autonomy include evaluating the ability of the patient to understand and process information, ensuring that the patient is provided the necessary information or resources to make a decision, and supporting the patient's informed choice: "Each nurse has an obligation to be knowledgeable about the moral and legal rights of all patients to self-determination" (ANA, 2001, p. 8). Legal considerations related to professional nursing are addressed in Chapter 11.

The principle of autonomy may also be difficult to apply in patient care when the nurse or other members of the health care team have a strong conviction that respecting self-determined choice is not in the best interests of the patient. In this type of situation, the nurse may need to consider the limits of individual patient autonomy and the criteria for justified paternalism on the part of the nurse. *Paternalism* is defined as the overriding of patient choices or intentional actions in order to benefit the patient (Beauchamp & Childress, 2008). Although paternalism is seldom justified in the care of patients, some situations may warrant overriding patient autonomy when the benefits to be realized are great and the harms that will be avoided are significant (Childress, 1982). When the risks from permitting autonomous choice are life-threatening or when it is not known whether the patient truly understands the seriousness of possible consequences, there is a legitimate reason to override patient autonomy. Heeding a principle of autonomy means that nurses should also respect a patient's choice to refuse treatments. The basic human right of all patients to refuse treatment was formally legislated by the Omnibus Budget Reconciliation Act of 1990.

The Patient Self-Determination Act (PSDA) (Box 12-3) became effective December 1, 1991, and requires all health care institutions receiving Medicare or Medicaid funds to inform patients that they have the right to refuse medical and surgical care and the right to initiate a written advance directive. An advance directive is a written or oral statement by which a competent person makes known his or her treatment preferences and/or designates a surrogate decision maker in the event that the person becomes unable to make medical decisions on his or her own behalf.

Honoring the principle of autonomy also means protecting a patient's privacy and treating his or her

BOX 12-3	**Requirements of the Patient Self-Determination Act**

- Provide written information to adult patients about their rights to make medical decisions, including the right to accept or refuse treatment and the right to formulate advance directives.
- Document in each patient's record whether the patient has previously executed an advance directive.
- Implement written policies regarding the various types of advance directives.
- Ensure compliance with state laws regarding medical treatment decisions and advance directives.
- Refrain from discrimination against individuals regarding their treatment decisions stipulated by an advance directive.
- Provide education for staff and the community on issues and the law concerning advance directives.

From Omnibus Reconciliation Act of 1990, Sections 4206 & 4751, P. L. 101-508, Nov. 5, 1990.

information as confidential: "A person's health care information can be used in negative ways that can harm the person" (Grace, 2009, p. 98). Most nurses are now familiar with the requirements of the Health Insurance and Portability and Accountability Act (HIPAA) of 1996 and its Privacy Rule, which went into effect in 2003.

> The privacy rule specifically covers all individually identifiable information including written, oral, or computerized …
> The problem with the privacy rule … is that it is impossible to delineate all possible scenarios related to privacy infringements … so ethical reflection is still needed for its interpretation in specific situations. (Grace, 2009, pp. 100–101)

Nurses must think of protecting a patient's medical information just as they would want their own health information protected. According to Grace (2005), "A rule of thumb for health care professionals related to sharing information with others is to disclose only as much information as is necessary to permit optimal care and only information that is pertinent to the situation" (p. 115).

Finally, the principle of autonomy applies to children in a limited sense—that is, they are considered to a greater or lesser degree capable of making their own decisions: "Research in the biological, social, cognitive, and psychological sciences has revealed that capacity for reasoning and decision-making is developmental and varies related to biological factors, the age of the child, the type of environment in which the child is raised, and the types of experiences" to which the child has been exposed (Grace, 2009, p. 175). It is considered important to include children in decisions and provide information in age-appropriate and developmentally appropriate ways throughout the entire consent process. Children may participate in decision making by assenting to treatments or interventions; by doing this, children are more likely to feel understood and probably more willing to comply with the intervention: "The person who is in the body, and *is* the body, can have unique insights that may be essential for informed decision making" (Alderson, Sutcliffe, & Curtis, 2006, p. 33). Parents or guardians are officially charged with consenting for a child, but they often require assistance and guidance from a health care professional in so doing. As nurses, we must help the child's decision maker to understand that decisions are not isolated incidents and may affect the child's self-identity for his or her lifetime (Aspinall, 2006).

Veracity. Veracity, like autonomy, is linked to the idea of informed consent. Patients have the right to "be given accurate, complete, and understandable information" (ANA, 2001, p. 8) in a manner that facilitates decision making that is in line with their beliefs, values, and lifestyle. The principle of veracity is defined as the obligation to tell the truth and to not lie or deceive others (Fry & Veatch, 2006). Truthfulness has long been regarded as fundamental to the existence of trust among individuals and has special significance in health care relationships (Fry & Grace, 2007). Veracity is necessary for the fiduciary relationship discussed earlier. A lack of trust may bring about undesirable consequences for future relationships with patients, who are vulnerable if their health needs are not met. When patients can trust that nurses will be honest with them, they are more likely to be open and provide us with the information we need in order to appropriately meet their needs.

Knowledge developed in nursing and other disciplines, such as psychology and sociology, has revealed that most, if not all, people need to be able to process the meaning that their condition holds, no matter how serious. When patients are seriously ill, nurses may sometimes withhold information. They also may be asked by relatives of the patient to withhold information because they worry that the patient may not want to know the truth or that the truth may harm him or her. This is often true for patients who are near death; however, only the patient can decide what he or she would want to know. For example, the wife of a middle-aged male who is diagnosed with malignant pancreatic cancer may request that the health care team withhold the severity of her husband's illness until he accomplishes his lifelong dream to sail around the world. The wife's rationale may be to encourage her husband to fulfill his dream, but what if this knowledge would change the husband's dreams and he would rather stay home and watch his new granddaughter take her first steps? Research studies have supported the idea that, despite illness, patients tend to want to know the full truth about their condition. Full disclosure of their condition allows terminally ill patients the right to organize their remaining days in a way that is appropriate and meaningful to them.

Additionally, it is often the case that the family member, rather than the patient, is the person who is struggling with the idea of death. Furthermore, cultural differences have a significant effect on ideas about dying and the concept of full-disclosure; these factors should always be taken into account. When we are knowledgeable about the literature on the needs of dying patients (refer to Website Resources at the end of this chapter), we can help family members cope with their feelings and interact appropriately with their ill relative. Nurses can also assist the family to access helpful resources, such as how to prepare a child for a parent's impending death.

Even in the case of children, evidence suggests that many patients would benefit from the acknowledgment of their condition. Of course, this must be done in a manner that is sensitive to the child's cognitive development and understanding of his or her condition as well as being responsive to the way in which the child questions what is happening (Dunlop, 2008).

Important Ethical Concepts in Nursing. Several other concepts that are important to good nursing practice are discussed briefly here. Having an understanding of more ethical concepts will enhance the decision-making process of a nurse in complex situations. In a previous edition of this book, Fry and Grace (2007) delineate "advocacy, accountability, cooperation, and caring" as "moral concepts" that "comprise part of the foundation for nursing ethics" (p. 279).

Advocacy. Advocacy has developed as an important concept and as a fundamental value in professional nursing (Hamric, 2000). The term *advocacy* can be traced to the 14th-century French word *advocacie,* meaning "the function of an advocate; the work of advocating; pleading for or supporting." In this definition, *advocate* is derived from the Latin word *advocatus,* meaning "one summoned or called to another, especially one called in to aid one's cause in a court of justice" (Oxford English Dictionary, 1989, p. 194). The implication is that because a person was unable to speak adequately on his or her own behalf in a situation

holding importance for that person, another person (an advocate) was needed. The term has evolved within legal settings and involves such concepts as the protection of human rights or the defense of one person against the criminal or civil charges of another. In health care settings, advocacy may mean a defense of a patient's rights, especially when these rights are being deliberately or accidentally ignored. For example, many institutions employ patient advocates who are expected to defend and speak for patients who cannot, by virtue of hospitalization or diminished autonomy as a result of illness, voice their own concerns or choices or assert their rights.

At least three different, yet related meanings of the concept of advocacy exist in contemporary nursing literature. In the first sense, the role of the nurse as patient advocate is to argue for the patient's needs, choices, or desires to be met when the patient is unable to argue for himself or herself. The nurse advocates in a similar manner to that of a lawyer who presents the case of a client, pleads for a particular interpretation of the case, and defends the client's rights. Many have argued that the defense of a patient's rights can be a risky endeavor for a nurse (Bernal, 1992; Gaylord & Grace, 1995; Mallik, 1998; Wheeler, 2000) and thus should not be undertaken without an assessment of the likely dangers and benefits. For example, if a nurse's advocacy results in the nurse being fired, he or she will no longer be able to serve the needs of that particular patient group.

A second interpretation of advocacy, called the *values-based decision model,* views the nurse as the person who helps the cognitively intact patient discuss his or her needs, interests, and choices consistent with values, lifestyle, or personal plan of action. The nurse does not impose decisions or values on the patient, but rather helps the patient explore the benefits and disadvantages of available options to make decisions most consistent with the patient's beliefs and values. When the patient is not able to comprehend information or articulate preferences, the nurse attempts to discover from other sources what actions are most likely to be in the patient's best interests on the basis of previously existing knowledge about the patient's values. For example, a woman who is nonresponsive and seriously ill in the ICU, with little chance of a meaningful recovery, needs a voice to enlighten the staff about her preferences. If the woman never developed an advance directive and has no living relatives, the nurse may need to talk with the woman's lifelong neighbor to determine what type of person the patient is and what she believed to be important in life and then relay this information back to the patient's health care team to aid in their treatment plan.

The broadest interpretation of advocacy incorporates the former two interpretations but includes the idea that all role-related actions of the professional nurse are advocacy actions when directed toward the goal of good patient care (Gaylord & Grace, 1995; Grace, 2001). Advocacy, in this sense, means utilizing nursing judgment to ensure those actions that will best serve the patient are done. This may mean something as simple but important as ensuring that care is coordinated. For example, after cardiac surgery the nurse monitors and addresses any conflicting orders from the surgeon who operated and the cardiologist who is responsible for medical management. It may also mean that the nurse takes action at the unit, institutional level, or professional association level when he or she sees recurring problems that interfere with patient care, such as inadequate staffing patterns. Snoball's (1996) study findings, among others, support this idea that nurses view advocacy as a role or practice responsibility to further the interests of patients. Benner, Hooper-Kyriakidis, and Stannard (1999) have studied and provided rich examples of nurses in the role of advocate. Further discussion of the advocacy role in professional nursing practice occurs in Chapter 4.

Accountability. The concept of accountability has two major related attributes: answerability and responsibility (Fry, 1994) and can be defined in terms of either of these attributes. The ANA's Code of Ethics for Nurses (2001) interprets accountability as being both the acceptance of responsibility and being "answerable to oneself and others for one's own actions" (p. 16). Accountability thus means being able to defend one's practice decisions and ensuing actions in light of the ability to address patient needs. It means to justify or to give an account of the decision-making process that resulted in a particular action or actions.

The terms of legal accountability are contained in licensing procedures and state nurse practice acts. The terms of moral accountability are contained in the ANA's Code of Ethics for Nurses (2001) and other standards of nursing practice in the form of norms set by the members of the profession. Accountability is a very important concept of professional nursing practice and should be emphasized in the educational process. It is a concept from which important values are derived and principles are frequently formulated. Along with advocacy, cooperation, and caring, accountability forms the conceptual framework for the moral dimensions of nursing practice and helps sustain the tradition of nursing by providing both the practice of nursing and the social role of nursing with a necessary historical context.

Cooperation and Collaboration. Cooperation is a concept that includes active participation with others to obtain quality care for patients, collaboration in designing approaches to nursing care, and reciprocity with those with whom nurses professionally identify. It means to consider the values and goals of those with whom one works, in the same manner that one treats his or her personal values and goals (Fry & Grace, 2007). The ANA's Code of Ethics for Nurses (2001) indicates support for cooperation as a moral value by its statement that "the nurse collaborates with other health professionals and the public in promoting community, national, and international efforts to meet health needs" (p. 23). Collaboration is also important in most patient situations in which a complex problem needs to be solved, as in ethics committee forums. Cooperation fosters networks of mutual support and close working relationships.

Cooperation is also an altruistic concept because it expresses the human bonds that grow from working together and spending time together. It can threaten patient care if one's relationships to members of the profession or co-workers become more important than the quality of patient care. The appropriate role for cooperation, instead, is the maintenance of working relationships and conditions that are mutually agreed upon and express obligations toward the patient.

Collaboration is another term for *cooperation* that is more specifically focused on people using their knowledge and talents and working together to accomplish a particular goal: "Physicians, nurses, and allied health care providers have different interactions with patients based on role responsibilities, personal characteristics, and time spent engaged with the patient" (Grace, Willis, & Jurchak, 2007, p. 7). For this reason, collaboration requires that everyone's perspective is heard and considered in light of resolving the problem at hand. Much has been written about the fact that nurses' perspectives are not always heard. Because nurses tend to spend the most time with patients, it should be expected that they have important information to contribute. Along with advocacy and accountability, cooperation helps form a strong conceptual framework that enables nurses to meet the requirements of professional practice.

Caring and the Ethic of Care. Caring is another concept of importance to the nursing profession. It "highlights the relational aspects of human interactions" (Grace, 2009, p. 56). As an ethic of practice, caring has its origins in feminist ethics and related research (Gilligan, 1982). Gilligan's research supported the idea that women do not simply rely on principle-based reasoning to determine good actions, but also understand that context and relationships should not be omitted from ethical decisions. For example, a nursing home patient, Mrs. Jackson, wants to be allowed to go to the bathroom on her own. She is a bit unsteady on her feet but is cognitively intact and fiercely independent. Principled reasoning might direct us to override her wish in order to act with beneficence and prevent her from harming herself in a fall. However, an ethic of caring would allow us to view the issue from Mrs. Jackson's perspective—that she is fiercely independent and that restricting her actions might cause psychological harm, especially because she already feels restricted by the nursing home environment. This ethic would direct us to find a means of honoring her independence while still lessening the likelihood of a fall. For example, we might show her how to ambulate with a cane or walker.

Thus "care as a facet of nursing requires engagement on the part of the nurse with the patient in a relationship that permits the meaning and contexts of the person's need to be exposed" (Grace, 2009, p. 57).

Care also requires the use of knowledge and skills on the part of the nurse to address those needs. Certain conditions can interfere with a nurse's ability to care in the sense of synthesizing his or her knowledge, skills, and understanding of the patient in order to address that person's real needs. Patient-related factors include whether it is difficult to care for or to communicate with the patient. Other factors that influence nurse caring include the time available for caring, administrative support for caring behaviors, and the physical environment where care takes place.

Some nurses have expressed concern about the extent to which nurses are expected to care for patients. For example, too much caring may cause nurses to become physically and emotionally drained, which can lead to "burnout" and unresolved nurse stress. Caring can involve a personal cost on the part of the nurse that has not been adequately understood or investigated. However, caring behaviors on the part of the nurse continue to be expected and valued by the profession and the public, and caring is universally considered fundamental to the nursing role (Grace, 2001).

USING CLINICAL AND ETHICAL JUDGMENT

The discussion above, combined with the decision-making considerations provided in Table 12-1 and the reader's own nursing knowledge and skills, should be adequate tools to gain clarity on a complex case situation and to envision possible routes of action. Box 12-4 presents a short but difficult case study. Read this scenario and then continue reading below to analyze what the most important issues are, what additional information is needed, and how the nurse might resolve the issue.

Case Analysis. How might Rachel go about resolving this issue? Within this case analysis, the decision-making considerations are italicized to help you work through the case. These will not necessarily follow the order presented in Table 12-1, because this case, like most, cannot be necessarily be analyzed in a linear, straightforward fashion. We must weave back and forth, asking questions of the data and seeking more information as we see the need. As a result of data

TABLE 12-1	**Ethical Decision Making in Difficult Situations: Important Considerations**
Steps	**Question**
Identify the major problem(s)—relate these to professional goals.	• What are the facts: Clinical, social, environmental? • What implicit assumptions are being made? • What ethical principles or perspectives are pertinent? Examples: autonomous decision making is in question, values are in conflict among providers and patient/significant others, economics versus patient good. • Are there power imbalances? What are these? Who has an interest in maintaining them?
Identify information gaps.	• Do you need more information? • From whom or where might you get this information?
Determine who is involved.	• Who is the main focus? Is there more than one important party? Who has (or thinks they have) an interest in the outcome (relatives, staff, others)? Who will be affected by the outcome?
Decide what the prevalent values are.	• Values held by patient, staff, institution? • Are there value conflicts? Interpersonal, interprofessional, personal versus professional, patient versus professional?
Determine whether an interpreter is necessary (for cultural or language issues). Who would be the most appropriate interpreter (knowledgeable and neutral)?	• Are there cultural perspectives? Who can help with these?
Identify possible courses of actions and probable consequences.	• Which course of action is likely to be the most beneficial and the least harmful to those involved, including you? • Can safeguards be put in place in case of unforeseen consequences?
Implement the selected course of action. Conduct an ongoing evaluation.	• Does the actual outcome correlate with the anticipated outcome? What was unexpected? Was this foreseeable given more data? • Do similar problems keep reoccurring? If so, why (requires a look at underlying environmental or societal issues, perhaps)? Does this point to the need for policy changes or development at the site, institution, or societal level? What further actions might be needed? • Are there continuing staff provider education needs related to the issue?
Engage in self-reflection, reflection on practice (individually, in an interdisciplinary group debriefing session, or in a specialty group forum).	• Could you have done things differently? What would you have liked to understand better? • Would a consultation with colleagues or an ethics resource person have altered your conception of the issue or the course of action taken? • What valuable insights did you gain that should be shared with others and may be applicable to the approach used for future problems?

From Grace, P. J. (2009). *Nursing ethics and professional responsibility in advanced practice.* Sudbury, MA: Jones and Bartlett. Reprinted with permission.

BOX 12-4	Case Study—Ethical Judgment in End-of-Life Care

Mrs. Petrovic is a 70-year-old woman from Croatia, a relatively small European country that has undergone a lot of turmoil in recent years. She moved to the United States with her daughter Gordana and son-in-law Andro 10 years ago because of Andro's job. Mrs. Petrovic does not speak much English but is able to communicate most of her basic needs.

Five years ago, Mrs. Petrovic was diagnosed with breast cancer. After a lumpectomy, radiation, and chemotherapy, she remained cancer-free for 3 years. However, during the past 2 years, her cancer has returned, proved resistant to further chemotherapy, and metastasized to the bones in her pelvis and spine. She also has severe pain that has worsened over the last few months.

Mrs. Petrovic is admitted to an oncology unit at a large metropolitan medical center for further evaluation and pain management. The medical team agrees that her condition is terminal, although radiation may lessen her symptoms and possibly give her a little more time. Gordana is very protective of her mother because she previously lost her father and a brother during the Croatian war for independence. Gordana works in the

morning at a grocery store and stays with her mother in the evening. Andro, the son-in-law, is also attentive but has been described by some of the nurses as "loud and demanding" at times. The oncologist and radiologist want to present the possibility that radiation may be helpful for alleviating some of Mrs. Petrovic's discomfort. They call a family meeting and explain the options. Present at the meeting are nurses Rachel and Moira, who have both cared for Mrs. Petrovic and know her family. Mrs. Petrovic is not present at the meeting because Gordana feels that it will be more alarming for her mother to watch the conversation while not understanding the discussion.

After the meeting Gordana says that she and Andro will discuss this more with Mrs. Petrovic and that they need time to think. Shortly after the meeting ends, Rachel (Mrs. Petrovic's nurse for the day) notices that there seems to be some family conflict and that Mrs. Petrovic is in tears. Rachel asks whether there is a problem, and Gordana says, "We want her to have the radiation. We told her it will help her, but she doesn't want any more treatment." Andro angrily says, "She has to have it. We can't lose any more of our family!"

gathering, seeking clarity, and exposing the hidden aspects of a complex or troubling situation, appropriate courses of action can often be revealed. Imagine that you are nurse Rachel. What will you do to help this patient and family?

The first step is always to consider what it is about the immediate issue that you find most troubling. The *major problem* here is that a decision needs to be made and Mrs. Petrovic has the right to make it *(autonomy)*. It is primarily her good *(main focus)* that is at stake *(beneficence)*. As long as Mrs. Petrovic meets the "understanding and voluntariness" criteria (Beauchamp & Childress, 2008), she is considered to have decision-making capacity. That is, as long as she is able to comprehend information, to process it, and to express how the resulting choices fit with her values, beliefs, and goals for herself (including a peaceful death)—and there is no reason to believe that outside influences are pushing her to select an option that she would not have chosen otherwise—she should

be allowed to determine for herself what to accept or refuse. However, in this scenario, these very criteria are in question.

Rachel did not directly provide Mrs. Petrovic with the information because of the language barrier. Her family provided the information; thus we do not know for sure exactly what she has been told. As a result, we are not able to correct erroneous *assumptions* or to support her in her decision. In fact, there is reason to suspect that Mrs. Petrovic's family members are *influencing* her to make the choice they want her to make. This is understandable, given the fact that they have a history full of losses (father, brother, and homeland) and they lack the clinical knowledge of the health care professionals. They may be hoping that Mrs. Petrovic can recover. We know from studies that people tend to believe what they want to hear, especially when there seems to be some uncertainty. Perhaps Mrs. Petrovic's daughter and son-in-law are *assuming* that Mrs. Petrovic can be cured (she was cancer-free for a period of time) or perhaps *they* are not ready to face her imminent death. At any rate, we have reason to believe there is a *power imbalance* here. Mrs. Petrovic is relying on her family to translate the options to her and to respect her choices. She is forced to rely on her family members to accurately convey information, and she could be influenced by their choices due to concern for what they want.

We need *more information,* and we need to obtain this from Mrs. Petrovic. Although we need to spend more time discussing with Gordana and Andro what the options mean (helping them to understand that neither course of action is curative and assisting them to access the resources they need), we also need to explain why it is important that their mother make this decision herself. In some *cultures,* autonomy is not as strongly valued as family decision making; in that case, our approach might need to be a little different. Regardless, the family members would still need help in deciding what is best for their mother given their knowledge of her past life trajectory and their understanding of her beliefs and values. Additionally, research has shown that many families who are required to make decisions for a loved one at the end of life (which is NOT the case for Mrs. Petrovic because she is capable of making her own decisions) experience decisional conflict in knowing which course of action is best. Therefore, even if the decisions were Gordana's and Andro's to make, they would still need our help and support in making the best decisions (Andershed, 2005).

What is really needed here is a *neutral translator* who has no *stake* in the outcome of the decision (see Website Resources for International Medical Interpreters Association). Mrs. Petrovic has a *right* to a translator, and Rachel could suggest this to Gordana and Andro in a way that is nonthreatening. Additionally, Rachel could provide them with information about what is known (research and literature) about how difficult it can be for family members to make good decisions for their loved one, when the family members themselves are emotionally involved and in need of support. It would be crucial to ensure that the family is supported in this process and to try to understand their point of view.

It is always possible that Mrs. Petrovic will decline the services of the translator, preferring her children

to make the decision for her, but we would need to obtain this information from the translator or from Mrs. Petrovic herself (if her limited English is sufficient for this purpose). All patients who have limited understanding of English have the right to a specially trained medical interpreter. Title VI of the Civil Rights Act, administered through the Office for Civil Rights of the Department of Health and Human Services, is the basis for the legal obligation to provide language access accommodations for persons who have limited English language proficiency while obtaining health care. This law applies to any health care provider who receives federal funds, including physicians who treat Medicaid or Medicare patients, as well as hospitals that receive federal funds (Romero, 2009).

In this situation the *immediate course of action* for Rachel was determined by the dual needs for more information and to provide support for all members of this very distressed family. She had developed a rapport both with Mrs. Petrovic and her children over the past few days since the patient's admission. As a course of action, Rachel first responded to Gordana, validating the family's understandable distress, and asked whether she could talk with Mrs. Petrovic by herself. Rachel also told Gordana and Andro that she would come out and talk with them afterwards. Despite Mrs. Petrovic's limited understanding of English, Rachel was able to convey her concern about the patient's obvious distress. She was also able to elicit from Mrs. Petrovic a desire for a more complete discussion. The patient agreed that an interpreter would be helpful and stated that she did not know that was possible. Mrs. Petrovic conveyed to Rachel her desire to speak directly to the health care team about her options with the help of an interpreter. She also told Rachel that she wanted her children to be present at that meeting because she believed that this would help them come to terms with her wishes.

Rachel was not scheduled to work on the day of the next family meeting with Mrs. Petrovic, the physicians, and the medical interpreter. However, Rachel believed it was very important as Mrs. Petrovic's most consistent caregiver to attend *(advocacy),* so she arranged to change her schedule with a colleague. The consequences of the meeting revealed that Mrs. Petrovic did not want the radiation treatment (she had experienced problematic side effects during her earlier treatments). It was determined that Mrs. Petrovic understood that radiation might alleviate her pain; however, she felt that her pain was being managed more effectively after consultation with the hospital pain team and she made it clear that she wanted no further interventions. Gordana and Andro were able to accept her decision once they realized that the goal of the radiation was only to relieve symptoms and would not actually lengthen her life. During the next few days, Rachel and Moira discussed with Gordana and Andro some resources that were available to them, such as pastoral care and bereavement counseling.

Because of a high influx of immigrants into the area of the city served by this medical center and the increasing number of patients with limited or no English language skills, Rachel and Moira realized that such problems were likely to become more common. These nurses conferred with the unit's clinical nurse specialist (CNS) about how to be proactive in such situations (collaboration). What could the unit do in terms of preventive ethics? Preventive ethics involves recognizing an emerging or potentially escalating issue and addressing it early. The CNS suggested involving the chair of the hospital's ethics committee to seek assistance in exploring this issue. A meeting was arranged with an ethics consultant, the CNS, and the unit nurses. As a group, they discussed this case and some other similar cases with the dual intent of formulating policy and informing themselves. As a result of this meeting, Rachel and Moira agreed to arrange monthly ethics rounds, in which nurses could discuss problem cases, support one another, and develop policy as necessary, consulting with members of the ethics committee or other ethics resources as necessary.

Contemporary Issues and Problems

Having reviewed what it means to be ethical, discussed different ethical principles, and analyzed an ethical problem using a decision-making process, let us explore some common ways you will utilize this information as a nurse.

This is a very exciting time in health care practice. Technological and biological advances have enormous potential to improve human life. However, the rapid development of innovations often outpaces our ability to accurately understand all of the implications of their use. Additionally, there are forces within the health care environment interested in making profits from these advances. As a result, nurses and others must be able to translate the benefits and risks of such advances and empower patients to ask the appropriate questions before accepting claims that are being made (Box 12-5).

The availability of a range of genetic tests and the fact that some tests are marketed directly to consumers, rather than being proposed by a person's health care provider, exemplifies this problem. The following section discusses the importance for nurses of what has been called *genetic literacy.*

GENETIC TESTING

A basic understanding of genetics is important for nurses because it is increasingly integrated into nursing care settings and nurses may be the first ones to whom patients turn for advice about the benefits of genetic testing. In recognition of the increasing role of genetics in health and disease, a consensus panel of nurses came together in 2005 and developed the *Essential Nursing Competencies and Curricula Guidelines for Genetics and Genomics* (Consensus Panel, 2006). The Competencies outline nursing professional responsibilities with regard to genetics and genomics, including identifying clients who could benefit from genetic testing and referral of clients for specialized genetic and genomic services as needed. Nurses should become familiar with the Competencies and with those aspects of genetic testing that they are likely to encounter in their particular settings. It is beyond the scope of this chapter to do a review of the molecular biology involved; however, at the end of Box 12-6 is a list of resources for further study. Additionally, issues related to genetics and genomics are addressed in Chapter 16. Perhaps the most important thing for nurses to recognize is the limit of their own knowledge and when and to whom one should refer. Nurses should, however, use their knowledge and

BOX 12-5	Direct-to-Consumer Marketing (DTCM) of Drugs and Tests

Definition: The advertising of prescription drugs, tests, vaccinations, and medical banking systems (e.g., cord blood banks) directly to the public.

Aim: A commercial enterprise to increase revenues from brand-name drugs and other technologies.

Potential benefits: Informational—encourages patients to visit their health care provider for symptoms or conditions. Accessibility—early treatment lessens side effects.

Potential dangers: People could be misled. No neutral counselors or educated clinicians to interpret the meaning of the information. Lack of balance in the information. Health care professionals pressured to give the patient what is requested. Uncertainty about the meaning of results and unforeseen consequences of results.

Example: Matloff and Kaplan (2008) studied the example of Myriad Genetics, the company that holds the patent for testing for the BRCA[1] and BRCA[2] genes. These genes are present only in a small proportion of the population (less than 1%). If a harmful mutation of BRCA[1] or BRCA[2] is found, there is an estimated 50% to 80% chance of developing breast cancer or a 15% to 75% chance of developing ovarian cancer over one's lifetime. According to Matloff and Kaplan, Myriad's DTCM campaign trades on misunderstanding and fear. Respondents to the advertisements are encouraged to talk with genetic counselors supplied by the company, given information packets, or told to discuss the issue with their physicians, who may or may not be knowledgeable about the field. It is questionable that Myriad's counselors will provide unbiased information in the same way that a neutral genetic counselor would. Additionally, negative tests do not mean that one is not at risk. Genetic testing requires a deliberative process whereby people are helped to think through what meaning the test results could have for them or their family members.

expertise to help people sort through the questions that need to be asked, determine the goals to be achieved, and access the resources needed. Box 12-6 delineates types of genetic testing and ethical considerations for the nurse in supporting patients.

A crucial point to remember is that although we have become very sophisticated in our ability to identify and isolate genetic information, what we can do with this information in terms of cure or treatments lags far behind. Additionally, although some genetic tests are reliable in terms of specificity (they identify a gene that is likely to cause a problem) and can give a relatively accurate probability of disease development, most genetic tests are not of this sort. Although genetic and genomic research are opening new doors for gene-based diagnostics and treatments that are specific to the individual—personalized medicine—we do not yet have cures or treatments for the majority of genetically implicated diseases.

A second important point is that although some inheritable diseases are caused by a single identifiable gene—for example, Huntington's disease, Tay Sachs disease, and some cancers (such as BRCA[1 & 2])—these are relatively rare. The majority of diseases that have a genetic component are caused by a combination of genetic changes and environmental influences.

Genetic problems can be inherited during the process of egg fertilization. In this process two sets of genetic instructions are passed to the embryo: one from the sperm and one from the egg. Genetic problems can also be acquired as a result of environmental insults such as exposure to toxins or other damage occurring either in utero or later in life and affecting the parts of the body where the environmental insult occurred. The study of the interrelationships among genes, the environment, and psychosocial factors is called *genomics*. Chapter 16 provides more detailed information about genetics and genomics and their integration into nursing practice.

Now let us suppose you are a pediatric nurse in an outpatient setting, where a very sick 15-month-old boy, Marco, is brought in by his parents. The pediatrician believes Marco is showing signs of having cystic fibrosis (a very serious genetic disease) and wants to have him tested. Marco's test is positive, and his parents are very upset. The parents mention that the wife is 2 months along in her second pregnancy, and they want to know what they should do. How has knowing this genetic information changed the family, and how can you, as their nurse, help them?

BOX 12-6	Genetic Testing: Supporting Patient Decision Making*

Types and Purposes of Genetic Tests

- A genetic test may be used to confirm *carrier* status. Carrier status means that a person carries a *recessive* gene, which is likely to pose problems if that person mates with another person who is also a carrier. When this happens, there is a 1:4 chance that each offspring will have the disease, a 1:2 chance that offspring will be carriers themselves, and a 1:4 chance that the offspring will be neither a carrier nor subject to disease.
  - Carrier status simply means that a person has a *recessive* gene on one of the chromosomes. Multiple genes lie along each chromosome.
  - We have 23 pairs of chromosomes in each body cell nucleus.
  - 22 pairs are somatic (body), the 23rd pair is the sex chromosomes (XX = female; XY = male).
  - The genes at corresponding sites on each of the chromosome pair "code" for the same protein. However, one gene is usually dominant, meaning it will be active. Thus the *recessive* trait will not be expressed unless present in corresponding genes on **both** chromosomes in the pair. That is, the person inherited two recessive genes: one on the maternally donated chromosome and one on the paternally donated chromosome.
- A genetic test can be used to *screen* for the presence of a known problem gene.
  - This can be carried out in the process of in vitro fertilization (IVF)—it permits the selection of an embryo that does not have the gene.
  - Newborn screening allows the identification of those at increased risk for genetic disease and in some cases permits disease-preventive actions (e.g., phenylketonuria, which requires dietary modifications).
- A genetic test can be used to *predict* the likelihood of developing a disease
  - In children—for early-onset diseases such as familial adenomatous polyposis, which if positive, require diligent screening for disease with the goal of early intervention
  - In adults with a family history of genetic disease— if early detection is possible and effective
  - In adults—for life-planning purposes (long process of informed consent required)
  - In adults—if preventive strategies are available

- A genetic test may be *diagnostic*; it can confirm a suspected diagnosis.
  - Useful when it will alter treatment
  - Allows other etiology to be pursued if negative

Important Questions

Perhaps the most important role of nurses in advising is to ensure that the following questions are asked and answered before proceeding. This may mean that the nurse prepares by seeking further information about what is known and what is not known or that the nurse refers the person for formal genetic counseling (see Resources at end of this box).

- What are the goals of the testing?
  - Use the testing types and purposes above as a guide.
- Does the person understand the goals?
  - Discover what the person thinks that testing will do for him or her.
- What is the meaning of a positive or negative result?
  - What is the probability that a positive result means disease will follow?
  - Can the person live with the knowledge of a positive result in the absence of a cure or treatment?
  - How will the person feel about a negative result if others in the family have tested positive (possibility of survivor guilt)?
  - A negative result means only that a particular mutation was not found. Many diseases such as cystic fibrosis have numerous mutations, but tests are done only for the most common.
- What will be done, given positive or negative results?
  - What are the anticipated courses of action?
  - Will this require more frequent screening for disease development?
  - Will a negative result have implications for health insurance?
  - A colleague told of someone who had been treated for breast cancer and had a family history, but when her genetic test was negative for the BRCA gene, the insurance company refused to pay for ongoing surveillance with MRI.
  - What if nothing can be done?

*For a more comprehensive description of genetics and genomics in nursing practice, refer to Chapter 16.

BOX 12-6	Genetic Testing: Supporting Patient Decision Making—cont'd

- Who, besides the person, might be affected by the results?
  - This means understanding the impact the information will likely have on others in the person's family; they may need help in determining when to disclose or when not to disclose to others.
- What is known about the affects of testing on people's quality of life (QOL)?
  - Research has indicated that some people become depressed when a result is positive and they cannot enjoy life. Others are relieved at having an explanation for symptoms. The implications are that we should help people to think about these possibilities.
- Is there a possibility of discrimination in health insurance, life insurance, job?
  - As of 2008 the Genetic Information Non-Discrimination Act (GINA) was signed into law. Its goal is to protect against employment and insurance loss as a result of genetic information. The health insurance provisions became effective May 21, 2009; the employment provisions became effective November 21, 2009 (http://www.genome.gov/10002328).
  - GINA does not protect against loss of life insurance, disability insurance, or long-term care insurance. Military personnel are also not protected by GINA. The Act does not mandate coverage for any particular test or treatment. GINA's employment provisions generally do not apply to employers with fewer than 15 employees

(http://www.genome.gov/Pages/PolicyEthics/GeneticDiscrimination/GINAInfoDoc.pdf). Although GINA provides certain protections, the program is far from perfect!

Special Considerations for Children

The general recommendation is that predictive genetic testing not be carried out on children, except in a case in which the gene to be identified signals the probability of an early-onset and serious disease and in which early identification permits effective treatment.

For most genetic testing, involving later-onset maladies, children should be allowed to wait until they are of an age when they can decide for themselves. It is important to remember that once a person has received knowledge of positive status, this knowledge is permanent.

Resources

American Nurses Association:
   http://www.nursingworld.org
ANA's Executive Summary: http://www.nursingworld.org/about/summary/sum99/genetics.htm
The National Society of Genetic Counselors:
   http://www.nsgc.org/
The U.S. government's genome information site:
   http://www.genome.gov/
Genetic Information Non-Discrimination Act:
   http://www.genome.gov/10002328
Government information on genetic testing: http://www.cancer.gov/cancertopics/understandingcancer/genetesting/

VACCINES

Increasingly, much attention has been paid in society to the efficacy of vaccines and their potential complications. Although the debate about childhood vaccines and a possible link to autism is still very tumultuous, let us consider another societal vaccine concern. In 2006, the FDA approved a vaccine to prevent certain forms of human papilloma viruses (HPV) (which have been found to cause genital and anal cancers, in particular cervical cancer in women). The vaccine does not work against all forms of HPV, just the most common. It has been placed on the market and highly encouraged

in adolescent females. The benefits of the HPV vaccine include decreasing the number of HPV infections and genital warts and reducing the number of cervical cancer cases linked to HPV. However, in order for it to be the most effective, the vaccine must be given before the first sexual experience (American Cancer Society, 2009). Therefore the vaccine is protecting against a disease that would not be contracted until, or if, the girl engages in future unprotected sexual activity (De Soto, 2007). Some states have tried to mandate the vaccine for girls for admittance into public schools. Many of these girls' parents have been outraged by this attempt to interfere in such a personal decision. One of the most problematic ethical issues regarding the HPV vaccine is that HPV is not spread in the same manner as most communicable diseases that have vaccines. Thus many question whether this issue should even be a concern for the public school system (Gostin & DeAngelis, 2007; Bennett, 2008).

Another issue that raised ethical concerns was the possibility of mandating the vaccine in adolescent boys as well (Bennett, 2008). Males can acquire and pass on HPV to their sexual partners, thereby passing the potential for cervical cancer to their female partners. According to the American Cancer Society (2009), the vaccine has been tested in males, but it is unknown whether males would reap the benefits of its protection against cancers (certainly not against cervical cancer, the intended benefit of the vaccine). Still, many believe that boys should be encouraged to receive the vaccine, even though it may have no direct benefit to them and could potentially cause them harm. These concerns do not even take into consideration the cost related to the vaccine for both boys and girls.

Now suppose you are working as a nurse in a public school that has mandated that all girls and boys, before entering the eighth grade, show documentation that they have received this vaccine. What would you do?

PREVENTIVE ETHICS

It would seem that the best way to avoid facing difficult ethical debates and problems would be to have a plan in place whereby such issues are less likely to develop; this notion has led to the term *preventive ethics*. One form of preventive ethics is to promote advance care planning. In 1996, 5 years after the PSDA was passed, Miles, Koepp, and Weber (1996) conducted a meta-analysis of studies and found that only 15% to 25% of people have discussed advance directives. These low percentages are not due to a lack of awareness about advance directives. Home health care agencies and managed care organizations are required to provide information about patient rights related to accepting treatment, in writing, at the time the patient comes under an agency's care. The most common reasons for not having advance directives are apathy, procrastination, and discomfort with the topic. Gillick (2009) highlights several other

reasons having to do with the complexity of the decision-making involved. Certain cultural groups, such as African Americans, are especially wary of providing advance directives (Waters, 2000) for a variety of reasons, including mistrust of the system.

In spite of the PSDA, and partly for the reasons given above, the majority of people still do not have advance directives (Fagerlin & Schneider, 2004). However, several relatively recent highly publicized cases, such as that of Terri Schiavo, have continued to make the issue of advanced planning for care an ongoing problem. Terri Schiavo had been in a persistent vegetative state (PVS) for many years as a result of a cardiac arrest. She did not require a mechanical ventilator to breathe but did have a feeding tube for nutrition and hydration. After several years of no improvement in her condition, her husband requested that her feeding tube be removed so that she could be allowed to die; he said that this action is what she would have wanted. Her parents disagreed. Terri had no advance directive to support the husband's request. The case entered a protracted legal battle in which her husband's wishes finally prevailed (Dresser, 2004). How could this scenario have ended better?

Nurses play a pivotal role in assisting patients with advance care planning. In 1991, in La Crosse, Wisconsin, the Gundersen Lutheran's Respecting Choices Organization & Community Advance Care Planning Course was developed to promote advance care planning in an entire community. This program still exists today and continues to improve patient care. The foundation from Respecting Choices has enlightened health care providers on the complexity of advance care planning for success. See Website Resources for useful links. Hickman, Hammes, Moss, and Tolles (2005) described the elements of a successful advance directive program to include a facilitated educative process, good timing, proper documentation, and a system in place to ensure the patient's wishes are fulfilled. In some situations, the nurse may need to assess whether an advance directive is an accurate statement of what the patient wants, whether a patient has fully taken into account the consequences of a treatment decision before completing an advance directive, and whether a surrogate decision maker is inappropriately making decisions for a patient with intact decision-making capacity (Mezey, Evans, Golub, Murphy, & White, 1994). Fins et al. (2005) investigated the complexities of being a health care proxy and reported that some proxies veered away from the direct word of the advance directive, for example, when the patient's directive was to "do everything" but attending clinicians agreed that there was an extremely poor prognosis. Instead some proxies used their own moral discretion given what they knew about the patient's beliefs and values. In this sense the: "… moral judgments made by proxies were superior to strict adherence to prior wishes" (p. 65). That is, the proxies deemed the interests of the patient were not served by prior wishes. Both health care proxies interpreting a patient's written preferences and patients developing their own advance directives require tremendous input from the skilled nurse to promote the good of the patient.

COMMUNICATION

An integral part of nursing is therapeutic communication, not only between patient and nurse, but also between the nurse and other health care providers. Unfortunately, it is often only when there is a *lapse* in communication that individuals realize how important it is for safe care. Inherent in good communication is making sure that all involved parties have a chance to relate their ideas and are ensured of a safe environment to discuss any differences in opinion. To be an ethical nurse, one must aim to understand the communication process and to encourage all involved parties to be heard.

When communicating with patients, the nurse needs to be very cognizant of the fact that the patient may be scared about the content or does not understand the premise of the conversation. This lack of understanding and feeling of vulnerability by the patient can result in an off-balance conversation in which the patient is not on the same level as the nurse. Fredriksson and Eriksson (2003) explored the meaning of a caring conversation between nurse and patient. From this study they found that nurses need to encourage patients to regain a sense of their selves in order for there to be an ethical balance of both parties in the conversation.

Likewise, nurses need to take into special consideration conversations with family members, especially when there is a cultural barrier. For example, a nurse was discharging a Portuguese-speaking patient who had just been diagnosed with lung cancer. The patient and family were not sure about what medications to resume at home. Unfortunately, a Portuguese-speaking interpreter was not available, and there was no effective communication among the parties. The patient was in a hurry to go home, but the family was concerned about the discharge instructions. Should the discharge be postponed until an interpreter is available to ensure no potential problems exist? What if the emergency room is overloaded with patients needing to be admitted? How could miscommunication be a potential harm to the patient and/or family?

What if this same scenario occurred, but instead of a cultural communication barrier, the patient being discharged was homeless and did not understand his discharge plans? This patient would have no available resources upon leaving the hospital. What would be the ethical course of action for this patient?

SUMMARY

Being an ethical nurse is a process that takes time and an understanding of ethics. The process may not provide answers but it will provide a better understanding of all the implications of the question being addressed and will provide a framework that helps nurses to proceed with a plan of action. Understanding moral philosophy, professional ethics, nursing professional values, and nursing ethics provides a foundation for ethical nursing practice and decision making. As highly trusted health care professionals, nurses play a key role in assisting patients and families struggling with major health care decisions. Preventive ethics is a strategy for addressing many of the contemporary ethical issues and problems faced by professional nurses in daily practice.

KEY POINTS

- Nursing ethics is both (1) a field of inquiry that uses philosophical analysis and empirical research to discover what constitutes good nursing practice, what is needed for good practice, and what are the characteristics of good nurses; and (2) an appraisal of the actual actions of nurses for their intent and ability to further an individual and social good and fulfill professional goals while trying to deliver good care.

- Professional responsibility is the extent to which nurses recognize that their practice is inherently ethical in nature because of the vulnerability of patients and aim to facilitate nursing goals.
- Ethical principles such as beneficence, justice, autonomy, veracity, and fidelity, along with nursing concepts such as advocacy, accountability, cooperation, and caring, have important moral dimensions. They serve as considerations in nurses' ethical decision making. The primary goal of ethical decision making is the good of the patients immediately in our care. Secondary goals are the good of family members and societal justice.
- Many ethical decision-making frameworks are available in the nursing literature. They provide a systematic approach to the ethical analysis of values conflicts and questions of what should be done in the nursing role. However, the way decision making proceeds is not always linear and depends on the problem and ongoing data gathering for direction.
- Nursing ethics research is ongoing and has developed from being mostly related to nurses' understanding of appropriate etiquette and personal conduct to its current broad field of inquiry. At presently, a variety of research methods are used, depending on the question to be answered. These include quantitative, qualitative, and philosophical methods; historical explorations; and feminist critiques of health care delivery systems.
- Nurses, who are consistently rated as among the most trustworthy professionals, are often relied on to provide advice and access to resources. For this reason, professional responsibility includes remaining current on biotechnological advances and the ways in which these advances affect nurses' practice populations.

CRITICAL THINKING EXERCISES

1. To what extent should one's personal code of ethics, integrated with religious beliefs and cultural values, influence moral decision making in nursing practice?
2. What personal characteristics do you think are essential to ethical nursing practice? In what ways are these characteristics likely to foster ethical practice?
3. If a terminally ill patient under your care asked you to help him end his life or assist him in dying, what would you do? Why?
4. Some ethicists have argued that nursing practice is not morally unique; that is, the same moral issues and questions arise in all health professionals' practices. Do you agree or disagree with this statement? Why?
5. The term *applied ethics* means the application of ethical theory, principles, and reasoning to a realm of practice. How do you apply ethics to your own area of nursing practice?
6. If a nurse notices that certain types of problems that interfere with good nursing care keep recurring, such as inadequate staffing, what are his or her responsibilities (if any)?
7. What would you do if a patient asked your advice about a test such as the BRCA[1] or BRCA[2], which is advertised directly to the public, also known as *direct-to-consumer-marketing?* (This is a good topic to explore for in-class presentation.)

WEBSITE RESOURCES

American Medical Association—*Principles of Medical Ethics* (2001): http://www.ama-assn.org/ama/pub/category/2512.html

American Nurses Association: http://www.nursingworld.org/EthicsHumanRights

A. Ethics and Human Rights Position Statements: Foregoing Nutrition and Hydration (1992)

B. Ethics and Human Rights Position Statements: Nursing and the Patient Self-Determination Acts (1991)

C. Ethics and Human Rights Position Statements: Assisted Suicide (1994)

D. Mechanisms Through Which SNAs Consider Ethical/Human Rights Issues (1994)

E. The Nonnegotiable Nature of the ANA Code for Nurses with Interpretive Statements, (1994)

F. Position Statement: Nursing Care and Do Not Resuscitate Decisions (2003)

G. Position Statement: Pain Management and Control of Distressing Symptoms in Dying Patients (2003)

International Medical Interpreters Association (IMIA) Code of Ethics (2006): http://www.imiaweb.org/code/default.asp

National Association of Social Work Code of Ethics (1999): http://www.socialworkers.org/pubs/code/code.asp

National Institute of Health—State of Science Conference Statement on Improving End of Life Care (2004): http://sccmcms.sccm.org/SCCM/Publications/Critical+Connections/References/December+2005/

Society of Critical Care Medicine—Statement on End of Life Decisions (2006): http://sccmcms.sccm.org/SCCM/Professional+Resources/Critical+Care+Ethics/EndOfLifeCare.htm

Respecting Choices: http://www.respectingchoices.org/index.asp

REFERENCES

Abma, T. A., Widdershoven, G. A., Frederiks, B. J. M., van Hooren, R. H., van Wijmen, F., & Curf, P. L.M.G. (2008). Dialogical nursing ethics: The quality of freedom restrictions. *Nursing Ethics, 15*, 789–802.

Alderson, P., Sutcliffe, K., & Curtis, K. (2006). Children's competence to consent to medical treatment. *Hastings Center Report, 36*(6), 25–34.

American Cancer Society. (2009). *Human papilloma virus (HPV), cancer, and HPV vaccines—Frequently asked questions.* Retrieved on May 4, 2009, from http://www.cancer.org/docroot/CRI/content/CRI_2_6x_FAQ_HPV_Vaccines.asp

American Nurses Association. (2001). *Code of ethics for nurses with interpretive statements.* Silver Springs, MD: Author.

American Nurses Association. (2003). *Nursing's social policy statement* (2nd ed.). Silver Spring, MD: Author.

Andershed, B. (2005). Relatives in end-of-life care—part 1: a systematic review of the literature the five last years, January 1999-February 2004. *Journal of Clinical Nursing, 15*, 1158–1169.

Aspinall, C. (2006). Another voice: Children and parents and medical decisions. *Hastings Center Report, 36*(6), 3.

Beauchamp, T. L., & Childress, J. F. (2008). *Principles of biomedical ethics* (6th ed.). New York: Oxford University Press.

Benner, P., Hooper-Kyriakidis, P., & Stannard, D. (1999). *Clinical wisdom and interventions in critical care.* Philadelphia: Saunders.

Bennett, M. P. (2008). Ethics and the HPV vaccine: Considerations for school nurses. *The Journal of School Nursing, 24*, 275–283.

Bernal, E. W. (1992). The nurse as patient advocate. *Hastings Center Report, 22*(4), 18–23.

Childress, J. F. (1982). *Who should decide? Paternalism in healthcare.* New York: Oxford.

Consensus Panel (2006). *Essential nursing competencies and curricula guidelines for genetics and genomics.* Silver Springs, MD: American Nurses Association.

Corley, M. C. (2002). Nurses' moral distress: A proposed theory and research agenda. *Nursing Ethics, 9*(6), 636–650.

Corley, M. C., Minnick, P., Elswick, R. K., & Jacobs, M. (2005). Nurses moral distress and the ethical work environment. *Nursing Ethics, 12*(4), 381–390.

DeNavas-Walt, C., Proctor, B. D., & Smith, J. C. (2008). *U.S. Census Bureau, Current Population Reports—Income, poverty, and health insurance coverage in the United States: 2007.* Washington, DC: U.S. Government Printing Office.

De Soto, J. (2007). Should HPV vaccine be mandatory: Should we force drug therapy because patients might get the disease based on future behavior? *Journal of Family Practice, 56*(4), 1–2.

Dresser, R. (2004). Schiavo: A hard case makes questionable law. *Hastings Center Report, 34*(3), 8–9.

Dunlop, S. (2008). The dying child: Should we tell the truth? *Pediatric Nursing, 20*(6), 28–32.

Eizenberg, M. M., Desivilya, H. S., & Hirschfeld, M. J. (2009). Moral distress questionnaire for clinical nurses: Instrument development. *Journal of Advanced Nursing, 65*(4), 885–892.

Fagerlin, A., & Schneider, C. E. (2004). Enough. The failure of the living will. *Hastings Center Report, 34*(2), 30–42.

Fins, J., Maltby, B., Friedmann, E., Greene, M., Norris, K., & Adelman, R. (2005). Contracts, covenants, and advance care planning: An empirical study of the moral obligations of patient and proxy. *Journal of Pain and Symptom Management, 29*(1), 55–68.

Fowler, M. (1997). Nursing's ethics. In A. J. Davis, M. A. Aroskar, J. Liaschenko, & T. S. Drought (Eds.), *Ethical dilemmas and nursing practice* (4th ed.). Stamford, CT: Appleton & Lange.

Fredriksson, L., & Eriksson, K. (2003). The ethics of the caring conversation. *Nursing Ethics, 10*(2), 138–148.

Fry, S. T. (1994). *Ethics in nursing practice: A guide to ethical decision making.* Geneva, Switzerland: International Council of Nurses.

Fry, S. T. (2002). Guest editorial: Defining nurses' ethical practices in the 21st century. *ICN International Nursing Review, 49*, 1–3.

Fry, S. T., & Grace, P. J. (2007). Ethical dimensions of nursing and health care. In J. L. Creasia, & B. J. Parker (Eds.), *Conceptual foundations: The bridge to professional nursing practice* (4th ed, pp. 273–299). St. Louis: Mosby.

Fry, S. T., & Veatch, R. M. (2006). *Case studies in nursing ethics* (3rd ed.). Sudbury, MA: Jones & Bartlett.

Gaylord, N., & Grace, P. (1995). Nursing advocacy: An ethic of practice. *Nursing Ethics, 2*(1), 11–18.

Gillick, M. R. (2009). Decision making near life's end: A prescription for change. *Journal of Palliative Medicine, 12*(2), 121–125.

Gilligan, C. (1982). *In a different voice: Psychological theory and women's development.* Cambridge, MA: Harvard University.

Gostin, L. O., & DeAngelis, C. D. (2007). Mandatory HPV vaccination: Public health vs. private wealth. *Journal of the American Medical Association, 297*(17), 1921–1923.

Grace, P. J. (1998). *A philosophical analysis of the concept 'advocacy': Implications for professional-patient relationships.* Unpublished doctoral dissertation, University of Tennessee Knoxville.Available at http://proquest.umi.com. Publication No. AAT9923287, Proquest Document ID No. 734421751.

Grace, P. J. (2001). Professional advocacy: Widening the scope of professional responsibility. *Nursing Philosophy, 2*(2), 151–162.

Grace, P. J. (2004). Patient safety and the limits of confidentiality. *American Journal of Nursing, 104*(11), 33–37.

Grace, P. J., Fry, S. T., & Schultz, G. S. (2003). Ethics and human rights issues experienced by psychiatric-mental health and substance abuse registered nurses. *American Psychiatric Nurses Association, 9*(1), 17–24.

Grace, P. J. (2005). Ethical issues relevant to health promotion. InC. Edelman, & C. L. Mandle (Eds.), *Health promotion through the lifespan* (6th ed, pp. 107–137). St. Louis: Mosby.

Grace, P. J. (2009). *Nursing ethics and professional responsibility in advanced practice.* Sudbury, MA: Jones & Bartlett.

Grace, P. J., & McLaughlin, M. (2005). Ethical issues: When consent isn't informed enough. *American Journal of Nursing, 105*(4), 79–84.

Grace, P. J., Willis, D. G., & Jurchak, M. (2007). Good patient care: Egalitarian interprofessional collaboration as a moral imperative. *American Society of Bioethics and Humanities Exchange, 10*(1), 8–9.

Hamric, A. (2000). What is happening to advocacy? *Nursing Outlook, 48*(3), 103–104.

Hickman, S. E., Hammes, B. J., Moss, A. H., & Tolles, S. W. (2005). Hope for the future: Achieving the original intent of advance directives. *Hastings Center Report, 35*(6), s26–s30.

International Council of Nurses (2006). *The ICN code of ethics for nurses.* Retrieved April 20, 2009, from http://www.icn.ch/ethics.htm

Jameton, A. (1984). *Nursing practice: The ethical issues.* Upper Saddle River, NJ: Prentice-Hall.

Mallik, M. (1998). Advocacy in nursing: Perceptions and attitudes of the nursing elite in the United Kingdom. *Journal of Advanced Nursing, 28*(5), 1000–1011.

Matloff, E., & Kaplan, A. (2008). Direct to confusion: Lessons learned from marketing BRCA testing. *American Journal of Bioethics, 8*(6), 5–8.

Mezey, M., Evans, L. K., Golub, Z. D., Murphy, E., & White, G. B. (1994). The patient self-determination act: Sources of concern for nurses. *Nursing Outlook, 42*(1), 30–38.

Miles, S. H., Koepp, R., & Webber, E. P. (1996). Advance end-of-life treatment planning. *Archives of Internal Medicine, 156,* 1062–1068.

Mohr, W. K., & Mahon, M. M. (1996). Dirty hands: The underside of marketplace healthcare. *Advances in Nursing Science, 19*(1), 28–37.

National Institutes of Health, Office of Human Subjects Research (1979). *The Belmont report: Ethical principles and guidelines for the protection of human subjects of research.* Retrieved May 6, 2009, from http://ohsr.od.nih.gov/guidelines/belmont.html

Nightingale, F. (1969). *Notes on nursing: What it is and what it is not* (rev. ed). New York: Dover Publications.

Oxford English Dictionary (1989). (2nd ed.). Oxford, UK: Clarendon.

Rachels, S. (2007). *The elements of moral philosophy* (5th ed.). New York: McGraw-Hill.

Rawls., J. (1971). *A theory of justice.* Cambridge, MA: Belknap, Harvard.

Romero, C. M. (2009). *Using medical interpreters.* Retrieved April 24, 2009, from http://www.translatorsbase.com/articles/37.aspx

Snoball, J. (1996). Asking nurses about advocating for patients: Reactive and proactive accounts. *Journal of Advanced Nursing, 24*(1), 67–75.

Spenceley, S. M., Reutter, L., & Allen, M. N. (2006). The road less traveled: Advocacy at the policy level. *Policy, Politics, and Nursing Practice, 7*(3), 180–194.

Thompson, I. E., Melia, K. M., & Boyd, K. M. (2000). *Nursing ethics* (4th ed.). New York: Churchill Livingstone.

Tschudin, V. (2006). How nursing ethics as a subject changes: An analysis of the first 11 years of publication of the journal of Nursing Ethics. *Nursing Ethics, 13*(1), 65–85.

Waters, C. M. (2000). End-of-life care directives among African-Americans: Lessons learned-a need for community-centered discussions and education. *Journal of Community Health Nursing, 17*(1), 25–37.

Wheeler, P. (2000). Is advocacy at the heart of professional practice? *Nursing Standard, 14*(36), 39–41.

Zaner, R. M. (1991). The phenomenon of trust and the physician-patient relationship. In E. D. Pellegrino, R. M. Veatch, & J. P. Langan (Eds.), *Ethics, trust and the professions* (pp. 45–67). Washington, DC: Georgetown University Press.

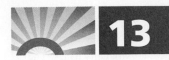

Health Care Informatics

TERESA L. PANNIERS, PhD, RN
SUSAN KAPLAN JACOBS, MLS, MA, RN, AHIP

OBJECTIVES

At the completion of this chapter, the reader will be able to:

- Discuss the implications of health care informatics for nursing practice.
- Outline, with examples, the use of advanced health care technologies used to support patient care.
- Describe components of the electronic health record.
- Discuss the issues of privacy, confidentiality, and security in data management.
- Compare the various nursing taxonomies used to document nursing's contribution to patient care.
- Discuss the evolution of the specialty of nursing informatics.
- Recognize that evidence-based nursing considers both internal and external sources of evidence as a foundation for best practice.
- Understand that scholarly information is gathered and arranged in standard formats and accessed by print or electronic indexes.
- Recognize that the Internet contains both scholarly and nonscholarly information and that critical evaluation is crucial.

PROFILE IN PRACTICE

Elizabeth A. Drew, MSN, RN
Critical Care Nurse, Inova Fairfax Hospital and The Inova Heart and Vascular Institute, Falls Church, Virginia

As a member of the bridge generation between Generation X and the Millennials, or the Digital Generation, I grew up as technology boomed and have little difficulty adjusting to its continued evolution. I was lucky to have an elder sibling who was a "computer whiz," and as a result, I had a more enriched exposure to computers than most of my peers. However, my passion was not technology. My heart and hands were always meant for caring. I dreamed of being a teacher or a doctor from a young age, but destiny led me to nursing, where I could simultaneously teach and heal. My ease with technology has followed me through life. Through high school and college and into my career as a nurse, I have always been seen as the go-to person for mentoring colleagues in new computer programs. My thirst for knowledge and my passion for nursing led me to seek a master's degree in nursing with a focus on administration. It was through this program that I became aware of the extensive opportunities for advanced practice in nursing, including informatics.

Nursing informatics links the caring of nursing with the effectiveness of technology. I have a vision of a future where health information systems are well accepted at the bedside, leading to greater efficacy in care and improved patient outcomes, where the bedside nurse is no longer hindered by technology's complexity but rather aided by its ability to improve time management. I have seen technology's influence

from applications that improve documentation at the bedside, translate trends of labs and vital signs into early sepsis identifiers, reduce wrong patient–wrong medication/lab/procedure errors, and more. In addition to these technologies, I believe that the electronic health record holds great potential for improving safety and the quality of patient care. Integrating informatics into the mainstream of education and practice is one of my goals for nursing. The inclusion of informatics in the practice arena offers great possibilities for the future of nursing.

Introduction

Professional nurses face two practice challenges in the 21st century: (1) the delivery of high technology client care and (2) the management and synthesis of vast amounts of health care information to formulate plans of care. Health care informatics provides a framework for evaluating technologies. Nursing informatics has emerged as a specialty practice area in an environment of interdisciplinary teams and patient-centered care. Although health care delivery and quality is greatly enhanced by the arrival of point-of-care technology, the electronic health record, and telehealth and clinical decision support systems, new challenges maintaining the privacy, confidentiality, and security of individual health care information have emerged. Additionally, these new technologies have advanced the development of nursing languages to support the classification of nursing's contributions to health care outcomes such as the nursing minimum data set and nursing taxonomies. Information literacy and evidence-based practice are the foundation for practice application and lifelong learning. Professional nurses must develop skills in accessing, synthesizing, and evaluating information from a variety of resources such as library searches, aggregate databases, and the Internet. This chapter provides an overview of these topics and basic skill sets for professional nurses to manage the advancements of the information age.

Health Care Informatics: A Driving Force for Nursing Practice

Mandel (1993) describes *health care informatics* as an umbrella term used to encompass the rapidly evolving discipline of using computing, networking, and communications—methodology and technology—to support the health-related fields, such as medicine, nursing, pharmacy, and dentistry. Health care informatics has evolved dramatically since the inception of computerization of data in the early 1960s. For example, hospital information systems were the mainstay of systems used in the 1970s. These systems were developed in response to a concern for reimbursement of the costs incurred by hospitalized individuals. Financial, charge-capture, and communication activities were carried out using mainframe computers that processed information in a centralized manner. In the 1980s, with the advent of personal computers, information was able to be processed in a decentralized manner. Nurses found that data related to critical elements of care could be captured and that the information gleaned could be used to improve nursing practice. A greater emphasis was placed on nursing information systems that defined and supported nursing care delivered at the bedside. Systems for care plans, documentation, and quality assurance were developed to support nursing practice. During the 1980s, systems also became more comprehensive, and attempts were made to integrate nursing data with data from other departmental systems.

The 1990s heralded the era of telecommunications, with the trend being one of open systems and communication over wide-area networks. The term *open systems* refers to the ability of different types of computers to communicate with one another. *Wide-area networks* refers to the linkage of computers located in different buildings in the same geographic area or, more broadly, across the country and around the world. As the 21st century progresses, ownership of information about health care options is increasingly being taken by consumers. In fact, Lynch (1999) describes a cultural revolution wherein the technologies of networked information will provide the enabling tools to allow consumers to have access not only to public information, but to most of the same information resources used by health care professionals. Increasingly, consumers will demand such information and will use it to make more informed choices about their health care options.

Nanotechnology is the next wave of technological revolution that will be seen in the field of health care. Staggers, McCasky, Brazelton, and Kennedy (2008) define *nanotechnology* as the use of atomic and molecular structures to create new health care treatments using therapeutic agents that are so tiny that it is difficult to imagine their actual size, approximately one hundredth the thickness of a sheet of paper at their largest. An example of a nanotechnological application in health care is the use of nanopatterned substrates to encourage the growth, regeneration, and repair of tissues (Taylor, 2002). In health care, the most immediate applications appear to be external tissue grafts, dental and bone replacements, internal tissue implants, and nanotechnologies embedded in medical devices and in vivo testing devices (Taylor, 2002). Although nanotechnology holds much promise for improved health care delivery, nurses caution that these new technologies must be tested thoroughly for safety because nanoparticles can be inhaled or absorbed through the skin (McCarthy, 2009). Nanotechnologies offer the opportunity for enhanced health care, and nurses are positioned at the forefront in the responsible use of these new applications.

THE SPECIALTY OF NURSING INFORMATICS

Within the field of health care informatics, nursing has developed the specialty of nursing informatics to delineate the contribution made by nurses in an environment of interdisciplinary teams and patient-centered care. *Nursing informatics* has been defined as a combination of computer science, information science, and nursing science designed to assist in the management and processing of nursing data, information, and knowledge to support the practice of nursing and the delivery of nursing care (Graves & Corcoran, 1989).

Staggers and Thompson (2002) note that in the three decades since the inception of the specialty of nursing informatics, several definitions to describe the specialty have been proposed, including definitions that are technology oriented, those that are conceptual in nature, and ones that focus on the role of nurses practicing nursing informatics. From this comprehensive analysis, Staggers and Thompson added to the definition of nursing informatics to include the concepts of integration of data, information, and knowledge to support patients. In addition, the authors recognized the importance of using technologies to support nurses' decision making (Staggers and Thomson, 2002, p. 260).

Most recently, the American Nurses Association (2008) has endorsed the concepts from informatics pioneers and describes the field of nursing informatics as follows:

> Nursing informatics (NI) integrates nursing science, computer and information science, and cognitive science to manage, communicate, and expand the data, information, knowledge, and wisdom of nursing practice. Nurses trained in NI support improved patient outcomes through their expertise in information processes, structures, and technologies, thus helping nurses and other care providers to create and record the evidence of their practice. (p. 1, para. 1)

As nurses interact with consumers and other health care providers, they use a vast array of information technologies to support and enhance the care provided to clients. Consider the following case study:

Mr. Lazarus has been undergoing cancer chemotherapy for treatment of lymphoma in an outpatient oncology center. Mr. Lazarus has been experiencing cancer-related fatigue for which he is being treated with erythropoietin–alpha (Visovsky & Schneider, 2003). In the past 24 hours, he has developed fever, chills, and pleuritic chest pain and is experiencing a productive cough. He has been admitted to the hospital for suspected pneumonia. On admission, the history of Mr. Lazarus's condition and the treatment regimen at the outpatient center are transferred electronically to establish an electronic client record.

On initial examination in the medical unit, the previous history and physical data are available to the resident physician, Dr. Cassidy, allowing him to update the client record with the information required to care for Mr. Lazarus during this acute episode of his illness. Following the initial workup, a chest x-ray is obtained and blood is drawn. While Mr. Lazarus is being evaluated by Nurse Matthews, the radiologist is reading the x-ray film and subsequently enters the results directly, using a point-of-care application that is part of a larger point-to-point integrated clinical information system. At the same time, the technician in the clinical laboratory is entering the results of the culture and sensitivity testing of the sputum sample directly into the integrated system.

Nurse Matthews and Dr. Cassidy are able to retrieve these results using the point-of-care system at the patient's bedside. Dr. Cassidy confirms the diagnosis and prescribes the appropriate antibiotic by entering it directly into the point-of-care system. The order is transmitted to the pharmacy, where it is immediately filled and transported to the unit, allowing Nurse Matthews to begin the antibiotic treatment. Nurse Matthews has been entering Mr. Lazarus's vital signs using a hand-held computer throughout the shift and is able to access a graphical depiction of the temperature, blood pressure, pulse, and respirations. She notes that his temperature is slowly returning to normal and his respirations are less rapid. In providing comprehensive care, Nurse Matthews logs into the database and queries the Nursing Interventions Classification related to care for patients receiving chemotherapy and receives information about nursing activities appropriate to this clinical condition.

Mr. Lazarus's pneumonia has subsided, and he has recovered enough to return home; yet he continues to experience cancer-related fatigue. Because he lives alone, a community health nurse initially follows his care at home. In addition to monitoring Mr. Lazarus's pulmonary and hematologic status through use of a point-of-care communication device that connects directly to the medical center, the community health nurse institutes therapies to combat the cancer-related fatigue. These interventions include receiving aromatherapy and foot soaks (Kohara et al., 2004), engaging in bedside physical therapy to prevent deconditioning (Crannell & Stone, 2008), setting priorities for essential activities, pacing his activities, and napping for short intervals as needed (Visovsky & Schneider, 2003). When Mr. Lazarus no longer requires the personal services of the community health nurse, he will be followed through a telehealth application for clinical consultations with specialists at the medical center. Mr. Lazarus makes use of a videophone that connects him directly to the medical center to receive medical and nursing care and advice. Mr. Lazarus continues to be treated directly at the medical center when needed, but his visits to the center are less frequent because he has gained access to the center via videophone.

This case study shows the seamless depiction, transmittal, and storage of data that are needed to provide the sophisticated level of care for Mr. Lazarus. Let's take a closer look at some of the many health care informatics applications integral to nursing that support this level of care.

POINT-OF-CARE COMPUTING

Point-of-care computing allows the health care practitioner to process patient care data at the point where the service is being provided. In Mr. Lazarus's case, the point-of-care computing took place in a variety of settings, including his bedside, the pharmacy, and the radiology department. Using point-of-care computing increases the accuracy of data capture, affords rapid processing, and decreases redundancy in record keeping. Point-of-care applications are becoming routine applications in health care settings. All point-of-care technologies rely on the concept of networking. *Networking* means that communications equipment is used to connect two or more computers and their resources (Capron & Johnson, 2004). Networks can be classified as local-area networks (LANs) or wide-area networks (WANs). A *local-area network* is a computer network in a hospital, a clinic, or an office. A *wide-area network* is a network that provides communication services to more than one hospital, clinic, or office.

As the use of point-of-care technologies increases, nurses are concerned with how these technologies affect their workflow patterns. For example, Whittemore and Moll (2008) analyzed nurses' opinions of the use of computers on wheels (COWs) as compared with workstations on wheels (WOWs) at All Children's Hospital in Florida. Nurses found many workflow problems with the COWs, including the small screen size; the heavy, burdensome equipment; the lack of adequate battery power; and finally, the lack of the ability to discern how much battery life was left in the computer. The technological and ergonomic problems with the COWs led to nurses avoiding the use of the computers on wheels altogether. After asking nurses what they look for in a mobile computer, overwhelmingly, the nurses asked for "mobile workstations that had a smaller footprint, a height-adjustable work surface, the ability to add or upgrade components as needed, and the ability to provide on-screen battery-charge status" (Whittemore & Moll, 2008, p. 34). When the information technology (IT) department installed the workstations on wheels (WOWs), nurses were quick to use the system and wanted to have a system at their fingertips at all times. In a similar vein, Anderson (2009) describes how mobile carts using networking as a point-of-care technology give nurses easy access to information systems, diagnostic equipment, bar code readers, laboratory specimen analysis, and diagnostic equipment. Nationally, nurses in a number of hospitals are using mobile systems, some consisting of tablets on carts to ease use on the patient unit. Lights over the mobile system's medication drawer enable nurses to retrieve drugs at night without turning on the light in the patient's room. These point-of-care systems offer nurses the ability to provide care at the patient's bedside while accessing all the relevant information needed to meet the patient's needs and to document the impact that nursing practice has on patient outcomes. Ultimately, the use of point-of-care computing enables a more efficient means of patient assessment and treatment. Using these technologies,

patients such as Mr. Lazarus have an increased likelihood of receiving quality, cost-effective care.

THE ELECTRONIC HEALTH RECORD

According to the Health Information Management Systems Society (HIMSS) (www.himss.org/ASP/topics_ehr.asp), the electronic health record (EHR) is a longitudinal electronic record of patient health information generated by one or more encounters in any care delivery setting. Included in this information are patient demographics, progress notes, problems, medication, vital signs, past medical history, immunizations, laboratory data, and radiology reports. The EHR automates and streamlines the clinician's workflow. It has the ability to generate a complete record of a clinical patient encounter, while also supporting other care-related activities directly or indirectly via interface, including evidence-based decision support, quality management, and outcomes reporting. All EHRs include administrative components. In addition, most commercial EHRs combine data from large ancillary services such as pharmacy, laboratory, and radiology. The EHR also contains clinical care components, including nursing plans, medication administration records (MAR), and computerized patient order entry (CPOE) (MITRE Corporation, 2006). Clinical decision support can also be built into the EHR. The administrative components of the EHR include such things as registration, discharge, and transfer (RADT) data. These data are key components of the EHR and can uniquely identify an individual based on name, demographics, next of kin, employer information, chief complaint, patient disposition, and other identifying data (MITRE Corporation, 2006).

Laboratory systems are designed to interface with the EHR using a unique identifier for each patient. Radiology systems tie together patient radiology data and images. Pharmacy systems are highly automated systems that provide medications in a streamlined way to patients. The pharmacy system has built-in alerts and can be used to prevent occurrences of adverse medication interaction and decrease the chance of a patient receiving the incorrect medication or incorrect dose of a medication. Computerized physician order entry allows physicians and other care providers to order laboratory, pharmacy, and radiology services electronically (MITRE Corporation, 2006). Clinical documentation is a valuable component of the EHR and can increase the quality of care received by patients while streamlining the workflow process for care providers. Some examples of clinical documentation include physician, nurse, and other clinician notes; flow sheets; perioperative notes; discharge summaries, advance directives or living wills; and medical record/chart tracking (MITRE Corporation, 2006). Medical devices can also be integrated into the EHR and can be used to provide patient alerts and up-to-date physiological data.

A major issue in the successful implementation of the EHR is the use of standards to describe, code, and translate each piece of data residing in the EHR. Because many EHR systems use modules or systems that interact with one another, it is imperative that data be coded using a standard format so that they are interoperable—that is, data can move seamlessly within the EHR and between and among the systems that interface with the EHR. Key standards needed within the EHR are "clinical vocabularies, healthcare message exchanges, and EHR ontologies (i.e., content and structure of the data entities in relation to each other)" (MITRE Corporation, 2006, p. 9). Several clinical vocabularies play a strategic role in providing access to computerized clinical information. In a subsequent section of this chapter, a description of nursing languages and vocabularies is provided to illustrate how standards are formulated for use within the EHR. Other clinical vocabularies that are standardized for use in the EHR include the International Classification of Disease (ICD), the Systematized Nomenclature of Medicine (SNOMED), and Health Level 7. In practical terms, once the data are organized and structured in a standardized manner for the EHR, these data are then available to support health care delivery, to enhance clinician workflow, and to document patient outcomes.

Electronic health records are implemented in a variety of ways in health care settings. In Mr. Lazarus's case, while he is being treated in the hospital, Nurse Matthews can access his EHR using a handheld device. At the same time the nurse can use other technologies such as a pulse oximeter and a blood analyzing system to ascertain physiological measures that can assist in her assessment of his health status. These technologies can be integrated in such a way that all data are automatically uploaded into Mr. Lazarus's EHR, which is maintained in a central location accessible through a hard-wired network.

Privacy, Confidentiality, and Security in the Electronic Health Record. Nurse Matthews uses the EHR with the understanding that Health Insurance Portability and Accountability Act (HIPAA) requirements must be met. The HIPAA Act of 1996 (Flores & Dodier, 2005) requires the development of privacy rules for the use of technologies that incorporate electronic data exchanges such as those in the EHR. Although HIPAA, as a regulatory mechanism for use of technologies, has been in existence since 1996, it remains a work in progress with nurses "at the forefront in the resolution of the dilemma of patient privacy versus health care expediency" (Flores & Dodier, 2005, p. 2). One of the intents of HIPAA was to construct a framework of protections around personal information in such a way as to increase public confidence in and support of EHRs (Williams et al., 2008). Components of care essential to compliance with HIPAA include "standardization of electronic health care transactions, identifiers for health care providers, and [enforcement of] a "Privacy Rule" that has an impact on all health care providers and health care plans that transmit health care information in electronic form" (Flores & Dodier, 2005, p. 2). More information about HIPAA is available online (www.hhs.gov/ocr/hipaa).

Privacy is an essential component of the EHR. Patient data are sensitive and, if breached, can have a negative impact on an individual's health and well-being. According to the Nurses Code of Ethics, "the need for health care does not justify unwanted intrusion into the patient's life" (American Nurses Association, 2001, p. 12; American Nurses Association, 2005, Provision 3.1). This statement forms the foundation for the issue of *privacy* in the electronic health record. Similarly, the Nurses Code of Ethics notes that "the nurse has the duty to maintain confidentiality of all patient information" (American Nurses Association, 2001, p. 12; American Nurses Association, 2005, Provision 3.2).

Security refers to putting in place mechanisms that protect health care data from being accessed willfully by unauthorized individuals and from being breached by accident. Electronic data systems are in some ways easier to protect than paper records, because authentication, authorization, and auditing (the key components of patient identity and data access management) are all facilitated (Myers, Frieden, Bherwani, & Henning, 2008). Authentication is the process of determining whether or not the person attempting to access data is authorized to do so. Authorization deals with levels of access to data; in the EHR, these levels can be restricted based on the need to access information in order to meet patients' needs. For example, highly sensitive data, such as HIV/AIDS information or substance abuse data can be restricted to the appropriate clinicians who need this information to provide appropriate care to the patient. The audit trail strengthens the EHR because it can reveal who has accessed data automatically in an electronic system, a capability that is not available with paper records.

Myriad methods exist for ensuring privacy, confidentiality, and security of data in the EHR. For example, Myers et al. (2008) suggest that for routine sensitive data, several security measures be employed, including having a high-level individual designated to oversee the confidentiality and security issues, creating a comprehensive agency confidentiality policy, conducting a periodic audit of data safety procedures, establishing a policy for provision and revocation of passwords, and encrypting data, monitoring use of printers, and requiring password protection on all wireless devices, portable media, desktops, laptops, and shared user drives. For highly sensitive data, the security issues are heightened. Some suggestions include performing a background check on all personnel handling highly sensitive data, maintaining highly sensitive data on stand-alone workstations, restricting access, performing video surveillance, and regularly auditing both user access and activity on computers containing sensitive information (Myers et al., 2008).

In summary, the provision of health care is greatly enhanced with the use of the electronic health record. However, using electronic data requires a high level of responsibility on the part of the patient, the care provider, and the institutions housing electronic data.

In our case study, Nurse Matthews works with Mr. Lazarus to use his health care data appropriately while maintaining security and confidentiality when using the data. Above all, Nurse Matthews respects Mr. Lazarus's privacy at all times and treats his personal data as part of his complete care plan, a plan that is handled with the greatest of care.

TELEHEALTH

Demiris, Doorenbos, and Towle (2009) define *telehealth* as "the use of videoconferencing and/or other telecommunication technologies to enable communication between patients and health care providers separated by geographical distance" (p. 128). Two primary modes of telehealth transmission are available: (1) interactive live video and (2) the store-and-forward method. The live method is much more costly than the store-and-forward method; this is a consideration in any telehealth application. Equipment required for telehealth includes a *computer platform,* which is the hardware and software combination that makes up the basic functionality of a computer; a *network protocol,* which is a set of rules for the exchange of data between two or more computers; and an LAN and/or a WAN that allows practitioners to share data and resources among several computers over a local or wide geographical area (Capron & Johnson, 2004). Patients such as Mr. Lazarus can benefit from telehealth applications that aim at promoting independence and empowerment (Demiris et al., 2009).

Many examples of successful telehealth applications have been developed by health care practitioners. For instance, Walsh and Coleman (2005) launched a pilot telehealth program for individuals with the diagnoses of heart disease and diabetes who reside in an area within a radius of approximately 20 miles from the main office of a visiting nurse association (VNA). Initially, patients were taught to use monitoring equipment to assess daily blood pressure, glucose, and other physiological measures related to their chronic conditions. The physiological measures gathered by the patient were used as the basis for health assessment during each telehealth encounter. Video with magnifying capabilities was used to assess wounds and to monitor healing and, furthermore, to allow a nurse to view the label on medication bottles currently being used by patients in their homes while the nurse remained in the VNA main office. A unique aspect of the system is the empowerment of older adult patients to participate actively in their care from the comfort of their own homes. The telehealth system used in this pilot project demonstrated cost savings, increased patient satisfaction, and maintenance of a level of independence that, ultimately, translates into improved health status and quality of life for older adult patients experiencing chronic health problems.

Switzer et al. (2009) describe a web-based telestroke system called Remote Evaluation of Acute Ischemic Stroke (REACH) that assists in the evaluation and treatment of individuals living in rural areas in Georgia who present with symptoms of acute stroke. The web-based system allows a stroke specialist to obtain a medical history, examine the patient with live video, and review computed tomography studies. The use of this telesystem has afforded patients the opportunity to receive tissue plasminogen activator (tPA) before being transported to a tertiary medical center. The system allows physicians to make clinical decisions based on actual physiological data rather than rely on treatment using the telephone alone. As a result, outcomes for these stroke patients have been greatly enhanced.

In another telehealth application, Balamurugan et al. (2009) describe a pilot study using a telesystem to offer a diabetes self-management system for patients with diabetes living in rural Arkansas. The telehealth platform consisted of T-1 connections between the larger university hospital and the rural private hospital. The program itself utilized a tele-educational unit consisting of a combination of didactic presentation, demonstration, and interactive discussions using the American Diabetes Association–recommended curriculum for diabetes education (Balamurugan et al., 2009). The program comprised six biweekly group sessions; of the 38 enrollees in the study, 25 individuals completed the program. These individuals demonstrated improved knowledge about their diabetes, indicated more self-efficacy, and reported more frequent self-care practices to manage their diabetes. The program demonstrated that education and disease management for chronic illnesses can be achieved through a telehealth application.

Returning once again to our case study, we can see how telehealth applications could assist Mr. Lazarus to obtain high-quality care, including interactions with specialists, by means of telecommunications and the efficient receipt and transfer of data to support the nursing care he is receiving at home. Also, Mr. Lazarus can receive support by communicating with a cancer support group using technologies such as an electronic chat room wherein cancer patients share information and advice with one another.

CLINICAL DECISION SUPPORT SYSTEMS

A *clinical decision support system* (CDSS) is another health care informatics application that assists nurses in providing quality patient care. Anderson and Willson (2008) described a CDSS as a computer application that matches patient characteristics with an expert knowledge base to provide a solution to a clinical problem using specific recommendations embedded in the system. A CDSS increases the nurse's decision-making effectiveness when he or she is faced with a complex clinical situation that has more than one plausible choice of treatment and a certain amount of risk associated with each of the treatment choices. CDSS may address a single complex problem, or it can be embedded within a clinical information system or an EHR to broadly address patients' clinical problems.

Anderson and Willson (2008) reviewed nursing CDSS to determine those systems that support evidenced-based practice for nursing care. Examples of systems that support evidenced-based care include a computerized emergency triage system called the Toowoomba Adult Triage Trauma Tool (TATTT) (Ely et al., 2005); a 24-hour telephone advice line developed for advising individuals to appropriate levels of health care in the United Kingdom (O'Cathain, Sampson, Munor, Thomas, & Nicholl, 2004); and a computer-assisted system for implementing clinical practice guidelines for pressure ulcer treatment (Clark et al., 2005).

The TATTT (Ely et al., 2005) was developed to provide an evidence-based method of triage assessment and classification of patients presenting for care in an emergency setting. The system used the Australasian

Triage Scale (ATS), which categorizes patients into five groups based on how severe and/or life-threatening the patient's presenting condition is. Using this scale, patients are triaged by indicating immediately life-threatening conditions (immediate care) to less urgent (care within 120 minutes). Ten triage nurses who used the computerized TATTT (Ely et al., 2005) in a simulated setting reported that the tool accurately assessed patients, was easy to use, and increased their confidence in triaging patients in an emergency setting.

In the United Kingdom, 24 nurses were studied using a CDSS system among 12 health care sites (O'Cathain et al., 2004). The system was devised to provide safe, consistent health care recommendations regarding the most appropriate health care service to contact or to advise self-care. Nurses in the study reported that the system provided consistency in decision making among nurses with different clinical backgrounds. However, nurses noted that the system was not able to consider contextual information such as chronicity of a health problem or past medical history. In this case, if deemed appropriate, nurses were able to override the software based on their own clinical decision-making skills. Overall, the study nurses felt that both the software and the nurse were essential to clinical decision making. They described a process of "dual decision making," with the nurse as active decision maker seeking confirmation or looking for agreement with the suggestions provided by the system.

The CDSS described by Clark et al. (2005) was aimed at addressing the specific complex problem of pressure ulcers, a clinical condition associated with a high level of patient suffering, as well as high health care costs. The automated CDSS implemented evidence-based clinical practice guidelines for treating pressure ulcers. The study was conducted among primary, secondary, and tertiary health care settings in a large urban health region in Canada. Nurses used the CDSS in seven health facilities (one acute, one extended care, four intermediate care, and one home care) to select optimal, evidence-based care strategies for treating pressure ulcers, as well as to record, analyze, and aggregate data related to the quality and costs of pressure ulcer treatment. The findings of

the study showed that although the system was perceived as helpful related to assessing risk for pressure ulcers and developing the appropriate plan of care, nurses experienced some technical difficulties with the system and these difficulties lowered the nurses' perception of the usability of the system. The authors concluded that with support from nursing leadership and attendance to mitigating technical difficulties, the system has potential for augmenting nurses' decision making in caring for patients with pressure ulcer and for providing data to guide evidence-based practice.

Although the systems described here demonstrate some of the positive aspects, as well as challenges, for nursing when engaging technology in the form of CDSS, with regard to Mr. Lazarus's case, it is likely that Nurse Matthews will use a broad CDSS for assistance in clinical decision making. Suppose Mr. Lazarus continues to experience fever, chills, and pleuritic chest pain despite the treatment for pneumonia that has been instituted. Nurse Matthews could use a clinical decision support system that is embedded in Mr. Lazarus's EHR to relate these specific clinical findings to the condition of lymphoma. In essence, Nurse Matthews would have available the combined knowledge of many experts in the field and would be able to get immediate, specific feedback to augment her own intuitive skills. A CDSS would provide Nurse Matthews with evidence-based, objective data to assist her in understanding how a differential diagnosis is made related to these new symptoms exhibited by Mr. Lazarus.

NURSING LANGUAGES

When considering applications such as point-of-care computing and telehealth, it is imperative that nurses record patient data using a standard language. Although the data, information, and knowledge required to provide client care may be derived from a number of sources, nursing leaders have begun to distinguish those elements that describe the unique contributions of nursing to the promotion of health of individuals, families, and communities. The Nursing Minimum Data Set and established nursing taxonomies are examples of the progress made toward defining the diagnoses, interventions, and outcomes that are directly attributable to nursing and provide input to health care informatics databases.

The Nursing Minimum Data Set. The Nursing Minimum Data Set (NMDS), developed at the University of Wisconsin–Milwaukee, was generated to acknowledge the contribution of nursing to client outcomes. As the importance of nationwide health databases increases, it is essential that a minimum number of essential nursing elements be included in those databases. The NMDS is defined as "a minimum set of items of information with uniform definitions and categories concerning the specific dimension of professional nursing, which meet the information needs of multiple data users in the health care system" (Werley, 1988, p. 7). The NMDS comprises a nursing diagnosis, nursing intervention, nursing outcome, intensity of nursing care measure, and health record number. The system also includes a unique identifier for the nurse provider and data elements in common with the Uniform Hospital Discharge Data Set (UHDDS). Because this system is compatible with the UHDDS, there is great potential for documenting nursing's contributions to health care to insurers, hospital decision makers, nurse administrators, chief information officers, chief nursing officers, and informatics nurse specialists. A major purpose of the NMDS is to establish a comparison of client-centered data that can be used to evaluate the effectiveness of nursing care among practice settings and geographic boundaries. The NMDS recognizes personnel delivering care, the type of nursing care provided, the impact of that care on client outcomes, and the costs of nursing care. This system can enhance greatly the ability of nursing to conduct research and to create health policy.

Nursing Taxonomies. Nursing taxonomies are languages that provide data that can complete the NMDS framework. In other words, the NMDS provides the structure for what data are needed to describe nursing practice, and the nursing taxonomies provide the specific data, which fall into large categories such as nursing diagnosis, interventions, and outcomes. Examples of the taxonomies that have been developed in nursing and that are recognized by the American Nurses Association (American Nurses Association,

2009a; Lundberg et al., 2008; Lunney, Delaney, Duffy, Moorhead, & Welton, 2005) include the North American Nursing Diagnosis Association (NANDA) taxonomy, the Nursing Interventions Classification (NIC), the Nursing Outcomes Classification (NOC), the Omaha Problem Classification, and the Clinical Care Classification System (CCCS). Information on other ANA-recognized taxonomies that may be useful for your specific area of clinical practice can be found online (www.nursingworld.org/MainMenuCategories/ThePracticeofProfessionalNursing/NursingStandards/DocumentationInformatics/NIDSEC/RecognizedLanguagesforursing.aspx).

The *NANDA classification system* was developed to standardize nomenclature for nursing diagnoses. The work began initially in 1973 when a group of nurses met at the first national conference. In 1982, after several national conferences, the North American Nursing Diagnosis Association was formalized (www.nanda.org). Development of NANDA diagnoses is an ongoing process as evidenced by the continued review and identification of new diagnoses for review including *allergy response* and *family anticipatory grieving* (Meyer, 2009).

Moorhead (2008) stated that "the Nursing Interventions Classification (NIC) is a comprehensive, research-based, standardized classification of interventions that nurses perform" (p. 27). The taxonomy consists of levels that classify nursing interventions initially as abstract domains, then as related sets of interventions, and finally as a very concrete set of intervention labels. Background readings are also provided to nurses for each of the interventions. Examples of interventions from the 5th edition of *Nursing Interventions Classification* that would assist Nurse Matthews in providing care for Mr. Lazarus (our case study) are provided in Table 13-1.

The *Nursing Outcomes Classification* (NOC) is a comprehensive, standardized classification of patient outcomes developed to evaluate the effects of nursing interventions (Moorhead, 2008). The 4th edition of the NOC is composed of 385 NOC outcomes grouped into 31 classes and 7 domains. Each outcome has a definition and a list of indicators to evaluate the effects of nursing care. The new edition includes 58 new outcomes, including examples such as burn healing, knowledge of

TABLE 13-1	Examples of Nursing Interventions Appropriate for Mr. Lazarus's Care Using the *Nursing Interventions Classification* (NIC) 5th Edition[*]
Nursing Intervention	**Definition**
Active listening	Attending closely to and attaching significance to a patient's verbal and nonverbal messages
Anxiety reduction	Minimizing apprehension, dread, foreboding, or uneasiness related to an unidentified source of anticipated danger
Case management	Coordinating care and advocating for specified individuals and patient populations among settings to reduce cost, reduce resource use, improve quality of health care, and achieve desired outcomes
Chemotherapy management	Assisting the patient and family to understand the action and minimize the side effects of antineoplastic agents
Coping enhancement	Assisting a patient to adapt to perceived stressors, changes, or threats that interfere with meeting life demands and roles
Environmental management: safety	Mentoring and manipulation of the physical environment to promote safety
Music therapy	Using music to help achieve a specific change in behavior, feeling, or physiology
Respiratory monitoring	Collection and analysis of patient data to ensure airway patency and adequate gas exchange
Infection protection	Prevention and early detection of infection in a patient at risk
Teaching: individual	Planning, implementation, and evaluation of a teaching program designed to address a patient's particular needs

From Bulechek, G. M., Butcher, H. K., & Dochertman, J. M. (2008). *Nursing Interventions Classification (NIC)*, 5th edition. St. Louis: Mosby.
[*]Interventions represent a sample from the list of 542 research-based nursing interventions.

preterm infant care, and community disaster response (Moorhead, 2008). Each of the outcomes included under a domain has a unique code for input into automated clinical information systems that can be used to provide evidence of the quality of care provided by nurses.

The *Omaha Problem Classification,* commonly referred to as the *Omaha System,* is a classification scheme used with clients treated in a community health setting. It consists of three components: the Problem Classification Scheme, the Intervention Scheme, and the Problem Rating Scale for Outcomes. Insofar as nurses provide the majority of community health care, this system has a direct impact on the provision of that care (Lundberg, et al., 2008; Martin & Norris, 1996; Martin & Scheet, 1992).

Saba's Clinical Care Classification (CCCS; formerly called the Home Health Care Classification System) consists of two interrelated terminologies: (1) nursing diagnoses and outcomes and (2) nursing interventions (Saba, 2009). The CCCS uses a framework of 21 care components that classify and code nursing diagnoses and interventions for assessing, documenting, and classifying home health and ambulatory care (www.sabacare.com). The major purpose of CCCS is to classify clients, predict resource requirements, and measure outcomes of care in the area of home health and ambulatory care.

Recently, nurses have found that in order to communicate their impact on patient care provided in a multidisciplinary manner, they must use standardized terminology within the EHR (Lundberg et al., 2008). Returning to our case study, Nurse Matthews can incorporate the standardized terms embedded in the various nursing taxonomies into Mr. Lazarus's EHR to demonstrate the impact of nursing care on the patient's outcomes of care. At the same time, Nurse

Matthews can communicate to other members of the health care team and to administrators the impact of nursing-related patient outcomes on the quality and costs of care.

Library Information Resources to Support Nursing Practice

In addition to the previously mentioned informatics technologies, Nurse Matthews has a world of information resources available to support her practice through health sciences library gateways. The principles set forth by the Institute of Medicine's *Crossing the Quality Chasm: A New Health System for the 21st Century* include 10 rules aimed at efforts to redesign the health system, including decision making that is "evidence-based" (Institute of Medicine, 2001). An understanding of how information is arranged, accessed, evaluated, and cited ("information literacy") is critical to connecting nursing research to practice. Basic computer competencies and information management skills are needed by all nurses practicing in the information environment that will include EHRs (Tiger Initiative, 2007; 2009).

Information resources may be accessible from remote sites, on the patient unit, from a personal computer, or from a hand-held device. Searching the journal literature and library catalogues is expedited by the use of information technology. Electronic databases, mostly accessed by subscription, are powerful tools for searching the journal literature by subject. A wide variety of documents, data, graphics, sound, video, and social networking tools are available on the Internet.

When Nurse Matthews leaves Mr. Lazarus's bedside she has the option of exploring these sources to retrieve information relevant to his nursing care. A literature search may be conducted to find research-based journal articles. Her institution may allow her to retrieve the full text of some of these electronically. She may already subscribe to electronic mailing lists or table-of-contents services and participate in online chat rooms or support groups for oncology nurses. She may access a web portal that integrates access to her e-mail, retrieves information from both free and fee-based databases, and assists her in organizing information. She may use the Internet to take advantage of distance learning opportunities to earn continuing education credits. The following sections explain more about using technology to retrieve and organize information.

Any discussion of information retrieval must begin with the concept of *information literacy:* understanding the basic architecture of information and the need for critical evaluation. Although nurses may be comfortable with computer applications for word processing, e-mail, presentation software, spreadsheets, and other applications, specialized skills are needed for effectively using electronic search tools.

Primary sources (e.g., research articles, books, dissertations) are those that contain original information, not previously published, and include the peer-reviewed journal literature. Secondary sources provide a synthesis of information published elsewhere (e.g., textbooks, newspaper articles, comments, letters, review articles, meta-analyses). Bibliographical databases (e.g., CINAHL, MEDLINE, PsycINFO) index the primary and secondary sources. Aggregated point-of-care resources may bundle both primary and secondary sources in one search interface.

USING LIBRARY ONLINE CATALOGUES AND READY REFERENCE INFORMATION

Library holdings are generally accessed by using online catalogues. In addition to titles of books owned, users may also ascertain the newspaper and journal titles to which a library subscribes. Information in published books is usually at least several years old and should be considered for *background* information in health topics. A nurse in search of a book-length history of palliative care, background on nursing ethics, leadership or trends, nursing theories, and so forth should start by using the library catalogue to locate background sources. Ready reference materials such as handbooks, manuals, directories, dictionaries, and encyclopedias can provide information on drugs, disease, history, trends, anatomy, and physiology and may be available in hard copy or via electronic books or a library's "e-book" collection. Another source of ready reference information is the Internet. Every day, more and more background information is readily available online. A metasite that evaluates and aggregates links for nurses, such as the Essential Nursing Resources list (Interagency Council on Information Resources in Nursing, 2007) or a consumer health site such as MedlinePlus (www.medlineplus.gov), can lead Nurse Matthews to dictionaries, patient teaching materials, illustrated encyclopedias, links to organizations, support groups, and much more.

USING JOURNAL ARTICLE DATABASES

A database is defined as "a usually large collection of data organized especially for rapid search and retrieval (as by a computer)" (Merriam Webster, 2009). Bibliographical or journal article databases contain records of journal articles, as well as selected book chapters, practice guidelines, research instruments, patient education materials, and other formats. The journal literature contains the most up-to-date findings of scholarly research and is crucial to supplement the background information gathered from books, as discussed above. Methods of access to article databases vary among institutions, but these resources are generally accessed through institutional license agreements. The most comprehensive coverage of nursing journals and journals aimed at the nursing audience is the CINAHL database (www.cinahl.com), which provides electronic access to more than 4000 journals in nursing, allied health disciplines, and alternative and complementary therapy journals dating from 1937 to the present. Selected journals are also indexed in the areas of consumer health and biomedicine, many with abstracts (CINAHL Information Systems, 2009). Although primarily a database of citations and abstracts, CINAHL also provides full text for selected state nursing journals and some newsletters, standards of practice, practice acts, government publications, research instruments, and patient education material. A sample search is detailed later in this chapter.

MEDLINE, the premier biomedical database (produced by the U.S. National Library of Medicine), indexes more than 5200 journals in medicine, nursing, dentistry, veterinary medicine, the health care system, and the preclinical sciences. Containing more than 16 million records dating back to 1949 (with some older citations), MEDLINE is available from a number of

commercial vendors and is also free online as PubMed (www.pubmed.gov). MEDLINE includes journals that are not indexed in CINAHL and is a necessary adjunct to CINAHL for comprehensive searching of the nursing literature.

When selecting any database, searchers should consider the period covered and how often a database is updated, as well as the type of literature indexed. PsycINFO, the database that indexes the literature of psychology (in some cases dating back to the 19th century), is a valuable adjunct to CINAHL and MEDLINE for many of the psychosocial aspects of health care. For example, information about a topic in palliative care might be related to ethical, legal, theological, economic, or historical literature, as well as the biomedical and psychosocial sciences. Many nursing topics encompass qualitative aspects of health that are not easily measured, such as anxiety, coping, attitudes, quality of life, and so forth. Consult with a librarian to identify databases that access interdisciplinary information and to find full-text collections licensed by institution. Other specialized databases useful to nurses include those presented in Table 13-2.

Database Citations. The building block of a database is the citation (or record), which has separate searchable fields (Box 13-1). The citation includes enough information for the searcher to locate the full article; specialized features of databases index selected additional information. The subject heading field displays the assigned descriptors or subject headings, which may be classified as "major" or "minor." These terms are assigned by professional indexers who review the articles. MEDLINE is based on the hierarchical MeSH vocabulary (the National Library of Medicine's Medical Subject Headings). CINAHL uses MeSH as the model for its thesaurus, but CINAHL also incorporates unique headings and publication types for concepts in nursing and allied health, including nursing specialties. MeSH descriptors are updated on a yearly basis by the National Library of Medicine as new concepts appear in the literature. For example, *telemedicine* was added to MeSH in 1993, and *palliative care* was introduced in 1996. Thesauri embedded in database programs are

TABLE 13-2	Key Bibliographical Databases for Nursing
Database/Years Covered/Producer	**Description**
CINAHL Database/1937–present Ebsco Information Services www.ebscohost.com/cinahl	Citations to articles in more than 4000 nursing, allied health disciplines, and alternative/complementary therapy journals, along with the publications of the American Nurses Association and the National League for Nursing. Full text for selected research instruments, journals, critical paths, and more. By subscription.
Cochrane Library/1993–present Cochrane Collaboration www.cochrane.org	Regularly updated databases include systematic reviews prepared and maintained by collaborative review groups. Also included are protocols for reviews currently being prepared (background, objectives, and methods of reviews in preparation). Abstracts are searchable free of charge. Full text by subscription.
MEDLINE/1966–present National Library of Medicine www.ncbi.nlm.nin.gov/pubmed	Premier biomedical database, with more than 16 million citations to articles on all health-related topics from more than 5200 journals. Free access from pubmed.gov and from many vendors.
PsycINFO/1887–present American Psychological Association www.apa.org/psycinfo	Covers the professional and academic literature in psychology and related disciplines. Includes records from the printed Psychological Abstracts plus material from Dissertation Abstracts International and other sources.
Social Sciences Citation Index (Part of the Web of Science) (SSCI)/1956–present Institute for Scientific Information www.isinet.com	International multidisciplinary index to the literature of the social, behavioral, and related sciences, including many nursing topics. Features the ability to search cited references to track literature forward in time.
Virginia Henderson International/1983–present www.nursinglibrary.org	Searchable abstracts for the Registry of Nursing Research database, contributed by nurse researchers internationally. Includes contact information for principal investigators, connecting library users with other nurses with similar research interests.

used to help searchers translate or "map" language to the preferred term. A searcher who enters the term *end-of-life care* is directed to the MeSH or CINAHL term *terminal care*. Scope notes (definitions of terms) are also available online and may suggest related terms to expand a search, such as *hospice care* or *palliative care*. Searchers have the option of selecting broader terms, or they may choose to "explode" the search to include narrower terms. For example, narrower terms under the CINAHL heading *fatigue* include *cancer fatigue* and *fatigue syndrome, chronic*.

In addition to the assigned MeSH or CINAHL terms, subheadings are often attached. In the CINAHL example shown in Box 13-1, the subheading *adverse effects* has been appended to the subject heading *chemotherapy, cancer*. Other access points or fields

(e.g., author, words in the title or abstract, journal title, institution) may be used for retrieval. In the 2003 record shown, *cancer-related fatigue* is searchable as a key word in the title and abstract fields.

Search Strategies. A search strategy begins by stating a problem in the form of a question. For example: *What are the research-based strategies for management of cancer chemotherapy-related fatigue?* The main concepts in the question relate to the problem: the patient with chemotherapy/cancer-related fatigue. This question must next be translated into appropriate search terms in the database. Boolean operators (connectors) serve as powerful tools to shape retrieval: these connectors are *AND* and *OR* (Figure 13-1, *A, B*). A search command that uses the word *AND* between two terms

BOX 13-1	A Sample Record from CINAHL

The search command *chemotherapy, cancer AND fatigue* would retrieve this citation because both terms are present as CINAHL subject headings. A key word search on *cancer-related fatigue* would also retrieve this citation because the phrase is found in the title as well as in the abstract.

Title: Cancer-related fatigue

Authors: Visovsky C; Schneider SM

Source: Online Journal of Issues in Nursing (ONLINE J ISSUES NURS), 2003 Sep 30; 8(3).

Publication type: journal article—research, systematic review, tables/charts

Major Subjects
Fatigue
Neoplasms—Complications

Minor Subjects
Anemia—Complications
Anemia—Etiology
Anxiety
Attention
Cancer Pain—Complications
Chemotherapy, Cancer—Adverse Effects
Combined Modality Therapy—Adverse Effects
Coping; Energy Conservation
Fatigue—Prevention and Control
Fatigue—Psychosocial Factors
Fatigue—Symptoms
Fatigue—Therapy

Information Needs
Nursing Practice, Evidence-Based
Patient Assessment
Patient Education
Quality of Life
Questionnaires
Radiotherapy—Adverse Effects
Self-Care
Sleep Disorders
Therapeutic Exercise

Abstract
Approximately 1.3 million people in the United States will be diagnosed with cancer in 2003, and millions of other individuals are already living with the disease. Fatigue continues to be the most prevalent and disruptive symptom of cancer and its treatment regimens. Fatigue was the most frequent and distressing cancer-related symptom occurring in women with lung cancer, two times greater than the next symptom, pain, and remains one of the most common symptoms in newly diagnosed lung cancer patients at any stage of the disease. There are many causes of cancer-related fatigue, including preexisting conditions, physical and psychological symptoms caused by cancer, and the consequences of cancer treatment. High levels of fatigue decrease quality of life, physical functional status, and symptom management. This article presents an evidence-based review of cancer-related fatigue, strategies for the management of cancer-related fatigue, and recommendations for clinical practice.

dictates that *both* terms must be in the retrieved record. In this example, a search for *chemotherapy, cancer AND fatigue* would retrieve the record shown in Box 13-1, along with other citations. Use of the *OR* connector retrieves records that contain *either* term and is often used with synonyms to expand the search results; for example, *fatigue OR lethargy OR sleepiness* (Figure 13-1, *C*).

Search strategies for limiting retrieval in databases such as MEDLINE and CINAHL include using the focus feature to retrieve articles that have been determined to have the subject heading as a major focus of the article. In the example shown, both *fatigue* and *neoplasms* are classified as "major subjects" of the citation. "Publication type" can be a powerful indicator of the level of evidence retrieved. Look for

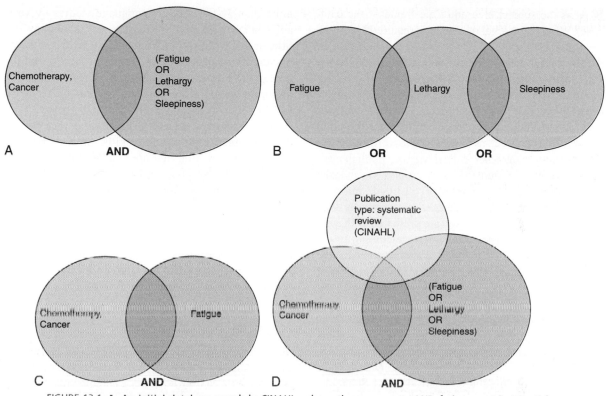

FIGURE 13-1 **A,** An initial database search in CINAHL—*chemotherapy, cancer AND fatigue*—retrieves articles with both terms present in the citation. See Box 13-1. **B,** An expanded search uses *OR* to string synonyms together. *Fatigue OR lethargy OR sleepiness* broadens the search to include articles with any of the terms in the citation. **C,** A search on *chemotherapy, cancer AND (fatigue OR lethargy OR sleepiness)* retrieves results with *chemotherapy, cancer AND* any of the synonyms that are connected by *OR*. **D,** The search results may be further reduced by other categorical limits, such as "publication type: systematic review," in CINAHL.

the database feature to "revise a search" or "limit a search." Limiting search results will filter for a higher level of evidence—for example, limit by publication type ("research" or "systematic review" in CINAHL), by article type ("clinical trial" or "meta-analysis" in MEDLINE), or by using the PubMed version of MEDLINE ("special queries" or the "find systematic reviews" feature). The sample citation indicates that the article is "research" and a "systematic review," meaning that it provides a strong level of evidence. Thus a CINAHL search on *chemotherapy, cancer AND fatigue,* limited to the publication type "systematic review" would retrieve the citation shown in Box 13-1, along with other citations that meet the search criteria (Figure 13-1, *D*) (Visovsky & Schneider, 2003).

Year of publication and age groups are other attributes that may be used to limit searches. An effective strategy is to locate an article that is highly relevant and make note of the other subject headings describing it to generate ideas for a new search. For instance, if a searcher views records retrieved and notices the subject headings *chemotherapy, cancer/adverse effects,* the searcher can then use that search string to search for related articles. Related subjects for searching might include *energy conservation, coping, quality of life, anemia, lethargy, sleepiness,* or *sleep disorders.* The literature search process is iterative—that is, often a literature search is revised several times on the basis of the information gained from the initial retrieval. Remember to reassess: What database was searched?

What is the subject area and time frame of the database? What is the level of evidence required?

Aggregated Information Resources for Nursing and Biomedical Information. Searching the databases described above will retrieve primary research studies, as well as higher levels of evidence such as presynthesized sources suitable for the point of care. Journals such as *Evidence-Based Nursing* and *Worldviews on Evidence-Based Nursing* publish evaluated abstracts of studies. These articles are indexed in CINAHL and are examples of "distilled" information sources; the original studies meet rigorous criteria based on research methods and are presented with evaluated abstracts by expert clinicians (McKibbon, 1998). Some specialized databases contain consolidated information sources, which synthesize the findings of many studies (e.g., systematic reviews or meta analyses). The *Cochrane Database of Systematic Reviews* includes many nursing topics and is the result of an international collaboration (Cochrane Collaboration, 2009). Systematic review articles are also published by other journals (e.g., the article in the *Online Journal of Issues in Nursing* by Visovsky and Schneider in Box 13-1). Clinical practice guidelines (statements published by many organizations to provide synthesized evidence for specific clinical circumstances) are often available on the Internet. The National Guideline Clearinghouse is a repository for guidelines that provides syntheses and expert commentaries, as well as the ability to compare several guidelines on similar topics (National Guideline Clearinghouse, 2009). A search on *chemotherapy fatigue* retrieves results that include a guideline published by the American Cancer Society, including measures to counteract chemotherapy fatigue (National Guideline Clearinghouse, 2006). See Table 13-2 for additional sources.

Another way to locate clinical practice guidelines is to search CINAHL and limit results by publication type ("practice guideline") or search MEDLINE and limit results by article type ("practice guideline"). The Sigma Theta Tau Registry of Nursing Research is a unique resource that contains abstracts of studies (submitted by nurse researchers) that may be unpublished or in progress. Available from the Virginia Henderson International Nursing Library, this resource indexes more than 11,000 English-language studies by variables or phenomenon of study, as well as by author, title, or key words provided by the researchers (www.nursinglibrary.org). Studies are not peer reviewed for quality. The individual registrant is responsible for providing enough information about his or her work to allow users to evaluate relevance and quality.

Aggregated resources are also available as collections of nursing procedures, skills, links to articles, and drug information that are bundled into one interface, licensed by your institution's library. Ebsco's *Nursing Reference Center* and Lippincott's *Nursing Procedures and Skills* are two examples. This type of "one-stop shopping" is useful but may be limited to one collection of articles, drug lists, or tools. Nurses should pay particular attention to notice when a resource was last updated. A search for evidence often requires the thoughtful exploration of many types of resources.

Links to Full Text. Whether free on the World Wide Web or available for a fee, bibliographical databases may include selected links to the full text of journal articles. Selected articles may be freely available online at sites such as PubMedCentral (PMC) (www.pubmedcentral.nih.gov), the U.S. National Institutes of Health digital archive (http://publicaccess.nih.gov), or the Directory of Open Access Journals (www.doaj.org). Consult a librarian at your institution to explore access to full-text links and full-text electronic journals and archives, as well as options for interlibrary loan and document delivery.

Critical Appraisal. The final step in the search for evidence is to critically appraise the evidence retrieved. Often a searcher will determine the usefulness of an article from viewing the citation and the abstract. However, reading the full text of an article is necessary to adequately evaluate therapeutic interventions, outcomes, and strength of the evidence presented. Critical appraisal of evidence includes viewing the Methods section of a paper and addressing the following issues: Was the study original? About whom is the study? Was the design of the study sensible? Was the study adequately controlled? Was the study large enough? Was it continued for long enough? Was follow-up complete? (Greenhalgh, 2006)

Tools for critical appraisal are freely available on the Internet and can assist nurses in the critical evaluation process. Examples include the CASP tools (www. phru.nhs.uk/Pages/PHD/CASP.htm), a set of appraisal tools for specific types of research articles, and the AGREE tool (www.agreecollaboration.org/pdf/agreei nstrumentfinal.pdf), an appraisal instrument for clinical practice guidelines.

Evidence-Based Practice. Evidence-based nursing is defined as "the application of valid, relevant, research-based information in nurse decision-making ... used alongside our knowledge of our patients (their symptoms, diagnoses, and expressed preferences) and the context in which the decision is taking place (including the care setting and available resources), and in processing this information we use our expertise and judgement" (Cullum, 2008, p. 2).

The database citations and article information we have discussed above are sources of *external* evidence, published resources such as articles, synopses, practice guidelines, and government or association websites. In addition to the external evidence that informs decision making, *internal* evidence, consisting of local data, patient circumstances, resources, and experience of clinicians, also inform practice (Stetler, 2001). The best external evidence may be superseded by the individual circumstances of a patient, the available resources, and the judgment of the clinician. Information-literate consumers are able to view any piece of evidence in the larger context of both the internal and external evidence.

CONSUMER HEALTH INFORMATION

In their role as health educators, nurses encounter clients who have become more proactive about retrieving information. Nurses "support and educate consumers to be effective participants in their own care" and need to respond to more informed consumers (Lamm, 1998, p. 92). CINAHL, MEDLINE, and other bibliographical databases of scholarly literature are *not* the optimal databases for consumers in search of health information. Patients are often in need of reassurance (good news) and are not likely to differentiate a case study from a clinical trial. The National Library of Medicine's site MedlinePlus (www.medlineplus.gov)

provides a mediated interface to selected topics in MEDLINE; this is an example of one site to which consumers should be directed rather than to MEDLINE.

The Internet

The above section has emphasized the importance of using bibliographical databases as the first step to accessing scholarly information. However, information oriented toward health care professionals may be unsuitable, misleading, or even potentially harmful for a lay audience. Non–peer-reviewed materials lack quality control and may be out of date or incorrect.

Many users share the misperception that everything is available on the Internet and that everything is free. Users frequently use the terms or phrases "on the Internet," "online," and "available electronically" interchangeably, but the discussion of bibliographical databases earlier in this chapter illustrates that all digital resources are not equal—and users will not find most of the databases of the peer-reviewed scholarly literature freely available. Although the Internet may be its mode of transmission, scholarly, peer-reviewed literature is expensive to produce and organize, and most bibliographical databases and full-text electronic journals are only obtained by license arrangements as institutional subscriptions. Many journal publishers offer free online versions of their continuing education articles or partial access to current or archived titles, but comprehensive searchers cannot rely on this fraction of the literature. Unlike library catalogues and other databases, the web is not organized according to any one scheme (although the information contained at any individual site may be an organized database). No individual organization owns, monitors, or controls the Internet. No controlled vocabulary exists. As a result, finding information can be challenging and requires combining strategies.

NAVIGATING THE WEB

Consumers, as well as professionals, are faced with a daily barrage of media attention focused on the Internet. Ever-present how-to articles in popular magazines and newspapers (as well as in the scholarly literature) offer tips for users and also provide warnings. One strategy for searching the Internet is to find sites where respected searchers have evaluated the content. Selected metasites for nursing information, such as the Hardin Meta Directory of Nursing Internet Sites (www.lib.uiowa.edu/hardin/md/nurs.html), Essential Nursing Resources (Interagency Council on Information Resources in Nursing, 2009), or Nursing on the Net from the National Library of Medicine (http://nnlm.gov/training/nursing/sampler.html), provide a starting point for subject-oriented sites.

Search engines (e.g., Bing, Google, the subset http://scholar.google.com) use software "spiders" or "robots" that crawl electronically to collect websites and then add them to a catalogue. Using a search engine is similar to searching the index of a book. The searcher enters a word, and the engine retrieves records with key words matching the term entered. Although valuable for obscure terms, key word searching may result in large, unwieldy lists, and terms may be retrieved out of context. For instance, a search on the term "nursing" may retrieve links to organizations such as the American Nurses Association, as well as random links to sites for medical uniforms or the word "nursing" in another context (e.g., breastfeeding, nursing homes). Each search engine has its own rules for determining how sites are indexed and how the results are ranked (listed) according to relevance. Some give a higher ranking to sites based on a term's frequency of occurrence in the retrieved document; others may consider whether the term is found in a title versus in the body of the page. Search engines have different rules for entering a search string, for using Boolean connectors, and for using quotation marks for phrases, truncation symbols, and so forth. Some search engines also include a subject directory of the included sites (e.g., http://directory.google.com); such a directory presents a searchable menu of subjects, similar to browsing the table of contents of a book. The user should look for a "Help" link on the search engine's home page to determine how to enter a search. Searchers should always consider using several search tools because no individual search engine covers the entire contents of the Internet.

The web contains many rich sources of information that are not accessed by search engines. This is a category referred to as the "deep web" or the "invisible web." In addition to "gated" sites, which are accessed only by authentication as a subscriber, many free sites and contents of free databases are invisible to standard search engines. Although a known citation to a journal article might be located using a tool such as Google, a comprehensive search for scholarly literature is best done using the full functionality available with specialized databases such as MEDLINE, CINAHL, and related sources described earlier.

EVALUATING THE WEB

Critical evaluation is a crucial step in any search for information on the World Wide Web. Unlike the scholarly peer-reviewed literature organized into journals and cited in standard records by the bibliographical databases, the web contains documents in many nonstandard formats contributed by nonscreened sources and unevaluated for quality. As the web evolves, steps are being taken to ensure consistency and establish standards. The Health on the Net (HON) Foundation, a not-for-profit international collaboration, has published a code of conduct that suggests standards for producers of health information websites (www.hon.ch/HONcode/Conduct.html).

Basic, agreed-upon criteria for evaluating websites exist. As health professionals interacting with patients, nurses need to be alert to the context in which information is presented. Patients reading information intended for professionals may misinterpret information; the information may not be false, but it may still do harm (Eysenbach & Diepgen, 1998). Also, even though a website may have been modified recently, the information may still not be up to date. Nurses should approach all information critically and use criteria such as that in Table 13-3 to evaluate websites.

Strategies for Managing Information

Electronic access to information for both professionals and consumers provides a rich resource for up-to-date access, as well as a way to deal with the challenge of managing information overload. An effective strategy for nurses is to begin by subscribing to several relevant

TABLE 13-3	Criteria for Evaluating Health Information on the Internet
Content	What is the scope of the site?
	What does it purport to cover?
	If it's a database, what years are covered?
Audience	Who is the intended audience? Health professionals? Health consumers?
	What is the context?
Authority	Who is the creator?
	What are the creator's credentials?
	Is the site based at or affiliated with an institution?
Accuracy	Is the author qualified to write this document?
	Are references cited?
	Can the same information be verified elsewhere?
Purpose/Objective	Is the site an opinion? For profit? For education? For self-promotion?
	For advertising? What is the bias?
Structure/Organization	What does the site look like?
	Is it readable and well organized?
	Can users get to linked information in three clicks or fewer?
Currency	When was the site last updated?
	When was the content updated?
	Are the links active and up to date?

Data from Goldsborough, R. (1999). Net savvy. Information on the net often needs checking. *RN, 62*(5), 22, 24; Hodson-Carlton, K., & Dorner, J. L. (1999). An electronic approach to evaluating healthcare web resources. *Nurse Educator, 24*(5), 21; Kapoun, J. (1998). Teaching undergrads WEB evaluation: A guide for library instruction. *College and Research Libraries News, 59*(7), 522-523; Silberg, W. M., Lundberg, G. D., & Musacchio, R. A. (1997). Assessing, controlling, and assuring the quality of medical information on the internet: Caveant lector et viewor—let the reader and viewer beware. *JAMA, 277*(15), 1244–1245; Walther, J. H., & Speisser, N. (1997). Developing and delivering medical reference source instruction in a special library. Retrieved from www.library.ucsb.edu/istl/97-fall/article2.html.

electronic mailing lists or discussion forums in a relevant specialty (University at Buffalo School of Nursing, 2009). The American Nurses Association provides free online resources for nursing students (American Nurses Association, 2009b). Current news on nursing and health care issues can be delivered directly to your e-mail in-box. As patient advocates, nurses can use Internet directories to locate support groups for patients, including online support groups for homebound patients. Journal table-of-contents services (which send a journal's table of contents by e-mail) may be available from individual websites, journal publishers, or by subscription. Blogs such as "In Our Own Words: Medscape Nursing" (http://blogs.medscape.com/nurses/) allow nurses to post entries and share professional experiences. RSS feeds can be subscribed

from many sites of interest, such as the National Guideline Clearinghouse (mentioned earlier). Also widely available are guidelines for setting up a "feed reader," such as those found at the Lippincott website (www.nursingcenter.com/rss/rssfeed.asp). Options for customizing a web portal or news reader (e.g., www.reader.google.com) are available at many institutions or search engine sites. Online social networks such as Nurse Connect (www.nurseconnect.com) may offer job information, networking opportunities continuing education opportunities, and support.

As nurses explore available content on the web, both free and fee based, it is wise to "bookmark" websites that are helpful (i.e., mark them as favorites) as a way to begin to customize an information gateway. Portals provide users with multiple services (e.g., e-mail, blogs, chat rooms, journals and databases, news links). One example is WebMD, a site that blends peer-reviewed content with news items, "sponsored content," and advertising (www.webmd.com/about-webmd-policies/about-editorial-policy).

CITING SOURCES

Acknowledging and properly citing literature retrieved are essential to demonstrate information literacy competency. Avoiding plagiarism requires citing the source of any thoughts, ideas, and writing that are not your own. Review the code of conduct posted on your institution's website; be sure you understand the habits to avoid plagiarism; and learn how and when to properly attribute material to secondary sources. A free web tool such as Noodle Tools (www.noodletools.com) can be used to format and generate references to adhere to particular style elements such as those required by MLA (Modern Language Association) or APA (American Psychological Association, 2009). More advanced bibliographical management tools (e.g., EndNote, Reference Manager, Refworks) may be available at your institution or can be purchased to assist nurses in building a personal database of articles and information retrieved and formatting bibliographies in standard styles. A free web tool such as Zotero (www.zotero.org) can provide similar functionality.

SUMMARY

In this age of high-technology client care, nursing practice makes use of sophisticated technologies to provide care and also requires vast amounts of information to formulate plans of care. Nurses must synthesize information efficiently to support and enhance their practice. To strengthen nursing practice, nurses must evaluate technologies within the framework of health care informatics to discern the effects of these technologies in producing high-quality outcomes for patients. Nurses must be educated consumers of information resources and active participants in developing practice innovations resulting from the use of information technology. Information technology has dramatically changed the environment of information retrieval and will no doubt

continue to evolve. Nurses need a foundation in the principles of information literacy and evidence-based practice to continue to apply new forms of technology and to build on them for lifelong learning. By undertaking these actions, nurses will be sought to fill leadership positions in the provision of client care in the information age.

KEY POINTS

- Health care informatics will be used to support and enhance nursing practice in the 21st century.
- Nurses will use advanced technologies such as point-of-care systems, telehealth, and decision support systems to provide comprehensive care to clients.
- Consumers will use networking technology to gain access to information that will enable them to make informed choices about their health care options.
- The use of the electronic health record will proliferate, and nurses will be challenged to maintain the privacy, confidentiality, and security of patients' health data.
- Nursing will experience rapid developments in information technology and will need to integrate these developments into practice.
- Nursing will continue to be challenged to develop its nursing language through systems such as the Nursing Minimum Data Set, the North American Nursing Diagnosis Association Taxonomy, the Nursing Interventions Classification, the Nursing Outcomes Classification, the Perioperative Classification System, the Omaha Problem Classification, and the Home Health Care Classification of Nursing Diagnoses and Interventions.
- Information systems are used to support nurses' clinical decision making and critical thinking.
- Integrated management systems are used to support the effective administration of nursing practice in a variety of settings.
- Nurses will continue to communicate globally by using the Internet to enhance education, practice, and research.
- Evidence-based practice brings together both external and internal sources of information as the basis for patient care, with improved outcomes as its goal.
- Information retrieved online requires careful critical evaluation. No formal peer-review process regulates the quality or accuracy of what is posted online.
- Online information is available for free or for a fee. Most of the full-text scholarly literature is accessible in specialized databases available by institutional subscription or for a fee.

CRITICAL THINKING EXERCISES

1. Consider how you would use the electronic health record (EHR) to access, process, retrieve, and store patient care data in your agency. How would using the EHR affect your workflow and patient outcomes?
2. Review the nursing taxonomies in this chapter. Which of these taxonomies best fits with your own practice? Why?
3. Conduct a search in a bibliographical database such as CINAHL. Compare results with those found through a similar search in another database such as PubMed. Based on your comparison, consider how coverage for nursing topics varies among databases.
4. Use an Internet search engine (e.g., www.google.com) to search for a phrase. Evaluate several of the retrieved sites based on the evaluation criteria provided in Table 13-3.
5. Compare the information found at a website with that found in a scholarly journal article. How is it organized, cited, and arranged?

REFERENCES

American Nurses Association. (2001). *Nurses Code of Ethics with Interpretive Statements.* Washington, DC: Author.

American Nurses Association. (2005). *Nurses Code of Ethics with Interpretive Statements.* Retrieved July 19, 2009, from http://www.nursingworld.org/ethics/code/protected/_nwcoe813.htm

American Nurses Association. (2008). *Nursing informatics: Scope and standards of practice.* Washington, DC: Author.

American Nurses Association. (2009a). *Recognized languages for nursing.* Retrieved July 15, 2009, from http://www.nursingworld.org/MainMenuCategories/ThePracticeofProfessionalNursing/NursingStandards/DocumentationInformatics/NIDSEC/RecognizedLanguagesfornursing.aspx

American Nurses Association. (2009b). *Student nurses.* Retrieved May 6, 2009, from http://www.nursingworld.org/EspeciallyForYou/NursingStudents.aspx

American Psychological Association. (2009). *Homepage APA style.* Retrieved May 7, 2009, from http://www.apastyle.org

Anderson, H. J. (2009). Hospital tune up cart strategies. *Health Data Management 17*(2), 34, 36, 38.

Anderson, J. A., & Willson, P. (2008). Clinical decision support systems in nursing. *CIN: Computers, Informatics, Nursing, 26*(3), 151–158.

Balamurugan, A., Hall-Barrow, J., Blevins, M. A., Brech, D., Phillips, M., Holley, E., & Bittle, K. (2009). A pilot study of diabetes education via telemedicine in a rural underserved community opportunities and challenges: A continuous quality improvement process. *The Diabetes Educator, 35*(1), 147–154.

Bulechek, G. M., Butcher, H. K., & Dochterman, J. M. (2008). *Nursing Interventions Classification (NIC)* (5th ed.). St. Louis: Mosby.

Capron, H. L., & Johnson, J. A. (2004). *Computers: Tools for an information age* (8th ed.). Upper Saddle River, NJ: Pearson Education.

CINAHL Information Systems. (2009). *CINAHL database.* Retrieved May 30, 2009, from http://www.ebscohost.com/cinahl

Clark, H. F., Bradley, C., Whytock, S., Handfield, S., van der Wal, R., & Gundry, S. (2005). Pressure ulcers: Implementation of evidence-based nursing practice. *Journal of Advanced Nursing, 49*(6), 578–590.

Cochrane Collaboration. (2009). *The Cochrane Library.* Retrieved May 6, 2009, from http://cochrane.org

Crannell, C. E., & Stone, E. (2008). Bedside physical therapy project to prevent deconditioning in hospitalized patients with cancer. *Oncology Nursing Forum, 35*(3), 343–345.

Cullum, N. (2008). *Evidence-based nursing: An introduction.* Oxford: Blackwell.

database. (2009). In Merriam-Webster Online Dictionary. Retrieved August 24, 2009, from http://www.merriam-webster.com/dictionary/database

Demiris, G., Doorenbos, A. Z., & Towle, C. (2009). Ethical considerations regarding the use of technology for older adults. The case of telehealth. *Research In Gerontological Nursing, 2*(2), 128–136.

Ely, D., Hegney, D., Wollaston, A., Fahey, P., Miller, P., McKay, M., & Wollaston, J. (2005). Triage nurse perceptions of the use, reliability and acceptability of the Toowoomba Adult Triage Trauma Tool (TATTT). *Accident and Emergency Nursing, 13,* 54–60.

Eysenbach, G., & Diepgen, T. L. (1998). Towards quality management of medical information on the internet: Evaluation, labelling, and filtering of information. *BMJ, 317*(7171), 1496–1502.

Flores, J. A., & Dodier, A. (2005). HIPAA: Past, present and future implications for nurses. *Online Journal of Issues in Nursing, 10*(2). Retrieved August 1, 2009, from http://www.nursingworld.org/MainMenuCategories/ANAMarketplace/ANAPeriodicals/OJIN/TableofContents/Volume102005/No2May05/tpc27_416020.aspx

Goldsborough, R. (1999). Net savvy. Information on the net often needs checking. *RN, 62*(5), 22, 24.

Graves, J., & Corcoran, S. (1989). The study of nursing informatics. *Image: Journal of Nursing Scholarship, 21,* 227–231.

Greenhalgh, T. (2006). *How to read a paper: The basics of evidence-based medicine* (2nd ed.). London: BMJ.

Hodson-Carlton, K., & Dorner, J. L. (1999). An electronic approach to evaluating healthcare web resources. *Nurse Educator, 24*(5), 21.

Institute of Medicine. (2001). Committee on Quality of Health Care in America. *Crossing the quality chasm: A new health system for the 21st century.* Retrieved March 29, 2009, from http://www.iom.edu/File.aspx?ID=27184

Interagency Council on Information Resources in Nursing. (2009). *Essential nursing resources.* Retrieved March 15, 2010, from http://www.icirn.org

Kapoun, J. (1998). Teaching undergrads WEB evaluation: A guide for library instruction. *College and Research Libraries News 59*(7), 522–523.

Kohara, H., Miyauchi, T., Suehiro, Y., Ueoka, H., Takeyama, H., Morita, T. (2004). Combined modality treatment of aromatherapy, footsoak, and reflexology relieves fatigue in patients with cancer. *Journal of Palliative Medicine, 7*(6), 791–796.

Lamm, R. (1998). Final report of the National League for Nursing Commission on a workforce for a restructured health care system. *Nursing & Health Care Perspectives 19*(2), 91–93.

Lundberg, C., Brokel, J. M., Bulechek, G. M., Butcher, H. K., Martin, K. S., Moorehead, S., et al. (2008). Selecting a standardized terminology for the electronic health record that reveals that impact of nursing on patient care. *Online Journal of Nursing Informatics, 12*(2). Retrieved August 1, 2009, from http://ojni.org/12_2/index.html

Lunney, M., Delaney, C., Duffy, M., Moorhead, S., & Welton, J. (2005). Advocating for standardized nursing languages in electronic health records. *Journal of Nursing Administration, 35*(1), 1–3.

Lynch, C. (1999). Medical libraries, bioinformatics, and networked information: A coming convergence? *Bulletin of the Medical Library Association, 87,* 408–414.

Mandel, S. H. (1993). A global perspective of informatics in health in developing countries. In S. H. Mandel, M. Korpela, D. Forster, K. Moidi, & P. Byass (Eds.), *Health informatics in Africa-HELINA 93* (pp. 3–8). Amsterdam: Excerpta Medica.

Martin, K. S., & Norris, J. (1996). The Omaha System: A model for describing practice. *Holistic Nursing Practice, 11*(1), 75–83.

Martin, K. S., & Scheet, N. J. (1992). *The Omaha system: Applications for community health nursing.* Philadelphia: Saunders.

McCarthy, A. (2009). Call to regulate nanotechnology. *Australian Nursing Journal, 16*(11), 21.

McKibbon, K. A. (1998). Evidence-based practice. *Bulletin of the Medical Library Association, 86*(3), 396–401.

Meyer, G. (2009). Diagnosis development committee. *International Journal of Nursing Terminologies and Classifications, 20*(2), 101–102.

MITRE Corporation. (2006). *Electronic Health Records Overview.* Retrieved August 1, 2009, from http://www.ncrr.nih.gov/publications/informatics/EHR.pdf

Moorhead, S. (2008). New editions of nursing interventions classification and nursing outcomes classification in 2008. *International Journal of Nursing Terminologies and Classifications, 19*(3), 127–128.

Myers, J., Frieden, T. R., Bherwani, K. M., & Henning, K. J. (2008). Privacy and public health at risk: Public health confidentiality in the digital age. *American Journal of Public Health, 98*(5), 793–801.

National Guideline Clearinghouse. (2006). *Nutrition and physical activity during and after cancer treatment: An American Cancer Society guide for informed choices.* Retrieved May 6, 2009, from http://www.guideline.gov/summary/summary.aspx?doc_id=11877&;nbr=006079&string=chemotherapy+AND+fatigue

National Guideline Clearinghouse. (2009). Retrieved May 6, 2009, from http://www.guideline.gov

O'Cathain, A., Sampson, F. C., Munro, J. F., Thomas, K. J., & Nicholl, J. P. (2004). Nurses' views of using computerized decision support software in NHS direct. *Journal of Advanced Nursing, 45*(3), 280–286.

Saba, V. (2009). Clinical care classification system (CCCS). Retrieved August 1, 2009, from http://www.sabacare.com

Silberg, W. M., Lundberg, G. D., & Musacchio, R. A. (1997). Assessing, controlling, and assuring the quality of medical information on the internet: Caveant lector et viewor—let the reader and viewer beware. *JAMA, 277*(15), 1244–1245.

Staggers, N., McCasky, T., Brazelton, N., & Kennedy, R. (2008). Nanotechnology: The coming revolution and its implications for consumers, clinicians, and informatics. *Nursing Outlook, 56*(5), 268–274.

Staggers, N., & Thompson, C. B. (2002). The evolution of definitions of nursing informatics: A critical analysis and revised definition. *Journal of the American Medical Informatics Association, 9*(3), 255–261.

Stetler, C. B. (2001). Updating the Stetler model of research utilization to facilitate evidence-based practice. *Nursing Outlook, 49*(6), 272.

Switzer, J. A., Hall, C., Gross, H., Waller, J., Nichols, F. T., Wang, S., et al. (2009). A web-based telestroke system facilitates rapid treatment of acute ischemic stroke patients in rural emergency departments. *The Journal of Emergency Medicine, 36*(1), 12–18.

Taylor, J. (2002). *New dimensions for manufacturing: A UK strategy for nanotechnology.* Retrieved August 1, 2009, from http://www.azonano.com/details.asp?ArticleID=1291

Tiger Initiative. (2007). *Evidence and informatics transforming nursing: 3-year action steps toward a 10-year vision.* Retrieved April 23, 2009, from http://www.tigersummit.com

Tiger Initiative. (2009). *Collaborating to integrate evidence and informatics into nursing practice and education: An executive summary.* Retrieved April 23, 2009, from http://www.tigersummit.com

University at Buffalo School of Nursing. *Nursing discussion forums.* Retrieved May 4, 2009, from http://nursing.buffalo.edu/mccartny/nursing_discussion_forums.html#1

Visovsky, C., & Schneider, S. M. (2003). Cancer-related fatigue. *Online Journal of Issues in Nursing, 8*(3), 17.

Walsh, M. & Coleman, J. R. (2005). Developing a pilot telehealth program: One agency's experience. *Home Healthcare Nurse, 23*(3), 188–191.

Walther, J. H., & Speisser, N. (1997). Developing and delivering medical reference source instruction in a special library. Retrieved from http://www.library.ucsb.edu/istl/97-fall/article2.html

Werley, H. H. (1988). *Identification of the nursing minimum data set.* New York: Springer.

Whittemore, D., & Moll. J. (2008). COWs and WOWs, oh my! *Health Management Technology, 29*(7), 32, 34.

Williams, A. R., Herman, D. C., Moriarty, J. P., Beebe, T. J., Bruggeman, S. K., Klavetter, E. W., et al. (2008). *HIPAA* Costs and patient perceptions of privacy safeguards at Mayo Clinic, *The Joint Commission on Quality and Patient Safety, 34*(1), 27–35.

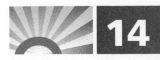

14

Diversity in Health and Illness

CATHY L. CAMPBELL , PhD, APN-BC
ISHAN C. WILLIAMS, PhD

The authors have updated the work done by Dr. Courtney Lyder in the 4th edition of this text.

OBJECTIVES

At the completion of this chapter, the reader will be able to:

- Describe nursing care strategies that may be used to provide care to a diverse patient population.
- Describe methods used to become culturally competent.
- Identify societal factors affecting the delivery of culturally responsive nursing care in the United States.
- Identify barriers to and resources for minority access to care in the United States.
- Describe the differences in the concepts of race, culture, and ethnicity.
- Discuss strategies to approach diverse populations in the provision of culturally relevant care.

PROFILE IN PRACTICE: NURSING STUDENTS WITHOUT BORDERS

Anne Harrington, BSN, RN, and Lindsey Wilson, BSN, RN
University of Virginia School of Nursing, Charlottesville, Virginia

Established in 1999, Nursing Students Without Borders (NSWB) is a student-run organization at the University of Virginia School of Nursing. The goal of the founding members was to organize the concept of global community service into a health care program that had a sustainable impact on underserved communities. While expanding the perspectives and experiences of nursing students, the mission of NSWB is to launch health education initiatives, outline a network to access health care resources within the community, and distribute material donations.

The UVA chapter of NSWB is currently focused on building a primary care clinic for the Red Cross in

San Sebastián, El Salvador, which will serve the town and surrounding *cantones,* or rural communities. The region, home to 19,000 people, still suffers from the economic and developmental devastation incurred during a 12-year civil war that ended in 1992. A current clinic operates out of a two-room rented house and provides basic primary care services by a local physician during the day and emergency care at night by volunteers. As the sole free-of-cost, 24-hour clinic in the area, the Red Cross clinic offers an invaluable service to people who could not otherwise afford health care.

When NSWB began working with the community in 1999, members developed a 3-year education campaign in the San Sebastián schools that concentrated on first aid, hygiene, nutrition, and reproductive health. Other objectives for the co-op included independent research studies for the NSWB students, providing contemporary medical information and supplies to the town clinic and midwives, holding advanced first aid courses for the Red Cross volunteers, and training them to continue the educational drive. Over time, many of these objectives were met or became sustainable by the community. For example, Red Cross volunteers are now able to train younger members using a system based on the one developed by former NSWB educators.

As these previous objectives were met, a new need was identified when it became clear the Red Cross could no longer effectively provide care in their current structure. Although the current clinic does not lack skilled providers, the work is greatly constrained by an unsterile environment and limited resources. NSWB collaborated with the Red Cross and local community leaders to make plans to build a new larger facility that would permit the Red Cross to provide a broader spectrum of care to a greater number of people.

As this project has unfolded over the past several years, a reciprocal learning partnership developed as NSWB team members interacted with the San Sebastián leadership—each encountering and learning from the differences in approach that team members from both cultures brought to the project of creating sustainable and affordable access to improved health care.

Initially, in an attempt to build a clinic facility designed to meet the specific needs of the population, NSWB brought an American architect to San Sebastián to meet with the physician and Red Cross volunteers in their environment. Together, they discussed common goals for the new building and developed architectural plans that were practical for the staff and feasible to build. The local environment, which has a fairly temperate climate, played a large role in the design, and the new clinic will have outdoor access from each room, providing natural ventilation and eliminating the cost of an expensive central air system. By working collaboratively and using local architecture as an example, the clinic was designed on an affordable budget without compromising the integrity of the space.

Another important aspect was the inclusion of a library and conference room. In a desire to continue and promote further learning, NSWB and the Red Cross members decided that a space dedicated to further training promoted the values of members from both groups and would serve as a reminder of the mission for the clinic. Including the input of both NSWB and Red Cross members allowed for a design that would improve upon current conditions and allow the Red Cross to meet its potential while being appropriate for the specific community.

The location of the clinic was an important decision that required cultural sensitivity. A piece of land was purchased in a central location in town, easily accessible to those utilizing and providing the services. As was typical in El Salvadoran culture, the deed was placed in the name of a neutral third party, who was also a trusted official in the community. Because the Roman Catholic Church is regarded so highly in El Salvador, the priest of the local church was chosen to serve this purpose, despite there being no connection between the Red Cross and the Catholic Church. By choosing to include the Church, NSWB gained credibility within the community and acquired a deeper understanding of the importance of religion in the local culture.

In the fall of 2008, when NSWB broke ground on the clinic, the Church once again played an important role in the community ceremony and celebration. When working with Red Cross members to plan the details of the ground-breaking, it was requested that a benediction of the clinic site by a priest begin the ceremony, which also included speeches by a number of community leaders, most notably San Sebastián's mayor, before the El Salvadorian tradition of pouring the first bit of cement for the foundation took place, marking the official beginning of construction.

The close communication between NSWB team members and the Red Cross leadership resulted in inclusion of the priest and local government officials, who do not regularly participate in clinic business. This was a key element in building a foundation of support for this ambitious project among the rest of the local community. If the importance of bringing in these trusted key officials had been overlooked, the project would have lost critical support among community members and some residents might have been reluctant to accept the new building as part of their community.

Construction blueprints and ceremonial details are just two examples of the many aspects of this project through which NSWB has learned the importance of working collaboratively to create a sustainable project that is culturally relevant and supported by the local community. Time and again, relationships and friendships built on trust have been proven to be the most effective—and the only way to work in San Sebastián. Nursing students are placed outside their comfort level

and societal norms as they adapt to a system in which community consent dictates the success of a project.

NSWB trips to El Salvador are designed to include exposure to political, historical, religious, and economic issues, all of which have significant impact on the delivery of care to the impoverished town of San Sebastián. By creating a lasting partnership built on a foundation of cultural competence and reciprocal learning, NSWB and the Red Cross continue to work to provide health care to the community, while teaching nursing students how to work in a global society.

PROFILE IN PRACTICE: HEALTH CARE NEEDS IN RURAL APPALACHIA

Audrey Snyder, PhD, RN, ACNP-BC, CEN, FAANP
Assistant Professor, University of Virginia School of Nursing, Charlottesville, Virginia

I have had the privilege of coordinating the nursing volunteers for the Remote Area Medical (RAM) Clinic in Wise, Virginia, over the last 10 years through Community Outreach and Service at the University of Virginia Health System. Having worked as an emergency department (ED) nurse for many years, I understand that the ED has become the safety net for many of our patients. In fact, many vulnerable and underserved populations rely on the ED as their primary source of health care. Often, by the time patients are seen in the ED, they are in very poor health because they did not seek health care earlier for a minor complaint, which has now worsened. Poor socioeconomic status is the primary predictor of poor health status. Continually seeing the plight of these patients was a motivator behind my decision to begin volunteering with the RAM clinic.

The majority of the patients served at RAM live in the rural Appalachian mountainous region. The population of this area is higher than the national average in several categories: persons greater than 65, persons younger than 18, and persons living below the poverty line. These factors make the people we serve through RAM a particularly vulnerable population. Culturally, this very rural population has a strong sense of independence based on their geographic isolation, economic hardships, and the lack of health care sources of usual health care, especially in specialty practices.

Many residents lack health insurance or coverage for preventative health screenings, including dental or eye care. Travel to areas where these individuals could receive free or reduced-fee specialty care can be difficult or impossible because of logistical and economic hardships. Initially, the RAM clinic focused on vision screenings and dental care. From an aesthetic perspective, if a person has poor dentition, it diminishes employment opportunities, thus meaning the person is less likely to have health insurance. Even if this person has health insurance, it is unlikely to cover dental care, and since everyday survival is given higher priority than dental care, a vicious cycle of poor health is perpetuated. From a medical perspective, patients with poor dentition are less likely to eat fruits and vegetables and more likely to eat soft, nonnutritious foods, thus aggravating conditions such as diabetes and obesity. In turn, these medical conditions become the primary focus, and dentition again takes a back seat, continuing the cycle.

To address this problem, in the second year of RAM, a medical clinic was added. The population living in this region has a higher incidence of heart disease, pulmonary disease, diabetes, and hypertension. Because of the high incidence of diabetes, endocrinologists recommended that we perform routine fingerstick glucose screenings on all patients who present to the clinic. For many patients, a visit to the RAM clinic will serve as their yearly physician check-up, and they will see no other provider unless they become acutely ill.

A mobile "health wagon" managed by a nurse practitioner provides primary care based on ability to pay ($3 per visit) for one area in southwest Virginia. The health wagon is the yearly financial sponsor of the RAM clinic. Every summer, more than 5000 patients are cared for in 2.5 days at the county fairgrounds. All test results are reviewed, and all abnormal tests and lab data are followed by attempts to help patients identify a primary care provider or to refer patients to specialists as needed. The University of Virginia has partnered with the health care providers in southwest Virginia to strategize development of a plan to improve access to health care for patients in this region.

Rural communities are often reluctant to receive services from people outside of their communities. Thus the health wagon meets with stakeholders on a monthly basis in preparation for the summer clinic. Telemedicine sites now dot the map of southwest Virginia and provide access to specialty care providers. Providers working with patients at these clinics must understand the patient's culture, including the social context and significance in the patient's life, since these factors affect the patient's ability to comply with physician's instructions or patient education. For example, consider a rural patient who has diabetes and is

overweight. Simply telling this person to increase physical activity by walking a mile a day may not be helpful if the person lives on the side of a mountain and walking down the road increases the risk of being hit by a car. On the other hand, encouraging such patients to walk a certain number of minutes inside their home or around the outside of their house, weather permitting, is a more realistic instruction and demonstrates an understanding of the patient's environment. Another realistic option would be walking the perimeter of a store parking lot when the patient goes to buy groceries or other goods. Because of geographic isolation, the lack of access to health care, and limited financial resources, these rural patients and their family members often need to perform tasks and learn skills that may in other settings and situations be provided by a professional and/or covered by insurance. Thus family members must be incorporated into the patient's plan of care. For example, identifying the person who prepares the meals in the home will facilitate nutrition education. The team takes advantage of such episodic encounters to provide as much teaching as possible to help these patients facilitate self-care and to build on the cultural value of self-reliance. The patients we work with at the RAM clinic are gracious and have taught us much about their culture and their challenges in managing their health care.

Introduction

America is more of "mixed salad" than a "melting pot" and is composed of diverse groups of individuals. Yet the nursing profession in the United States does not reflect the diversity of the population it serves. This is a significant challenge for the nursing profession and for the 88% of nurses that are non-Hispanic whites. The nursing profession needs to address recruitment of a diverse workforce and the preparation of professional nurses who are competent to deliver culturally responsive care. Professional nurses must develop the knowledge, skills, and values to provide culturally responsive care. Professional nursing is also uniquely positioned to address health care disparities within the

health care delivery system. This chapter explores the relationship between diversity and health and offers frameworks for exploring culture and care. Specific nursing-related barriers, strategies, and resources are identified for developing cultural competency in health care delivery.

Diversity and Health

We live in a pluralistic society, and it is becoming more evident that cultural differences, if not acknowledged, will increasingly serve to isolate and alienate us from one another. It is not enough to simply educate people about cultural differences; one must also confront these competing standards of truth. Given that health care professionals learn from their culture the "art" of being healthy or ill, it is imperative for health professionals to treat each patient with respect to his or her own cultural background. *Culture* can be defined in multiple ways. In general, most definitions encompass socially inherited and shared beliefs, practices, habits, customs, language, and rituals. Culture shapes how people view their world and how they function within that world. Culture can transcend generations. The one unifying theme in defining culture is that it is *learned.* Much of what we believe, think, and act is attributable to culture. Hence one's culture can profoundly determine what is perceived as health versus illness. There are also numerous definitions for diversity. Many people define *diversity* simply as racial or ethnic differences. This chapter considers diversity more broadly to encompass differences that may be rooted not only in culture, but also in age, health status, gender, sexual orientation, racial or ethnic identity, geographical location, or other aspects of sociocultural description and socioeconomic position (Kennedy, Fisher, Fontaine, & Martin-Holland, 2008). Given the importance of culture in how we define ourselves and our environment, each person must be treated with respect and his or her cultural sensitivity must be valued.

How nurses incorporate the patient's cultural diversity in their general plans of care can mean the difference between success and failure (Seidel, Ball, Dains, & Benedict, 2006). Kleinman and Benson (2006) notes that cultural issues are crucial to all clinical care and management of illness, because culture shapes health-related beliefs, values, and behaviors. Thus providing culturally responsive care requires that the nurse, when confronted with culturally diverse patients, is attuned to the cultural cues presented while balancing sensitivity, knowledge, and skills to accommodate social, cultural, biological, psychosocial, and spiritual needs of the client respectfully. When clinicians are focused only on the disease without a context, there is a distortion of reality.

The importance of being sensitive to cultural diversity cannot be overemphasized. The ability to build on the strengths of diverse communities and to understand and respect other cultures results in interventions that can lead to healthy practices and behaviors. Health

and illness can be perceived in a variety of ways, and acknowledging the significance of culture in people's problems as well as their solutions is essential. Moreover, numerous expectations exist of what is considered appropriate treatment and care. Cultural values and social norms are major influences and can greatly affect the interaction and outcomes for both nurses and patients (Box 14-1).

As the United States continues to increase in diversity, nurses will be providing care for patients from many backgrounds different from their own. It would not be feasible or realistic for nurses to try to memorize cultural traits from every diverse cultural group (Engebretson, Mahoney, & Carlson, 2008). Instead, nurses must have an appreciation of the cultural differences among his or her clients, respect each client's culture, and behave in a way that demonstrates this respect.

Many theoretical frameworks exist to provide nurses with a contextual basis for understanding and providing culturally *and* linguistically appropriate care. Leininger's (1991) theoretical framework for transcultural nursing emphasizes the commonalities and differences among world views that reflect various aspects of society to diverse health systems (Figure 14-1). This depiction of the many interrelated dimensions of culture and care is useful for exploring important meanings and patterns of care. The theoretical framework is focused on comparative culture care examined through a holistic and multidimensional lens (Leininger, 2002). The purpose of the theory is to provide culturally congruent, safe, and meaningful care to clients from different or similar cultures. Furthermore, the theory posits that world view, cultural, and social structures and others influence care outcomes related to culturally congruent care; generic emic (folk) practices (an attempt to understand the viewpoint of the people themselves) and professional ethic nursing practices (according to the principles, methods, and interests of the observer) influence outcomes; and the three modes for transcultural care actions and decisions are culture preservation and/or maintenance, cultural care accommodation and/or negotiation, and cultural care repatterning and/or restructuring to provide culturally congruent care (Leininger, 2002). When nurses work

---

BOX 14-1	Case Study: Visiting

When Ellen began her clinical rotation on a large American Indian (Lakota) reservation, her thinking revolved around what she could teach the community workers there. She spent days traveling many miles with various community health representatives (CHRs). These were American Indian men and women who had approximately 1 month's training (sometimes in addition to other training and student experiences). They then assumed roles as providers, visiting homes of other tribe members, doing routine and basic care, and acting as liaisons between the American Indian population and the biomedical system. Slowly, Ellen realized how Lakota culture shaped the CHRs' and other residents' perceptions of health, illness, and their expectations for treatment and care. As the weeks went on and Ellen learned to be open to new ways of knowing and doing things, her interpretations changed, as her following journal entries indicate:

Week 1: "The CHRs don't really do anything. They just go and drink coffee and sit down and visit."

Week 2: "I think they just visit because they don't know what else to do. They even talk about themselves there and the problems their own kids are having. And they are all quiet a lot. Sometimes they hardly talk about the patient's problem."

Week 3: "You know, something happens when the CHRs visit, but I don't know what it is. I don't see how their visiting works, but I see that people appreciate it."

Week 4: "The patients do what the CHRs want them to do. Something goes on, but I don't get it; they never actually tell the patients what to do."

Week 5: "I still don't see how the visiting works when the CHRs don't do much instruction. They do other things—wash the quadriplegic man's long hair, dress decubitus ulcers, weigh babies—but mostly they visit. Somehow it works."

Week 6: "I've got it. Visiting is what the CHRs do. That is what is important and how they intervene. It is because of the visiting that the patients respond, not because of what the CHRs do when they visit."

---

with patients who have cultural orientations that are different in minor or major ways from their own, those considerations are particularly significant. Further discussion of Leininger's framework occurs in Chapter 5.

Another model for examining cultural competence in nursing care is the Campinha-Bacote Model of Cultural Competence (Campinha-Bacote, 2002). In this model, nurses continuously work toward cultural competence by addressing five constructs: cultural awareness, cultural knowledge, cultural skill, cultural encounters, and cultural desire. The final—and perhaps the most important—concept in the model is cultural desire: "Cultural desire is the spiritual and pivotal construct that provides the energy source and foundation for the health care provider's journey toward cultural competence" (Campinha-Bacote, 2002). Thus cultural competence can be illustrated as a volcano, depicting how cultural desire stimulates the process of cultural competence.

The Campinha-Bacote Model of Cultural Competence is an interactional dynamic model of cultural competence, requiring that all five identified constructs be achieved. The process of cultural awareness occurs when the nurse is able to examine his or her own values, biases, and stereotypes. Cultural awareness also requires the nurse to examine the potential cultural biases (racism) that may exist within the health care setting. The process of cultural knowledge occurs when nurses educate themselves about the world views of other cultures and ethnic groups. This cultural knowledge may include learning how disease processes and management may vary depending on the cultural group. Cultural skill occurs when the nurse can conduct a relevant cultural assessment. Hence cultural skill is achieved when cultural data are used to develop and implement a culturally relevant treatment plan. Cultural encounters encourage the nurse to engage directly with patients from different ethnic and cultural backgrounds to modify existing beliefs about a cultural group and prevent potential stereotyping. Finally, cultural desire addresses the motivation of the health care provider to acquire new knowledge about different cultures. This last construct is based solely on the nurse's intrinsic need to acquire new cultural knowledge and cannot be driven by external regulations or requirements.

Similar to the Campinha-Bacote model, the U.S. Health Resources Services Administration attempted to identify the critical domains of cultural competence for health care providers and organizations (USDHHS, 2006). These nine domains are value and attitudes,

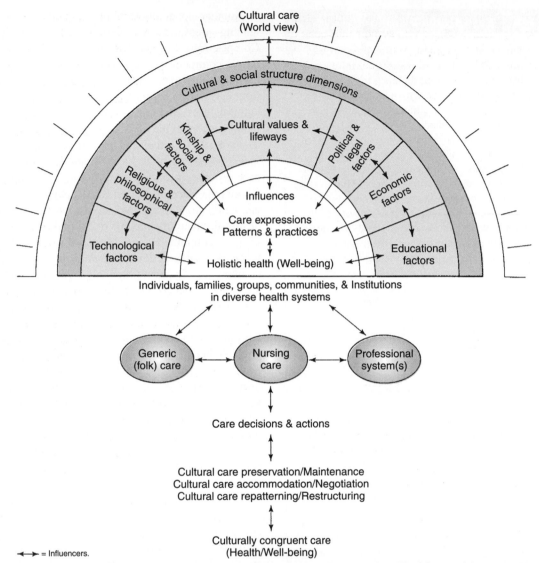

FIGURE 14-1 A modification of Leininger's model of transcultural nursing. (Modified from Leininger, M. M. [1991]. *Culture care diversity and universality: A theory of nursing.* New York: National League for Nursing; with permission of the National League for Nursing, New York, NY.)

cultural sensitivity, communication, policies and procedures, training and development, facility characteristics, intervention and treatment models, family and community participation, and monitoring and evaluation. By addressing all nine domains, both health care providers and organizations can achieve cultural competence.

VALUES THAT SHAPE HEALTH CARE AND NURSING

The discipline of nursing reflects the values and norms of a society; in the United States these values and norms are predominantly Eurocentric, middle class, Christian, and androcentric in view. In general, the American culture tends to value personal freedom and independence (Shaw & Degazon, 2008), as well as individual achievement over the common good (Seidel et al., 2006). For example, the concept of a single autonomous decision maker that is the hallmark of a Eurocentric world view does not accurately capture the involvement of family members and other significant people in health care decision making (Campbell, 2007). The notion that everyone be treated exactly the same is idealized and unrealistic. Traditionally, health care providers are presumed to know more about their patients' needs than patients themselves do. This concept, known as *paternalism,* is discussed further in Chapter 12. Although there is a growing movement to listen to patients' goals and beliefs and incorporate such goals and beliefs as resources in their care, this continues to be a challenge when patients' beliefs differ greatly from those of the providers of health care.

NURSING'S CHALLENGE

Nursing is in a strategic position to provide care to diverse groups with diverse expectations, problems, and goals. Not surprisingly, nurses manage patients who are generally underserved. Today's nurses attend to both population-based and individual patterns and needs. Many nurses realize that respectful encounters with topics such as race, ethnicity, religion, politics, gender, sexual orientation, and belief systems outside biomedicine are essential to providing effective nursing care (Shaw & Degazon, 2008). However, some nurses still practice with the inherent belief that patients who disagree with them are wrong. Others acknowledge the diversity they encounter but are overwhelmed by its complexity. Despite these perceived difficulties, the integration of patients' beliefs and values can result in effective nursing care (Seidel et al., 2006).

The paucity of nurses prepared in nursing school to manage diversity effectively is daunting. A commitment to diversity is a value in many schools of nursing; however, faculty members may lack the skills and resources to incorporate diversity into their syllabi, teaching strategies, and course evaluation (Kennedy et al., 2008). Moreover, the lack of diversity among nursing faculty and students in nursing schools further compounds this issue. The Sullivan Commission (2004) report on diversity in the health care work force underscored the scarcity of minority faculty and students in nursing. A report by the American Association of Colleges of Nursing (AACN), Enrollment and Graduations in Baccalaureate and Graduate Programs in Nursing 2007-2008 (AACN, 2008), provides descriptive information about minority nursing students and faculty. Students from minority backgrounds represented 26% of students in entry-level baccalaureate programs, a 3% increase from the 1995 data. In terms of gender breakdown, men accounted for 10.5% of students in baccalaureate programs in 2008. Although a 3% increase in minority students enrolling in baccalaureate nursing education is promising, the future still looks bleak for minority faculty. The majority of faculty members in schools of nursing are not minorities either. In fact, it is estimated that only 10.8% of full-time nursing school faculty come from minority backgrounds, and only 5.7% are male (AACN, 2008). Without representation from diverse ethnic, racial, and gender perspectives, the potential for disseminating alternate views on providing culturally responsive care diminishes. For the first time, the lack of diversity in the educational experience of health care professionals and in the work force has been linked to issues of quality and patient safety. Patient safety is explored in more detail in Chapter 20. The scarcity of diverse perspectives in race, ethnicity, culture, and language in health care settings increases the possibility for discordance during health care visits. Racial and language discordance can have an impact on patient and family health care literacy and negatively affect the safe, timely, and effective use of medications and other treatments (Ho, Brady, & Clancy, 2008).

Members of diverse groups are increasingly acknowledged to have rights to their own distinct lifestyles, values, and norms. In nursing, the ability to communicate and work interculturally and to understand culture-based care and caring practices is viewed as essential to providing high-quality, effective care. Our education must reflect the diversity of the individuals and communities we serve.

DECREASING BIASES

The concepts of race and ethnicity are commonly thought to be dominant elements of culture. However, culture, as defined above, is much broader than this, and each concept has a different meaning. No one definition can encompass the meaning of race. The most widely used methods for defining races are those based on skin color, facial features, ancestry, and national origin. Many social scientists argue that most racial definitions are imprecise, arbitrary, derived from custom, and vary among cultures. Hence defining human beings on the basis of race is related more to sociopolitical constructs than to science. The U.S. Office of Management and Budget (1997) responded to criticism and revised its standards for classifying federal data on race and ethnicity. The new standards set five categories for data on race, including (1) American Indian or Alaska Native, (2) Asian, (3) Black or African American, (4) Native Hawaiian or other Pacific Islander, and (5) White. A separate designation for data on ethnicity includes two categories: (1) Hispanic or Latino and (2) not Hispanic or Latino. Racial and ethnic categories set forth in the standards should not be interpreted as being primarily biological or genetic in reference. Race and ethnicity may be thought of in terms of social and cultural characteristics as well as ancestry. Often people fail to consider other factors that influence culture and determine how people think and behave—for instance, age, educational level, income level, geographical residence, length of residency in the United States, and specific health care beliefs about time, personal space, and eye contact, to name just a few.

Ethnicity is usually defined as membership of a person to a particular cultural group. Ethnic groups usually have a sense of shared common origins, distinct history, or collective cultural individuality (Spector, 2004). Thus people may be in the same ethnic group, yet have different nationalities. Ethnicity appears to be a more viable mechanism than race for examining similarities and differences. However, in the United States, race still influences everyday social experience; it is one major issue that today's nurses must confront to manage diversity effectively.

More than 3000 different cultural groups exist in the world. Regardless of their ability to interact with 20 or 200 patients, nurses must be sensitive to recognize and confront their own biases that may hinder their ability to provide quality care. A *bias* can be defined as influence in a particular, typically unfair direction (prejudice). To manage diversity effectively, nurses

must be sensitive to both differences and similarities, knowledgeable about expected patterns of behavior, and skillful at integrating their sensitivity and knowledge into appropriate assessment and interventions. Information about acceptable patterns of behavior and their interpretation should always be tested against an individual's perception of a specific situation. Not verifying one's own perception with that of the individual may lead to biases and stereotyping.

Nurses should identify their own personal prejudices and biases because these biases may distort the level of care that is provided. Self-awareness or cultural awareness is the first step toward becoming culturally competent (Leininger, 2002; Purnell & Paulanka, 2003). Biases can be so intrinsic that the nurse is unaware of them. Research studies have found that health care providers can unknowingly bias the care provided to patients on the basis of race or gender (Campesino, 2008; Cully, 2006; Fiscella & Franks, 2005; Kirk et al., 2005). With open communication and changing prejudgments of a person's cultural beliefs and customs, intrinsic biases can be mitigated. Figure 14-2 illustrates the positive and negative consequences to biases. (See chapter 19 for further discussion.)

"COLORBLIND" AND OTHER OXYMORONS

National data suggest that the health care of minorities has improved in the United States This is evident in longer life expectancies and decreases in infant mortality (Centers for Disease Control, 2007). The National Healthcare Disparities Report (NHDR) produced by the Agency for Healthcare Research and Quality (AHRQ) on behalf of the U.S. Department of Health and Human Services (HHS) reported that two disparities were eliminated in 2004: the disparity in access to adequate dialysis services between African Americans and whites with end-stage renal disease and the disparity between Asians and whites who had a usual primary care provider (Agency for Healthcare Research and Quality, 2007).

However, many other health disparities remain. Compared with incidence among whites, the incidence of new HIV cases for African Americans and Hispanics was 10 and 3.5 times higher, respectively (AHRQ 2007). In fact, when compared with all other racial

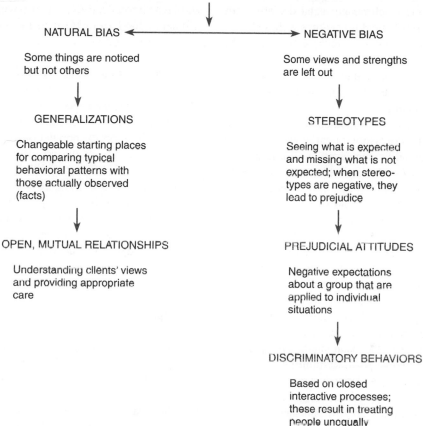

OBSERVATIONS AND INFORMATION PROCESSING

NATURAL BIAS ← → NEGATIVE BIAS

Some things are noticed but not others

Some views and strengths are left out

GENERALIZATIONS

STEREOTYPES

Changeable starting places for comparing typical behavioral patterns with those actually observed (facts)

Seeing what is expected and missing what is not expected; when stereotypes are negative, they lead to prejudice

OPEN, MUTUAL RELATIONSHIPS

PREJUDICIAL ATTITUDES

Understanding clients' views and providing appropriate care

Negative expectations about a group that are applied to individual situations

DISCRIMINATORY BEHAVIORS

Based on closed interactive processes; these result in treating people unequally

FIGURE 14-2 Open versus closed information processing.

or ethnic groups, African Americans experienced the highest incidence of new HIV cases, especially African American men in 2006 (CDC, 2008). American Indians and Alaska Native mothers were twice as likely to have lacked prenatal care and experienced high mortality rates in comparison with white mothers (CDC, 2007), and poor children were more than 28% more likely than high-income children to experience poor communication with their health care providers (AHRQ, 2007). The issue of health disparities is also addressed in Chapter 12 and Chapter 19.

Clearly, access to health care varies greatly for African Americans, Hispanics, and other racial/ethnic minorities compared with whites, as well as for poor communities compared with more higher-income populations. This may be partly attributable to minority populations having higher rates of unemployment and jobs without health benefits. The factor that is consistently associated with access to health care and the quality of care is having health insurance (AHRQ, 2007). However, what is startling is the large number of studies that find race-based differences in the receipt of primary health care and therapeutic procedures for a broad range of conditions, including pain management, even after adjusting for insurance status and severity of disease (Agoston et al., 2003; Green et al., 2003; Kandzari et al., 2004; Pathman, Fowler-Brown, & Corbie-Smith, 2006). In a study investigating the effectiveness of local and national initiatives to reduce surgical procedural differences between African American and white older adults, data were culled from Medicare beneficiaries from 1992 to 2001.

This study found that over a 10-year period both local and national efforts to eliminate racial disparities in the use of high-cost surgical procedures were not successful (Jha, Fisher, Li, Orav, & Epstein, 2005). In fact, access to five surgical procedures significantly differed between African American and white older adults. Differentiated care still exists within the American health care system.

One easy but ineffective method for avoiding the difficult work of addressing racial issues is to be "colorblind." Pretending that everyone in society is equal and that issues of disparate access are in the past perpetuates societal patterns of differential treatment based on race, culture, and so forth (Campbell, 2007; Hassouneh, 2006). This approach in health care simply denies that variations in life experiences exist. For example, the disparities that exist between African Americans and whites in their use of hospice services at the present time have been linked to the different social realities for these populations during the period when hospice was first introduced in the United States. The hospice movement had its genesis in the late 1960s and early 1970s as an alternative to hospital-based care for people with life-limiting illness. At this same time, African Americans were not looking for an alternative to hospital-based end-of-life care; they were seeking equal access to the services available to whites in their communities. For them, the hospice alternative was perceived as second-rate care—a myth that persists today in many minority communities (Campbell, 2007; Taxis, 2006). This is just one example of how patients can become resentful when their unique experiences are ignored. Many aspects of racism and other biases can be institutionalized such that individuals fail to recognize that there are societal structures that have created the environment for disparities to exist. The failure to consider the unique experiences of minorities further perpetuates and condones the behavior (Hassouneh, 2006). Acknowledging and challenging the biases that exist within oneself and the health care institutions designed to care for the sick are first steps in eliminating those biases. Simply increasing one's knowledge about different cultural groups of people does not necessarily negate biased attitudes that may be internalized, nor does increasing one's knowledge about the cultural beliefs and practices mean that the health professional will be able to effectively interact with someone from another cultural group (Campesino, 2008).

Diversification of America

The United States has become increasingly diverse in the last century. According to the U.S. Census Bureau, the nation's minority population reached 102.5 million in 2007, 34% of the estimated total U.S. population of 301.6 million. California had a minority population of 20.9 million, 20% of the nation's total, and Texas had a minority population of 12.5 million, 12% of the U.S. total. Hispanics remained the largest minority group and African Americans (single race or multiracial) were second at 40.7 million in 2007. African Americans were the largest minority group in 24 states, compared with 20 states in which Hispanics were the largest minority group. The African American population was followed by Asians, who totaled 15.2 million; American Indians and Alaska Natives, who totaled 4.5 million; and Native Hawaiians and other Pacific Islanders, with 1 million (U.S. Census Bureau, 2008).

The U.S. Census Bureau predicts that within the next 90 years non-Hispanic whites will account for 40% of the U.S. population. Simply stated, in less than a century racial and ethnic minorities will become the majority in the United States. In 2007, four states and the District of Columbia were found to be "majority-minority." Majority-minority states are those where more than 50% of the population is made up of people other than single-race non-Hispanic whites. Hawaii led the nation with a population that was 75% minority in 2007, followed by the District of Columbia (68%), New Mexico (58%), California (57%), and Texas (52%). Next in line, although not majority-minority states, were Nevada, Maryland, and Georgia, each with a minority population of 42% (U.S. Census Bureau, 2008).

As the racial and ethnic diversity of the U.S. population continues to increase, so does the need for health care professionals to acquire knowledge about such populations to provide culturally responsive care. Although some people may find these projections threatening and others may find them hopeful, nursing at times seems to be stuck between "fight and flight" in managing such realities. Demanding conformity to a single set of norms is no longer acceptable. Social variation continues despite a homogenized culture that permeates every household with standardized fast food and consumer expectations. As a society, the United States is moving toward a truer democracy, and nursing must adapt to this reality.

INDIVIDUAL VERSUS GROUP IDENTITY

The delivery of nursing care is usually individualized to the patient. However, for many cultures the nurse must be more cognizant of the influence of the patient's family. In fact, in some cultures nursing care decisions are not considered solely the wishes of the patient (the American way) but must take into consideration the wishes and decisions of all family members. In many Asian and African cultures, decisions are made by groups or by heads of groups. Although care may be individualized for each patient, nurses must become comfortable with managing patients in the collective terms of their families. Also, nurses must recognize that the process of acculturation differs for everyone. That is, acculturation may occur at different rates among families of the same cultural background, as well as among members of the same family. In fact, each community, whether grouped by culture, ethnicity, religion, sexual orientation, or another self-identified category, will have its own variations within the group (Agar, 2006; Engebretson et al., 2008), including treatment preferences or health-related behaviors. Ignoring these issues will perpetuate the problems of stereotyping and prejudice, which can lead to misdiagnosis and culturally incompetent care.

CARE BARRIERS AND RESOURCES

Although the diversity within the American population should be celebrated, this factor can pose barriers to health care delivery because of issues related to language, economics, and potential distrust of health providers (Box 14-2). For example, many older African Americans have a general distrust of health care providers, an opinion rooted, at least partly, in the Tuskegee syphilis study in which 399 poor African American

sharecroppers in Macon County, Alabama, were denied treatment for syphilis and deceived by physicians of the U.S. Public Health Service from 1932 to 1972 (Brandon, Isaac, & La Veist, 2005). One goal of the Tuskegee syphilis study was to chronicle the natural evolution of syphilis in the African American community to see whether it differed from the same disease process in the white community. Hence these poor, uneducated African American men were told they were being treated for "bad blood." However, government officials went to extraordinary measures to block the men from receiving treatment for their syphilis. Many argue that the distrust engendered by this study is a significant factor in the low participation of African Americans in clinical trials, organ donation efforts, and routine preventive care.

Differences in ideas about relationships may facilitate or discourage resource utilization. Nurses' expectations that patients will want to care for themselves or have personal involvement in decision making may be perceived as an inappropriate imposition in some cultures. Moreover, cultural perceptions may be that illness results in a sick role that is characterized by dependence on others. For example, in Japan elders may spend several weeks to months in hospitals because the cultural expectation is that they will only leave the hospital after they are completely recovered and require no more nursing care.

Resources

The increasing racial and ethnic diversity of the U.S. population makes it essential that nurses acquire knowledge and develop a skill set to provide care that is culturally responsive. The Office of Minority Health (U.S. Department of Health and Human Services, 2007) has developed several excellent resources for health care providers, including a three-module training series on cultural competence called Culturally Competent Nursing Modules. Introduced in 2007, the training program consists of an introduction followed by the three modules. Modules can be studied separately or as a group, and nurses can earn up to 9 hours of continuing education credit. The content is based on the National Standards for Culturally and Linguistically Appropriate Care (CLAS). The modules are self-directed, interactive, and web-based. A DVD version is available so that the content can be used in a group setting. Case studies and reflective exercises provide an opportunity for nurses to explore issues of diversity in the health care setting, such as honoring religious beliefs and practices, incorporating alternative and complementary treatments into the plan of care, and creating a health care environment that is truly inclusive (Carol, 2008; USDHHS, 2007).

Another resource sponsored by the Office of Minority Health is the Think Cultural Health website (USD-HHS, 2009). The site (www.thinkculturalhealth.hhs.gov) offers the latest resources and tools to promote cultural competence in health care and includes free online courses accredited for continuing education credit as well as additional resources to help providers and organizations promote respectful, culturally congruent, high-quality care to an increasingly diverse patient population. Additional content includes online courses such as "A Physician's Practical Guide to Culturally Competent Care" and "Culturally Competent Nursing Care," as well as interactive tools such as the "Health Care Language Services Implementation Guide" (Carol, 2008; USDHHS, 2009).

Nurses are in a unique position because they often function as the gatekeepers between the patient and the health care system. Thus they are in a unique position to facilitate flow of information from patients to health care providers while maintaining the dignity of the patient. Nurses must have a good knowledge of the health behaviors and beliefs of a diverse group of patients. This knowledge can be acquired from a variety of methods (e.g., listening to patients and families, reading books, accessing computer-based programs). Hassouneh cautions nursing students, practicing nurses, and nursing faculty about relying solely on a "cookbook" approach to learning culturally responsive care (Hassouneh, 2006, p. 256). Cultural assessment is a dynamic process that begins with willingness of the student to explore not only the person's cultural, but also biases in the student's own perspective that might prevent a full exploration. The placement of unique value on holism positions nurses to understand, respect, and protect the individual differences within the patient populations served.

BOX 14-2	**Case Study: Barriers to Care**

Joy, a community health nurse (CHN), prepared to visit an older American Indian man, Mr. Murphy, who had been hospitalized with bronchitis, and an elderly American Indian woman, Mrs. Bird, who was characterized as "noncompliant" with her dialysis treatment and who consumed alcohol. Joy had numerous other clients who could use home visits, but in the rural area in which they lived, homes were miles apart and difficult to locate, roads were often treacherous, and few people had phones for verifying availability. Each attempted visit involved the time of a translator as well as the CHN.

When Joy and the translator arrived at the home of Mrs. Bird, she was away having a healing ceremony. Joy interpreted this as a good sign; perhaps she would return to dialysis after the ceremony. "What else can I do?" Joy asked herself. "I can't leave her a note; she does not read English." Next, Joy and the translator moved on to the small home of Mr. Murphy. They asked whether he was taking his medicine, and he showed them several bottles of pills, still full. They ask whether he had eaten breakfast. He described bacon

and eggs. But the unwashed dishes in the sink lacked evidence, and the wood stove that served both to heat the tiny dwelling and for cooking was not warm. "One order of Meals on Wheels coming up," quipped Joy to the translator when they returned to the car, "at least when they can get back there. But the pills? Mr. Murphy knows I want him to take them. He says he has them for when he needs them. I will try to visit him more often and have others check on him, but I must respect his choices."

1. If you had been that visiting nurse, how would you have responded to each of the clients? In your response, make sure that you demonstrate your understanding of the culture.
2. How could the knowledge of cultural practices have been used to help patients be successful with their treatment plan?
3. How might it have been possible to incorporate traditional healing or folk remedies with mainstream Western medicine when developing a treatment plan for Mr. Murphy and Mrs. Bird?

BOX 14-3	Cultural Competency in Healthcare Delivery: Have I "ASKED" Myself the Right Questions?"

Awareness: Am I aware of my biases and prejudices toward other cultural groups, as well as racism in health care?

Skill: Do I have the skill of conducting a cultural assessment in a sensitive manner?

Knowledge: Am I knowledgeable about the worldviews of different cultural and ethnic groups, as well as knowledge in the field of biocultural ecology?

Encounters: Do I seek out face-to-face and other types of interactions with individuals who are different from myself?

Desire: Do I really "want to" become culturally competent?

Copyrighted by Josepha Campinha-Bacote (2002) and reprinted with permission from Transcultural C A.R.E. Associates.

Cultural Assessment Strategies

Cultural assessment has two aspects: the desire to acquire knowledge of a different culture and the strategies for acquiring knowledge of that different culture. The desire to acquire knowledge of a new culture is an intrinsic process. No one can force the nurse to acquire this knowledge. To assist with the continuous appraisal of cultural competence, the acronym ASKED, based on the Campinha-Bacote Model of Cultural Competence (Campinha-Bacote, 2002), was developed (Box 14-3). This is an excellent model to examine desire for cultural knowledge acquisition.

Once the desire for obtaining cultural knowledge is present, developing a framework of strategies to acquire the knowledge is important. Categories of strategies for a basic cultural assessment are presented in Box 14-4. These strategies are helpful in

BOX 14-4	Approaches Recommended for All Cultural Groups

- Provide a feeling of acceptance.
- Establish open communication.
- Present yourself with confidence. Introduce yourself. Shake hands if it is appropriate.
- Strive to gain your client's trust, but don't be resentful if you don't get it.
- Understand what members of the cultural or subcultural group consider to be "caring," both attitudinally and behaviorally.
- Understand the perceived relationship between your client and authority.
- Understand your client's desire to please you and his or her motivations to comply or not comply.
- Anticipate diversity. Avoid stereotypes based on sex, age, ethnicity, socioeconomic status, and so forth.
- Do not make assumptions about where people come from. Let them tell you.
- Understand the client's goals and expectations.
- Make your goals realistic.
- Emphasize positive points and strengths of health beliefs and practices.
- Show respect, especially for men, even if you are interested in the women or children. Men are often decision makers about follow-up.

- Be prepared for the fact that children go everywhere with some cultural groups as well as with poorer families, who may have few child care options. Include them.
- Know the traditional, health-related practices common to the group with whom you are working. Do not discredit them unless you know they are harmful.
- Know the folk illnesses and remedies common to the group with whom you are working.
- Try to make the clinic setting comfortable. Consider colors, music, atmosphere, scheduling expectations, pace, tone, seating arrangements, and so forth.
- Whenever possible and appropriate, involve the leaders of the local group. Confidentiality is important, but the leaders know the problems and often can suggest acceptable interventions.
- Respect values, beliefs, rights, and practices. Some may conflict with your own or with your determination to make changes. But every group and individual wants respect, above all else.
- Learn to appreciate the richness of diversity as an asset, rather than a hindrance, in your work.

identifying general lifestyles and health patterns that may help in nursing care planning and interventions. Nurses should never assume that particular beliefs, practices, or supports do or do not exist. Expected patterns must always be contrasted with actual, individual situations. Finally, it is important to recognize that the process of becoming culturally competent and being sensitive to others' cultural beliefs occurs along a continuum. Nurses will be at different points on the continuum—and each individual nurse may be at a different point of the continuum with each minority group served.

SUMMARY

America is composed of a diverse group of individuals; yet 88% of nursing professionals are non-Hispanic whites. Thus there is a great need for nurses to engage in learning experiences that create new ways of examining culture and diversity. Many note that the United States is not so much a melting pot as a tossed salad. If this is true, nurses must strive to understand the similarities and dissimilarities among the patient populations served. Remaining cognizant of personal intrinsic biases and those that permeate throughout the health system is vital.

Because nurses serve as gatekeepers to the health care system, they are in a unique position to help bridge the gap in the disparities that exist for diverse patients. As nurses acquire cultural competencies, they in turn will help break down the barriers that divide in the health care system.

A quote from Dr. Josepha Campinha-Bacote speaks to our progress toward cultural competence in nursing education: "I contend that nursing is on a progressive course toward successfully answering the question, 'How do we effectively teach cultural competence in nursing education?' We must realize that it is a journey that reflects an ongoing transformational process" (Campinha-Bacote, 2006, p. 244).

KEY POINTS

- Cultural views of individuals and groups influence perception of health and health care.
- Diversity management uses affirmation and encouragement to move toward development of the client's full potential.

- Open and honest communication can facilitate nurse-client relationships to provide a better understanding of clients' perspectives of health and illness.
- Health care professionals and institutions may possess intrinsic biases against differing cultures; thus nurses must remain hypervigilant to identify and correct those biases.
- Culturally congruent care incorporates those cultural characteristics (e.g., religion, social relations, education, language) deemed important by the client.
- Cultural assessment in nursing involves systematic appraisal of beliefs, values, and practices of the client.
- Nurses must remain mindful not to make automatic assumptions about patients based on their cultural affiliation.
- Nurses must remain motivated to learn about different cultures to provide culturally relevant care.
- Nurses will either learn to manage diversity or be managed by it.

CRITICAL THINKING EXERCISES

1. Discuss strategies nurses could implement to promote culturally sensitive care.
2. Discuss current barriers within health care institutions that hinder culturally appropriate care.
3. How could a nurse develop the requisite balance of cultural sensitivity, knowledge, and skills needed to manage diverse clients effectively?
4. In your experience, what strategies work well for practice of culturally acceptable nursing assessment, communication, and intervention?

REFERENCES

Agar, M. (2006). Culture: Can you take it anywhere? *International Journal of Qualitative Methods, 5(2)*. Retrieved January 30, 2009, from https://ejournals.library.ualberta.ca/index.php/IJQM/article/view/4384/3513

Agency for Healthcare Research and Quality. (2007). *National Healthcare Disparities Report, 2007*. Retrieved January 24, 2009, from http://www.ahrq.gov/qual/nhdr07/nhdr07.pdf

Agoston, I., Cameron, C. S., Yao, D., De La Rosa, A., Mann, D. L., & Deswal, A. (2004). Comparison of outcomes of white versus black patients hospitalized with heart failure and preserved ejection fraction. *American Journal of Cardiology, 94,* 1003–1007.

American Association of Colleges of Nursing. (2008). Fact Sheet: Enhancing diversity in the nursing work force. Retrieved January 3, 2009, from http://www.aacn.nche.edu/Media/FactSheets/diversity.htm

Brandon, D. T., Isaac, L. A., & La Veist, T. A. (2005). The legacy of Tuskegee and trust in medical care: Is Tuskegee responsible for race differences in mistrust of medical care? *Journal of the National Medical Association, 97*, 951–956.

Campbell, C. (2007). Respect for persons: Engaging African-Americans in end-of-life research. *Journal of Hospice and Palliative Care Nursing, 9*(2), 74–78.

Campesino, M. (2008). Beyond transculturalism: Critiques of cultural education in nursing. *Journal of Nursing Education, 47*(7), 298–304.

Campinha-Bacote, J. (2002). *A culturally competent model of care*. Retrieved from http://www.transcultural care.net

Campinha-Bacote, J. (2006). Cultural competence in nursing curricula: How are we doing 20 years later? *Journal of Nursing Education 45*(7), 243–4.

Carol, R. (2008). Click here for cultural competence. *Minority Nurse, Summer 2008*, 38–41.

Centers for Disease Control, National Center for Health Statistics. (2007). Health, United States, 2007 (With Chartbook on Trends in the Health of Americans). Hyattsville, MD. Retrieved from http://www.cdc.gov/nchs/data/hus/hus07.pdf

Centers for Disease Control. (2008). *MMWR Analysis Provides New Details on HIV Incidence in U.S. Populations* (September 2008). Retrieved from http://www.cdc.gov/hiv/topics/surveillance/resources/factsheets/MMWR-incidence.htm

Cully, L. (2006).Transcending transculturalism? Race, ethnicity and health care. *Nursing Inquiry, 13*, 144–153.

Engebretson, J., Mahoney, J., & Carlson, E. (2008). Cultural competence in the era of evidence-based practice. *Journal of Professional Nursing, 24*(3), 172–178.

Fiscella, K., & Franks, P. (2005). Is patient HMO insurance or physician HMO participation related to racial disparities in primary care? *American Journal of Managed Care, 11*, 397–402.

Green, C. R., Anderson, K. O., Baker, T. A., Campbell, L. C., Decker, S., Fillingim, R. B., et al. (2003). The unequal burden of pain: Confronting racial and ethnic disparities in Pain. *Pain Medicine, 4*, 277–294.

Hassouneh, D. (2006). Anti-racist pedagogy: Challenges faced by faculty of color in predominantly white schools of Nursing. *Journal of Nursing Education, 45*(7), 255–262.

Ho, K., Brady, J. & Clancy, C. (2008). Improving quality and reducing health disparities. *Journal of Nursing Care Quality, 23*(3), 185–188.

Jha, A. K., Fisher, E. S., Li, Z., Orav, J. E., & Epstein, A. M. (2005). Racial trends in the use of major procedures among the elderly. *New England Journal of Medicine, 353*, 683–691.

Kandzari, D. E., Tcheng, J. E., Grines, C. L., Cox, D. A., Stuckey, T., Griffin, J. J. (2004). Influence of admission and discharge aspirin use on survival after primary coronary angioplasty for acute myocardial infarction. *American Journal of Cardiology, 94*, 1029–1033.

Kennedy, H. P., Fisher, L., Fontaine, D., & Martin-Holland, J. (2008). Evaluating diversity in nursing education. *Journal of Transcultural Nursing, 19*(4), 363–370.

Kirk, J. K., Bell, R. A., Bertoni, A. G., Arcury, T. A., Quandt, S. A., Goff, D. C. (2005). A qualitative review of studies of diabetes preventive care among minority patients in the United States, 1993-2003. *American Journal of Managed Care, 11*, 349–360.

Kleinman, A., & Benson, P. (2006). Anthropology in the clinic: The problem of cultural competency and how to fix it. *PLOS Medicine, 3*(10): e294 *doi:10.1371/journal.pmed.0030294.*

Leininger, M. (2002). Culture care theory: A major contribution to advance transcultural nursing knowledge and practices. *Journal of Transcultural Nursing, 13*, 189–192.

Leininger, M. M. (1991). The theory of culture care diversity and universality. In M. M. Leininger (Ed.). *Culture and diversity and universality: A theory of nursing* (NLN Publication No. 15-2402) (pp. 5–68). New York: National League of Nursing.

Office of Management and Budget. (1997). Revisions to the standards for the classification of federal data on race and ethnicity. Retrieved from http://www.whitehouse.gov/omb/fedreg/1997standards.html

Pathman, D. E., Fowler-Brown, A., Corbie-Smith, G. (2006). Differences in access to outpatient medical care for Black and White adults in the rural south. *Medical Care, 44*(5), 429–438.

Purnell, L. D., & Paulanka, B. J. (2003). *Transcultural health care: A culturally competent approach*. Philadelphia: Davis.

Seidel, H. M., Ball, J. W., Dains, J. E., & Benedict, G. W. (2006). *Mosby's guide to physical exam*. Cultural Awareness (Chapter 2, pp. 38–50). St. Louis: Mosby.

Shaw, H. K., & Degazon, C. (2008). Integrating the core professional values of nursing: A profession, not just a career. *Journal of Cultural Diversity, 15*(1), 44–50.

Spector, R. E. (2004). *Cultural diversity in health and illness* (6th ed.). Upper Saddle River, NJ: Pearson/Prentice-Hall.

The Sullivan Commission. (2004). *Missing persons: Minorities in the health professions.* Retrieved from http://www.aacn.nche.edu/Media/pdf/SullivanReport.pdf

Taxis, J. C. (2006). Attitudes, values, and questions of African Americans regarding participation in hospice programs. *The Journal of Hospice and Palliative Care Nursing, 8*(2),77–85.

U.S. Census Bureau, U.S. Department of Commerce. (2008). *U.S. Hispanic Population Surpasses 45 Million.* Retrieved March 27, 2011, from http://www.census.gov/newsroom/releases/archives/population/cb08-67.html

U.S. Department of Health and Human Services, Health Resources and Services Administration. (2006). *Indicators of Cultural Competence in Health Care Delivery Organizations.* Retrieved from http://www.hrsa.gov/culturalcompetence/healthdlvr.pdf

U.S. Department of Health and Human Services, Office of Minority Health. (2007). *Culturally Competent Nursing Modules.* Retrieved from https://www.thinkculturalhealth.hhs.gov/CCNM

U.S. Department of Health and Human Services, Office of Minority Health (2009). *Think Cultural Health.* Retrieved from https://www.thinkculturalhealth.hhs.gov

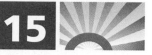

15

Health and Health Promotion

SANDRA P. THOMAS, PhD, RN, FAAN

OBJECTIVES

At the completion of this chapter, the reader will be able to:

- Compare several definitions and models of health.
- Compare several models of health behavior.
- Describe psychological, behavioral, and environmental factors related to wellness.
- Apply the stages of change model to a selected health behavior.
- Apply the health belief model to a selected health behavior.
- Describe the use of evidence-based interventions to promote behavior change.
- Describe the goals of *Healthy People 2010*.
- Compare several types of community-level health promotion programs.

PROFILE IN PRACTICE

Leslie El-Sayad, MSN, RN, FNP
Nurse Practitioner, Morgan County Medical Center, Wartburg, Tennessee

During my 20 years in primary care in rural eastern Tennessee, I have tried to avoid burnout and becoming jaded concerning my patients' motivations or lack thereof. But questions flit across my mind, unbidden, when patients make decisions that adversely affect their health. I think to myself, "Isn't it as plain as the nose on her face what she should do? Haven't I discussed that with her enough times?" Two principles have helped remind me to respect the patient's viewpoint on health.

First, no one sets out deliberately to make a wrong decision. This idea is based on one of nursing theorist Ernestine Wiedenbach's beliefs about the individual: whatever the individual does represents his or her

best judgment at the moment of doing it. Given their immediate circumstances (and rural poor populations are more affected by immediate circumstances than those with more available options), past experiences, knowledge base, physical and mental state, and social or economic pressures at the time a decision is made, patients will make the best decisions they are capable of making. Therefore there is no looking back or chastising—only going forward with new knowledge. We cannot presume to know what is best for another person.

Second, symptoms by themselves may have no meaning to a person unless they have a significant effect on his or her life. A person may have no wish to change anything. Long lectures about the benefits of better health habits are demeaning and will not be helpful. A person may walk around with large tumors, constant dyspepsia, extreme dyspnea, or gnarled and painful joints, but an ingrown toenail will bring him to the provider because he could not wear his boots. Risk factors do not have a one-to-one relationship to disease. They are risk factors, not guarantees of poor outcomes. Despite scientifically based predictions, patients will not buy into your suggested preventative measures if they see no gain. It is difficult to promote health, but it is my job. Keeping the above principles in mind saves my sanity and helps me respect my patients' abilities on behalf of their health.

Introduction

Ricky Jones is a 45-year-old long-distance truck driver who once used amphetamines heavily to help him stay awake while driving. He presently weighs 205 pounds (height of 5 feet 8 inches, medium frame [BMI 31.2]) and expresses disgust with his weight and lack of physical fitness. After his annual physical examination, the nurse practitioner collaboratively sets initial goals of increasing Ricky's level of exercise and achieving a 10-pound weight loss. As Ricky departs, he wryly expresses a wish that amphetamines were still readily available so that he could diet more easily.

Many Americans share Ricky's longing for an easy way to lose weight or become fit. Millions of dollars are spent on books, tapes, pills, and exercise machines. But the outcomes Ricky seeks are not easy to achieve. Changing health behavior is difficult. Nurses, such as the family nurse practitioner profiled above, know how difficult it is to motivate well people to undertake behaviors that lessen the likelihood of future illness. Some health professionals have a mistaken notion that the mere provision of didactic information will bring about health-promoting actions. But studies show that although individuals are often aware of the risks associated with behaviors such as alcohol use and smoking, they modify their thinking about these risks rather than taking the more difficult route of changing the behaviors (Leffingwell, Neumann, Leedy, & Babitzke, 2007). Information is the solution only when ignorance is the problem. Health care providers need a more sophisticated understanding of the principles of behavior change to help their patients make health-promoting decisions. This chapter explores a variety of evidence-based interventions to change health behavior.

Concept of Health

Before discussing specific health behaviors, it is important to define *health,* a concept that remains something of an enigma. Is health a state, a process, or a goal? Gadamer (1996) pointed out that health "is not something that is revealed through investigation but rather something that manifests itself precisely by virtue of escaping our attention" (p. 96). To the average layperson, it is *illness* that compels attention, a departure from taken-for-granted smooth functioning. Likewise, traditional medical and nursing curricula have prepared health professionals to care for the acutely ill. Many textbooks still place greater emphasis on morbidity and mortality than on health promotion.

In contemporary nursing literature, many authors assert that nursing has a mandate to promote holistic health. What does this mean? Unfortunately, some people think that *holistic* means "new age" or "alternative," something outside traditional beliefs or practices. Because the term is frequently misused, it may be useful to trace its origin. The word *holism* was first used in a 1926 book by Jan Smuts (p. 99), the first prime minister of South Africa and a lifelong student of biological evolution. Smuts rejected the mechanistic explanation of the world that was pervasive in his time. He saw physical matter and the mind as inseparable, and he believed that holism, a dynamic striving toward integration, was the ultimate principle of the universe. Not until the late 1950s and 1960s did these ideas begin to infiltrate the American health care delivery system. In medicine, Halbert Dunn began to speak of "high level wellness," the ultimate integration of body, mind, and spirit as an interdependent whole (1959, 1971). In nursing, Martha Rogers (1970) wrote about unitary human beings who are not reducible to parts or symptoms. She also emphasized the indivisible whole of person and environment.

Concurrent with the gradually shifting perspective of health professionals, a consumer wellness movement burgeoned that was linked to the other human liberation movements of the 1960s and 1970s such as the civil rights and women's movements. Public dissatisfaction with paternalistic medical treatment and mystifying medical terms, along with a better educated, more affluent populace, contributed to a thirst for information about holistic therapies and self-care. Americans became preoccupied with self-care clinics, self-help groups, and the tantalizing potential of peak wellness and self-actualization. One prominent nursing theorist, Dorothea Orem, began to emphasize patients' self-care agency, recommending nursing intervention only when a self care deficit is detected (1983). Education of the public for self-care became an important element of federal government policies and public health initiatives, such as the Healthy People initiative, first begun in 1979 and reformulated each succeeding decade. Motivated by escalating costs of care for sick workers, corporations began to demand that employees assume more responsibility for their health and provided them incentives such as exercise rooms, walking trails, and low-fat meal options in the employee cafeteria. Several of the nursing theorists noted here and elsewhere in this chapter are also discussed in Chapter 5.

Evolving Conceptions of Health

Nursing interventions to promote health are guided by ideas about human beings and the meaning of the concept of health. Smith (1983) traced evolving conceptions of health across the centuries, categorizing them into four models (Table 15-1).

CLINICAL MODEL

Listed first is the narrowest view of health, the clinical model, perhaps more readily recognizable to nurses as the "medical model." Health is simply the absence of disease or disability in this model. On examination of

TABLE 15-1	Models of Health
Model	**Conception of Health**
Clinical	Elimination of disease as identified through medical science
Role performance	Ability to perform social, occupational, and other roles
Adaptive	Ability to engage in effective interaction with environment
Eudaemonistic	Self-actualization of individual; optimal well being

Modified from Smith, J. (1983). *The idea of health: Implications for the nursing profession.* New York: Teachers College Press.

the physiochemical system of the patient, the health care provider would declare "health" if no signs of any incipient illnesses were detected. Unfortunately, this narrow conceptualization of health is still dominant in many health care settings.

ROLE PERFORMANCE MODEL

The role performance model depicts health as the ability to fulfill one's customary social roles. Thus if a young mother is able to adequately carry out her childcare activities, she would be deemed healthy. If she cannot perform these activities, she would be considered ill. The problem with this view of health is the distressful and stultifying nature of many people's occupational or familial roles. Scholars are now placing emphasis on the quality of experience in social roles and the degree of choice about occupancy of these roles (Thomas, 1997a). Can individuals trapped in unsatisfying jobs or marriages achieve optimal health? What is the health impact of juggling multiple roles or experiencing role conflict? What if performance in one role (worker, for example) so dominates one's existence that performance in another role (parent) is compromised?

ADAPTIVE MODEL

Based largely on the ideas of Dubos (1965), the adaptive model emphasizes the ability to adapt flexibly to ever-changing environments and challenges.

Continuous readjustment to life's stressful demands is necessary. Healthy people are resilient and hardy. Disease is viewed as a failure of adaptation. Although the adaptive model achieved popularity in nursing, as exemplified in the work of theorists such as Callista Roy (1970), there is a still broader conceptualization of health.

EUDAEMONISTIC MODEL

Drawn from the Greek philosophers and from the humanistic psychologist Abraham Maslow (1961), the eudaemonistic model depicts health as the complete development of the individual's potential, an exuberant well-being. Clearly, this model emphasizes the human capacity for growth. Within nursing, theorist Margaret Newman (1978, 1994) has proposed that health is expanding consciousness.

For this chapter, a broad concept of health was selected, consistent with the broader view exemplified in Smith's adaptive and eudaemonistic models and Dunn's description of high-level wellness. Adopting a broader view of health has several implications for nursing practice. For one thing, separating mind, body, and spirit becomes impossible. Moreover, the patient's embeddedness in family, friendships, culture, and the environment cannot be ignored. Also, the patient's own power for healing is recognized. The role of the nurse is that of *facilitator* of the patient's own innate capabilities for healing and growth. Skilled counseling is as important as technical competence. Chapter 4 discusses roles in more detail.

Health Promotion and Disease Prevention

The terms *health promotion* and *disease prevention,* although often used synonymously, actually have different meanings. Flowing logically from adaptive or eudaemonistic views of health, health promotion refers to activities that protect good health and take people beyond their present level of wellness. By achieving lean and fit bodies and well-managed stress levels, individuals have a greater likelihood of achieving a high quality of life and reaching the goal

BOX 15-1	The 15 Leading Causes of Death in the United States, 2005

1. Heart disease
2. Malignant neoplasms
3. Cerebrovascular diseases
4. Chronic lower respiratory diseases
5. Accidents
6. Diabetes mellitus
7. Alzheimer's disease
8. Influenza and pneumonia
9. Nephritis, nephrosis
10. Septicemia
11. Suicide
12. Chronic liver disease and cirrhosis
13. Essential hypertension and hypertensive renal disease
14. Parkinson's disease
15. Assault (homicide)

From Kung, H-C., Hoyert, D. L., Xu, J., & Murphy, S. L. (2008). Deaths: Final data for 2005. *National Vital Statistics Reports* (Vol. 56, No. 10). Hyattsville, MD: National Center for Health Statistics.

of self-actualization. In contrast, disease prevention efforts are derived from the clinical model of health. Emphasis is frequently placed on avoidance, deprivation, or restraint. Behaviors are undertaken to prevent specific diseases. The importance of preventive efforts becomes obvious when reviewing statistics showing that men lose the equivalent of 11.5 well-years of life and women lose the equivalent of 15.6 well-years from morbidity (Kaplan, Anderson, & Wingard, 1991). Mortality statistics likewise demonstrate the importance of lifestyle modifications to prevent premature death. The chief causes of death in the United States are strongly related to unhealthy behaviors such as smoking and overeating (Box 15-1).

Modification of Health Attitudes and Behaviors

Convincing empirical evidence shows that healthy lifestyles can significantly reduce the mortality rate from cardiovascular diseases, cancer, obesity, diabetes, and human immunodeficiency virus/acquired

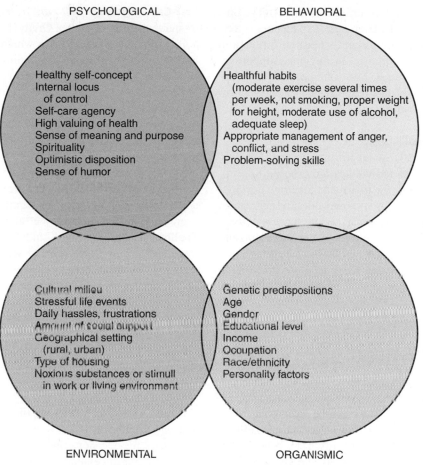

PSYCHOLOGICAL

Healthy self-concept
Internal locus
  of control
Self-care agency
High valuing of health
Sense of meaning and purpose
Spirituality
Optimistic disposition
Sense of humor

BEHAVIORAL

Healthful habits
  (moderate exercise several times
  per week, not smoking, proper weight
  for height, moderate use of alcohol,
  adequate sleep)
Appropriate management of anger,
  conflict, and stress
Problem-solving skills

Cultural milieu
Stressful life events
Daily hassles, frustrations
Amount of social support
Geographical setting
  (rural, urban)
Type of housing
Noxious substances or stimuli
  in work or living environment

Genetic predispositions
Age
Gender
Educational level
Income
Occupation
Race/ethnicity
Personality factors

ENVIRONMENTAL

ORGANISMIC

FIGURE 15-1 A comprehensive model of wellness.

immunodeficiency syndrome (HIV/AIDS). Therefore the modification of health attitudes and behavior is one of the most important responsibilities of every nurse. As shown in Figure 15-1, a comprehensive model of wellness includes interacting factors such as psychological characteristics, health-promoting behaviors, and aspects of the environments in which people live and work. Both attitudes and behaviors are modifiable by health care providers, as well as some (but not all) aspects of environments. The sections that follow examine a number of these modifiable factors. Although a comprehensive wellness model includes organismic variables (e.g., genetic predispositions) and demographic characteristics (e.g., age, income, gender), these are not amenable to modification by

health care providers. We instead emphasize the factors that can be affected by nurses.

PSYCHOLOGICAL ATTITUDES AND CHARACTERISTICS ASSOCIATED WITH WELLNESS

Self-Concept. Many theorists consider a healthy self-concept (and closely related concepts such as self-acceptance or self-esteem) essential for wellness. Persons who feel better about themselves are more inclined to enact self-care behaviors that promote good health. Abundant data demonstrate that self-destructive habits such as drug abuse are linked to lower self-worth. Although experiences with parents, teachers, and peers all contribute to initial development of self-concept, later life experiences offer opportunities to alter it. A client's negative evaluation of the self can be altered in an ongoing, supportive relationship with a nurse. For example, the nurse can guide the client to recall strengths, such as persistence in confronting life stressors.

Locus of Control. Locus of control is a construct from Rotter's (1954) social learning theory. According to this theory, as individuals are exposed to reinforcements (rewards) for their behavior, they develop beliefs about their ability to control desired outcomes or rewards. Eventually, most people have a stable, general expectancy that reinforcements are contingent on their own behavior (termed *internal locus of control*) or an expectancy that rewards are received on a purely random basis or dispensed by powerful others (called *external locus of control*). This stable, general expectancy has been given a variety of other names by researchers. For example, locus of control is subsumed in Kobasa's (1979) multidimensional hardiness construct and Antonovsky's (1984) sense of coherence. What does locus of control have to do with wellness? Rotter's theory was modified for health by researchers such as Wallston (1989). Logically, individuals who have an internal locus of control are more likely to engage in positive health behaviors. They believe that the reinforcement (good health) is directly related to their own actions, not controlled by powerful others (e.g., doctors) or by the vicissitudes of fate. Although questionnaires are available to measure locus of control, a nurse can easily assess it by asking questions such as the following: "What do you think caused you to have this heart attack? Who do you think knows best what you really need? Do you normally follow instructions pretty well, or do you prefer to work things out your own way?" Nursing interventions can be tailored accordingly. If the person has an internal locus of control, a nurse should allow a high degree of client participation in goal setting and selection of reinforcers. If the person has an external locus of control, providing plenty of concrete guidance and support is important. For example, if the goal is weight loss, suggest involvement in a program with regular group meetings, such as Weight Watchers.

Self-Care Agency. *Self-care agency,* a term coined by nurse theorist Dorothea Orem (1995), refers to the ability to care for oneself, for which the person must have knowledge, skills, understanding, and willingness. In working with a client, assessment of all these factors is necessary. A parallel concept from social cognitive theory called *self-efficacy* (Bandura, 1997) has generated a sizable body of health psychology and nursing literature. According to Bandura's theory, when people perceive that they have efficacy to accomplish a specific behavior (e.g., breast self-examination), they are predisposed to undertake the behavior. Studies of older adults found that self-efficacy significantly influenced exercise behavior (McAuley et al., 2008; Resnick & Spellbring, 2000). Other studies have established links between self-efficacy and weight management, smoking cessation, chronic disease management, and medication adherence (Anderson & Anderson, 2003). This empirical evidence suggests that a nurse's first step in working with many clients is to enhance their belief in personal capability. Research shows that self-efficacy is modifiable through strategies such as anticipatory guidance and persuasive motivational messages (Bandura, 1997).

Values. Values are elements that show how a person has decided to use his or her life. Values serve as a basis for decisions and choices. The nurse must assess the reinforcement value of health to an individual compared with other life values such as pleasure, excitement, or social recognition. Jackson, Tucker, and Herman (2007) found that individuals who place a higher value on health also display greater involvement in a health-promoting lifestyle. Of course, some people declare that they highly value health, but their behaviors contradict this declaration. A value system may contain conflicting values. For example, highly valuing achievement and financial prosperity may result in overwork and neglect of health. Assisting a client to clarify conflicting values can be a useful intervention. The chapter on ethics (Chapter 12) discusses values in more detail.

Sense of Purpose. Having a sense of meaning and purpose for one's life may be an important factor in individuals' responsiveness to health providers' instructions. Purpose in life includes having goals for the future and a sense of directedness. Exploring whether clients aim to follow a particular career trajectory, pursue an enjoyable hobby or avocation, or see their children and grandchildren grow and mature is often helpful. In what way does each person aim to make a difference or leave a legacy? Persons with clear goals may devote more effort to health maintenance because most goals cannot be achieved without good health. Empirical evidence shows that purpose in life is correlated with good health habits (Williams, Thomas, Young, Jozwiak, & Hector, 1991).

Spirituality. Health researchers and clinicians are increasingly recognizing that spirituality is an integral component of holistic health and wellness. Spirituality is not synonymous with involvement in organized religion, but the sense of connection with a divine wisdom or higher power often motivates practices such as meditation, prayer, and attendance at religious services. Studies have examined the relationship of spirituality and/or religious practice with disease conditions (e.g., heart disease, cancer, mental illness) as well as health risk behaviors (e.g., smoking, drinking, using drugs) (Hart, 2008). Rapidly burgeoning research shows that religious people are less anxious and depressed and are more adept at coping with illness and tragedy than are nonreligious individuals (Koenig, cited in Paul, 2005). Clients may be motivated to take health-promoting actions by a belief that the body is a temple for the spirit.

Optimism. An optimistic disposition has been shown to be important to health in studies conducted for more than two decades. Carver and Scheier (2002) assert that optimism is a stable personality characteristic with important implications for the manner in which people regulate their actions, particularly actions relevant to health. The construct of optimism includes tendencies to expect the best, look on the bright side, and anticipate good things in the future. It is important to note that the presence of optimism is not dependent on a person's particular locus of control; expectations of favorable outcomes could be derived from perceptions of being lucky or blessed (external locus of control) or from convictions of personal control (internal locus of

control). Higher levels of optimism have been associated with positive health outcomes such as completion of an alcohol treatment program and faster recovery after coronary bypass surgery, bone marrow transplant, and traumatic injury (Carver & Scheier, 2002). An optimistic outlook can be cultivated if it does not come naturally (Seligman, 1998).

Sense of Humor. Although a sense of humor is a socially appealing trait, it also conveys health benefits. The physical effects of mirth have been compared with the effects of exercise. For example, laughing 100 times expends the same number of calories as 10 minutes on a rowing machine (Godfrey, 2004). The efficiency of the respiratory system increases, and the cardiovascular and muscular systems relax (Kennedy, 1995). Humor and laughter have been linked to higher levels of endorphins and immunoglobulin A and lower levels of cortisol (Berk et al., 1989; Godfrey, 2004). Laughter is an excellent way to dispel stress and tension as well. Perhaps that is why laughter clubs quickly became popular across the globe after an Indian physician started the first one in 1995 (Perry, 2005).

HEALTH BEHAVIORS ASSOCIATED WITH WELLNESS

Behaviors associated with wellness are listed in Figure 15-1. The first research about health behaviors was done in the 1950s by social psychologists who sought to explain the public's perplexingly low response to screening programs that were free or low in cost (Hochbaum, 1958). From this work, a model emerged that can be used to predict preventive health action. According to the health belief model (HBM), an individual's perceptions of his or her susceptibility to a disease (and the severity of that disease), the perceived benefits of taking action, and cues to action (from media, health professionals, or family) contribute to the likelihood of taking preventive actions—provided that barriers are not too great (Becker et al., 1977). Subsequent research with the HBM found barriers to be the most useful element of the model in predicting behavior such as physical exercise (Janz & Becker, 1984). Typical barriers are time, expense, and inconvenience.

In the 1980s, nurse researcher Nola Pender presented a model with similarities to the HBM but with greater emphasis on health-promoting behaviors. Based on research that tested Pender's health promotion model, the model was revised, deleting constructs with insufficient predictive power (Figure 15-2).

Individual characteristics and prior behavior are theorized to affect perceptions of self-efficacy, benefits and barriers to action, and a variable called "activity-related affect," which refers to the feelings about the behavior in question. For example, is exercise fun or unpleasant? All these factors, as well as interpersonal

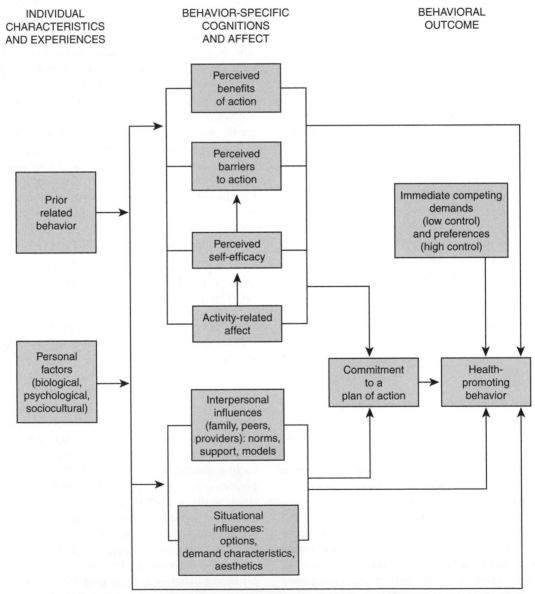

FIGURE 15-2 Pender's revised health promotion model. (From Pender, N., Murdaugh, C. L., & Parsons, M. A. [2002]. Health promotion in nursing practice [4th ed.]. Upper Saddle River, NJ: Prentice-Hall.)

and situational variables, can influence commitment to a plan of action. Additionally, competing demands such as work or family care responsibilities are taken into account in the prediction of health-promoting behavior, the outcome variable of the model. The best predictors of health-promoting behavior, according to a synopsis of 38 studies, are perceived self-efficacy, perceived barriers, and prior behavior (Pender, Murdaugh, & Parsons, 2002).

Most health behavior models fail to acknowledge the powerful role of *affect*. Lawton, Conner, and McEachan (2009) found that affect (the enjoyment of the activity) was a better predictor than cognitive attitude (harm or benefit of the activity) for four risky behaviors (e.g., drinking) and five health-promoting behaviors (e.g., eating fruits and vegetables). The researchers concluded that "many of the behaviors that most threaten our health and safety may not be reasoned or planned but depend, at least to some extent, on whether they make us feel happy or sad, relaxed or tense" (Lawton et al., 2009, pp. 63–64).

Health Habits. More than 30 years ago, longitudinal studies established that good health habits, such as regular exercise, are correlated with better health status and longevity (Belloc & Breslow, 1972; Breslow & Enstrom, 1980). Given that the benefits of healthful habits are well established, the average American's lack of adherence to the recommended lifestyle regimen is discouraging. We focus here on exercise, diet, tobacco use, sleep, and emotion management.

Exercise. Most adults (75%) do not engage in 30 minutes of daily exercise, and one third are completely sedentary (Physical activity trends—United States, 2001). Sedentarism has increased in both children and adults with the escalation of hours spent using computers, television, and hand-held electronic devices for entertainment as well as business purposes (Ricciardi, 2005). The prevalence of inactivity rises with age, and women are more likely than men to be inactive at all ages (Wang, Pratt, Macera, Zheng, & Heath, 2004). Analyzing data from a nationally representative sample, researchers found a strong relationship between inactivity and cardiovascular disease, resulting in medical expenses of more than $23 billion dollars (Wang et al., 2004). Even when an exercise program is started, the usual rate of dropout is 50% in the first 3 to 6 months (Pender, 1996). Many people have an aversion to exercise, mentally associating it with competitive sports or regimented calisthenics. Even as health club membership climbs—at least among the more affluent—too many Americans pay someone else to wash the car, use riding mowers to mow the lawn, and treat their treadmills as clothes racks.

Nurses need to spread the word that gym membership and expensive equipment are not necessary for regular physical workouts. Research shows that long-term adherence to an exercise program is more likely when the regimen is home based rather than dependent on participation in a group class at a gym (King et al., 1997). If finances preclude purchasing a set of weights, soup cans and other household items can be substituted. Although fear of crime inhibits outdoor exercise, especially among women and older adults (Roman & Chalfin, 2008), nearly everyone can find some safe place to walk (shopping malls are a good alternative for those who live in unsafe neighborhoods). Studies show that walking provides almost all the benefits of more vigorous activity, requires no equipment or fees, and can be done alone or with a companion (Norman & Mills, 2004). Gardening, dancing, and biking are pleasurable activities that are also beneficial to the heart and muscle tone. A person raking leaves burns 288 calories per hour—while also enjoying fresh air and fall colors. Clients may be more motivated to exercise when informed of immediate benefits, such as increased energy and improved mood. Exercise can lift spirits for as long as 2 to 4 hours (Kaplan, 1997).

Because so many clients are completely sedentary, professionals must remember to begin with realistic and achievable goals, such as 5 to 10 minutes of walking. In an experiment with healthy young college women, aimed at enhancing their exercise self-efficacy, some women dropped out of the study at the time of the pretest because they perceived that a "step test" was frightening and aversive. They were afraid that the subsequent exercise sessions (step aerobics, dancing, and kickboxing) would be far too difficult for them to perform (D'Alonzo, Stevenson, & Davis, 2004). If such apprehensions are present in healthy young women, consider how they could be magnified in older adults. Effective exercise interventions must be tailored carefully. On a positive note, emphasize to clients that as little as 10 minutes a day of moderate exercise can reduce risk for disease and improve quality of life (Listfield, 2009).

Healthy Eating. The United States is in the midst of an alarming obesity epidemic, in which more than one third of adults are obese (Ogden, Carroll, McDowell, & Flegal, 2007). Not only is obesity (a body mass index greater than 30) rapidly rising, but so is morbid obesity (defined as a BMI greater than 40). Between 2000 and 2005, the number of individuals with a BMI greater than 40 increased by 50% (and those with a BMI greater than 50 increased by 75%) (Sturm, 2007). By 2030, the global burden of obesity will be staggering: 2.16 billion adults are predicted to be overweight and 1.12 billion obese (Kelly, Yang, Chen, Reynolds, & He, 2008). Childhood obesity has reached such unparalleled proportions that the Centers for Disease Control and Prevention has launched a $60 million prevention program (Holloway, 2005). It is clear that the "happy meals" children consume today will have unhappy consequences for their health tomorrow. The prevalence of obesity in school-age children has quadrupled since the 1970s (Estabrooks, Fisher, & Hayman, 2008), and an obese child has a 70% to 75% chance of becoming an obese adult (Clarke & Lauer, 1993). Some obese children already have the arteries of 45-year-old adults. Among the consequences of the rapidly rising incidence of obesity in the United States is the increased number of adults with hypertension (65 million now compared with 50 million in 1994). Millions more are prehypertensive (Kluger, 2004), prompting the government to recommend the low-fat, low-salt, low-sweets DASH diet (Dietary Approaches to Stop Hypertension).

Despite widespread media promotion of the USDA's Food Guide Pyramid (MyPyramid) and the plant-based Mediterranean diet, Americans consume nowhere near the recommended daily servings of fruits and vegetables. Current intake of flour, grains, and beans is only two thirds of what society consumed in 1910. Each person, on average, consumes 150 pounds of sweeteners (mostly sugar and corn syrup) per year, 25 pounds more than in 1984. Americans drink twice as much carbonated soda as milk. And society still consumes too much fat (U.S. Department of Agriculture, 2008). Falling consumption of fish is another problem, resulting in inadequate intake of omega-3 fatty acids, which could reduce heart attack risk (Campos, Baylin, & Willett, 2008) and improve mood and mental health (Hallahan & Garland, 2005). Human beings are not genetically adapted for this type of diet. In fact, people should be eating like hunter-gatherers, who had no atherosclerosis even when they lived to advanced ages (Cordain, Eaton, Brand Miller, Mann, & Hill, 2002). This would mean replacing carbohydrates (especially foods with a high glycemic index, such as bread and potatoes) with proteins.

Food is laden with emotional and social significance, complicating attempts at dietary modification. Therefore targeting interventions to children while their eating habits are still developing makes good sense. When she learned that one third of school-age children in her state were overweight or obese, the Texas agriculture commissioner (a mother of three) banned junk food from school cafeterias (Booth-Thomas, 2004). Grain bars, nuts, and baked chips replaced candy in the school vending machines. Fresh produce, yogurt, and low-sugar drinks became available to the students. Nurses could become involved in similar efforts to combat childhood obesity in their own communities.

Complicating nurses' efforts to combat the obesity epidemic is their own predilection to be overweight or obese; more than half of nurses weigh too much (Miller, Alpert, & Cross, 2008). Research shows that laypersons have less confidence in nurses' ability to provide health education when nurses themselves are overweight (Hicks et al., 2008).

Tobacco Use. According to the World Health Organization, 20% of the world's people smoke; in 2008 smoking killed more than 5 million people (WHO, 2008). In the United States, public smoking has been discouraged by bans in offices, restaurants, and airports. Many Americans have kicked the habit. But smoking prevalence remains high among lower-income groups, and it is rising among girls and women, with a concomitant increase in female lung cancer. Another disturbing trend is waterpipe (hookah)

TABLE 15-2	Prochaska's Transtheoretical Model of Change Applied to Smoking Cessation
Stage 1: Precontemplation	Smokers do not see their smoking as a problem and do not intend to stop within the next 6 months.
Stage 2: Contemplation	Smokers see their smoking as a problem and think about quitting but are not ready to change.
Stage 3: Preparation	Smokers intend to take action in the next month; some have made small changes, such as cutting down on the number smoked or delaying the first smoke of the day.
Stage 4: Action	Smokers adopt a goal of smoking cessation and make an attempt to quit, involving overt behavior change and environmental modification.
Stage 5: Maintenance	Smokers work to prevent relapse and maintain abstinence.

Modified from Prochaska, J. O., DiClemente, C. C., & Norcross, J. C. (1992). In search of how people change: Applications to addictive behaviors. *American Psychologist, 47,* 1102–1114.

smoking, which is becoming popular among college students because of the pleasant flavorings (e.g., apple, coffee) and sweeteners added to the tobacco (Primack et al., 2008). Approximately 90% of new smokers are teenagers; 3000 begin smoking every day (Lindell & Reinke, 1999). More adolescents are smoking today than at any time since the 1970s. Some 35% of today's high school students smoke cigarettes, compared with 28% in 1991 (Centers for Disease Control and Prevention, 1996). Some youngsters have their first smoke in middle school or earlier. These youngsters do not know they are exposed to more than 4000 chemicals each time they light up, including arsenic and radioactive compounds such as polonium (Ruppert, 1999). Some of them have the mistaken belief that water-pipes, cigars, clove cigarettes, or chewing tobacco are healthy alternatives to cigarettes. The statistics on youth tobacco use are deeply disturbing given the addictive potential of nicotine. In addition, adolescent smoking is a powerful predictor of adult smoking (Chassin, Presson, Rose, & Sherman, 1996).

Studies have shown that nurse-delivered smoking cessation counseling is effective even when relatively brief; only a few minutes are necessary for a nurse to ask about smoking status, assess a client's desire to quit, and provide evidence-based advice about tactics (Bialous & Sarna, 2004). Approximately 76% of smokers say they want to quit, but they lack specific plans to do so (Herzog & Blagg, 2007). There are many barriers to quitting: withdrawal symptoms, missing the companionship of cigarettes, less control

of stress and moods, fear of weight gain, and lack of encouragement from family and friends. Some of the barriers can be dispelled by clear, strong, and personalized advice from clinicians; "Continuing to smoke makes your asthma worse" or "Quitting smoking may reduce the number of ear infections your child has" (Fiore et al., 2008, p. 163). Some parents are surprised to learn that their children are still exposed to the toxins in tobacco smoke even if the parent smokes only while the children are sleeping. "Third-hand smoke" lingers in the home, contaminating surfaces where children crawl and play (Third-Hand Smoke: Another Reason to Quit Smoking, 2008).

Motivating a client to stop smoking is always a challenge. James Prochaska and his research team have studied the stages of change in addictive behaviors (Prochaska, DiClemente, & Norcross, 1992). In working with a client, the Prochaska model is helpful in assessing the client's stage. The Prochaska model is applied to smoking cessation in Table 15-2. Health professionals can promote client movement to subsequent stages by interventions that raise consciousness. For example, a middle-age man in a high-stress job may be startled to learn that smoking does *not* improve mood on stressful days; smoking actually worsens mood (Aronson, Almeida, Stawski, Klein, & Kozlowski, 2008). An adolescent girl who uses smoking for weight control may consider cessation when she learns of its negative effects on the skin. Interventions to promote smoking cessation can be guided by the HBM, as shown in Table 15-3. Medication

TABLE 15-3	Application of the Health Belief Model in Interventions to Promote Smoking Cessation
Factor	**Interventions**
Perceived susceptibility	Teach about morbidity and mortality statistics of smokers versus nonsmokers.
Perceived severity	Illustrate what happens to lungs and other organs when smoking; show pictures of diseased lungs and wrinkled skin.
Perceived barriers	Identify barriers unique to the individual and counsel regarding common fears about weight gain, greater stress, and irritability.
Perceived benefits	Identify benefits, such as more pleasant breath and body odor; increased energy; decreased cough; improved circulation; enhanced ability to taste; and reduced risk of heart disease and stroke and cancers of the mouth, throat, esophagus, lungs, bladder, and cervix.
Cues to action	Use telephone calls and postcard reminders. Provide pamphlets about cessation strategies. Organize support groups and buddy systems.

should be prescribed, unless contraindicated; nicotine replacement therapy combats withdrawal symptoms such as irritability and craving. Research by Judith Prochaska's team showed that exercise during smoking cessation not only improves mood but also increases the probability of staying smoke-free (Prochaska et al., 2008). During cessation, smokers must break the associations between smoking and familiar environments (e.g., the living room couch) that stimulate craving (Stambor, 2006), so alterations in the environment and daily routines are recommended. Lapses in abstinence are common, and clients must be encouraged to resume the strategies that initially helped them to quit. Successful quitters usually make several tries.

Sleep. Sleep does not receive sufficient attention from health care providers, but it is essential to physical and mental health. It affects concentration, productivity, and mood. Research shows that a good night's sleep improves thinking and memory (Gorman, 2004). Unfortunately, millions of Americans are sleep deprived. The 2005 "Sleep in America" poll showed that 75% of adults had symptoms of a sleep problem a few nights per week (or more) within the past year; 60% of drivers say they drove while drowsy within the past year; and sleep-related issues constituted the primary reason people were late for work (National Sleep Foundation, 2005). Even children are sleeping less than experts recommend. For example, preschoolers should sleep 11 to 13 hours, but a survey showed an average of only 10.4 hours; school-age children should sleep 10 to 11 hours but average only 9.5 hours (National Sleep Foundation, 2004). Many parents are unaware of the recommended amount of sleep for their children. Nurses' health promotion efforts must include education about sleep hygiene and sleep disorders.

Emotion Management. Appropriate management of emotions (particularly anger and hostility) has been recognized as essential to wellness for several decades, spurred by the research linking the angry, competitive type A behavior pattern to coronary heart disease (Shoham, Ragland, Brand, & Syme, 1988).

Over the years, anger has proven to be the most toxic element of the type A pattern. Links have been documented between anger and hostility and coronary artery calcification, increased cardiovascular reactivity, elevated lipid levels, lower pulmonary function, poorer general health, and early death (Bunde & Suls, 2006; Harburg, Julius, Kaciroti, Gleiberman, & Schork, 2003; Holt-Lunstad, Smith, & Uchino, 2008; Iribarren et al., 2000; Jackson, Cohen, Kubzansky, Jacobs, & Wright, 2007; Merjonen, Pulkki-Raback, & Keltikangas-Jarvinen, 2007; Pollitt et al., 2005; Suarez, Bates, & Harralson, 1998). Research by immunologists showed that intensely hostile interactions, such as arguments with a spouse, lower one's immunocompetence (Kiecolt-Glaser et al., 1993).

Although anger is a normal human emotion, it is pathogenic when it is too frequent, too intense, too prolonged, or managed ineffectively. Habitual suppression is just as problematic as the tendency to have explosive outbursts because suppression of emotion requires great effort. Suppressed anger is associated with higher blood pressure and eventual development of hypertension (Harburg et al., 2003; Perini, Muller, & Buhler, 1991; Thomas, 1997b). Anger also contributes to disease by causing increased consumption of food, cigarettes, alcohol, and other mood-altering drugs.

The health-promoting way of managing anger is to wait until the initial physiological arousal abates, then discuss the anger-provoking incident with the provocateur or a confidant and, finally, take constructive action to resolve the problem. Persons who regularly discuss their anger in this way have lower blood pressure and better health (Thomas, 1997c). When resentment about an old grievance has become chronic, it should be released by forgiving the offender. If the offender is deceased or far away, forgiveness can still be accomplished through reflective journaling or a healing ritual. Extensive research by psychologist James Pennebaker (1990) demonstrates the healing power of expressing emotions through confiding in others or writing about painful events. Health promotion efforts by nurses should include instruction about healthy emotional disclosure and anger management. Guidelines for teaching anger management to community groups may be found in Thomas (2001). Interventions should be tailored with regard to gender, culture, and customary expression style (whether volatile or suppressive) (Thomas, 2006, 2007).

Problem Solving. Problem-solving skills must be taught to clients who do not know systematic strategies and techniques for enacting healthful habits or making changes in health behavior. For example, recovering alcoholics need to learn ways to slowly sip on nonalcoholic beverages at a party; dieters must practice polite refusal of foods at a family gathering. Middle school students may benefit from role playing a scenario in which they refuse illicit drugs at a party. Individuals who lack assertiveness may need to rehearse firm insistence that sex partners use condoms. Assertiveness can also empower underserved groups to request needed community services or assistance from other members of the health care team. When giving exercise or diet prescriptions to clients, health care providers should ask what problems or barriers they envision; this will point the way to the skills that need to be taught. Some clients benefit from problem-solving activities in groups, such as groups conducted with dieters (Hollis et al., 2008).

Evidence-Based Interventions to Promote Behavior Change

Health professionals often use threats of future disease when urging behavior change. However, when people are frightened, they use denial to convince themselves that the threatening event (e.g., HIV/AIDS, cancer) is not likely to happen to them. Research shows that such threats of distant adverse outcomes are not as likely to be as successful as approaches that confer immediate benefits and rewards or reduce denial (Eitel & Friend, 1999). Motivational enhancement counseling is effective in producing lifestyle change (Burke, Arkowitz, & Menchola, 2003). Components of the motivational counseling approach are provider empathy, a spirit of collaboration with the client, avoidance of lecturing or arguing, and support of client self-efficacy (Riegel et al., 2006). Nurses should remember that many laypersons hold unfavorable views of the medical establishment and are skeptical about medical practitioners' advice because of prior negative experiences (Hughner & Kleine, 2008). Therefore establishing a collaborative relationship with clients is the first priority (Thomas & Pollio, 2002). Then readiness to change can be assessed. Surprising readiness to change may be evident when the nurse simply asks screening questions during routine primary care visits, such as "Do you drink more than you should?" For example, a high percentage (75%) of outpatients who screened positive for alcohol misuse indicated readiness to change (Williams et al., 2006). When promoting behavior change, be aware that "approach goals" (e.g., increasing consumption of fruits and vegetables) are easier for clients to work on than "avoidance goals" (e.g., decreasing snacks or sweets) (Sullivan & Rothman, 2008).

A health risk appraisal (HRA) is a tool that can be used to provide clients with an estimate of biological age versus chronological age, an assessment of risk factors that may lead to health problems, and specific recommendations for behavioral changes that may lengthen their lives. A variety of computerized HRA instruments are available, as well as paper-and-pencil versions of the tests. Some health risk appraisal tools are limited in scope, focusing only on a specific area, such as risk for coronary heart disease. Others assess broad areas, including the environment, education, stress, family history, and health behavior. These surveys are often administered during health fairs at community centers and shopping malls. An HRA instrument is best used in conjunction with laboratory tests (e.g., cholesterol, triglycerides) and the on-site measurement of some variables by professionals (e.g., blood pressure, triceps skin-fold thickness). Nurses should bear in mind that the accuracy of HRA mortality predictions has been called into question, so focusing on the client's life expectancy is not recommended. Individuals who are given the results of their risk assessment along with a supportive educational process benefit more than persons who simply receive the test results.

The selection of incremental, achievable goals is also essential because clients can be overwhelmed by the prospect of drastic changes such as sweeping dietary modifications. One research team asked overweight adults to make only one small change in food choice and one small change in physical activity per week; significant improvements in waist circumference, intra-abdominal fat, and weight resulted (Lutes et al., 2008).

Nurse practitioner Lynda Carpenito asks obese clients whether they want to lose weight; if the answer is yes, she then asks, "How much?" The client's goal becomes her goal. Next, with the client, two or three areas are chosen to work on (e.g., replacing bologna with low-fat/low-salt chicken or tuna) (Carpenito, 1998). Such an approach is far more likely to result in compliance than stringent calorie restriction. Clients should be taught that slow weight loss is preferable to rapid loss from fad diets, which can produce ketosis, gout, and other adverse consequences. Inspiration can be derived from the participants in the National Weight Control Registry, who have lost 30 pounds or more, and kept it off for at least a year. Their success is attributed to (1) limiting calories to 1300 to 1500 per day; (2) starting the day with breakfast; (3) weighing regularly; and (4) engaging in 60 to 90 minutes of physical activity per day (Hill & Wing, 2003). Even small changes may increase quality of life. For example, overweight women who lost as little as 5 pounds handled everyday activities more easily and had fewer aches and pains (Fine et al., 1999). Older adults (ages 70 to 82) who simply expended energy in routine daily activities, such as household chores and climbing stairs, had a 32% lower risk of mortality over the 6 years of a longitudinal study by Manini et al. (2006). Achieving an extra decade of life may be a significant motivator of healthful habits for some individuals. According to longitudinal studies of more than 360,000 patients, people who did not smoke and maintained low cholesterol levels (200 mg/dL or below) and blood pressure (120/80 mm Hg or less) can live up to 9.5 years longer than those less careful about their health (Stamler et al., 1999). Death from cardiovascular disease, as well as from all other causes, was substantially reduced among adults with this desirable risk profile.

In contrast to interventions that target a single deleterious behavior, success was achieved by one team of researchers who delivered a multiple-behavior intervention to college students. PowerPoint slides were used to enhance the verbal messages. Despite the brevity of the behavioral counseling (25 minutes), significant improvements were found in sleep and health-related quality of life, along with reduced alcohol and marijuana use (Werch et al., 2008).

When health care providers write prescriptions for exercise or diet, adherence improves (Dobson, 2008). Another strategy with proven effectiveness is contracting. The purpose of writing a contract is to arrange a favorable, positively reinforcing experience when the client performs the desirable health behavior. Elements of a good contract are depicted in Box 15-2. A sample contract for weight loss appears in Figure 15-3.

BOX 15-2	Elements of a Good Contract for Behavior Change

- The behavior must be carefully selected and explicitly described.
- The behavior must be measurable (e.g., number of cigarettes smoked, minutes of exercise).
- A data collection plan must be developed (e.g., calendar, log, chart, graph, diary).
- Client and nurse agree on the goals (short-term and long-term) and time frame.
- Client and nurse agree on the reinforcers (extrinsic and intrinsic).
- Reinforcers are specified for step-by-step approximations of the desired behavior.
- Client and nurse sign the written contract and both keep a copy.
- Client and nurse evaluate effectiveness of the plan.
- The plan is revised as needed.

Keeping a log or diary also contributes to successful behavior change, especially when attempting to lose weight. In a 2008 study by Hollis and colleagues, food diary keepers lost twice as much weight as those who did not keep food diaries.

An impediment to the use of written prescriptions and contracts is the low functional literacy of Americans. According to a 2004 report from the Institute of Medicine, 90 million American adults have difficulty understanding and acting on the information given to them by their health care providers (Nielsen-Bohlman, Panzer, & Kindig, 2004). Literacy levels are lower among minorities, the poor, older adults, and those with less education. The implication of the Institute of Medicine report is clear: If giving written materials to clients, use simple, everyday vocabulary. Ascertain clients' comprehension of the behavior change instructions and invite questions before they leave the clinical area.

Desired outcome:	Weight loss of 10 lb
Long-term goal:	To lose 2½ lb. per week for 4 weeks
Short-term goals:	1. Maintain 1200 calorie/day diet 2. Increase water consumption to eight glasses per day 3. Avoid skipping meals 4. Ride exercise machine: 　　Week 1: 15 minutes 3 times per week 　　Week 2: 20 minutes 3 times per week 　　Week 3: 25 minutes 3 times per week 　　Week 4: 30 minutes 3 times per week 5. Weigh self on Monday mornings. Record weight on flow sheet.
Intrinsic rewards:	Increased self-esteem and confidence Clothes fit better Improved physical fitness and appearance
Extrinsic rewards:	Upon successful completion of each day's regimen, a 20-minute bubble bath At end of each week, movie with a friend At end of contract, purchase of a new outfit

Signature of nurse _____ Signature of client _____ Date _____

FIGURE 15-3 Example of a health behavior change contract.

Environmental Factors That Affect Wellness

Nurses must look beyond individual capabilities in the quest to help clients become healthier. The range of health-promoting choices available to individuals may be drastically limited by societal forces, structures, and policies (Butterfield, 1990). As depicted in Figure 15-1, numerous environmental factors affect wellness.

CULTURE

The cultural milieu in which a person develops and resides has a profound influence. In successful health promotion initiatives, the help of cultural insiders is solicited so that professionals can be aware of cultural norms and traditions before interventions are developed. Customs, laws, novels, films, television, and other cultural forces shape ideas about health and how to achieve it. Culture determines whether an individual thinks healthful body movement should take the form of tai chi or jogging, or whether aging should involve accepting wrinkles or having face lifts. Culture can also convey conflicting messages. Paradoxically, Americans are saturated with media images of toned, sleek bodies, while fast-food restaurants beckon at every intersection. A visitor from another planet, confronted with our highly health-conscious but overweight, sedentary population, might conclude that most Americans have a death wish. This topic is also addressed in Chapter 14.

ENVIRONMENTAL INFLUENCES

Nurses' attention to environmental hazards was heightened when the American Nurses Association adopted the Precautionary Principle in 2004. Thousands of new chemicals have been introduced in recent years, but research regarding their effects on human beings is often lacking. Many products commonly used in agriculture, industry, and the home are proving to be harmful. If adverse health effects are suspected, the Precautionary Principle mandates that nurses take precautionary measures even if cause-effect relationships have not been scientifically demonstrated. Nurses are also urged to include an environmental exposure history in routine health assessments (Buchanan, 2005). Clients should be queried about exposures where they live, play, and work.

Many people are exposed to noxious substances or stimuli in the workplace. Asbestos, mercury, radiation, and toxic chemicals such as pesticides are just a few of the hazards workers may encounter. Social and psychological hazards must be considered as well. Racial or sexual discrimination on the job may present a health risk equivalent to (or even greater than) environmental factors such as excessive workplace noise. Queries about a client's place of residence may reveal proximity to polluting industries or hazardous waste sites. Many Americans reside in substandard housing in neighborhoods where crime and violence are commonplace. Some lack the security provided by a close-knit community of solicitous neighbors. They may have limited coping resources to withstand the daily bombardment of stressful events and hassles.

STRESS

What happens when the environment bombards individuals with stressors? Researchers now know that stress is not simply a physiological reaction to environmental stimuli, as conceptualized by Selye (1956), but is instead a psychological appraisal that the environmental demands exceed one's coping resources (Lazarus, 1991). Early stress research focused on major life events such as foreclosure of a mortgage, bereavement, divorce, or job loss, demonstrating that an accumulation of such events could be detrimental to health (Holmes & Rahe, 1967). These major life events are undoubtedly disruptive, but minor daily hassles such as traffic jams and rude salespersons tax frustration tolerance as well (Kanner, Coyne, Schaefer, & Lazarus, 1981). Allostasis (the continual adjustment of our bodies to stressors) can slide into health-damaging *allostatic load* when stress lasts too long or the body's response is too strong (McEwen & Lasley, 2003). Chronic stress increases vulnerability to disease and accelerates the aging process by shortening the life span of cells (Epel et al., 2004). Stress can undermine enactment of health-promoting behavior. For example, during weeks with a high frequency of stressful events, people tend to exercise fewer days and for less time (Stetson, Rahn, Dubbert, Wilner, & Mercury, 1997). Fortunately, stress management modalities, ranging from meditation to yoga to breathing techniques, are widely available. However, health care providers must, once again, keep the environmental context in mind. Individuals in highly stressful environments may choose health-damaging behaviors to help them cope. One study showed that British working-class mothers smoked in full knowledge of the deleterious consequences because smoking was one of the few coping strategies available to them (Graham, 1984). One of every eight Americans lives in conditions of poverty, with an income below the federal poverty level (U.S. Census Bureau, 2000). People living in poverty are not likely to perceive that they can master stress. In fact, when poverty is chronic and resources scant, individuals are likely to have pervasive feelings of powerlessness and a fatalistic outlook.

SOCIAL SUPPORT

Loving relationships with significant others may buffer or moderate stress. Connectedness to others is a central element in health throughout life. Considerable empirical evidence shows that social support produces improved resistance to disease and even influences recovery from myocardial infarction (Lett et al., 2007) and longevity. How does social support result in improved health? Both emotional and instrumental types of support have been identified (Finfgeld-Connett, 2005). Support from relatives and friends can include concrete material help (e.g., money, provision of health information and advice) as well as affirmation of self-worth and encouragement to maintain good self-care practices. Extrafamilial support groups and health professionals can also play a vital role in encouraging exercise, smoking cessation, dieting, and other health-promoting actions. The value of a dieting or jogging "buddy" is well known. Stigmatized and marginalized client populations, such as the homeless, may lack a supportive network. Mobilizing social support can be an essential nursing intervention in such cases.

National Health Promotion Goals

Nurses' health promotion efforts must be supported and guided by an adequate understanding of U.S. public policy. The Healthy People documents published in 1979, 1990, and 2000 by the U.S. Public Health Service (USPHS), Department of Health and Human Services, have focused on both individual and societal influences on health. These widely disseminated publications have drawn attention to health disparities among Americans and provided guidance to state and local planners of public health programs. Health promotion and disease prevention objectives are precisely stated and measurable. The precisely delineated objectives in the Healthy People documents have enabled measurement of the nation's progress.

The *Healthy People 2000 Review* showed considerable progress in reaching more than half of the nation's 300 objectives for the final decade of the twentieth century (USPHS, 1999). For example, outbreaks of waterborne diseases and foodborne infections were reduced. However, the report showed that movement was going in the wrong direction for one fifth of the objectives. Of note, little improvement had been made in reducing the number of overweight individuals. Other disturbing trends included an increase in heavy drinking by high school seniors and increased deaths from falls and motor vehicle crashes (USPHS, 1999). In *Healthy People 2010,* many objectives focused on interventions to reduce illness, disability, and premature death, whereas others aimed at strengthening public health services and improving dissemination of health-related information (USPHS, 2000). Selected objectives and their targets are shown in Table 15-4. Currently, regional meetings are taking place to determine the goals for *Healthy People 2020,* after which public comment will be solicited. Updates on nurses' involvement in the process may be obtained at www.nursingworld.org. Comments may be offered at www.healthypeople.gov/hp2020/comments/default/asp. The national health care goals and Healthy People are discussed further in Chapter 19.

TABLE 15-4	Selected Examples of National Health Promotion Objectives as Identified in *Healthy People 2010*		
Focus Area	**Goal**	**Objective**	**Target**
15. Injury and violence prevention	Reduce disabilities, injuries, and deaths due to unintentional injuries and violence	15-15. Reduce deaths caused by motor vehicle crashes	By 2010: 9 deaths per 100,000 (reduced from 15.8)
19. Nutrition and overweight	Promote health and reduce chronic disease associated with diet and weight	19-3c. Reduce the proportion of children and adolescents who are overweight or obese	By 2010: 5% overweight or obese children and adolescents aged 6 to 19 years (reduced from 11%)
25. Sexually transmitted diseases	Promote responsible sexual behaviors, strengthen community capacity, and increase access to quality services to prevent sexually transmitted diseases and their complications	25-11. Increase the proportion of adolescents who abstain from sexual intercourse or use condoms if sexually active	By 2010: 95% of adolescents in grades 9 to 12 (increased from 85%)

Community Health Promotion

Health professionals are collaborating increasingly with community leaders to design interventions such as youth activity programs, nutrition classes, school-based clinics, and health screenings. Community health is difficult to define, but it is more than the sum of the health states of individual members (Pender, 1996). Among the indicators of a community's health are communication patterns, ability to take organized action, level of social functioning (work and school attendance), proportion of individuals at the poverty level, crime rates, and traditional morbidity and mortality statistics. One type of community intervention has focused on improving the cardiovascular health status of entire communities. Examples include the Stanford Five City Project, the Pawtucket Heart Health Program, and the Minnesota Heart Health Program (National Heart, Lung, and Blood Institute, 1990). These programs attempt to reduce risk factors such as obesity, hypertension, smoking, sedentary lifestyles, and serum cholesterol levels. Community members become involved in media campaigns. Distinct programs are set up for different groups within the community. Points of contact with community residents include churches, stores, schools, and work sites. The results of these programs are varied, but many have been successful in reducing cholesterol levels, tobacco use, and weight gain and in lowering blood pressure and coronary heart disease risks in general (Mittelmark, Hunt, Heath, & Schmid, 1993; Salonen, Tuomilehto, Nissinen, Kaplan, & Puska, 1989). Competition between "teams" is encouraged in the popular Lighten Up weight loss programs, such as Lighten Up Iowa and Lighten Up Wisconsin. Interstate competition also takes place (Norman & Mills, 2004).

A second type of community program is the Healthy Cities initiatives, first developed in Canada and Europe. The first site in the United States, the Indiana Healthy Community Project, was developed by a nurse (Flynn, Rider, & Bailey, 1992). Rather than focusing on a predetermined health problem such as cardiovascular risk, the Healthy Cities initiatives address a broad range of concerns that are identified by community members, such as gang violence and job creation. Coalitions of community groups are formed to develop programming. The California Healthy Cities Project (1994) has initiated programs on environmental protection, healthy behavior, and economic development. For individuals who live in rural areas rather than cities, county-based programs involving county extension agents, such as Walk Kansas, have proven successful (Estabrooks, Bradshaw, Dzewaltowski, & Smith-Ray, 2008).

Another type of programming considers members of a health maintenance organization (HMO) as a community. Curry, Ludman, and Wagner (1996) developed a useful model for health behavior change in an HMO with 400,000 members. Interventions take place at multiple levels. At the level of the organization, activities include developing consensus on the health behavior targets, careful planning, and allocation of resources. At the practice level, roles are developed for all members of the practice team. At the individual level, client motivation and readiness to change are addressed. Also included in the model are client teaching (by group classes and self-help materials), telephone counseling, support, and follow-up.

This model was successfully implemented, first targeting tobacco use. At the individual level the HMO offered a comprehensive stop-smoking program called Free and Clear. At the practice level all primary care providers were given the protocol of the National Cancer Institute, and chart audits monitored provider implementation. Finally, at the organizational level decisions were made to provide coverage for both the Free and Clear program and nicotine replacement therapy. The HMO joined in community efforts to defeat a smoker's rights bill in the state legislature and to convince the *Seattle Times* to stop accepting tobacco advertisements. The result was that smoking prevalence among the HMO's adult members dropped from 25% to 17%. The model is currently being used for other targeted behavior changes such as cancer screening and diet modification.

School-based interventions, especially those involving contemporary media used by youth, are achieving success in smoking prevention and cessation. For example, Canadian researchers created an interactive website called the Smoking Zine (www.smokingzine.org:81/start), which was supplemented by motivational groups in the classroom and 6 months of e-mail messages to the adolescent students. The intervention provided cessation motivation to the smokers who were most resistant to quitting and prevented nonsmokers from taking up the habit (Norman, Maley, Li, & Skinner, 2008).

Interventions at the neighborhood level are also proving efficacious. Researchers in Portland, Oregon, conducted a neighborhood walking program aimed at improving quality of life in older adults (Fisher & Li, 2004). Neighbors walked together, led by a researcher-trained leader, three times a week for 6 months. Physical functioning, mental well-being, and life satisfaction were significantly improved in the 56 intervention neighborhoods compared with control neighborhoods in which residents only received informational materials about aging. This low-cost intervention could be replicated easily with other age groups. The benefits of replication could be enormous. According to Rutledge and Loh (2004), regular exercise by Americans could save more than $6 billion in health care costs.

Nurses teamed up with community health workers in the "Sister to Sister" project, which assisted low-socioeconomic African American women in subsidized housing to quit smoking (Andrews, Felton, Wewers, Waller, & Humbles, 2005). The community workers were residents of the community and former smokers themselves. They shared their own experiences in smoking cessation during individual sessions and group meetings with the study participants. The project achieved a 2-month abstinence rate of 60%, with study participants showing significant increases in self-efficacy. The support of the community health workers was an important component of the intervention.

Canadian researchers are studying the role of the family as an intermediary between community health promotion programs and subsequent desired changes in family members' risk behaviors. In the Quebec Heart Health Demonstration Project, four types of families (balanced, traditional, disconnected, and emotionally strained) were examined. Balanced families (characterized by a balance between focus on interior of the family and presence in the extrafamilial world) scored highest of the four types on valuing of health and were predicted to be more responsive to community health promotion programming (Fisher et al., 1998). Yet to be determined are ways to increase responsiveness of the more poorly functioning families. The greatest challenge of health promotion in the 21st century may be reaching the more vulnerable and disenfranchised members of society and involving them in strategies to enhance and prolong their lives.

SUMMARY

Changing health behavior is difficult even when doing so would lessen the likelihood of future illness. Although individuals are often aware of the risks associated with poor health behaviors, they modify their thinking about these risks rather than changing the behaviors. Information is the solution only when ignorance is the problem. Understanding the principles of behavior change helps patients make health-promoting decisions. Using a comprehensive model of wellness identifies the behavioral, psychological, environmental, and organismic factors of attitude and behaviors associated with wellness. Pender's health promotion model assists in predicting health—promoting behavior change based on personal factors and prior related behavior. Health risk appraisals and contracting are useful to fostering health promotion behaviors. Environmental factors also affect wellness. National health promotion goals to guide health plicy are defined in the *Healthy People* initiative.

KEY POINTS

- Conceptualizing health more broadly than "the absence of disease" has significant implications for nursing practice.
- Health promotion and disease prevention have different foci, in that health promotion activities aim to take people beyond their present level of wellness, whereas disease prevention efforts are undertaken to prevent specific diseases.
- The major causes of death in the United States are related to lifestyle.
- A comprehensive model of wellness includes modifiable attitudinal and behavioral variables as well as environmental factors and nonmodifiable organismic characteristics.
- The health belief model and Pender's health promotion model are useful in guiding health promotion research and practice.
- Prochaska's transtheoretical model can be used to assess client readiness to change health behavior.
- Motivational interventions are more likely to promote health behavior change than threats of future disease or distant adverse outcomes.
- Health care providers should make greater use of written prescriptions, contracting, and other evidence-based interventions.

- Nurses' health promotion efforts should be guided by national health promotion goals, such as those articulated in *Healthy People 2010*.
- Health promotion initiatives must target families and communities as well as individuals.

CRITICAL THINKING EXERCISES

1. Interview three persons regarding their definition of health. Compare their definitions with the various theories and models presented in the chapter.
2. Assess your own health behavior; then select a behavior that you desire to change. It can be something that you wish to increase (e.g., aerobic exercise, meditation, flossing teeth), decrease (e.g., eating junk food), or stop (e.g., smoking, nail biting). Develop a plan to change the behavior, then implement the plan for 1 month. Critically assess factors that facilitated or hindered achievement of your behavior change.
3. Select one detrimental health behavior, such as excessive drinking. Review the research literature regarding interventions to change this behavior. Identify gaps in this literature. For example, is it clear which interventions are most effective? Is sufficient information available about changing the behavior in women? In various ethnic and minority groups? In persons of diverse ages, sexual orientation, and socioeconomic status? Develop at least three questions for future research.

WEBSITE RESOURCES

Center for the Advancement of Health: www.cfah.org
The World Health Report 2002: Reducing Risks, Promoting Healthy Life: www.who.int/whr/2002/en/
The Collaborative on Health and the Environment: www.cheforhealth.org
For models of health behavior change: www.med.usf. edu/~kmbrown/hlth_beh_models.htm
For weight control information: www.win.niddk.nih. gov/index.htm
For treatment of obesity: Agency for Healthcare Research and Quality: www.ahrq.gov/clinic/epcsums/ obesphsum.pdf
For tips on achieving better sleep: www.sleepfoundation.org
For the new food pyramid guidelines: www.mypyramid.gov
For calculating calories in food and calories burned in activities of daily living: www.caloriesperhour.com
For general tips on smoking cessation: www. ahrq.gov/consumer/index.html#smoking www.smokingzine.org:81/start

Center for Tobacco Cessation: www.ctcinfo.org
For nurses who smoke: www.tobaccofreenurses.org

REFERENCES

Anderson, N. B., & Anderson, P. E. (2003). *Emotional longevity.* New York: Penguin.

Andrews, J. O., Felton, G., Wewers, M. E., Waller, J., & Humbles, P. (2005). Sister to sister: A pilot study to assist African American women in subsidized housing to quit smoking. *Southern Online Journal of Nursing Research, 6*(1), 1–20.

Antonovsky, A. (1984). The sense of coherence as a determinant of health. In J. D. Matarazzo, S. M. Weiss, J. A. Herd, N. E. Miller, & S. M. Weiss (Eds.), *Behavioral health: A handbook of health enhancement and disease prevention* (pp. 114–129). New York: Wiley.

Aronson, K. R., Almeida, D. M., Stawski, R. S., Klein, L. S., & Kozlowski, L. T. (2008). Smoking is associated with worse mood on stressful days: Results from a national diary study. *Annals of Behavioral Medicine, 36,* 259–269.

Bandura, A. (1997). *Self-efficacy: The exercise of control.* New York: W.H. Freeman.

Becker, M. H., Haefner, D. P., Kasl, S. V., Kirscht, J. P., Maiman, L. A., & Rosenstock, I. M. (1977). Selected psychosocial models and correlates of individual health-related behaviors. *Medical Care, 15*(5), 27–46.

Belloc, N. B., & Breslow, L. (1972). Relationship of physical health status and health practices. *Preventive Medicine, 1,* 409–421.

Berk, L., Tan, S., Fry, W., Napier, B., Lee, J., & Hubbard, R. (1989). Neuroendocrine and stress hormone changes during mirthful laughter. *The American Journal of the Medical Sciences, 289,* 390–396.

Bialous, S. A., & Sarna, L. (2004). Sparing a few minutes for tobacco cessation. *American Journal of Nursing, 104*(12), 54–60.

Booth-Thomas, C. (2004). The cafeteria crusader. *Time, 164*(24), 36–37.

Breslow, L., & Enstrom, J. E. (1980). Persistence of health habits and their relationship to mortality. *Preventive Medicine, 9,* 469–483.

Buchanan, M. (2005). Rebuilding the bridge. *American Journal of Nursing, 105*(4), 104.

Bunde, J., & Suls, J. (2006). A quantitative analysis of the relationship between the Cook-Medley Hostility Scale and traditional coronary heart disease risk factors. *Health Psychology, 25,* 493–500.

Burke, B., Arkowitz, H., & Menchola, M. (2003). The efficacy of motivational interviewing: A meta-analysis of controlled clinical trials. *Journal of Consulting and Clinical Psychology, 71,* 843–861.

Butterfield, P. G. (1990). Thinking upstream: Nurturing a conceptual understanding of the societal context of health behavior. *Advances in Nursing Science, 12*(2), 1–8.

California Healthy Cities Project. (1994). *Connections, 6*(2), 1–5.

Campos, H., Baylin, A., & Willett, W. C. (2008). Alpha-linolenic acid and risk of nonfatal acute myocardial infarction. *Circulation, 118,* 323–324.

Carpenito, L. J. (1998). When clients teach me about noncompliance. *Nursing Forum, 33*(1), 3–4.

Carver, C. S., & Scheier, M. F. (2002). Optimism. In C. R. Snyder, & S. J. Lopes (Eds.), *The handbook of positive psychology* (pp. 231–243). New York: Oxford University Press.

Centers for Disease Control and Prevention. (1996). Tobacco use and usual source of cigarettes among high school students-United States, 1995. *Morbidity and Mortality Weekly Report, 45,* 413–418.

Chassin, L., Presson, C. C., Rose, J. S., & Sherman, S. J. (1996). The natural history of cigarette smoking from adolescence to adulthood: Demographic predictors of continuity and change. *Health Psychology, 15,* 478–484.

Clarke, W. R., & Lauer, R. M. (1993). Does childhood obesity track into adulthood? *Critical Reviews in Food Science and Nutrition, 33,* 423–430.

Cordain, L., Eaton, S. B., Brand Miller, J., Mann, N., & Hill, K. (2002). The paradoxical nature of hunter-gatherer diets: Meat-based, yet non-atherogenic. *European Journal of Clinical Nutrition, 56* (Suppl. 1), S42–S52.

Curry, S. J., Ludman, E., & Wagner, E. H. (1996). A model for health behavior change in managed care. *Outlook: Newsletter of the Society of Behavioral Medicine, Summer,* 5–6.

D'Alonzo, K. T., Stevenson, J. S., & Davis, S. E. (2004). Outcomes of a program to enhance exercise self-efficacy and improve fitness in Black and Hispanic college-age women. *Research in Nursing and Health, 27,* 357–369.

Dobson, R. (2008). Half of patients given exercise prescriptions are more active. *British Medical Journal, 337,* 894–895.

Dubos, R. (1965). *Man adapting.* New Haven, CT: Yale University Press.

Dunn, H. (1959). High level wellness for man and society. *American Journal of Public Health, 49,* 88.

Dunn, H. (1971). *High level wellness.* Arlington, VA: Beatty.

Eitel, P., & Friend, R. (1999). Reducing denial and sexual risk behaviors in college students: Comparison of a cognitive and a motivational approach. *Annals of Behavioral Medicine, 21*(1), 12–19.

Epel, E. S., Blackburn, E. H., Lin, J., Dhabhar, F. S., Adler, N. E., & Morrow, J. D. (2004). Accelerated telomere shortening in response to life stress. *Proceedings of the National Academy of Sciences, 101*(49), 17312–17315.

Estabrooks, P., Bradshaw, M., Dzewaltowski, D., & Smith-Ray, R. (2008). Determining the impact of Walk Kansas: Applying a team-building approach to community physical activity promotion. *Annals of Behavioral Medicine, 36*, 1–12.

Estabrooks, P., Fisher, E. B., & Hayman, L. L. (2008). What is needed to reverse the trends in childhood obesity? A call to action. *Annals of Behavioral Medicine, 36*, 209–216.

Fine, J. T., Colditz, G. A., Coakley, E. H., Moseley, G., Manson, J. E., & Willett, W. C. (1999). A prospective study of weight change and health-related quality of life in women. *Journal of the American Medical Association, 282*, 2136–2142.

Finfgeld-Connett, D. (2005). Clarification of social support. *Journal of Nursing Scholarship, 37*(1), 4–9.

Fiore, M. C., Jaen, C. R., Baker, T. B., Bailey, W. C., Bennett, G., Benowitz, N. L., et al. (2008). A clinical practice guideline for treating tobacco use and dependence: 2008 update. A U.S. Public Health Service Report. *American Journal of Preventive Medicine, 35*, 158–176.

Fisher, K. J., & Li, F. (2004). A community-based walking trial to improve neighborhood quality of life in older adults: A multilevel analysis. *Annals of Behavioral Medicine, 28*, 186–194.

Fisher, L., Soubhi, H., Mansi, O., Paradis, G., Gauvin, L., & Potvin, L. (1998). Family process in health research: Extending a family typology to a new cultural context. *Health Psychology, 17*, 358–366.

Flynn, B. C., Rider, M. S., & Bailey, W. W. (1992). Developing community leadership in healthy cities: The Indiana model. *Nursing Outlook, 49*(3), 121–126.

Gadamer, H. G. (1996). *The enigma of health: The art of healing in a scientific age* (F. Gaiger & N. Walker, Trans.) Stanford, CA: Stanford University Press.

Godfrey, J. R. (2004). Toward optimal health: The experts discuss therapeutic humor. *Journal of Women's Health, 13*, 474–479.

Gorman, C. (2004). Why we sleep. *Time, 164*(25), 46–56.

Graham, H. (1984). *Women, health, and family*. Brighton, England: Harvester Press.

Hallahan, B., & Garland, M. (2005). Essential fatty acids and mental health. *British Journal of Psychiatry, 186*, 275–277.

Harburg, E., Julius, M., Kaciroti, N., Gleiberman, L., & Schork, M. A. (2003). Expressive/ suppressive anger-coping responses, gender, and types of mortality: A 17-year follow-up (Tecumseh, Michigan, 1971-1988). *Psychosomatic Medicine, 65*, 588–597.

Hart, J. (2008). Spirituality and health. *Alternative and Complementary Therapies, 14*, 189–193.

Herzog, T. A., & Blagg, C. O. (2007). Are most precontemplators contemplating smoking cessation? Assessing the validity of the stages of change. *Health Psychology, 26*, 222–231.

Hicks, M., McDermott, L. L., Rouhana, N., Schmidt, M., Seymour, M., & Sullivan, T. (2008). Nurses' body size and public confidence in ability to provide health education. *Journal of Nursing Scholarship, 40*, 349–354.

Hill, J., & Wing, R. (2003). The National Weight Control Registry. *Permanente Journal, 7*(3), 34–37.

Hochbaum, G. M. (1958). *Public participation in medical screening programs: A sociopsychological study. U.S. Public Health Service* Publication No. 572. Washington, DC: U.S. Department of Health and Human Services.

Hollis, J. F., Gullion, C. M., Stevens, V. J., Brantley, P. J., Appel, L. J., Ard, J. D., et al. (2008). Weight loss during the intensive intervention phase of the Weight-Loss Maintenance Trial. *American Journal of Preventive Medicine, 35*, 118–126.

Holloway, J. W. (2005). Health funding for prevention on the rise. *Monitor on Psychology, 36*(2), 66–67.

Holmes, T. H., & Rahe, R. H. (1967). The Social Readjustment Rating Scale. *Journal of Psychosomatic Research, 11*, 213–218.

Holt-Lunstad, J., Smith, T. W., & Uchino, B. (2008). Can hostility interfere with the health benefits of giving and receiving social support? The impact of cynical hostility on cardiovascular reactivity during social support interactions among friends. *Annals of Behavioral Medicine, 35*, 319–330.

Hughner, R. S., & Kleine, S. S. (2008). Variations in lay health theories: Implications for consumer health care decision making. *Qualitative Health Research, 18*, 1687–1703.

Iribarren, C., Sidney, S., Bild, D. E., Liu, K., Markovitz, J. H., & Roseman, J. M. (2000). Association of hostility with coronary artery calcification in young adults: The CARDIA study. *Journal of the American Medical Association, 283*, 2546–2551.

Jackson, B., Cohen, S., Kubzansky, L., Jacobs, D. R., & Wright, R. J. (2007). Does harboring hostility hurt? Associations between hostility and pulmonary function in the Coronary Artery Risk Development in (Young) Adults (CARDIA) Study. *Health Psychology, 26,* 333–340.

Jackson, E. S., Tucker, C. M., & Herman, K. C. (2007). Health value, perceived social support, and health self-efficacy as factors in a health-promoting lifestyle. *Journal of American College Health, 56*(1), 69–74.

Janz, N. K., & Becker, M. H. (1984). The health belief model: A decade later. *Health Education Quarterly, 11*(1), 1–47.

Kanner, A., Coyne, J., Schaefer, C., & Lazarus, R. (1981). Comparison of two modes of stress measurement: Daily hassles and uplifts versus major life events. *Journal of Behavioral Medicine, 4,* 1–39.

Kaplan, D. (1997). When less is more. *Psychology Today, 30*(3), 14.

Kaplan, R., Anderson, J., & Wingard, D. (1991). Gender differences in health-related quality of life. *Health Psychology, 10,* 86–93.

Kelly, T., Yang, W., Chen, C. S., Reynolds, K., & He, J. (2008). Global burden of obesity in 2005 and projections to 2030. *International Journal of Obesity, 32,* 1431–1437.

Kennedy, K. D. (1995). Invest in yourself: Have a laugh! Have a healthy laugh! *Nursing Forum, 30*(1), 25–30.

Kiecolt-Glaser, J., Malarkey, W., Chee, M. A., Newton, T., Cacioppo, J., & Mao, H. (1993). Negative behavior during marital conflict is associated with immunological down-regulation. *Psychosomatic Medicine, 55,* 395–409.

King, A. C., Kiernan, M., Oman, R., Kraemer, H. C., Hull, M., & Ahn, D. (1997). Can we identify who will adhere to long-term physical activity? Signal detection methodology as a potential aid to clinical decision-making. *Health Psychology, 16,* 380–389.

Kluger, J. (2004). Blowing a gasket. *Time, 164*(23), 73–80.

Kobasa, S. C. (1979). Stressful life events, personality and health: An inquiry into hardiness. *Journal of Personality and Social Psychology, 37,* 1–11.

Lawton, R., Conner, M., & McEachan, R. (2009). Desire or reason: Predicting health behaviors from affective and cognitive attitudes. *Health Psychology, 28,* 56–65.

Lazarus, R. (1991). *Emotion and adaptation.* New York: Oxford University Press.

Leffingwell, T. R., Neumann, C., Leedy, M. J., & Babitzke, A. C. (2007). Defensively biased responding to risk information among alcohol-using college students. *Addictive Behaviors, 32,* 158–165.

Lett, H. S., Blumenthal, J. A., Babyak, M. A., Catellier, D. J., Carney, R. M., Berkman, L. F., et al. (2007). Social support and prognosis in patients at increased psychosocial risk recovering from myocardial infarction. *Health Psychology, 26,* 418–427.

Lindell, K., & Reinke, L. F. (1999). Nursing strategies for smoking cessation. *The American Nurse, 31,* A2–A6.

Listfield, E. (2009, August 9). 10 minutes to better health. *Parade,* 19.

Lutes, L. D., Winett, R. A., Barger, S. D., Wojcik, J. R., Herbert, W. G., Nickols-Richardson, S. M., et al. (2008). Small changes in nutrition and physical activity promote weight loss and maintenance: 3-month evidence from the ASPIRE randomized trial. *Annals of Behavioral Medicine, 35,* 351 357.

Manini, T. M., Everhart, J. E., Patel, K. V., Schoeller, D. A., Colbert, L. H., Visser, M., et al. (2006). Daily activity energy expenditure and mortality among older adults. *Journal of the American Medical Association, 296,* 171–179.

Maslow, A. (1961). Health as transcendence of environment. *Journal of Humanistic Psychology, 1,* 1–7.

McAuley, E., Doerksen, S., Morris, K., Motl, R., Hu, L., Wojcicki T., et al. (2008). Pathways from physical activity to quality of life in older women. *Annals of Behavioral Medicine, 36,* 13–20.

McEwen, B., & Lasley, E. N. (2003). Allostatic load: When protection gives way to damage. *Advances, 19*(1), 28–33.

Merjonen, P., Pulkki-Raback, L., & Keltikangas-Jarvinen, L. (2007). Anger and cardiovascular health. In E. I. Clausen (Ed.), *Psychology of anger* (pp. 71–106). New York: Nova Sciences.

Miller, S. K., Alpert, P. T., & Cross, C. L. (2008). Overweight and obesity in nurses, advanced practice nurses, and nurse educators. *Journal of the American Academy of Nurse Practitioners, 20,* 259–265.

Mittelmark, M. B., Hunt, M. K., Heath, G. W., & Schmid, T. L. (1993). Realistic outcomes: Lessons from community-based research and demonstration programs for the prevention of cardiovascular diseases. *Journal of Public Health Policy, 14,* 437–461.

National Heart, Lung, and Blood Institute. (1990). *Three community programs change heart health across the nation* [Special edition]. Infomemo. Washington, DC: Author.

National Sleep Foundation. (2004). "Sleep in America" 2004 poll [Online]. Retrieved from http://www.sleepfoundation.org/_content//hottopics/2004SleepPollFinalReport.pdf

National Sleep Foundation. (2005). "Sleep in America" 2005 poll [Online]. Retrieved from http://www.sleepfoundation. org/_content/hottopics/2005_summary_of_findings.pdf

Newman, M. (1978). Toward a theory of health. Presented at Nurse Educator Conference, New York, NY.

Newman, M. (1994). *Health as expanding consciousness* (2nd ed.). New York: National League for Nursing Press.

Nielsen-Bohlman, L., Panzer, A. M., & Kindig, D. A. (Eds.). (2004). *Executive summary: Health literacy: A prescription to end confusion.* Washington, DC: The National Academies Press.

Norman, C. D., Maley, O., Li, X., & Skinner, H. A. (2008). Using the Internet to assist smoking prevention and cessation in schools: A randomized, controlled trial. *Health Psychology, 27,* 799–810.

Norman, G. J., & Mills, P. J. (2004). Keeping it simple: Encouraging walking as a means to active living. *Annals of Behavioral Medicine, 28,* 149–151.

Ogden, C. L., Carroll, M., McDowell, M., & Flegal, K. (2007). *Obesity among adults in the United States–No statistically significant change since 2003-2004.* Hyatts-ville, MD: U.S. Dept. of Health and Human Services, Centers for Disease Control and Prevention, National Center for Health Statistics.

Orem, D. E. (1983). The self-care deficit theory of nursing: A general theory. In I. W. Clements, & F. B. Roberts (Eds.), *Family health: A theoretical approach to nursing care* (pp. 205–217). New York: Wiley.

Orem, D. E. (1995). *Nursing concepts of practice* (5th ed.). St. Louis: Mosby.

Paul, P. (2005). The power to uplift. *Time, 165*(3), A46–A48.

Pender, N. (1996). *Health promotion in nursing practice* (3rd ed.). Stamford, CT: Appleton & Lange.

Pender, N., Murdaugh, C. L., & Parsons, M. A. (2002). *Health promotion in nursing practice* (4th ed.). Upper Saddle River, NJ: Prentice-Hall.

Pennebaker, J. W. (1990). *Opening up: The healing power of confiding in others.* New York: Morrow.

Perini, C., Muller, F., & Buhler, F. (1991). Suppressed aggression accelerates early development of essential hypertension. *Journal of Hypertension, 9,* 499–503.

Perry, A. (2005). Learning the yoga way of laughter. *Time, 165*(3), A26.

Physical activity trends—United States, 1990-1998. (2001). *Morbidity and Mortality Weekly Report, 50,* 166–169.

Pollitt, R. A., Daniel, M., Kaufmann, J. S., Lynch, J. W., Salonen, J. T., & Kaplan, G. A. (2005). Mediation and modification of the association between hopelessness, hostility, and progression of carotid atherosclerosis. *Journal of Behavioral Medicine, 28,* 53–64.

Primack, B. A., Sidani, J., Agarwal, A., Shadel, W., Donny, E., & Eissenberg, T. (2008). Prevalence of and associations with waterpipe tobacco smoking among U.S. university students. *Annals of Behavioral Medicine, 36,* 81–86.

Prochaska, J. J., Hall, S. M., Humfleet, G., Munoz, R., Reus, V., Gorecki, J., et al. (2008). Promoting physical activity for maintaining non-smoking: A randomized controlled trial. *Annals of Behavioral Medicine, 35,* S102.

Prochaska, J. O., DiClemente, C. C., & Norcross, J. C. (1992). In search of how people change: Applications to addictive behaviors. *American Psychologist, 47,* 1102–1114.

Resnick, B., & Spellbring, A. M. (2000). Understanding what motivates older adults to exercise. *Journal of Gerontological Nursing, 26*(3), 34–42.

Ricciardi, R. (2005). Sedentarism: A concept analysis. *Nursing Forum, 40*(3), 79–87.

Riegel, B., Dickson, V. V., Hoke, L., McMahon, J., Reis, B., & Sayers, S. (2006). A motivational counseling approach to improving heart failure self-care: Mechanisms of effec-tiveness. *Journal of Cardiovascular Nursing, 21,* 232–241.

Rogers, M. (1970). *An introduction to the theoretical basis of nursing.* Philadelphia: Davis.

Roman, C. G., & Chalfin, A. (2008). Fear of walking outdoors: A multilevel ecologic analysis of crime and disorder. *American Journal of Preventive Medicine, 34,* 306–312.

Rotter, J. B. (1954). *Social learning and clinical psychology.* Englewood Cliffs, NJ: Prentice-Hall.

Roy, C. (1970). Adaptation: A conceptual framework for nursing. *Nursing Outlook, 18*(3), 42–45.

Ruppert, R. A. (1999). The last smoke. *American Journal of Nursing, 99*(11), 26–32.

Rutledge, T., & Loh, C. (2004). Effect sizes and statistical testing in the determination of clinical significance in behavioral medicine research. *Annals of Behavioral Medicine, 27,* 138–145.

Salonen, J. T., Tuomilehto, J., Nissinen, A., Kaplan, G. A., & Puska, P. (1989). Contribution of risk factor changes to the decline in coronary incidence during the North Karelia project: A within community analysis. *International Journal of Epidemiology, 18,* 595–601.

Third-hand smoke: another reason to quit smoking. (2008). *Science Daily* (December 31, 2008). Retrieved January 15, 2009, from http://www.sciencedaily.com/releases/ 2008/12/081229105037.htm

Seligman, M. (1998). *Learned optimism.* New York: Pocket Books.

Selye, H. (1956). *The stress of life.* New York: McGraw-Hill.

Shoham, Y., Ragland, D. R., Brand, R. J., & Syme, S. L. (1988). Type A behavior pattern and health status after 22 years of follow-up in the Western Collaborative Group Study. *American Journal of Epidemiology, 128,* 579–588.

Smith, J. (1983). *The idea of health: Implications for the nursing profession.* New York: Teachers College Press.

Smuts, J. (1926). *Holism and evolution.* New York: Macmillan.

Stambor, Z. (2006). Specific environments alone can trigger smokers' cigarette cravings. *APA Monitor, 37*(3), 15.

Stamler, J., Stamler, R., Neaton, J. D., Wentworth, D., Daviglus, M. L., & Garside, D. (1999). Low risk-factor profile and long-term cardiovascular and noncardiovascular mortality and life expectancy: Findings for 5 large cohorts of young adult and middle aged men and women. *Journal of the American Medical Association, 282,* 2012–2018.

Stetson, B. A., Rahn, J. M., Dubbert, P. M., Wilner, B. I., & Mercury, M. G. (1997). Prospective evaluation of the effects of stress on exercise adherence in community-residing women. *Health Psychology, 16,* 515–520.

Sturm, R. (2007). Increases in morbid obesity in the USA: 2000-2005. *Public Health, 121,* 492–496.

Suarez, E. C., Bates, M. P., & Harralson, T. L. (1998). The relation of hostility to lipids and lipoproteins in women: Evidence for the role of antagonistic hostility. *Annals of Behavioral Medicine, 20*(2), 59–63.

Sullivan, H. W., & Rothman, A. J. (2008). When planning is needed: Implementation intentions and attainment of approach versus avoidance health goals. *Health Psychology, 27,* 438–444.

Thomas, S. P. (1997a). Distressing aspects of women's roles, vicarious stress, and health consequences. *Issues in Mental Health Nursing, 18,* 539–557.

Thomas, S. P. (1997b). Women's anger: Relationship of suppression to blood pressure. *Nursing Research, 46,* 324–330.

Thomas, S. P. (1997c). Angry? Let's talk about it! *Applied Nursing Research, 10*(2), 80–85.

Thomas, S. P. (2001). Teaching healthy anger management. *Perspectives in Psychiatric Care, 37,* 41–48.

Thomas, S. P. (2006). Cultural and gender considerations in the assessment and treatment of anger-related disorders. In E. L. Feindler (Ed.), *Anger-related disorders: A practitioner's guide to comparative treatments.* New York: Springer.

Thomas, S. P. (2007). Trait anger, anger expression, and themes of anger incidents in contemporary undergraduate students. In E. I. Clausen (Ed.), *Psychology of anger* (pp. 23–69). New York: Nova Science.

Thomas, S. P., & Pollio, H. R. (2002). *Listening to patients.* New York: Springer.

U.S. Census Bureau (2000). Census 2000 at demographic profile highlights [Online]. Available at http://factfinder. census.gov/servlet/SAFFFactsfi_sse=on

U.S. Department of Agriculture. (2008, August). Diet quality of Americans in 1994-96 and 2001-02 as measured by the Healthy Eating Index-2005. Nutrition Insight 37. Retrieved January 15, 2009, from http://www.cnpp.usda.gov

U.S. Public Health Service. (1979). *Healthy People: The Surgeon General's report on health promotion and disease prevention.* Washington, DC: U.S. Department of Health, Education, & Welfare.

U.S. Public Health Service. (1990). *Healthy People 2000.* Washington, DC: U.S. Department of Health and Human Services.

U.S. Public Health Service. (1999). *Healthy People 2000 review 1998-99.* Washington, DC: U.S. Department of Health and Human Services.

U.S. Public Health Service. (2000). *Healthy People 2010* [Online]. Available at http://www.health.gov/ healthypeople. Washington, DC: U.S. Department of Health and Human Services.

Wallston, K. A. (1989). Assessment of control in health care settings. In A. Steptoe, & A. Appels (Eds.), *Stress, personal control, and health* (pp. 85-106). New York: Wiley.

Wang, G., Pratt, M., Macera, C. A., Zheng, Z.-J., & Heath, G. (2004). Physical activity, cardiovascular disease, and medical expenditures in U.S. adults. *Annals of Behavioral Medicine, 28,* 88–94.

Werch, C. E., Moore, M. J., Bian, H., DiClemente, C., Ames, S. C., Weiler, R. M., et al. (2008). Efficacy of a brief image-based multiple-behavior intervention for college students. *Annals of Behavioral Medicine, 36,* 149–157.

Williams, E. C., Kivlahan, D. R., Saitz, R., Merrill, J. O., Achtmeyer, C. E., McCormick, K. A., et al. (2006). Readiness to change in primary care patients who screened positive for alcohol misuse. *Annals of Family Medicine, 4,* 213–220.

Williams, R. L., Thomas, S. P., Young, D. O., Jozwiak, J. J., & Hector, M. A. (1991). Development of a health habits scale. *Research in Nursing and Health, 14,* 145–153.

World Health Organization. (2008). *WHO Report on the global tobacco epidemic, 2008.* Geneva: Author.

Genetics and Genomics in Professional Nursing

DALE HALSEY LEA, MPH, RN, CGC, FAAN

OBJECTIVES

After completion of this chapter, the reader will be able to:

● Define genomic health care.

● Discuss the importance of the *Essentials of Genetic and Genomic Nursing: Competencies, Curricula Guidelines, and Outcome Indicators* to nursing practice.

● Discuss the nursing role in family history assessment.

● Describe nursing roles in genetic testing.

● Explain the nursing role in referral of patients and families for specialized genetic and genomic services.

● List two new ways that genetic testing is being used in clinical practice.

● Identify ethical issues of concern with regard to genomic health care.

PROFILE IN PRACTICE

Barbara J. Ganster, RN, BSN
Nurse Case Manager, Breast Care Center, National Naval Medical Center, Bethesda, Maryland

I work in the breast care center at a military treatment facility (MTF). Every week we hold a multidisciplinary clinic in which newly diagnosed breast cancer patients are seen by the team who will be involved in their care and treatment. I complete a family "pedigree" as part of our evaluation, looking for factors that may indicate a need for genetic counseling and possible genetic testing.

I was completing the pedigree on a patient who, for support, had brought along a friend, a survivor of breast cancer who had been diagnosed in her 30s. While I do a pedigree, I provide education and explain

why I am asking the questions. As we spoke, I mentioned to the friend that she had probably already had this conversation with her oncologist. She responded that she had not, but she added that since she had undergone bilateral mastectomies, it wasn't an issue for her. As I continued with the pedigree, I noted several times the friend giving nonverbal clues that had me increasingly concerned that there was more going on in her own family tree.

After I completed my patient's pedigree, I asked to speak with the friend. She did not want to take the focus off my patient, but I was able to reassure her that while the patient met with our social worker, I could spend a few minutes with her. Since this woman was not my patient and was not eligible for care at a military treatment facility, I had to balance educational needs and not do actual counseling.

I offered to do a family pedigree, which revealed several more maternal family members with histories of breast cancer and at least one with ovarian cancer. Also, the woman was of Ashkenazi Jewish ancestry. I encouraged her to take the pedigree to her oncologist, whom she was scheduled to see that week for follow-up. I explained that although she had decreased her risk for breast cancer by having bilateral mastectomies, other cancers were also associated with BRCA mutation, ovarian

cancer being the most concerning because survival rates are low, there are no good screening measures, and it usually is not detected early. If she was found to have a mutation, genetic counseling would include additional screening and possible risk-reduction measures.

My patient subsequently let me know her friend was referred to a genetic counselor and that she had tested positive for a BRCA mutation and was being seen by a gynecologist. The friend later contacted me to say thank you. Her pathology from the bilateral oophorectomies had shown a "precancerous" lesion on one ovary, and her gynecologist said that she had been destined for full-blown ovarian cancer if the surgery had not been done when it was.

PROFILE IN PRACTICE

Jean Jenkins, PhD, RN, FAAN
National Institutes of Health, National Human Genome Research Institute, Bethesda, Maryland

Kathleen Calzone, MSN, RN, APNG, FAAN
National Institutes of Health, National Cancer Institute, Center for Cancer Research, Genetics Branch, Bethesda, Maryland

As cancer nurses, we began our journey together to integrate genetics and genomics into nursing practice and patient care in 1995, when a genetic counselor colleague suggested that we put together a workshop for nurses to explore the need for genetic education. At that time, genetic research was opening new doors to understanding the underlying genetics of an inherited susceptibility to breast cancer and influencing risk management, diagnosis, and treatment. We realized that these genetic discoveries would have a significant impact on oncology nursing practice and that nurses, including ourselves, were not prepared for this revolution in health care. We have since become "joined at the hip" and continue to work to move genetics and genomics into all nursing education and practice.

Our initial meeting was the Workshop on Genetics Education in Nursing, held at the National Institutes of Health in September 1995. Since then, we have collaborated to create the core competencies in cancer genetics for advanced practice nurses, to initiate a nursing genetics and ethics study, and to publish books and articles on these topics. One of our proudest accomplishments has been the publication of a series of peer-reviewed

articles by genetics nurse specialists on genetics and genomics science and health care applications, showcasing important implications for nursing practice in the *Journal of Nursing Scholarship* over a 2-year period. This article series is now available as an educational resource for nurses (www.genome.gov/17515679) (Jenkins, 2007).

Another of our exciting endeavors was a 2-year initiative to establish essential competencies in genetics and genomics for all nurses. This culminated with an invitational consensus conference that brought together key nursing organizations at the American Nursing Association headquarters in September 2005 to finalize these competencies. This foundational meeting of 50 nursing organizations led to the consensus and publication of the *Essentials of Genetic and Genomic Nursing: Competencies, Curricula Guidelines, and Outcome Indicators* in 2005 and a second edition in 2008 (Consensus Panel on Genetic/Genomic Nursing Competencies, 2008) which defined the minimum genetics and genomics competencies needed by all registered nurses regardless of their educational preparation, clinical specialty, or role. To date, 49 nursing organizations have endorsed the *Essential Nursing*

Competencies, many of which are developing their own genetic and genomic educational and outreach efforts.

The next steps in the competency initiative focused on making the *Essential Nursing Competencies* a living, useful document. In October 2006, we convened the group of endorsing organizations and some key stakeholders to develop a 5-year, multifaceted strategic implementation plan for the integration of the genetics and genomics competencies into nursing curricula, NCLEX, specialty certifications, continuing education, and accreditation, a process that involves collaboration among nursing and academic organizations and federal agencies both nationally and internationally.

A "toolkit" for academic faculty was developed, launched disseminated in February 2010 and can be accessed at www.g-2-c-2.com. As the toolkit is developed and disseminated, we are also working to establish an interdisciplinary consortium because achieving competency in genetics and genomics is an issue for all members of the health care community. In the next year we will be working with the American Academy of Nursing to hold meetings that will help to establish a national nursing research outcomes agenda for genetic and genomic nursing.

Our vision for all nurses is (1) that they become fluent in genetics and genomics so that they can communicate with their patients, families, and communities, and (2) that they competently use genetic and genomic information to develop personalized plans to improve health care outcomes. Nurses are the keystone of the health care community and, as such, are fundamental to closing the gap between patients and the genetic and genomic discoveries that could optimize their health care.

☀ Introduction: Why Genetics and Genomics?

The human genome was completely mapped and sequenced in 2003. Discoveries from this human genome research are increasing our understanding of the role genes play in health and both rare and common diseases. A new era of health care—called *genomic health care*—is rapidly advancing. Genomic health care means that health care providers now have accessible new tools for tailoring health care to the individual by using a person's unique genomic information to design and prescribe the most effective treatment for each patient. These advances are ushering in new directions in the provision of health care and will have a significant impact on nurses and all other health care providers. Nurses in all practice settings will increasingly be expected to use genetic- and genomic-based approaches and technologies in their patient care. In recognition of the implications of genomic health care for nurses, the *Essentials of Genetic and Genomic Nursing: Competencies, Curricula Guideline, and Outcome Indicators* (Consensus Panel on Genetic/Genomic Nursing Competencies, 2008) was published. This chapter is founded on the *Essentials of Genetic and Genomic Nursing* and presents genetic and genomic discoveries and applications from yesterday to today, as well as for tomorrow. Applications of genetics and genomics to nursing and health care will be addressed, including family history assessment, genetic screening and testing, pharmacogenetics and pharmacogenomics, and direct-to-consumer (DTC) genetic testing. Ethical and social issues related to genetics and genomics will also be described. Genetics and genomics educational and clinical resources are provided to support the needs of all nurses wanting to learn more about and provide competent genomic health care. As noted in the *Essentials of Genetic and Genomic Nursing,*

> Because essentially all diseases and conditions have a genetic or genomic component, options for care for all persons will increasingly include genetic and genomic information along the pathways of prevention, screening, diagnostics, prognostics, selection of treatment, and monitoring of treatment effectiveness. The clinical application of genetic and genomic knowledge has major implications for the entire nursing profession regardless of academic preparation, role or practice setting. (Consensus Panel, 2008, p. 7)

Box 16-1 provides a listing of basic genetic terms and their definitions as a beginning step for nurses to

BOX 16-1	**Common Genetic and Genomic Terms**

Allele—One of the variant forms of a gene at a particular location on a chromosome. Different alleles create variation in inherited characteristics such as hair color or blood type.

Chromosome—One of the threadlike "packages" of genes and other DNA that are located in the nucleus of a cell. Humans have 23 pairs of chromosomes, 46 in all: 44 autosomes and 2 sex chromosomes. Each parent contributes one chromosome to each pair, so children get half of their chromosomes from their mothers and half from their fathers.

Deoxyribonucleic acid (DNA)—The chemical inside the nucleus of a cell that carries genetic instructions for making living organisms.

Double helix—The structural arrangement of DNA, which looks something like an immensely long ladder twisted into a helix, or coil. The sides of the "ladder" are formed by a backbone of sugar and phosphate molecules, and the "rungs" consist of nucleotide bases joined weakly in the middle by hydrogen bonds.

Gene—The functional and physical unit of heredity passed from parent to offspring. Genes are pieces of DNA, and most genes contain the information for making a specific protein.

Genetics—A term that refers to the study of genes and their role in inheritance; the way certain traits or conditions are passed down from one generation to another.

Genomics—A relatively new term that describes the study of all of a person's genes, including interactions of those genes with one another and with the person's environment.

Genetic disorders—A disease caused in whole or in part by a "variation" (a different form) or "mutation" (alteration) of a gene.

Mendelian inheritance—The way in which genes and traits are passed from parents to children. Examples of Mendelian inheritance include autosomal dominant, autosomal recessive, and sex-linked genes.

Protein—A large complex molecule consisting of one or more chains of amino acids. Proteins perform a wide variety of activities in the cell.

Ribonucleic acid (RNA)—A chemical similar to a single strand of DNA. In RNA, the letter U, which stands for "uracil" is substituted for T in the genetic code. RNA delivers DNA's genetic message to the cytoplasm of a cell, where proteins are made.

Data from National Human Genome Research Institute [2009b]. Genetics and Genomics for Patients and the Public. Retrieved from www.genome.gov/19016903; and National Human Genome Research Institute [2009f]. Talking Glossary of Genetic Terms. Retrieved from www.genome.gov/glossary.

become familiar with and knowledgeable about genetics and genomics.

YESTERDAY'S GENETICS

It was not until the late 1800s that scientists first began to discover the basic genetic structures—chromosomes—the threadlike structures inside of cells that contain genes. And it was not until the early 1900s that inherited diseases were linked to chromosomes. Scientific research and discoveries from the 1950s through the 1980s helped scientists to develop genetic tests for genetic conditions such as Down syndrome, cystic fibrosis, and Duchenne muscular dystrophy. During those years, genetic testing was used to confirm a diagnosis of a genetic condition and to screen newborns for conditions such as phenylketonuria (PKU) so that early treatments and interventions could

be administered (National Institutes of Health, 2009). Nurses practicing in neonatal and pediatric settings were therefore the first nurses to become informed about and involved with genetics in their practice with the advent of genetic testing for newborns and pediatric patients and their families. But were those nurses prepared with genetics knowledge so that they could provide competent and informed patient care? Not necessarily. The recognition that nurses did not have adequate knowledge of genetics to practice genetics health care was first documented in the nursing literature of 1979 (Cohen, 1979).

TODAY'S GENETICS AND GENOMICS

Mapping and sequencing of the entire human genome was completed in 2003, after 15 years of research. Knowledge of the human genome has opened new doors to understanding the role of genes in health and disease. As an example, genetic discoveries have led to the development of an increasing number of genetic tests that can be used to identify a trait, diagnose a genetic disorder, and/or identify individuals who have a genetic predisposition to diseases, such as cancer or heart disease. Our understanding of genes and their roles in health and disease has expanded beyond genetics, which involves the study of individual genes and their impact on relatively rare, single-gene disorders. A new field of research called *genomics* involves the study of all of the genes in the human genome together, including their interactions with one another, their interactions with the environment, and the influence of other cultural and psychosocial factors (Consensus Panel, 2008; Guttmacher & Collins, 2002). In the pre-genome era, health care providers used a "one size fits all" approach to treating their patients. In the post-genome era, health care providers will increasingly use genomic information to tailor treatments to the individual patient and to personalize their care (National Human Genome Research Institute, 2009c).

Genetics and genomics are therefore becoming an integral part of health care for patients from preconception to adulthood. Patients, families, and communities will increasingly expect all registered nurses and nurse specialists to be familiar with and use genetic and genomic information and technologies when providing care (Consensus Panel, 2008). Nurses at all levels and in all areas of practice will soon be taking an active role in risk assessment for genetic conditions and disorders, explaining genetic risk and genetic testing, and supporting informed health decisions and opportunities for early intervention (Skirton, Patch, & Williams, 2005).

Essentials of Genetic and Genomic Nursing

In recognition of the need for all nurses to become proficient in incorporating genetics and genomics into their practice, nursing leaders from clinical, research, and academic settings came together to create "the minimum basis by which to prepare the nursing workforce to deliver competent genetic- and genomic-focused nursing care" (Consensus Panel, 2008, p. 1). The *Essentials of Genetic and Genomic Nursing* was developed based on several sources and resources, including (1) review of peer-reviewed published work that has reported practice-based genetic and genomic competencies, guidelines, and recommendations; (2) input from nurses who were representatives to the National Coalition for Health Professional Education in Genetics (NCHPEG) in 2005; (3) public comment from the nursing community at large; and (4) statements during open comment periods from the nurses who attended a 2-day meeting of key stakeholders held in September 2005. The *Essentials of Genetic and Genomic Nursing* that were developed apply to the practice of all registered nurses regardless of their academic preparation, practice setting, role, or specialty. To date, more than 49 nursing organizations have endorsed the *Essentials of Genetic and Genomic Nursing* (Consensus Panel, 2008).

The *Essentials of Genetic and Genomic Nursing* is broken down into two categories: professional responsibilities and professional practice domain. The professional responsibilities are consistent with the nursing scope and standards of practice that were developed by the American Nurses Association (American Nurses Association, 2004). They include the incorporation of genetic and genomic technologies and information into registered nursing practice and the ability to tailor genetic and genomic information and services to clients based on their knowledge level, literacy, culture, religion, and preferred language. The professional practice domain includes the following: competencies in nursing assessment (applying and integrating genetic and genomic knowledge); identification of clients who could benefit from genetic and genomic information and services as well as reliable genetic and genomic resources; referral activities; and provision of education, care, and support, such as using genetic- and genomic-based interventions and information to improve client outcomes (Consensus Panel, 2008).

The *Essentials of Genetic and Genomic Nursing* document includes strategies to implement the competencies into nursing practice. These strategies include participating in the NCLEX test development process and working with the American Hospital Association and other regulatory agencies to incorporate genetics and genomics practice content. Another strategy is to have all certification exams include test items that measure the knowledge of genetic and genomic information specific to the specialty for which nurses are being certified. Practicing nurses are encouraged to pursue genetic and genomic continuing education. Accreditation programs are encouraged to evaluate whether the curriculum they are creating is designed to meet the essential nursing core genetic and genomic competencies. Nursing faculty members are given ideas and solutions regarding how they can incorporate genetics and genomics as a central science into their curricula. Resources to support the *Essentials of Genetic and Genomic Nursing* are also provided (Consensus Panel, 2008). Box 16-2 provides examples of currently available genetics and genomics educational resources for practicing nurses and nurse educators.

Applying Genetics and Genomics in Nursing Practice

This section focuses on several examples of how nurses are applying genetics and genomics in their practice. Two important clinical tools are now available to health care providers to personalize screening, prevention, diagnosis, and treatment of individuals and their families. These two tools are family history and genetic testing. Based on the *Essentials of Genetic and Genomic Nursing*, nurses will be involved with family history collection and pedigree construction and in offering and explaining genetic testing. Nurses will also refer individuals and families for genetic services and consultation.

FAMILY HISTORY

Knowing the role of family history in common and rare genetic conditions and disorders is an important first step in genetic and genomic risk assessment and early intervention. It is now known that individuals who have a family history of chronic diseases such as heart disease, diabetes, and cancer in close relatives are more likely to have a higher risk of developing

---

BOX 16-2 | Genetics and Genomics Educational Resources for Nurses

All About the Human Genome Project—National Human Genome Research Institute: www.genome.gov/10001772

Genetics Education Center—University of Kansas Medical Center: www.kumc.edu/gec

Genetics Education Program for Nurses—Cincinnati Children's Hospital: www.cincinnatichildrens.org/ed/clinical/gpnf/default.htm

Genetic Education Modules for Teachers—National Human Genome Research Institute: www.genome.gov/10005911

Genetics Home Reference: Your Guide to Understanding Genetic Conditions—National Library of Medicine: http://ghr.nlm.nih.gov

Genomics in Practice—Centers for Disease Control and Prevention, National Office of Public Health Genomics: www.cdc.gov/genomics/phpractice.htm

Human Genome Project Education Resources—Office of Science: U.S. Department of Energy: www.ornl.gov/sci/techresources/Human_Genome/education/education.shtml

Medicine and the New Genetics—Office of Science, U.S. Department of Energy: www.ornl.gov/sci/techresources/Human_Genome/medicine/medicine.shtml

Online Education Kit: Understanding the Human Genome Project—National Human Genome Research Institute: www.genome.gov/25019879

Online Genetics Resources—National Human Genome Research Institute: www.genome.gov/10000464

Online Multimedia Genomics Training—Centers for Disease Control and Prevention, National Office of Public Health Genomics: www.cdc.gov/genomics/training/presentations.htm

Talking Glossary of Genetic Terms—National Human Genome Research Institute: www.genome.gov/glossary

---

these diseases. Having a first-degree relative with any one of these disease has been shown to double that person's risk for developing the disease, with the risk increasing when there are more affected relatives or if the disease was diagnosed at an early age (National Human Genome Research Institute, 2009d). All health care providers, including nurses, have a responsibility

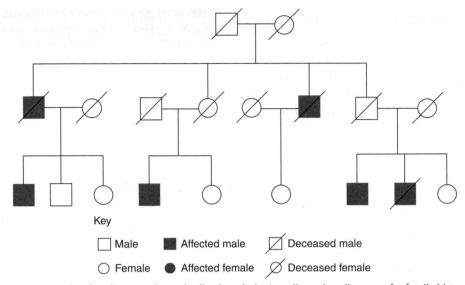

Key

☐ Male   ■ Affected male   ⊠ Deceased male

◯ Female   ● Affected female   ⊘ Deceased female

FIGURE 16-1 Example of pedigree and standardized symbols. A pedigree is a diagram of a family history that shows family members' relationships to each other and how a particular disease or trait is being passed on (inherited) in that family. For more information about how to construct a family history pedigree, go to the National Human Genome Research Institute, Your Family History, www.genome.gov/Pages/Education/Modules/YourFamilyHealthHistory.pdf. (From National Human Genome Research Institute, Talking Glossary of Genetic Terms, www.genome.gov/Pages/10002096.)

to collect family history information and could take advantage of this information to provide specific clinical prevention and management interventions for those diseases that run in the patient's family (National Human Genome Research Institute, 2009d).

In recognition of the importance of family history in health and disease, the U.S. Surgeon General, in cooperation with the U.S. Department of Health and Human Services and other government agencies, began a national public health campaign in 2004 called the *U.S. Surgeon General's Family History Initiative*. The Initiative encourages all American families to learn more about their family history and offers a computerized tool to help families create a portrait of their family health. (U.S. Department of Health and Human Services, 2009). Nurses need to be able to gather a minimum of three generations of family health history information in order to help families learn about their family health history. Nurses can offer individuals and families information about the *U.S. Surgeon General's Family History Initiative* to begin this process.

In accordance with the *Essentials of Genetic and Genomic Nursing*, nurses also need to be prepared to construct a pedigree from the collected family history information, using the standardized symbols and terminology (Consensus Panel, 2008). Figure 16-1 provides an example of a pedigree and standardized symbols. During the process of family history collection and pedigree construction, nurses need to be alert for clients who present with family histories with multiple generations affected with a particular disorder (e.g., autosomal dominant inheritance), those with multiple siblings who have a genetic disorder (e.g., autosomal recessive inheritance), and those affected with a disease or condition at an early age (e.g., multiple generations with early-onset breast or ovarian cancer). When a client is identified as having a family history of a possible inherited genetic disorder, the nurse discusses the family history with the health care team and lets the client know that he or she may have a risk factor for a specific disease. The nurse and health care team can then facilitate referrals for specialized genetic and genomic services (Consensus Panel, 2008).

GENETIC TESTING: WHAT IT IS AND HOW IT IS USED IN CLINICAL PRACTICE

One of the most significant applications of genomics to health care that has expanded rapidly since the mapping of the human genome is genetic testing. Genetic testing is now available for more than 1600 genetic disorders ranging from single-gene disorders, such as cystic fibrosis, to complex disorders, such as diabetes, cancer, and heart disease (GeneTests, 2009). A number of different types of genetic tests are used in health care today.

Carrier testing is a type of genetic testing that can tell individuals if they "carry" a genetic variation that can cause a disease. Carriers of the genetic variation do not usually show any signs of the disorder, because they carry one normal version of the gene. However, carriers can pass on the genetic variation to their children, who may develop the disorder or become carriers themselves. Thus testing may be offered or sought when couples are considering pregnancy or during early pregnancy. Carrier testing is offered to couples who are from particular ethnic or racial backgrounds and who have an increased risk for being carriers of an autosomal recessive gene for disorders. Examples include African American couples who have an increased chance to carry a gene for sickle cell anemia and couples of Ashkenazi Jewish ancestry who have an increased chance for being carriers of a gene for Tay-Sachs disease (Genetics Home Reference, 2009).

Diagnostic testing identifies a genetic variation that is either causing a person to have a genetic condition or disease now or may cause a condition in the future. Results of diagnostic genetic testing can help with treatment decisions and management of the disorder. Newborn screening is used to test infants in the first few days of life to determine whether they have a genetic disorder that will cause problems with health and development. Prenatal genetic testing is offered during pregnancy to help identify fetuses that have certain diseases. Preimplantation diagnostic genetic testing is carried out in conjunction with in vitro fertilization to determine whether embryos for implantation carry genes that could cause disease (Genetics Home Reference, 2009).

Research genetic testing helps scientists to learn more about how genes contribute to health and disease. Genetic and genomic research also helps with the development of gene-based treatments. The research genetic test results may not directly help the research participant; however, results may benefit others in the future by helping researchers expand their understanding of human genes and their roles in health and disease (National Human Genome Research Institute, 2009g).

Nurses will be increasingly involved in the genetic testing process and will need to become knowledgeable about the different types of genetic tests so that they can provide competent genetic- and genomic-based care. This knowledge will serve as the foundation to providing patients and families with interpretation of selective genetic and genomic information such as genetic testing results.

REFERRAL FOR GENETIC COUNSELING AND SUPPORT SERVICES

Nurses will benefit from knowing where to access specialized genetic and genomic services so that they are able to facilitate a genetics referral for clients who may have a genetic risk factor, abnormal genetic test result, or questions about a genetic or genomic condition or disorder. Genetics specialists are health care professionals who have specialized degrees and experience in medical genetics and counseling. Genetics professionals include medical geneticists, genetic counselors, and genetics nurses.

Genetic professionals work as members of health care teams to provide information and support to individuals and families who have genetic disorders or may be at risk for inherited conditions. Genetic professionals conduct the following activities during a genetic consultation:

- Assess the risk of a genetic disorder by evaluating and researching a family's history and evaluating medical records
- Consider the medical, social, and ethical decisions surrounding genetic testing
- Provide support and information to help a person make a decision about genetic testing

- Help to interpret the results of genetic tests and medical data
- Provide counseling and refer individuals and families to support services as needed
- Act as patient advocates
- Discuss and explain the possible treatments or preventive measures
- Review and discuss reproductive options (National Human Genome Research Institute, 2009a)

A number of online resources provide comprehensive listings of genetics services that nurses can use to locate genetics professionals and services in their practice area. These include GeneTests (2009), which has a searchable genetics clinic directory, and the University of Kansas (2009), which offers a listing of genetics centers, clinics, and departments.

☀ Tomorrow's Genetics and Genomics: Personalized Medicine

Genetic and genomic research is revealing more every day about the role of genetics in how each person's body metabolizes and responds to certain medicines. This section describes new directions in utilization of genetic testing results for selection of treatments that are leading to more individualized health care, called *personalized medicine*. Pharmacogenetics and pharmacogenomics will be defined and described. A new wave in personal genetic testing, called *direct-to-consumer genetic testing,* is also discussed.

PHARMACOGENETICS AND PHARMACOGENOMICS

There are now two new fields of research and applications of genetics and genomics for medical treatment of disease—pharmacogenetics and pharmacogenomics. *Pharmacogenetics* is the field of research that looks at the difference in each individual's response to medications based on genetic variation. This field investigates how an individual's genetic information affects the way in which drugs are transported and metabolized in the person's body as a result of

specific drug receptors. The goal of pharmacogenetics is to create an individualized drug treatment program that involves the best choice and dose of drugs for a particular patient. One example of the application of pharmacogenetics involves the drug warfarin, a blood thinner. Genetic testing can now be done for certain genes, called *CYP2C9* and *VKORC1,* that affect how warfarin is metabolized; this testing can guide the specific dosage and management to help prevent adverse side effects (Lea, Feero, & Jenkins, 2008).

Pharmacogenomics is the field of research that looks for genetic variations associated with drug discovery and development. Pharmacogenomic research is leading to the creation of new drugs that can be tailor-made for each specific patient and adapted to that person's particular genetic makeup. A person's diet, lifestyle, age, state of health, and environment can all affect that person's response to medicines. Now and in the future, in addition to considering these factors, an understanding of an individual's genetic makeup will increasingly help with the creation and prescription of personalized drugs that are most effective—and have fewer side-effects—for a specific person (National Human Genome Research Institute, 2009a). As an example, a test is now being used to determine whether a medicine called *trastuzumab* (Herceptin) will be effective in the treatment of breast cancer. The test determines whether a woman who has metastatic breast cancer also tests positive for human epidermal growth factor receptor 2 (HER2). Women who have a positive test result and have HER2-positive breast cancer have been found to have a more serious and aggressive form of the disease, with a greater chance of recurrence, poorer prognosis, and lower chance of survival, when compared with those women who have HER2-negative breast cancer. Herceptin, which is designed to target and block the function of HER2 protein overexpression, is now given to those women who test positive for HER2 (National Cancer Institute, 2008).

DIRECT-TO-CONSUMER GENETIC TESTING

Genomic research has also opened the door for a new approach to accessing genetic testing that allows people to order, via the Internet, genetic testing by sending a sample of their saliva or tissue to a laboratory that will perform the test. A growing number of for-profit companies offer this type of genetic testing, known as direct-to-consumer (DTC) genetic testing, to assess genetic status. The company analyzes the individual's gene-sequence data, interprets it for the risk information it reveals, and develops a report. The report is then sent directly to the consumer. Often a health care provider is not involved in this process. This means that individuals who have DTC genetic testing may bring the results to their health care providers, including nurses, to ask for their help in interpreting the complex genetic test results for common diseases. Most health care providers will have insufficient knowledge, training, or clear guidelines on how to interpret and use these genetic test results (Hunter, Khoury, & Drazen, 2008). Other concerns raised by DTC genetic testing include the possibility that individuals may misinterpret the genetic information that is given directly to them or the possibility that they may order genetic tests that are inappropriate. Several organizations, including the National Institutes of Health, are developing programs and resources to educate the general public and health care professionals about genetic testing (Feero, Guttmacher, & Collins, 2008).

Nursing practice will increasingly include these new directions in health care. Nurses will need to expand their knowledge and skills in tailoring genetic and genomic information and testing to their patients. Having knowledge of both the benefits and limitations of emerging genetic tests will enable nurses to assist their patients to be informed health care decision makers (Lea et al., 2008). Box 16-3 provides a listing of clinical genetics resources that nurses and their patients can use to learn more about genetic testing.

Ethical Issues in Genetics and Genomics

The nursing profession has long recognized the importance of ethics as an integral component of professional nursing practice. In recognition of the importance of an ethical foundation in nursing practice, the American Nurses Association created the *Code of Ethics for Nurses*. The Code of Ethics "makes explicit the primary goals, values and obligations of the profession" (American Nurses Association, 2001, p. 5). Genetics and genomics raise a number of ethical issues of concern for nurses. These include informed decision making and consent; privacy and confidentiality of genetic and genomic information; social, cultural, and religious issues in genomic research; and concerns about insurance and employment discrimination based on a person's genetic and genomic information. This section provides information about social, cultural, and religious issues in genomic research, misuse of genetic and genomic information, and discrimination based on genetic information. The Code of Ethics for Nurses provides a foundation and guide for nurses when confronting these ethical issues in genetics and genomics. Readers are directed to Chapter 12 for an overview of ethical issues for nurses, including more information on informed decision making and consent, as well as privacy and confidentiality of medical information.

SOCIAL, CULTURAL, AND RELIGIOUS ISSUES IN GENOMIC RESEARCH

Human genome research raises some difficult questions related to scientific, biomedical, and legal issues. Some of the most difficult questions, however, are related to social, cultural, or religious implications of new genetic knowledge and technology. Emerging knowledge about the history of our evolution and the small variations within an individual's genomes has the potential to affect concepts of race, ethnicity, and even gender. To address the challenges associated with the relationships among genomics, race, and ethnicity, researchers have now moved into the areas of social science and psychology to learn about genetic effects on behavior, as well as explore new dimensions of religious or philosophical concepts about identity, potentially redefining what it means to be human (Bonham, Warshauer-Baker, & Collins, 2005).

In recognition of the potential for misuse of genetic and genomic information, the National Human Genome Research Institute (NHGRI) created the Ethical, Legal and Social Implications (ELSI) program

BOX 16-3   Genetics and Genomics Clinical Resources

Centers for Disease Control and Prevention (CDC)—Offers online resources for credible health information. One of their online resources is a "Diseases & Conditions A-Z Index" that includes genetic disorders: www.cdc.gov/DiseasesConditions

Genetic Alliance—Provides individuals and organizations with dynamic resources that emphasize expanded access to quality, vetted information, including information about specific diseases, support groups for specific diseases, family history, and other resources: www.geneticalliance.org

Genetics and Rare Diseases Information Center (GARD)—Established by the National Human Genome Research Institute (NHGR) and the Office of Rare Diseases (ORD) to help members of the general public, including patients and their families, health professionals, and biomedical researchers find useful information about genetic and rare diseases. GARD has a website (http://rarediseases.info.nih.gov/GARD) and also provides immediate, virtually round-the-clock access to experienced information specialists who can furnish current and accurate information (in both English and Spanish) about genetic and rare diseases: www.genome.gov/10000409

Genetics and Genomics for Patients and the Public—Created by the National Human Genome Research Institute; provides detailed information about genetic disorders, background on genetic and genomic science, the new science of pharmacogenomics, tools to create your own family health history, and a list of online health resources: www.genome.gov/19016903

Genetics Home Reference—Provides consumer-friendly information about the effects of genetic variations on human health: http://ghr.nlm.nih.gov

GeneTests—Features expert-authored, peer-reviewed, current disease descriptions that apply genetic testing to the diagnosis, management, and genetic counseling of patients and families with specific inherited conditions. GeneTests also provides a directory of genetic clinics in the United States: www.genetests.org

National Institutes of Mental Health (NIMH)—Looking at My Genes: What Can They Tell Me? Frequently Asked Questions About Genome Scans and Genetic Testing: www.nimh.nih.gov/health/publications/looking-at-my-genes-what-can-they-tell-me.shtml

National Society of Genetic Counselors (NSGC)—The NSGC has a ResourceLink has to assist individuals and health professionals in locating genetic counseling services. Genetic counselors can be searched by state, city, counselor's name, institution, or areas of practice or specialization: www.nsgc.org/resourcelink.cfm

Office of Rare Diseases Research (ORDR)—Coordinates research and information on rare diseases at the NIH and for the rare diseases community. The ORDR website provides information for patients and their families with rare diseases and about NIH- and ORDR-sponsored biomedical research and scientific conferences: http://rarediseases.info.nih.gov

Personalized Medicine—Provides up-to-date information about a new era in health care, personalized medicine, which is creating new methods for earlier diagnoses and individualized interventions: www.ageofpersonalizedmedicine.org/index.asp

U.S. Surgeon General's Family History Initiative, Family History Tool—This web-based tool helps users organize family history information and then print it out for presentation to the family doctor. In addition, the tool helps users save their family history information to their own computer and even share family history information with other family members: https://familyhistory.hhs.gov

---

in 1990 as an important component of the Human Genome Project. Insights gained through the ELSI research help to inform development of regulations and legislation to safeguard against misuse of genetic information. ELSI-funded activities have included multiple research and education projects, books, articles, newsletters, websites, and television and radio programs, as well as conferences and other activities that focus on translating ELSI research into clinical and public health practices (NHGRI, 2009e). Nurses need to become familiar with ELSI research and be able to identify these social, cultural, and religious issues related to genetic and genomic information and technologies so that they can provide guidance and understanding to their patients, families, and communities (Consensus Panel, 2008).

DISCRIMINATION BASED ON GENETIC AND GENOMIC INFORMATION

Until recently, many individuals and families were worried about the possibility of insurance and employment discrimination based on their genetic test results and information. These concerns have led many people who could benefit from genetic testing to decide not to have the testing at all, or to pay for genetic testing on their own outside of their insurance company so that they would not be denied future health care coverage or employment (Genetics and Public Policy Center, 2009).

In May 2008, then-President George W. Bush signed the Genetic Information Nondiscrimination Act, called *GINA*. GINA gives U.S. citizens protection from health insurance and employment discrimination based on their genetic information. GINA is a major breakthrough for today's health care and has important implications for all health care providers, especially nurses. Nurses will need to become familiar with what protections GINA does and does not cover so that they can educate patients, families, and communities about this new federal protection law. Regulations interpreting GINA must first be drafted, and once these have been completed, health insurance and employment provisions will become available. The period of implementation will continue through May 2010.

GINA prevents health insurers from denying coverage, adjusting premiums, or otherwise discriminating on the basis of a person's genetic information. Health insurers may not request that a person have a genetic test. Employers are prohibited from using genetic information to make decisions to hire, fire, compensate, or promote an individual. The law also significantly limits a health insurer's or employer's right to request, require, or purchase someone's genetic information. The new GINA legislation does not allow insurers and employers to use research participants' genetic information against them (Genetics and Public Policy Center, 2008).

GINA also has important limitations that nurses should understand. The law does not prevent health care providers from recommending genetic tests to their patients. GINA does not mandate coverage for any particular test or treatment, and it does not prohibit medical underwriting based on current health status. GINA does not cover life, disability, and long-term care insurance, nor does it apply to members of the military (Hudson, Holohan, & Collins, 2008).

SUMMARY

Genetic and genomic research that has evolved since the human genome was mapped and sequenced is ushering in a new era of health care, genomic health care. Genomic health care involves the use of new knowledge and tools to tailor health care at the individual level by using a person's unique genetic and genomic information to guide care. This means that health care will be more personalized and will include the use of more effective gene-based screening, diagnostic, and treatment measures. Nurses in all practice settings will increasingly be called upon to use genetic- and genomic-based approaches and technologies in their patient care. Nursing leaders created the *Essentials of Genetic and Genomic Nursing: Competencies, Curriculum Guidelines, and Outcome Indicators* (Consensus Panel, 2008) in recognition of the implications of genomic health care for nurses. Having genetic and genomic knowledge and competency will enable nurses to provide the most effective and meaningful patient care.

KEY POINTS

- Genetic and genomic research has ushered in a new era of health care, called *genomic health care*.
- Genomic health care involves the use of new knowledge and tools to tailor health care to the individual by using a person's unique genetic and genomic information to guide care.
- Health care is becoming more personalized and includes the use of more gene-based screening, diagnostic, and treatment measures.
- All registered nurses in all areas of practice will increasingly be expected to use genetic- and genomic-based approaches and technologies in the care of patients, families, and communities.
- Nursing leaders created the *Essentials of Genetic and Genomic Nursing: Competencies, Curricula Guidelines, and Outcome Indicators* as a necessary foundation to prepare all nurses to provide genetic- and genomic-based nursing care.

- Two important tools that nurses will use to personalize screening, prevention, diagnosis and treatment of individuals and families are family history and genetic tests.
- Based on the *Essentials of Genetic and Genomic Nursing,* nurses will be involved in conducting family history collection and pedigree construction, as well as in offering and explaining genetic testing.
- Nurses will participate in the referral of individuals and families to genetics specialty services, where they can get more detailed genetic and genomic evaluation, diagnosis, and information.
- Nurses need to become knowledgeable about the ethical issues in genomic research and concerns about insurance and employment discrimination based on a person's genetic and genomic information.
- Nurses should become familiar with the scope and limitations of the Genetic Information Nondiscrimination Act (GINA) so that they can educate patients, families, and communities about the details of this new nondiscrimination legislation.

CRITICAL THINKING EXERCISES

1. As a nurse working in a family health clinic, you see a 40-year-old woman for a routine visit. During the visit, you update her family history. She informs you that she is concerned because her sister was just diagnosed with breast cancer at the age of 42. Since her sister's diagnosis, she has learned that one of her aunts (her father's sister) died of breast cancer at the age of 45. Also, that aunt's daughter, now 38, has a history of breast cancer. Her father's mother died at an early age from cancer as well. She tells you that her father's family has never wanted to talk about the family history of breast cancer; until recently, it was kept as a secret. The woman asks you, "What does this mean for me?" How would you answer her question? What resources would you make available to her?

2. At a cardiovascular clinic, two patients who are waiting to be seen begin a conversation about their history of having strokes. They talk about how they are being treated with the blood thinner warfarin. One of the patients is receiving a much lower dose of warfarin than the other patient. When this patient sees the nurse, he talks about his conversation with the other patient and asks the nurse why he is getting a lower dose: "Why don't I have the same higher dose as the other patient? If I have the lower dose, doesn't this increase my risk for having another stroke?" How would you answer this patient's question?

3. A young husband and wife come to the obstetric clinic where you work. They tell you that they are planning to have a baby. When taking their family history, you learn that both of them are of African American ancestry and that the husband's brother has a history of sickle cell anemia. The wife tells you, "We want to know what our risk is of having a baby with sickle cell anemia and whether there are any tests that can be done to help us find out." How would you respond to the couple's concerns? What resources could you make available to them to help answer their question?

4. A 50-year-old male patient has just learned that he has a history of early-onset colorectal cancer in his family. One of his brothers and a maternal uncle developed colorectal cancer at an early age. His physician has suggested that he and his family consider having genetic testing to determine whether they carry the gene that increases the risk for early-onset colorectal cancer. After seeing the physician, the patient tells you that he does not think he or his family members will want to have the genetic testing because "We don't want our insurance companies to deny us coverage." How would you respond to this patient's concerns about the possibility of his insurance company discriminating against him based on his genetic information?

REFERENCES

American Nurses Association. (2001). *Code of ethics for nurses with interpretive statements*. Silver Spring, MD: American Nurses Association.

American Nurses Association. (2004). *Nursing: Scope and standards of practice*. Washington, DC: American Nurses Association. Available online at http://nursesbooks.org

Bonham, V. L., Warshauer-Baker, E., & Collins, F. S. (2005). Race and ethnicity in the genome era: The complexity of the constructs. *American Psychologist*, *60*(1), 9–15.

Cohen, F. (1979). Genetic knowledge possessed by American nurses and students. *Journal of Advanced Nursing*, *4*(5), 493–501.

Consensus Panel on Genetic/Genomic Nursing Competencies. (2008). *Essentials of genetic and genomic nursing: Competencies, curricula guidelines, and outcome indicators*. Silver Spring, MD: American Nurses Association.

Feero, W. G., Guttmacher, A. E., & Collins, F. S. (2008). The genome gets personal—almost. *The Journal of the American Medical Association*, *299*(11), 1351–1352.

Genetics and Public Policy Center. (2008). *The Genetic Information Nondiscrimination Act.* [Online]. Retrieved from http://www.dnapolicy.org/policy.issue.php?action=detail&issuebrief_id=37

Genetics and Public Policy Center. (2009). *Genetic privacy & discrimination.* [Online]. Retrieved from http://www.dnapolicy.org/policy.privacy.php

Genetics Home Reference. (2009). *Genetic testing.* [Online]. Retrieved from http://ghr.nlm.nih.gov/handbook/testing

GeneTests. (2009). [Online]. Retrieved from www.genetests.org

Guttmacher, A. E., & Collins, F. S. (2002). Genomic medicine—a primer. *New England Journal of Medicine, 347,* 1512–1521.

Hudson, K. L., Holohan, M. K., & Collins, F. S. (2008). Keeping pace with the times: the Genetic Information Nondiscrimination Act. *New England Journal of Medicine, 358*(25), 2261–2263.

Hunter, D. J., Khoury, M. J., & Drazen, J. M. (2008). Letting the genome out of the bottle—will we get our wish? *New England Journal of Medicine, 358*(2), 105–107.

Jenkins, J. (Ed.). (2007). *Genetics in nursing and healthcare. nurseAdvance Collection series,* Indiana: Sigma Theta Tau International.

Lea, D. H., Feero, F., & Jenkins, J. F. (2008). Warfarin therapy and pharmacogenomics: A step toward personalized medicine. *American Nurse Today, 3*(5), 12–13.

National Cancer Institute. (2008). *Trastuzumab.* [Online]. Retrieved from http://www.cancer.gov/cancertopics/druginfo/trastuzumab

National Human Genome Research Institute. (2009a). *Frequently asked questions about genetic counseling.* [Online]. Retrieved from http://www.genome.gov/19016905

National Human Genome Research Institute. (2009b). *Genetics and genomics for patients and the public.* Retrieved from http://www.genome.gov/19016903

National Human Genome Research Institute. (2009c). *Genetics, genomics and patient management.* [Online]. Retrieved from http://www.genome.gov/27527600

National Human Genome Research Institute. (2009d). *Guidelines and tools to assess family history of common diseases: Value of family history.* [Online]. Retrieved from http://www.genome.gov/27527602

National Human Genome Research Institute. (2009e). *Social, cultural and religious issues in genetic research.* [Online]. Retrieved from http://www.genome.gov/10001848

National Human Genome Research Institute. (2009f). *Talking glossary of genetic terms.* Retrieved from http://www.genome.gov/glossary

National Human Genome Research Institute. (2009g). *Frequently asked questions about genetic research.* [Online]. Retrieved from http://www.genome.gov/19516792

National Institutes of Health. (2009). *Fact Sheet. Genetic testing: How it is used for healthcare,* [Online]. Retrieved from http://www.nih.gov/about/researchresultsforthepublic/genetictesting.pdf

Skirton, H., Patch, C., & Williams, J. (2005). *Applied genetics in healthcare: A handbook for specialist practitioners.* New York, NY: Taylor & Francis Group.

University of Kansas Medical Center. (2009). *Genetic centers, clinics and departments.* [Online]. Retrieved from http://www.kumc.edu/gec/prof/genecntr.html

U.S. Department of Health and Human Services. (2009). *My family health portrait: A tool from the surgeon general.* [Online]. Retrieved from https://familyhistory.hhs.gov

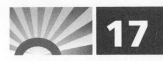

17

Rural Health Concepts

VICKIE H. SOUTHALL, MSN, RN

OBJECTIVES

After completion of this chapter, the reader will be able to:

- Discuss demographic characteristics of rural communities that have an impact on their health status.
- Identify leading health issues of rural areas.
- Compare the health status of rural and urban residents.
- Use characteristics of rural nursing to analyze the scope of rural nursing practice.
- Discuss how federal programs have affected rural health.
- Apply knowledge of rural health to develop effective strategies for rural nursing practice.

PROFILE IN PRACTICE

Melissa A. Sutherland, PhD, FNP-C
Nurse Practitioner, Broome County Health Department, New York

My interest in rural health care issues began when I earned my first bachelor's degree in rural sociology from Cornell University in 1995. After graduating, I worked for a year at the National Institutes of Health doing bench science research. My younger sister was in nursing school at the time, and I would hear stories about her clinical days and longed to work with more than anonymous blood samples. Returning to school a year later, I entered a second degree nursing program and was not sure how my first undergraduate degree would serve me in my new career. As a rural sociology major, I remembered learning about population statistics, social stratification, and vulnerable populations but little about health care. The year I spent in nursing school went quickly, and I found myself working on a

labor and delivery unit in North Carolina. On occasion I still wondered how my first undergraduate degree would serve me. What I did not realize at the time was that my rural sociology degree was influencing my work as a nurse. It provided a broad perspective and allowed me to step back and consider the societal factors that were affecting the lives and health care experiences of women and children.

During my master's program I connected my rural sociology background and nursing experiences. I had the opportunity to participate in the Helene Fuld Summer Institute for Rural Community Health Nursing. During the program I had the opportunity to work on a monograph, and I found myself gravitating to the chapter regarding women's health in rural areas.

Rural women face many barriers when seeking health care services. Access to health care may be limited by available services, socioeconomic status, and transportation issues. Rural areas often lack specialized services and providers for women, as well as an adequate number of providers in general. In particular, female providers are less likely to practice in rural areas, and provider gender has been shown to be important in a woman's decision to seek medical care and advice. Women needing second opinions or seeking out other options for specialized medical care find there are few options. Women who need testing for sexually transmitted diseases or HIV may find they need to travel to a more urban area or larger clinic to ensure their confidentiality as well as find a provider who offers the testing and counseling. Reproductive services are often more limited in rural areas with fewer options for birth control, resulting in higher rates of adolescent pregnancy.

Transportation issues are another challenge to health care access faced by women living in rural areas. Women may not have their own transportation, and with public transportation not available or very limited in rural areas, some women must depend on others for rides to and from health clinic appointments. The ride may not be reliable, and women may be late for or miss an appointment. If the clinic has a policy about late and missed appointments, the woman may not be allowed to reschedule or she may be charged a fee for missing an appointment. Policies such as these contribute to the challenges faced by rural women. In addition, the woman's confidentiality and privacy are compromised because of her dependence on others for transportation. Further, women may also not feel comfortable discussing sexual and substance use issues with their provider because of privacy issues when everyone in the community knows one another.

Access to health care is a major challenge for rural women. Those responsible for creating policies and providing resources related to rural women need to consider these barriers and seek feasible solutions to the problems. After completing my master's program, I worked as a primary care nurse practitioner serving uninsured rural women in a free clinic setting. My practice at the clinic led to a dissertation on the topic of health care for rural women. I want to improve the health care of rural women through research and the formation of policy. As I continue my career, the lives of rural women will remain a focus of my research and practice.

Introduction

According to a W.K. Kellogg Foundation (2001) survey of rural, urban, and suburban residents, 85% of Americans hold a strongly positive view of rural life. They characterize rural life as involving a strong sense of family, exhibiting a commitment to the community, being hardworking, possessing deeply held religious beliefs, and being self-sufficient. Rural life is seen as emblematic of the individualism and self-sufficiency that has often defined America. At the same time, these positive views are moderated by the serious economic and social challenges that are also ascribed to rural localities: low wages, poverty, decreased job opportunities, resistance to change, and a reluctance to accept outsiders.

Mention the word *rural* and the picture most people describe is that of an agricultural community. However, fewer than 10% of rural Americans live on farms, and only 2% earn their living from farming. Moreover, total agricultural employment—including farm workers, suppliers, processors, and marketers—account for less than 12% of rural employment (W.K. Kellogg Foundation, 2001). More than half of rural jobs are in the service industry, and manufacturing jobs also outnumber farming jobs. Because perception helps determine policy, the stereotypes held of rural America may be detrimental. For a further discussion of stereotypes, see the chapters on diversity (Chapter 14) and vulnerable populations (Chapter 19).

When rural health is mentioned, actions related to agricultural hazards are often proposed. Although these are needed, actions related to securing accessible health care services and increasing the availability of insurance are much higher priorities for rural residents. Understanding the most important rural needs can help policymakers develop the most effective health strategies and help rural residents identify lifestyle changes that can improve health. For example, many people, both urban and rural, perceive rural localities as being much "safer" than other areas. Although the crime rate is lower in most rural areas, the rate of death from accidents is much higher. Similarly, preconceptions of rural life may include visions of fresh vegetables and much physical labor. Although fresh vegetables may be more available in rural localities, rural residents now report some of the highest obesity rates.

Rural health care presents both challenges and opportunities. Many indicators of health status are less favorable than in other areas of the country. However, nurses have the potential to bring about change in a meaningful way because they are received with respect in rural areas. Nurses have opportunities to develop policies at the local level and influence health and fitness patterns in communities. The positive perceptions of rural communities can provide the foundation for building strategies to support and enhance rural health.

 ## What Is Rural?

A number of different classification systems exist for defining how rural a locality is. Some systems focus on actual population numbers, whereas others define rural areas by population density or distance from an urban center. People's perceptions of the definition of *rural* are relative; the term is often thought to mean "smaller than where I'm from." Someone from a large city may think of a town of 20,000 as rural, whereas residents of a remote farming community may consider the town of 20,000 to be a city. Depending on the criteria chosen, rural areas account for 17% to 25% of the American population.

The U.S. Census Bureau (2008) and the Office of Management and Budget (OMB, 2004) have established two of the most frequently used classification systems for determining what is rural and what areas qualify for rural federal programs. The classification system used by the OMB was significantly revised in June 2003, resulting in a decrease of the percentage of the population defined as rural. Previously, *metropolitan statistical areas* (MSAs) were designated as counties encompassing a central city or urbanized area of at least 50,000, whereas all other areas were designated as *nonmetropolitan areas*. Counties were included in MSAs if they were both economically tied to the central city by daily commuting and displayed a "metropolitan character" based on population density. The revised guidelines placed more emphasis on daily commuting. If 25% of a community's population commuted to a central city, then it was redesignated as *metropolitan*, no matter what its population density. The net effect of this change decreased the actual enumeration of *nonmetropolitan* (rural) population from 55 million to 49 million persons and the percentage of the U.S. population characterized as *nonmetropolitan* from 20% to 17%. The OMB also introduced the new category of *micropolitan*, an area with a small city of 10,000 (Cromartie & Bucholtz, 2008).

At approximately the same time, the Census Bureau, which classified rural areas as localities of fewer than 2500 residents, started to include the population of the areas immediately surrounding these localities in their population totals. For instance, in 1990 a small town of 2200 people with an adjacent suburb of 500 would have been designated as rural. Under the 2008 guidelines, the population of the two areas would be combined for a total of 2700 and designated as an urban cluster. The net effect of this definition change decreased the number of rural residents in the United States by 3 million by reclassifying them as urban. If these criteria had not been changed, the U.S. rural population would have actually increased by approximately 2 million from the 1990 to the 2000 census. The population in rural areas rose 0.4% per year from 2000 to 2006, primarily as a result of increased numbers of Hispanics moving there. Since then, the rural population has started to decline, partly because of rising energy prices and a slowing economy (National Advisory Committee on Rural Health and Human Services [NACRHHS], 2008; U.S. Department of Agriculture [USDA], 2008).

A third popular classification system uses population density as its determining characteristic. In this system, *urban* is defined as any area containing at least 99 persons per square mile, *rural* as containing 7 to 98 persons per square mile, and *frontier* as areas containing fewer than 6 persons per square mile (National Center for Frontier Communities, 2007). This system is particularly helpful in delineating the unique needs of sparsely populated, geographically isolated localities. Other definitions describe rural areas by their distance to urban centers (e.g., 30 miles, 60 minutes). Communities that are only 30 miles from an urban area have different health issues than communities whose residents must travel 2 hours to reach the nearest city (Frontier Education Center, 2004).

The 2004 Omnibus Appropriations Act simplified the definition of *rural* to include any incorporated city or town of 20,000 or fewer to broaden eligibility for many rural federal programs (Institute of Medicine [IOM], 2005). In general, the literature uses the term *rural* to describe localities of fewer than 20,000 to 50,000 inhabitants and fewer than 99 persons per square mile. No matter which definition is used, being rural and having fewer people in geographically extended areas affects both transportation and interactions with other people, as well as the availability and accessibility of health care services.

CHARACTERISTICS OF RURAL COMMUNITIES

Rural America includes so many diverse communities that making generalizations is difficult. A farming community in the Mississippi Delta can be quite different from a mining town in Montana or a Native American reservation in Arizona. History, cultural mix, weather, and geography help shape each community's identity. This individuality is usually highly valued among rural residents. Each community possesses unique characteristics so that generalizations of rural areas may not hold true for any individual community. However, certain trends and statistics help one understand the make-up of the rural population in the United States and what impact this has on rural health needs.

Sometimes described as "bipolar," rural communities tend to have higher proportions of the very old and the very young than their urban counterparts (National Center for Health Statistics [NCHS], 2001; Jones, Kandel & Parker, 2007). Fifteen percent of rural residents are at least 65 years of age, whereas only 11.7% of urban residents are 65 or older (USDA, 2007). The nonmetropolitan population has a median age of 40.1 years compared with 36.1 years for the metropolitan population (Miller, 2009). This demographic has implications for the prevalence of chronic disease in rural communities and the need for primary health care services. At the other end of the age spectrum, many rural communities, especially in the South and Midwest, also have a higher proportion of children younger than 18 years (Annie E. Casey Foundation, 2004; Rogers, 2005; Strong, Del Grosso, Burwick, Jethwani, & Ponza, 2005).

Minorities in general are underrepresented in rural areas when compared with other areas of the country, although rural America is becoming more diverse. Overall, minorities make up approximately 36% of the total U.S. population and 18% of the rural population (Jones et al., 2007). However, the rate of minority growth, particularly among Hispanic and American Indian populations, is increasing in rural areas (USDA, 2005). The prevalence of minorities is highly variable, and in many individual rural communities they make up a much larger percentage of the population. Minorities in rural areas are more likely to live in poverty than their white peers. In a study for the Office of Rural Health Policy, Probst and colleagues (2002) found that poor minorities are concentrated in certain regions and that the counties with high minority representation have incomes and assets worth less than two thirds of the national average. The six southern states of Alabama, Mississippi, Georgia, North Carolina, Louisiana, and South Carolina are home to 70% of the poor, rural African American population in this country. More than half of poor, rural American Indians live in New Mexico, Arizona, Oklahoma, Montana, and South Dakota, but their growth is increasing fastest along the East Coast. The Southwest is home to 73% of poor, rural Hispanics in the five states of Texas, New Mexico, Arizona, California, and Colorado (Probst et al., 2002), although the highest level of Hispanic growth and migration is now occurring in the Southeast and Midwest (USDA, 2005). Hispanics are the most rapidly growing segment of the rural population and face additional challenges in language barriers and the lack of qualified medical interpreters in rural areas (NACRHHS, 2008).

Poverty is more prevalent in rural communities, and lower-income families consistently have a higher rate of health problems (IOM, 2005). Per capita income is

$9555 lower than in urban areas (NACRHHS, 2008), and household income is 25% lower (IOM, 2005). However, these statistics can be slightly misleading because the cost of living is usually also somewhat lower for rural residents (IOM, 2005). On an annual basis, the federal government defines the threshold for determining poverty based on family size; this is referred to as the *poverty line*. Fourteen percent of rural and 11% of urban residents live below the poverty line. The disparity in income tends to be even greater among rural minorities and rural families with children (under age 18). The Annie E. Casey Foundation (2004) found the child poverty rate of 20% in rural areas is higher than the national average of 17%, but lower than that of large cities (26%).

Adults in rural areas are more likely to be married and less likely to have been divorced, and they have more children per family and fewer years of formal schooling (IOM, 2005). Families tend to be more morally and politically conservative, as evidenced by recent national elections. Rural residents report greater church attendance and involvement with religion, leading many health professionals to experience success in using churches as sites of health education or coordination of care. Rural residents are also strongly oriented toward work and self-sufficiency (Lee & McDonagh, 2006a; Long & Weinert, 1989). This self-reliance can manifest itself in self-care for health problems and distrust of government-run health care programs.

Overall, rural areas have higher rates of unemployment, especially in certain regions (USDA, 2008). The closing of one large industry or business in a small town can have a much greater impact on the overall unemployment rate of that rural area than a similar closing in a metropolitan area, which is likely to have a number of businesses and industries to buffer the loss. More important, rural residents are less likely to have private health insurance (NACRHHS, 2008). Having health insurance is a critical factor in determining a person's health status and access to health care. It can be used in predicting disability status and the likelihood of physician use, as well as the overall likelihood of health care treatment. This topic is covered in further detail in the chapter on vulnerable populations (Chapter 19).

Health Status of Rural Residents

The Department of Health and Human Services (Gamm, 2007) identified health insurance as a top-10 "health indicator" and a reliable predictor of overall health status. Rural residents are more often self-employed or employed in smaller, often family-run, businesses that are less likely to offer health insurance to their employees. However, the gap between urban and rural insurance coverage has decreased over the last 10 years, primarily as a result of increased utilization of government-sponsored insurance programs (IOM, 2005; NACRHHS, 2008). Most of the uninsured are full-time workers; businesses with fewer than 25 employees account for 38% of the uninsured workers in the United States (National Coalition on Health Care, 2009). Rural children are less likely to have insurance than children in urban areas, especially children of Hispanic or African descent (Martin, Probst, Moore, Patterson, & Elder, 2005). Migrant seasonal rural workers are unlikely to receive health benefits or even minimum wage. Seasonal migrant workers have the additional obstacle of establishing any level of continuity of care.

Conducted every 10 years, the *Rural Healthy People (RHP) 2010* project identified access to quality health services as the overwhelming top priority in rural areas (Bolin & Gamm, 2003). Residents of rural communities seem to have higher rates of chronic illness such as diabetes, hypertension, cardiovascular disease, cancer, and arthritis. However, when these disease rates are adjusted for age and the higher proportion of older residents in rural areas, the difference is erased (IOM, 2005; NACRHHS, 2008; Ricketts, 2000). Although living in a rural area does not increase the risk for developing chronic disease, a higher percentage of the rural population does cope with chronic illnesses. The resulting need for increased health services for these chronic diseases is coupled with the fact that fewer than 10% of physicians practice in rural communities even though 17% to 25% of the population lives there (Cromartie & Bucholtz, 2008; National Rural Health Association [NRHA], 2008; Ricketts, 2000). This disparity is likely to increase in the future

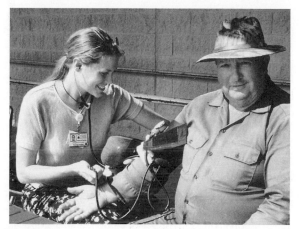

FIGURE 17-1 A nursing student checks blood pressure levels outside a rural grocery store during an outreach service activity.

as the proportion of female physicians in America increases. Female physicians are less likely to practice in rural areas than urban areas (Ballance, Kornegay, & Evans, 2009; Fordyce, Chen, Doescher, & Hart, 2007). However, nonphysician primary care providers such as nurse practitioners and nurse midwives are starting to fill the positions and serve the needs of rural communities (Lindsay, 2007) (Figure 17-1). In 2006, 27% of all employed nurse practitioners practiced in rural areas (Newland, 2006; Ricketts, 2005).

Although rates of coronary heart disease and stroke have fallen 50% during the past 30 years, these conditions were still the leading causes of death in 2000 and a top priority of rural health care providers (Zuniga, Anderson, & Alexander, 2003). Rural populations are particularly vulnerable to cardiac conditions because of their higher rate of smoking (unadjusted for age) and high-fat diets, as well as their greater distance from comprehensive cardiac rehabilitation facilities. Buczko (2001) found heart failure and stroke to be the most common discharge diagnoses for hospitalized rural Medicare beneficiaries.

According to the *Rural Healthy People 2010* survey, diabetes is the third-highest ranking health problem among rural residents, behind access to care and heart disease (cited in Gamm, 2007). The prevalence of diabetes seems to be somewhat higher in rural areas, but ethnic, socioeconomic, and lifestyle factors

are greater risk factors than geographical environment (Dabney & Gosschalk, 2003). For example, rates of diabetes are two to five times more common in certain minority groups; rural communities with high African American, Hispanic, or American Indian populations are particularly at risk. Limited resources for the management of diabetes and specialized care such as ophthalmological examinations compound the problem. The rate of hospital admissions due to diabetes increased 85% in recent years, and patients with diabetes from poor communities are 80% more likely to be hospitalized for diabetes (Agency for Healthcare Research and Quality [AHRQ], 2007).

Rural health leaders identify mental health and mental disorders as the fourth most important priority in rural health care (Gamm, 2007). Although both rural and urban areas report that approximately 20% of their residents are affected by mental disorders each year, suicide and severe psychological distress rates are higher in rural areas (Strong et al., 2005). Rural communities are far less likely to have sufficient mental health services. Almost 90% of the federally designated Mental Health Professional Shortage Areas in the United States are in nonmetropolitan counties, including 20% of nonmetropolitan counties that have no mental health services. Lengthy travel to mental health outpatient services is common and associated with fewer visits. Many insurance plans limit the number of visits to mental health professionals. However, rural residents report that they prefer discussing their psychological concerns with their primary care provider more than a psychiatrist. Frequently, specialized mental health services programs are only economically viable with grant funding and cease when the funding ends. Consequently, rural primary care physicians and nurse practitioners play a greater role in mental health care than do their metropolitan counterparts. Some studies have found that the treatment of rural residents with depression is more likely to be improved by enhancing the mental health education of primary care providers than by increasing the supply of specialty mental health providers in rural areas (Gale & Lambert, 2006; Sawyer, Gale, & Lambert, 2006). Hanrahan and Hartley (2008) propose a model of using advanced practice psychiatric nurses to ease the rural mental health workforce shortage.

Dental health is the fifth most identified health need in rural areas, according to the *Rural Healthy People 2010* survey. Dental caries are more prevalent in rural areas. Fewer than 20% of children covered by Medicaid receive preventive dental care each year. Tooth loss among senior citizens and lack of dental visits within the last year are much more common occurrences in rural areas. Shortages of dentists, lack of community-fluoridated water because of individual wells, decreased access to dental insurance, and increased rates of poverty in rural areas are all factors in the dental health status of rural communities (Martin, Wang, Probst, Hale, & Johnson, 2008; NACRHHS, 2008).

Substance abuse is recognized as a health problem in both rural and urban areas, with slightly higher rates of alcohol use among rural residents and slightly higher rates of illicit drug use among urban residents. However, the consequences may be greater in rural areas because of the lack of substance abuse treatment services, regional isolation, and the stigma associated with treatment in small localities (NACRHHS, 2007). Rates of driving under the influence of alcohol are greater in rural areas, possibly because of the greater distances traveled and greater reliance on automobile travel. Tobacco use is also significantly greater in rural areas, especially among adolescents. More recently, methamphetamine use has been recognized as a significant problem in rural America, where "meth labs" are easier to set up and escape detection (Gfroerer, Larson, & Colliver, 2007; NACRHHS, 2007). Prescription drug abuse, especially of OxyContin, has been found to be a greater problem in rural areas, particularly among rural youth and in mining communities. Approximately one in seven rural Americans report abuse or dependence problems (Duncan, Salant, & Colocousis, 2006).

Statistics on domestic violence tend to be conflicting but show no overall differences between rural and urban communities (Alexander & Castillo, 2004; Breiding, Ziembroski, & Black, 2009). However, with homes far apart, there may be fewer opportunities for domestic violence to be noticed and reported. Moreover, such behaviors may also be less likely to be identified as inappropriate by residents, particularly when support services are lacking. Fewer resources exist in rural areas for preventing intimate partner violence (Breiding et al., 2009).

Childhood immunization rates are similar among rural and metropolitan areas (NACRHHS, 2008; NCHS, 2007). This may be attributable, in part, to the positive health finding that rural residents are more likely to be able to report having a "usual source of health care," but they are less likely to report a health care visit within the previous 12 months (NCHS, 2007). Studies have found that rural residents are less likely to obtain some preventive health services such as mammograms (Casey, Call, & Klinger, 2001; Zhang, Tao, & Irwin, 2000), whereas other studies (Edwards & Tudiver, 2008; Pol, Rouse, Zyzanski, Rasmussen, & Crabtree, 2001) found that rural residents receive preventive services at rates as good as, or better than, their suburban and urban counterparts, as long as they visit a health care provider. Rural nurses have been noted to have a positive effect on the use of preventive health services (Butler, Kim-Godwin, & Fox, 2008).

Unintentional injuries or accidents are the fifth leading cause of death in the United States each year and are more prevalent in rural areas (NCHS, 2007; NRHA, 2008). Rates of motor vehicle–related injuries and death, in particular, are much higher. More than half of motor vehicle–related deaths occur in rural areas, and rural residents are 50% more likely to die from trauma than urban residents (Gonzalez, Cummings, Mulekar, & Rodning, 2006). Children in rural counties have a much higher rate of fatal injuries from all types of accidents.

Occupational injury rates are also much higher for workers employed in the agriculture, mining, and forestry industries. Most agricultural injuries involve tractors and farm machinery. Youth working in agriculture account for 40% of work-related fatalities, yet they make up only 8% of agricultural workers (Alexander & Castillo, 2004; Hill & Butterfield, 2006).

The problem of obesity and overweight has been described as our new national epidemic and a critical public health threat. The number of Americans who are overweight or obese has doubled in the last 20 years, and the number of overweight or obese children has tripled (Liu et al., 2007; Ogden et al., 2006; Trust for America's Health, 2008). Diet and activity patterns rank second only to tobacco as the leading "actual cause of death." The problem is particularly significant in rural areas because of higher self-reports of adult obesity than in urban areas. Numerous studies have also shown a considerably greater incidence of obesity and overweight in rural children and adolescents (Rogers, 2005; Trust for America's Health, 2008). Cultural patterns of eating increased calories—developed when rural residents historically were more engaged in heavy physical activity—may play a role. Rural communities with high percentages of African Americans or American Indians are especially at risk because of the high prevalence of obesity in these populations. Seventy percent of rural African American adolescents are obese (26%) or overweight (44%), as are 80% of rural African American adults (Trust for America's Health, 2008).

Characteristics of Rural Nursing Practice

Nurses practicing in rural areas experience unique opportunities and challenges. In a rural hospital, the nurse may help deliver a baby one morning, teach a family about pediatric postappendectomy home care later that morning, and provide care to an older patient with a hip fracture that afternoon. In addition, the rural nurse may perform skills such as starting IVs or administering respiratory treatments that support staff typically provide in larger hospitals.

Rural community health nurses routinely staff family planning and pediatric clinics, perform nursing home screenings, deliver health education at schools and senior centers, provide health care guidance to local governing boards, and provide case management to families with complex health care needs. A rural nurse needs to have general knowledge of a wide variety of nursing specialties and is often described as an "expert generalist" (Rosenthal, 2006; Scharff, 2006; Troyer & Lee, 2006).

Providing such diverse care can be both daunting and rewarding. Although much of nursing time may be spent taking care of patients less acutely ill and less complex than those in larger, more specialized facilities, rural nurses usually care for a wider variety of patients because patient volumes are too low to have specialty units. This variety of care can be exciting

but also less predictable because the workload falls on fewer individuals in rural settings. Adaptability, flexibility, and critical thinking are key characteristics for success. When crisis situations occur, rural nurses must be prepared to handle the situations on their own until other members of the health care team arrive (Rosenthal, 2006; Scharff, 2006). Rural nurses assume more diverse roles and must be prepared to take leadership roles in determining local policy and planning health services. A further discussion of the roles in nursing occurs in Chapter 4.

Greater autonomy and self-direction are described as benefits valued by rural nurses (Rosenthal, 2006; Scharff, 2006). With this independence the nurses perceive a greater degree of control and input in patient care, resulting in greater job satisfaction and lower rates of burnout. The downside is the potential for professional isolation and less guidance or backup during emergencies.

The hallmark of rural nursing is the development of close community ties and close relationships (Scharff, 2006). Rural nurses tend to know their patients more personally than do nurses in larger urban settings. They may have worked, socialized, and attended church with their families for years. In-depth knowledge of patients and families may provide greater insights into their health needs. Nurses working in rural areas identify continuity of care for individuals across the life span and the opportunity to practice holistic nursing as the most rewarding advantages of nursing in small communities.

This closeness can also lead to some of rural nursing's biggest challenges. Nurses in rural settings may have to care for family and friends. Making objective assessments can be difficult when relationships beyond the nurse-patient relationship exist. Hasty assumptions about patients can be made without thoroughly assessing each situation. Some patients may be hesitant to share certain personal information or may not be totally honest (Lee & McDonagh, 2006a). However, the rural nurse who develops an impeccable reputation for confidentiality may actually gain an advantage in securing confidential information.

Nurses are usually viewed with high esteem in rural communities (Bushy, 2009; Rosenthal, 2005). They may provide input and leadership in making health care decisions for the community. This positive visibility and respect can increase professional confidence and nursing power in influencing health policy. The lack of anonymity can also make it difficult to step out of the nursing role when not at work (Raph & Buehler, 2006). Getting stopped in the grocery store for health care advice or being sought out at a ball game to assess an injury can be frequent occurrences. As role models in the community, nurses may find themselves embarrassed if their own health habits fall short of what they recommend to patients.

☀ Rural Nursing Theory

Theories specifically related to rural nursing have evolved with time. The practice of rural nursing can be improved through understanding health perceptions and beliefs held by rural residents. Long and Weinert (1989) described several key concepts useful in understanding rural health needs and rural nursing practice. From these concepts, they developed three relational statements:

- Rural dwellers define health primarily as the ability to work, be productive, and perform usual tasks.
- Rural dwellers are self-reliant and resist accepting help or services from those seen as outsiders or from agencies seen as national or regional "welfare" programs.
- Health care providers in rural areas must deal with a lack of anonymity and much greater role diffusion than providers in urban or suburban settings (Long & Weinert, 1989, p. 120).

Lee and Winters (2004) later validated many of these concepts and added the concept of choice in understanding rural health. Choice involves the decision to live in a rural area and the choice of a health care provider. When rural residents were asked, they indicated they knew that their decision to live in a less-populated community would affect their health care choices and traveling distances. Acknowledging these limitations, they still choose rural life (Lee & McDonagh, 2006b; Lee & Winters, 2004).

Lee and McDonagh (2006b) further analyzed Long and Weinert's relational statements, finding that as rural America has changed, there is less emphasis by residents on defining health as the ability to do work

and more on the ability to do what they want to do and live life as they want. Rural residents remain self-reliant but have become more accepting of outside care, especially when caring for their infants and children (Lee & McDonough, 2006b).

Bales, Winters, and Lee (2006) further identified six major themes in analyzing rural needs and perceptions that affect rural nursing practice: self-reliance, hardiness, conscientious consumer, informed risk, inadequate insurance, and community support. Changes in health service technology, rural life, and national health care expectations may be changing rural residents' perceptions and the practice of rural nursing. Additional studies are needed to develop theory for rural nursing and a framework for practice.

☀ Rural Health Policy and Resources

A number of programs to support and enhance rural health have been developed during the last half-century. In the 1950s, the Hill-Burton Act helped finance construction of health care facilities in underserved communities, many of them rural. This decade also saw the initiation of special health services for American Indians. The Indian Health Service (IHS) today continues to pursue the goal of ensuring that "comprehensive, culturally acceptable personal and public health services are available and accessible to all American Indian and Alaska Native People" (IHS, 2008). IHS assists American Indian tribes in developing health programs, provides comprehensive health care services for both primary and acute care, and serves as an advocate for securing comprehensive health care. American Indians and Alaska Natives have treaty rights to federal health care services through the Department of Health and Human Services.

The unique needs of migrant workers were recognized in the 1960s. Grants to community nonprofit organizations have funded a number of culturally and linguistically competent medical and support services for migrant and seasonal farm workers and their families since then. Today, migrant health centers (MHCs) provide health services to more than 25% of all migrant workers, usually on a sliding-fee scale according to their ability to pay (Health Resources Services Adminstration, n.d.). Some MHCs are open year round, and others are seasonal. They also may offer environmental health services, infectious disease screening, and accident prevention programs. Migrant populations tend to be younger and have higher fertility rates than non-migrant populations, so family planning and children's health services are also needed (USDA, 2005).

In 1972, the National Health Service Corps (NHSC) was established to encourage health professionals to practice in health professional shortage areas (HPSAs), often rural areas, in return for repayment of educational loans. The NHSC has been responsible for placing many health professionals in rural areas but has been less successful in retaining them (Ricketts, 2000). In 1977, the Rural Health Clinics Service Act was passed to increase health care access to rural, underserved communities and to expand use of mid-level health care practitioners, such as nurse practitioners and nurse midwives, in these areas (Centers for Medicare and Medicaid Services [CMS], 2008c; Health Resources and Services Administration, 2005). The number of rural health clinics (RHCs) increased from 285 in 1980 to 2801 in 2006 (NACRHHS, 2008).

In 1989, the Omnibus Budget Reconciliation Act (OBRA) created the Federally Qualified Health Center (FQHC) program to provide health care to underserved populations by permitting recovery of reasonable costs for care to Medicare and Medicaid patients (CMS, 2008b). FQHCs provide similar services as RHCs but also must include preventive primary services and can be located in nonrural areas such as public housing projects or homeless facilities.

During a period of numerous health care financing changes in the 1990s, many large hospital systems bought out small hospitals and private primary care practices. Unfortunately, as the large systems found that the small facilities were less profitable, many closed or cut back services, worsening the access problem in already underserved areas (CMS, 2008a; Holmes, Pink, & Slifkin, 2006). Financial changes have created other unintended consequences in care delivery. When states began using managed care programs for Medicaid, some public health departments dropped many of their well-child clinics and services.

These cutbacks adversely affected rural communities, where a shortage of health care professionals already existed (Ricketts, 2000).

For many years, Medicare payments to rural hospitals were significantly less than those to urban ones for equivalent services because it was thought the cost of hospital care should be less in rural areas. However, rural hospitals argued that their costs were high because they had to offer salaries competitive with urban hospitals for health care professionals, and their low volumes could not compensate for patients whose care exceeded the reimbursement from prospective payment systems. Approximately 470 rural hospitals closed in 25 years (NACRHHS, 2008; NRHA, 2008). The Balanced Budget Act of 1997 created the Medicare Rural Hospital Flexibility Program to permit designation of critical access hospitals (CAHs) to help ameliorate this problem (CMS, 2008a; Holmes et al., 2006). The CAHs had to meet strict guidelines of having no more than 15 beds, providing 24-hour emergency care, and being at least a 35-mile drive from other hospitals. If a facility was designated as a CAH, it could receive cost-based reimbursement. The Medicare Prescription Drug Act of 2003 expanded the CAH program to include hospitals with as many as 25 beds, began to reimburse them at 101% of their reasonable costs rather than through a prospective payment system, and allowed them to operate psychiatric units and rehabilitation units (Center for Medicare & Medicaid Services, 2008a). As a result, in 2005 the IOM reported a "renaissance in rural health care" (p. 21) in some communities due to the cost-based care and the creation of new services, facilities, and networks. Although inpatient services have stabilized, quick access to emergency medical services remains a need in rural communities and has not appreciably improved in the last 20 years (NACRHHS, 2008).

See Box 17-1 for a listing of rural health resources.

Implications for Rural Nursing Practice

Nurses who want to prepare for rural nursing practice should get as broad a nursing education as possible. Both in community and hospital settings, rural nurses

BOX 17-1	Rural Health Resources

American Psychological Association Resource Center for Rural Behavioral Health: www.apa.org/rural

Center for International Rural and Environmental Health: www.public-health.uiowa.edu/Cireh

Indian Health Service (Department of Health and Human Services): www.ihs.gov

National Association of Rural Health Clinics: www.narhc.org

National Association for Rural Mental Health: www.narmh.org

National Center for Farmworker Health, Inc.: www.ncfh.org

National Resource Center on Native American Aging: http://ruralhealth.und.edu/projects/nrcnaa

National Rural Health Association: www.ruralhealthweb.org

Office of Rural Health Policy (Department of Health and Human Services): www.ruralhealth.hrsa.gov

Office of Rural Mental Health Research: www.nimh.nih.gov/about/organization/od/office-of-rural-mental-health-research-ormhr.shtml

Online Journal of Rural Nursing and Health Care: www.rno.org/journal/index.php/online-journal

Rural Assistance Center: www.raconline.org

Rural Health Research: www.ruralhealthresearch.org

Rural Health Research Centers: www.ruralhealthresearch.org/centers.php

Rural Healthy People 2010: www.srph.tamhsc.edu/centers/rhp2010/default.htm

Rural Information Center (Department of Agriculture): www.nal.usda.gov/ric

Rural Nurse Organization: www.rno.org

Rural Policy Research Institute: www.rupri.org

U.S. Department of Agriculture, Economic Research Service (Department of Agriculture): www.ers.usda.gov

assume many varied roles and care for all ages and types of patients. Nursing staff may have to perform ancillary skills that social workers, respiratory therapists, IV teams, laboratory technicians, and nutritionists might be responsible for in larger hospitals. At times, nurses function without a physician in the hospital (Rosenthal, 2006; Scharff 2006). When beginning practice, nurses should check their state's nurse practice act to determine exactly what actions are within the scope of practice. If they plan to practice in an area where a large number of citizens are employed in farming, mining, or forestry, nurses should become familiar with the health conditions unique to those occupations. Long and Weinert (1989) recommend that nurses also receive a strong base in change theory and leadership techniques because rural nurses are essential in developing local health policies.

Professional isolation and lack of health information resources, such as libraries and other health professionals, have been cited as challenges for rural nurses. The development of Internet-based information resources has helped ameliorate these problems. Online RN refresher courses, RN-BSN and BSN-MSN programs, rural nursing associations, professional meetings, interactive video conferencing, audio

conferencing, and telehealth networks are available to many rural nurses (Hendrickx, 2006; Shreffler-Grant & Reimer, 2006).

Because of rural residents' preference for "insiders," nurses new to a rural area need to allow time for acceptance. Involvement in community activities sponsored by civic, church-affiliated, or recreational groups may help the nurse become known and accepted. Health professionals have also found it helpful to identify key people who function as informal health informants or providers within rural communities. Developing positive relationships with community leaders can increase acceptance and effectiveness (Findholt, 2006; Long & Weinert, 1989; Rosenthal, 2005; Scharff, 2006).

Many rural communities do not have as many health care providers as they need. Some areas have increased access to care by opening rural health clinics staffed primarily by nurses and advanced practice nurses (Hanrahan & Hartley, 2008; O'Malley, Forrest, Politzer, Wulu, & Shi, 2005). However, the nursing shortage is often even greater in rural areas. Most health care professionals are educated in urban settings and have little exposure to rural culture, which can result in misunderstandings and mistrust by rural clients (Bushy, 2009; Conger & Plager, 2008; NRHA, 2005). A number of studies have shown that health care providers are more likely to choose to practice in a rural setting if they have grown up there or lived there previously (Bushy & Leipert, 2005; IOM, 2005; Lindsay, 2009; Manahan & Lavoie, 2008; Quinney, 2006). The IOM therefore recommends increased recruitment of health professional students from rural areas and greater use of rural areas as training and preceptor sites. The state of West Virginia mandates that all its health professional students in public institutions spend a minimum of 3 months doing clinical rotations in rural communities (Reynolds, 2009).

To plan health care that will be more accepted in rural areas, nurses can take advantage of the fact that residents tend to define their health care in terms of their ability to work or be productive (Bales, Winters, & Lee, 2006; Long & Weinert, 1989). In rural agricultural areas, health programs and clinics can be scheduled to avoid conflict with rural economic cycles such as planting or harvesting. Health promotion strategies can be developed to emphasize how they will prevent long-term disability and enhance the ability to remain productive. For example, diabetic education can emphasize how improved glucose control may decrease the risk for future vision problems or limb amputation.

Nurses can use the self-reliant nature of rural people to develop more effective health care approaches (Bales et al., 2006; Bushy, 2009; Lee & McDonagh, 2006a; Shreffler-Grant & Reimer, 2006). By anticipating which services people might need, nurses can teach them when and how to access those services. In teaching self-care, particular emphasis can be placed on signs and symptoms that require professional care and those that can be managed at home. Because of the distances that may be involved in traveling to medical specialists, local health care professionals can collaborate with distant specialists to provide follow-up care. Additionally, nurses can help identify the common informal health support systems found in rural communities (e.g., family, extended family, supportive neighbors, friends, volunteers) and encourage their involvement. Arrangements can be made for specialized services such as mammography and bone density testing to be brought directly to rural communities by a van or mobile clinic. To increase access, these services can be scheduled in conjunction with popular local events such as county fairs. New technologies in telehealth can bring the expertise of health care specialists to the rural setting. Rural hospitals may use high-speed Internet to have patient scans read by radiologists in urban medical centers (Quinney, 2006). Winters and Sullivan (2006) found that creation of an online support group for isolated rural women was beneficial in helping them cope with chronic illnesses.

Schools are often primary recreational and social centers in rural communities and can be good sites for health education and care programs (Bushy, 2009; Glover, 2006). Rural school nurses have the potential to play major roles in health education and services for youth. Because rural populations tend to report greater church attendance and involvement with religion, churches may also be successful sites for health teaching and care, as well as parish nursing. In addition, faith communities can be used to coordinate transportation for appointments distant from the community or to bridge gaps in home health between nurse visits, allowing residents to remain in their homes.

Recognition of confidentiality issues in rural populations can result in more effective health care planning and provision of service. Nurses may need to schedule services such as mental health or family planning clinics at particular times or plan them in conjunction with other clinics. In small towns, individuals are often recognized by their motor vehicles. Thus, for instance, the risk for being seen parked at a facility during an established sexually transmitted disease clinic time may hinder the seeking of treatment (Bushy, 2009).

Noting that rural areas have "a strong sense of community responsibility and propensity toward collaboration," the IOM (2005, p. 20) concluded that rural residents are skilled at formulating "unique and creative ways" to develop social systems and physical resources to meet their needs. Nurses can use these attributes to design programs that will improve rural health. However, they must first actively involve the community in designing the programs: "Don't go into a community to fix something unless you've asked them what they need. You can't fix people—you have to work with people" (AHRQ, 2003, p. 2).

Community members are more likely to support services that they participate in developing. Nurses can foster these partnerships by following the steps that Bushy (2009, p. 825) describes in a community decision-making model: (1) identify the problem area; (2) assess the community's perspective by determining the degree of public awareness and support of the problem, special interest groups, existing services, and potential barriers and resources; (3) analyze the data and determine local priorities; (4) develop a long-range plan with lists of potential target groups, resources, materials needed, and possible funding sources while creating awareness of the program; (5) take action after getting consensus; and (6) evaluate both short- and long-term outcomes.

SUMMARY

Rural communities possess many strengths as well as significant challenges in securing health care for their citizens. Building on community strengths produces much more success than focusing on drawbacks such as decreased transportation and shortage of resources. Nurses have a tremendous opportunity to improve the health of rural communities. Because of their respected status and multiple interactions, nurses working in rural settings can develop accepted health promotion and health care delivery programs that are accessible, affordable, and appropriate.

KEY POINTS

- Americans hold positive views of rural life, associating it with a strong sense of family, self-reliance, individualism, hard work, religious conviction, and commitment to community. Misperceptions that most of rural America is farm-oriented can hinder rural health policy.
- Several classification systems exist for defining *rural*; approximately one fifth of the country's population live in rural areas. Having fewer people in geographically extended areas affects transportation and interaction with other people; this, in turn, affects the availability and accessibility of health care services.
- Rural communities vary widely but generally have a greater percentage of elderly and children, fewer minorities, less educational achievement, more poverty, and higher rates of unemployment. Racial diversity is increasing, and rural areas with high percentages of minority populations experience much greater poverty.

- Access to health care and lack of insurance are identified as the most important issues in rural health, followed by cardiovascular disease, diabetes, mental health, dental health, substance abuse, and accidental injury. Obesity is described as the newest epidemic across the country, but this is particularly true in rural communities.
- Nurses working in rural communities need to have general knowledge of a wide variety of nursing specialties, be able to handle crisis situations until other members of the health care team arrive, and be prepared to assume leadership roles in determining local policy and planning health services.
- Autonomy, continuity of care, close community ties, high public esteem and respect, and holistic nursing characterize rural nursing practice; professional isolation, lack of anonymity, and issues of confidentiality are challenges related to rural nursing practice.
- Rural residents are self-reliant and tend to view health as the ability to work or be productive. These health perceptions and beliefs strongly influence the success of nursing interventions.
- Federal programs such as the IHS, MHCs, NHSC, RHCs, FQHCs, and CAHs have been developed to enhance rural health.
- Nurses preparing to practice in rural areas should have a broad educational background, gain an understanding of their community's strengths and limitations, and develop community partnerships and creative collaborations in planning effective health policy and services.

CRITICAL THINKING EXERCISES

1. The challenges of rural isolation, distance, and access to health care have a significant impact on maternal/child health care and prevention of disease. What creative strategies are available for a nurse in rural practice to bring about change and improve outcomes? What alternative sites or models of delivery might be successful?
2. Developing close relationships with patients, families, and groups is a positive aspect of rural nursing practice, but perceived confidentiality issues can be a challenge, especially in smaller communities. How should the nurse in rural practice manage perceptions of confidentiality? What interventions can the nurse use to educate clients and families about privacy issues?
3. Aging populations in rural areas often suffer from social isolation and lack of physical activity and mental stimulation. What nursing interventions would be effective in assisting this vulnerable group? Where could these services be provided?

4. In many rural communities the Hispanic population has increased greatly. What unique challenges and opportunities does this present for rural health departments staffed by health care professionals who do not speak Spanish and are unfamiliar with Hispanic culture?

5. Describe how schools of nursing might be able to increase the number and improve the preparations of rural nurses.

6. A rural public health nurse has discovered an extremely high rate of obesity and overweight among all age groups in a community. What strategies could be used to approach this problem? What creative community partnerships or collaborations could be developed?

REFERENCES

Agency for Healthcare Research and Quality. (2003). Creating partnerships, improving health: The role of community based participatory research. AHRQ Publication No. 03-0037. Washington, DC: U.S. Department of Health and Human Services.

Agency for Healthcare Research and Quality. (2007). Americans in poor communities are 80 percent more likely to be hospitalized for diabetes. AHRQ News and Numbers. Rockville, MD: Author. [Online]. Retrieved from http://www.ahrq.gov/news/nn/nn090507.htm

Alexander, J., & Castillo, G. (2004). Injury and violence prevention in rural areas: A literature review. In L. D. Gamm, L. L. Hutchison, B. J. Dabney, & A. M. Dorsey (Eds.). Rural Healthy People 2010: A companion document to Healthy People 2010, vol. 2 (pp. 89-106). College Station, TX: Texas A&M University.

Annie, E. (2004). Casey Foundation. City and rural kids count data book: Measures of child well-being in the nation's rural areas. Baltimore: Author.

Bales, R. L., Winters, C. A., & Lee, H. J. (2006). Health needs and perceptions of rural person. In H. J. Lee, & C. A. Winters (Eds.). Rural nursing: Concepts, theory, and practice (2nd ed., pp. 53-65). New York: Springer.

Ballance, D., Kornegay, D., & Evans, P. (2009). Factors that influence physicians to practice in rural locations: A review and commentary. The Journal of Rural Health, 25(3), 276-281.

Bolin, J., & Gamm, L. (2003). Access to quality health services in rural areas-insurance: A literature review. In L. Gamm (Ed.). Rural Healthy People 2010: A companion document to Healthy People 2010, vol. 2 (pp. 5-16). College Station, TX: Texas A&M University System Health Science Center, Southwest Rural Health Research Center.

Breiding, M. J., Ziembroski, J. S., & Black, M. C. (2009). Prevalence of rural intimate partner violence in 16 US states, 2005. The Journal of Rural Health, 25(3), 240-245.

Buczko, W. (2001). Rural Medicare beneficiaries' use of rural and urban hospitals. The Journal of Rural Health, 17(1), 53-58.

Bushy, A. (2009). Rural health. In F. A. Maurer, C. M. Smith, & 4th ed. (Eds.). Public health nursing practice: Health for families and populations (pp. 809-830). St. Louis: Saunders.

Bushy, A., & Leipert, B. (2005). Factors that influence students in choosing rural nursing practice: a pilot study. Rural and Remote Health 5, 387, [Online]. Retrieved from http://www.rrh.org.au/publishedarticles/article_print_387.pdf

Butler, C., Kim-Godwin, Y., & Fox, J. A. (2008). Exploration of health care concerns of Hispanic women in a rural southeastern North Carolina community. Online Journal of Rural Nursing & Health Care, 8(2), 22-32. [Online]. Retrieved from http://www.rno.org/journal/index.php/online-journal/article/viewFile/165/207

Casey, M. M., Call, K. T., & Klinger, J. M. (2001). Are rural residents less likely to obtain recommended preventive healthcare services? American Journal of Preventive Medicine, 21(3), 182-188.

Centers for Medicare and Medicaid Services. (2008a). Critical access hospital [Online]. Retrieved from http://www.cms.hhs.gov/MLNProducts/downloads/CritAccessHospfctsht.pdf

Centers for Medicare and Medicaid Services. (2008b). Federally qualified health centers [Online]. Retrieved from http://www.cms.hhs.gov/MLNProducts/downloads/fqhcfactsheet.pdf

Centers for Medicare and Medicaid Services. (2008c). Rural health clinic [Online]. Retrieved from http://www.cms.hhs.gov/MLNProducts/downloads/RuralHlthClinfctsht08.pdf

Conger, M. M., & Plager, K. A. (2008). Advanced nursing practice in rural areas: Connectedness versus disconnectedness. Online Journal of Rural Nursing and Health Care, 8(1) 24-38. [Online]. Retrieved from http://www.rno.org/journal/index.php/online-journal/article/viewFile/156/194.

Cromartie, J. & Bucholtz, S. (2008). Defining the "rural" in rural America. Amber Waves 6(3): 28-34. [Online]. Retrieved from http://www.ers.usda.gov/AmberWaves/June08/PDF/AW_June08.pdf

Dabney, B., & Gosschalk, A. (2003). Diabetes in rural America. In L. D. Gamm, L. L. Hutchison, B. J. Dabney, & A. M. Dorsey (Eds.). Rural Healthy People 2010: A companion document to Healthy People 2010, vol. 1 (pp. 109-116). College Station, TX: Texas A&M University.

Duncan, C. M., Salant, P., & Colocousis, C. (2006). Challenges and opportunities in rural America: looking at the data and listening to practitioners. Durham, NH: Carsey Institute. [Online]. Retrieved from http://www.carseyinstitute.unh.edu/documents/Ford_Report_2006.pdf

Edwards, J. B., & Tudiver, F. (2008). Women's preventive screening in rural health clinics. *Women's Health Issues*, *18*(2008), 155–166.

Findholt, N. (2006). The culture of rural communities: An examination of rural nursing concepts at the community level. In H. J. Lee, & C. A. Winters (Eds.). *Rural nursing: Concepts, theory, and practice* (2nd ed., pp. 301–310). New York: Springer.

Fordyce, M. A., Chen, F. M., Doescher, M. P., & Hart, L. G. (2007). 2005 Physician supply and distribution in rural areas of the United States. Seattle: Washington Rural Health Research Center. [Online]. Retrieved from http://depts.washington.edu/uwrhrc/uploads/RHRC%20FR116%20PB%20040908.pdf

Frontier Education Center. (2004). Addressing the nursing shortage: Impacts and innovations in frontier America. Retrieved from http://www.frontierus.org/documents/FINALNursing_shnal_rev.pdf

Gale, J. A., & Lambert, D. (2006). Mental health care in rural communities: The once and future role of primary care. *North Carolina Medical Journal*, *67*(1), 66–69.

Gamm, L. (2007). Rural Healthy People 2010 and sustaining rural populations. In L. L. Morgan, & P. S. Fahs (Eds.). *Conversations in the disciplines: Sustaining rural populations* (pp. 1–11). Binghamton, NY: Global Academic Publishing.

Gfroerer, B. A., Larson, S. L., & Colliver, J. D. (2007). Drug use patterns and trends in rural communities. *The Journal of Rural Health*, *23*(s1), 10–15.

Glover, L. B. (2006). Rural school health: Who covers for the rural school nurse when there is none? In H. J. Lee, & C. A. Winters (Eds.). *Rural nursing: Concepts, theory, and practice* (2nd ed., pp. 282–290). New York: Springer.

Gonzalez, R. P., Cummings, G., Mulekar, M., & Rodning, C. B. (2006). Increased mortality in rural vehicular trauma: Identifying contributing factors through data linkage. *Journal of Trauma*, *61*(2), 404–409.

Hanrahan, N. P., & Hartley, D. (2008). Employment of advanced-practice psychiatric nurses to stem rural mental health workforce shortages. *Psychiatric Services*, *59*(1), 109–111.

Health Resources and Services Administration. (2005). The health and well-being of children in rural areas: A portrait of the nation 2005. Rockville, MD: Author. [Online]. Retrieved from http://www.mchb.hrsa.gov/ruralhealth

Health Resources and Services Administration. (n.d.). The health center program: Special populations. Retrieved from http://bphc.hrsa.gov/about/specialpopulations.htm

Hendrickx, L. (2006). Continuing education and rural nurses. In H. J. Lee, & C. A. Winters (Eds.). *Rural nursing: Concepts, theory, and practice* (2nd ed., pp. 248–256). New York: Springer.

Hill, W. B., & Butterfield, P. (2006). Environmental risk reduction for rural children. In H. J. Lee, & C. A. Winters (Eds.). *Rural nursing: Concepts, theory, and practice* (2nd ed., pp. 270–281). New York: Springer.

Holmes, M., Pink, G. H., & Slifkin, R. T. (2006). Impact of conversion to critical access hospital status on hospital financial performance and condition. [Online]. Retrieved from http://www.flexmonitoring.org/documents/CAHFindingsBrief1.pdf

Indian Health Service. (2008). Federal basis for health services. [Online]. Retrieved from http://info.ihs.gov/BasisHlthSvcs.asp

Institute of Medicine. (2005). *Quality through collaboration: The future of rural health care.* Washington, DC: The National Academies Press.

Jones, C. A., Kandel, K., & Parker, T. (2007). Population dynamics are changing the profile of rural areas. *Amber Waves 5*(2), 30–35. [Online]. Retrieved from http://www.ers.usda.gov/AmberWaves/April07/PDF/Population.pdf

Lee, H. J., & McDonagh, M. K. (2006a). Examining the rural nursing theory base. In H. J. Lee, & C. A. Winters (Eds.). *Rural nursing: Concepts, theory, and practice* (2nd ed., pp. 17–26). New York: Springer.

Lee, H. J., & McDonagh, M. K. (2006b). Further development of the rural nursing theory base. In H. J. Lee, & C. A. Winters (Eds.). *Rural nursing: Concepts, theory, and practice* (2nd ed., pp. 313–321). New York: Springer.

Lee, H. J., & Winters, C. A. (2004). Testing rural nursing theory: Perceptions and needs of service providers. *Online Journal of Rural Nursing and Health Care, 4*(1). Retrieved from http://www.rno.org/journal/index.php/online-journal/article/viewFile/128/126

Lindsay, S. (2007). Gender differences in rural and urban practice location among mid-level health care providers. *The Journal of Rural Health*, *23*(1), 72–76.

Liu, J., Bennett, K. J., Harun, N., Zheng, X., Probst, J. C., & Pate, R. R. (2007). *Overweight and physical inactivity among rural children aged 10-17: A national and state portrait.* Columbia, SC: South Carolina Rural Health Research Center.

Long, K., & Weinert, C. (1989). Rural nursing: Developing the theory base. *Scholarly Inquiry for Nursing Practice*, *3*(2), 113–120.

Manahan, C., & Lavoie, J. (2008). Who stays in rural practice: An international review of the literature on factors influencing rural nurse retention. *Online Journal of Rural Nursing and Health Care*, *8*(2), 42–52.

Martin, A., Probst, J. C., Moore, C. G., Patterson, D., & Elder, K. (2005). *Trends in uninsurance among rural minority children*. Columbia, SC: South Carolina Rural Health Research Center.

Martin, A. B., Wang, E., Probst, J. C., Hale, N., & Johnson, A. O. (2008). *Dental health and access to care among rural children: A national and state portrait*. Columbia, SC: South Carolina Rural Health Research Center.

Miller, K. (2009). Demographic and economic profile: Nonmetropolitan America. Retried from http://www.rupri.org/Forms/Nonmetro2.pdf.

National Advisory Committee on Rural Health and Human Services. (2007). *The 2007 report to the Secretary: Rural health and human service issues*. Washington, DC: Department of Health and Human Services.

National Advisory Committee on Rural Health and Human Services. (2008). *The 2008 report to the Secretary: Rural health and human service issues*. Washington, DC: Department of Health and Human Services.

National Center for Frontier Communities. (2007). Developing the consensus definitions. [Online]. Retrieved from http://www.frontierus.org/defining.htm

National Center for Health Statistics. (2001). *Health, United States, 2001, with urban and rural health chartbook*. Hyattsville, MD: Author.

National Center for Health Statistics. (2007). *Health, United States, 2007, with chartbook on trends in the health of Americans*. Hyattsville, MD: Author.

National Coalition on Health Care. (2009). Health insurance coverage. [Online]. Retrieved from http://www.nchc.org/facts/coverage.shtml

National Rural Health Association. (2005). Recruitment and retention of a quality health workforce in rural areas: nursing. [Online]. Retrieved from http://www.ruralhealthweb.org/go/left/policy-and-advocacy/policy-documents-and-statements/official-policy-positions/official-policy-positions

National Rural Health Association. (2008). What's different about rural health care? [Online]. Retrieved from http://www.ruralhealthweb.org/go/left/about-rural-health/what-s-different-about-rural-health-care/what-s-different-about-rural-health-care

Newland, J. A. (2006). 2006 Nurse practitioner salary & survey. *The Nurse Practitioner: The American Journal of Primary Health Care*, *31*(5), 39–43.

Office of Management and Budget. (2004). Update of statistical area definitions and additional guidance on their uses. OMB Bulletin No. 04-03 [Online]. Retrieved from http://www.whitehouse.gov/omb/bulletins_fy04_b04-03/

Ogden, C. L., Carroll, M. D., Curtin, L. R., McDowell, M. A., Tabak, C. J., & Flegal, K. M. (2006). Prevalence of overweight and obesity in the United States, 1999-2004. *Journal of the American Medical Association*, *295*(13), 1549–1555.

O'Malley, A. S., Forrest, C. B., Politzer, R. M., Wulu, J. T., & Shi, L. (2005). Health center trends, 1994-2001: What do they portend for the federal growth initiative? *Health Affairs*, *24*(2), 465–472.

Pol, L. G., Rouse, J., Zyzanski, S., Rasmussen, D., & Crabtree, B. (2001). Rural, urban, and suburban comparisons of preventive services in family practice clinics. *The Journal of Rural Health*, *17*(2), 114–121.

Probst, J. C., Samuels, M. E., Jespersen, K. P., Wilbert, K., Swann, R. S., & McDuffie, J. A. (2002). *Minorities in rural America: An overview of population characteristics*. Columbia, SC: University of South Carolina Rural Research Center.

Quinney, D. (2006). Quality rural health care: The future is today. *Online Journal of Rural Nursing and Health Care*, *6*(1). [Online]. Retrieved from http://www.rno.org/journal/index.php/online-journal/article/viewFile/27/156

Raph, S. J., & Buehler, J. A. (2006). Rural health professionals' perceptions of lack of anonymity. In H. J. Lee, & C. A. Winters (Eds.). *Rural nursing: Concepts, theory, and practice* (2nd ed., pp. 197–204). New York: Springer.

Reynolds, P. J. (2009). Connecting interprofessional education to the community through service learning and community-based research. In C. B. Royeen, G. M. Jenson, & R. A. Harvan (Eds.). *Leadership in interprofessional health education and practice* (pp. 167–188). Sudbury, MA: Jones & Bartlett.

Ricketts, T. C. (2000). The changing nature of rural health care. *Annual Review of Public Health*, *21*, 639–657.

Ricketts, T. C. (2005). Workforce issues in rural areas: A focus on policy equity. *American Journal of Public Health*, *95*(1), 42–28.

Rogers, C. C. (2005). Rural children at a glance. U.S. Department of Agriculture, Economic Research Service, Economic Information Bulletin, Number 1.

Rosenthal, K. (2005). What rural nursing stories are you living? *Online Journal of Rural Nursing and Health Care, 5*(1). Retrieved from http://www.rno.org/journal/index.php/online-journal/article/viewFile/55/147

Rosenthal, K. A. (2006). The rural nursing generalist in the acute care setting: Flowing like a river. In H. J. Lee, & C. A. Winters (Eds.). *Rural nursing: Concepts, theory, and practice* (2nd ed., pp. 218–231). New York: Springer.

Sawyer, D., Gale, J., & Lambert, D. (2006). Rural and frontier mental and behavioral health care: barriers, effective policy strategies, best practices. National Association for Rural Mental Health. [Online]. Retrieved from http://www.narmh.org/pages/Rural%20and%20Frontier.pdf

Scharff, J. E. (2006). The distinctive nature and scope of rural nursing practice: Philosophical bases. In H. J. Lee, & C. A. Winters (Eds.). *Rural nursing: Concepts, theory, and practice* (2nd ed., pp. 179–196). New York: Springer.

Shreffler-Grant, J., & Reimer, M. A. (2006). Implications for education, practice, and policy. In H. J. Lee, & C. A. Winters (Eds.). *Rural nursing: Concepts, theory, and practice* (2nd ed., pp. 322–330). New York: Springer.

Strong, D. A., Del Grosso, P., Burwick, A., Jethwani, V., & Ponza, M. (2005). *Rural research needs and data sources for selected human services topics*. Washington, DC: Department of Health and Human Services.

Troyer, L. E., & Lee, H. J. (2006). The rural nursing generalist in community health. In H. J. Lee, & C. A. Winters (Eds.). *Rural nursing: Concepts, theory, and practice* (2nd ed., pp. 205–217). New York: Springer.

Trust for America's Health. (2008). F as in fat: how obesity policies are failing in America, 2008. Robert Wood Johnson Foundation. [Online]. Retrieved from http://healthyamericans.org/reports/obesity2008/Obesity2008Report.pdf

U.S. Census Bureau. (2008). The urban and rural classifications. [Online]. Retrieved from http://www.census.gov/geo/www/GARM/Ch12GARM.pdf

U.S. Department of Agriculture. (2005). Rural Hispanics at a glance. [Online]. Retrieved from http:\\www.ers.usda.gov/Publications/EIB8

U.S. Department of Agriculture. (2007). Nonmetro America faces challenges from an aging population. [Online]. Retrieved from http://www.ers.usda.gov/Briefing/Population/Challenges.htm

U.S. Department of Agriculture. (2008). Rural America at a glance: 2008 edition. [Online]. Retrieved from http://www.ers.usda.gov/Publications/EIB40

W.K. Kellogg Foundation. (2001). Perceptions of rural America. [Online]. Retrieved from http://www.wkkf.org/pubs/FoodRur/pub2973.pdf

Winters, C., & Sullivan, T. (2006). The chronic illness experience of isolated rural women: Use of an online support group intervention. In H. J. Lee, & C. A. Winters (Eds.). *Rural nursing: Concepts, theory, and practice* (2nd ed., pp. 153–165). New York: Springer.

Zhang, P., Tao, G., & Irwin, K. L. (2000). Utilization of preventive medical services in the United States: A comparison between rural and urban populations. *The Journal of Rural Health, 16*(4), 349–355.

Zuniga, M., Anderson, D., & Alexander, K. (2003). Health disease and stroke in rural America. In L. D. Gamm, L. L. Hutchison, B. J. Dabney, & A. M. Dorsey (Eds.). *Rural Healthy People 2010: A companion document to Healthy People 2010* (vol. 1, pp. 133–136). College Station, TX: Texas A&M University.

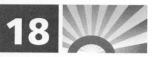

18

Intimate Partner Violence as a Health Care Problem

KATHRYN LAUGHON, PhD, RN

OBJECTIVES

At the completion of this chapter, the reader will be able to:

- Describe the role of the sexual assault nurse examiner.
- Describe intimate partner violence and intimate partners.
- Discuss the health consequences of intimate partner violence.
- Discuss the mental health consequences of intimate partner violence.
- Identify opportunities to assess intimate partner violence in health care settings.
- Describe assessment tools and techniques to screen patients for intimate partner violence.
- Describe the steps to take after a positive screen for intimate partner violence.

PROFILE IN PRACTICE

Natalie McClain, RN, PhD, CPNP
Northeastern University School of Nursing, Boston, Massachusetts

Various forms of violence, including intimate partner and sexual violence, are experienced by men, women, and children around the world each day. After experiencing sexual violence or intimate partner violence, survivors may seek medical care either for documentation of the assault or for treatment of injuries. Sexual assault nurse examiners (SANEs) are specially trained forensic nurses that provide health evaluations, treatment, and evidence collection to victims of sexual and intimate partner violence.

My first experience working as a SANE was in a clinic where children, adolescents, and young adults who were victims of sexual abuse were referred for forensic services, including medical examinations, treatment, and evidence collection. My role at the clinic included conducting examinations to document any injuries, treating health needs, collecting evidence, and providing expert testimony in both civil and criminal cases. Later, I worked as a SANE in an emergency department in a university teaching hospital, providing forensic services for adults and children who had experienced either sexual violence or intimate partner violence. In both of these settings I found that combining concepts essential to nursing—compassion and caring—with the need for detailed evidence collection and forensic documentation resulted in a more positive experience for survivors.

I find working with survivors of violence in their hour of need to be personally rewarding. Looking into the eyes of rape survivors, holding their hands, letting them know they are in a safe place, and listening to their words are the reasons I became a nurse. I wanted to care for others when they needed help. SANEs help make an uncomfortable and often embarrassing examination more kind and humane while obtaining evidence that is crucial to prosecuting the crime. Perhaps there is no other time in a person's life when he or she needs another person more than after surviving a violent attack.

In addition to the professional responsibilities of caring for survivors of sexual and physical violence, SANEs are also active in shaping the evolving practice. Much is still unknown about the best practices for evidence collection and physical injuries after sexual and physical assault. As a member of a SANE team and a nurse researcher, I have had opportunities to be active in research that will affect future practice and public policy for survivors of violence. As experts in the field, SANEs are essential to the growing science and debate over public policy that affects survivors of trauma.

The number of forensic nurses specializing in sexual and physical violence continues to grow. Nurses have successfully identified a wonderful way of using the nursing role to provide highly skilled and compassionate forensic care to survivors of trauma. As the specialty continues to grow, nurses may find themselves presented with an opportunity to work in forensic nursing. I encourage nurses to pursue interests working with survivors of violence. Although I found working with victims and survivors of sexual assault to be emotionally challenging, I believe working as a SANE allowed me to provide forensic service with the compassionate care that is at the heart of nursing.

Introduction

Intimate partner violence (IPV) happens to approximately one fourth of women in their lifetimes (Tjaden & Thoennes, 2000). IPV is defined by the Centers for Disease Control (CDC) as "either physical or sexual violence, both physical and sexual violence, or threats of either. Psychological and emotional abuse is also counted when there have been prior violence or a threat of violence. Intimate partners are current and former husbands and wives, same-sex partners, boyfriends, and girlfriends" (Saltzman, Fanslow, McMahon, & Shelley, 1999, p. 12).

In a given year, approximately 1.5 million women—approximately 2% of the population—are physically or sexually assaulted by an intimate partner. The health consequences of IPV include a wide range of poor health outcomes beyond the obvious dangers of injuries and death related to the assault. This chapter describes the epidemiology of IPV and its health consequences, the nurse's role in assessing for IPV, and guidelines for brief and more complete interventions. Also provided is a brief overview of the role of sexual assault nurse examiners (SANE) in addressing sexual assault and rape by intimate and nonintimate partners.

Background

Rates of physical abuse of women by intimate partners during their lifetimes ranges from 25% to 33%, according to two large nationally representative studies (Plichta, 1997; Tjaden & Thoennes, 2000). Between 3% and 12% of women have been physically assaulted in the past year. More than 7% of women have been sexually assaulted by an intimate partner in their lifetimes (Tjaden & Thoennes, 2000). Most IPV is perpetrated by men against women; approximately 85% of the victims of serious IPV are women (Rennison & Welchens, 2000). Although women can abuse men, the pattern of repeated violence in a context of coercive, controlling behaviors is most commonly directed against women. Abuse can also occur within same-sex couples, although little research has specifically focused on violence in same-sex couples (Renzetti, 1998). One of the few population-based studies of IPV that included same-sex couples suggests that the prevalence of IPV in male homosexual couples was similar to that of heterosexual couples and was slightly lower for female homosexual couples (Tjaden & Thoennes, 2000).

Consequences of Intimate Partner Violence

PHYSICAL HEALTH CONSEQUENCES

IPV has serious health consequences. The most obvious physical consequence is injury. Approximately 40% of assaults result in injury, and roughly 20% of women seek health care services related to the assault. The most severe outcome, death, is addressed in detail below. Other physical health problems include headaches, fainting, chronic pain syndromes, increased rates of upper respiratory problems, urinary tract infections, pelvic pain, painful intercourse, increased rates of sexually transmitted infections, and irritable bowel syndrome.

The cause of these health problems is not fully understood. Some indications are that the chronic stress of living with IPV may adversely alter immune function (Woods, 2005). Forced sex may result in cervical and pelvic injuries that could partially explain chronic pelvic pain. Abusive partners may also refuse to use condoms or have multiple sexual partners, thus placing their female partners at greater risk for sexually transmitted infections (El-Bassel et al., 2001; Neighbors, O'Leary, & Labouvie, 1999; Wingood & DiClemente, 1997).

MENTAL HEALTH CONSEQUENCES

IPV has been consistently associated with depression and posttraumatic stress disorder (PTSD) in the literature. In one large population-based study, women experiencing abuse were three times more likely than nonabused women to have experienced depression in the prior month and more than twice as likely to have been anxious (Hathaway et al., 2000). Women who are depressed may be more likely to enter into and stay in abusive relationships, but there is evidence that in some cases the depression did not occur until after the abuse. A relationship between the severity of the abuse and the severity of the depression has also been shown (Campbell & Soeken, 1999; Silva, McFarlane, Soeken, Parker, & Reel, 1997).

PTSD and its related symptoms are also associated with experiencing IPV (Campbell, 2002). One study of inhabitants of a shelter for battered women found that increasing levels of dangerousness are associated with increased numbers of PTSD symptoms (Sato-DiLorenzo & Sharps, 2007). Symptoms of PTSD include reexperiencing the trauma through memories of the event that will not go away (intrusive thoughts) or recurring dreams; avoidance behaviors such as a general numbing of emotions or avoiding places, sights, smells, or sounds that might trigger memories of the event; increased arousal and difficulty falling asleep; exaggerated startle responses; and irritability and other persistent, unpleasant feelings. Formal diagnosis of PTSD requires exposure to a traumatic event that places a person in fear of bodily harm or death. Many battered women are exposed to psychological trauma that does not meet the requirements of the formal diagnosis, but studies show that these women have similar symptom profiles to women experiencing severe physical and sexual trauma (Kaysen, Resick, & Wise, 2003). Additionally, the diagnosis of PTSD requires that the clinician screen for exposure to a traumatic event.

FEMICIDE

Death is the most severe outcome of IPV. Femicide (or the homicide of a woman) is the seventh leading cause of premature death for women overall in the United States and the second leading cause of death among African American women ages 15 to 34 years (CDC, 2005). As many as half of murdered women are killed by a current or former intimate partner (Langford, Isaac, & Kabat, 1998). Although intimate partner homicides have declined since the 1970s, the decline has mostly occurred among male victims, with the rate holding nearly steady for women (Campbell, Glass, Sharps, Laughon, & Bloom, 2007). Among those women, as many as 70% of IPV murder victims were previously battered by their partner (Campbell et al., 2007). Nearly half of these murder victims used the health care system—and thus might have had access to help, had someone asked the women about violence—before their deaths (Sharps et al., 2001; Wadman & Muelleman, 1999).

An 11-city case-control study of risk factors for intimate partner femicide found that specific risk factors are associated with victims of completed and attempted femicide, as compared with women who had been abused by an intimate partner but had not experienced lethal or near-lethal violence (Campbell et al., 2003). Victims of femicide or attempted femicide were more likely to have a partner who was unemployed but not looking for work, have a partner who had access to a gun, have been threatened with a weapon, have a child who was not the biological child of the perpetrator in the home, and be estranged or separated from the perpetrator.

Pregnancy and IPV

IPV rates during pregnancy appear to be about the same as IPV rates among all women (Sharps, Laughon, & Giangrande, 2007). Pregnancy is an important period for violence screening and intervention, however, and merits special attention. Almost all women seek health care during their pregnancies; thus pregnancy offers a unique opportunity for IPV screening. Experiencing IPV during pregnancy is associated with a number of poor pregnancy outcomes, including lower-birth-weight babies, more preterm labor, increased rates of smoking, and fetal trauma (Campbell et al., 2003; Silverman, Decker, Reed, & Raj, 2006). Pregnant women appear to have two to three times the risk for femicide compared with nonpregnant women (Krulewitch, Pierre-Louis, de Leon-Gomez, Guy, & Green, 2001; Krulewitch, Roberts, & Thompson, 2003; McFarlane, Campbell, Sharps, & Watson, 2002). Pregnant adolescents experiencing IPV are especially vulnerable to all these poor outcomes (Sharps et al., 2007).

Children and IPV

IPV can obviously put children in direct harm. They can be inadvertently injured as bystanders and can place themselves in harm's way if they try to intervene. Additionally, perhaps as many as 2500 children each year experience the death of one parent by the other (Laughon, Steeves, Parker, Sawin, & Knopp, 2008). Although little research has examined the specific

effects of this event, the children generally lose both parents in one sudden event: one is dead and the other in prison for many years or also dead (in the case of murder-suicides).

Far more children are exposed to the indirect effects of violence perpetrated against their mothers. Low weight gain in infants born to mothers abused during pregnancy can persist. Babies born to mothers who experience IPV during pregnancy are more likely to have low birth weight than their peers whose mothers did not experience IPV (El-Kady, Gilbert, Xing, & Smith, 2005; Silverman et al., 2006; Yost, Bloom, McIntire, & Leveno, 2005). Older children exposed to IPV have more behavioral problems, more difficulty in school, more social problems, and poorer health than do children who are not exposed (Dube, Felitti, Dong, Giles, & Anda, 2003; Kernic et al., 2002; McFarlane, Groff, O'Brien, & Watson, 2003). IPV in the home is also associated with a significant increase in child abuse (Campbell & Lewandowski, 1997). At least one study has shown, however, that assessment and interventions for the mother dramatically improve outcomes for her children (McFarlane et al., 2003).

Missed Opportunities in the Health Care System

Few women report being assessed for IPV at their health care visits (Glass, Dearwater, & Campbell, 2001). More than 40% of women who were murdered by an intimate partner used the health care system for an injury or mental health issue in the year before their deaths (Sharps et al., 2001). Assessment does work; women who screen positive for IPV are nine times more likely to experience physical violence in the year before their deaths than women who do not have a positive screen (Koziol-McLain, Coates, & Lowenstein, 2001). Findings from both quasi-experimental and experimental studies have shown that a nurse-delivered intervention significantly increases women's safety-promoting behaviors and reduces the severity and frequency of IPV experienced by women (Parker, McFarlane, Silva, Soeken, & Reel, 1999; McFarlane et al., 2004).

Assessment for Intimate Partner Violence

Nurses and other health care professionals should assess all women, not just women with identifiable risk factors. The Family Violence Prevention Fund's consensus guidelines recommend that women be screened at the following times:

- Primary care: first visit for new chief complaint, new patient encounter, new intimate relationship, and periodic exams
- Emergency department and urgent care: all visits
- Obstetrician/gynecologist: each prenatal and postpartum visit; new intimate relationship; all gynecological, family planning, sexually transmitted disease clinic, and abortion clinic visits
- Mental health: every initial assessment, each new intimate relationship, and annually if ongoing or periodic treatment
- Inpatient: as part of admission and discharge

Several tools are available for screening patients. The Abuse Assessment Screen (AAS) has been used in a variety of clinical settings. It includes a question about abuse during pregnancy that can be omitted if the woman is not pregnant. It also includes a body map for documenting areas of injury, if any. It has been found to be reliable and valid with white, African American, and Hispanic women (Soeken, McFarlane, Parker, & Lominack, 1998). It was recently updated to include strangulation behaviors, so the newest version of the instrument should be used (Laughon, Renker, Glass, & Parker, 2008). The Woman's Experience with Battering (WEB) scale is a longer, 10-item instrument. It screens for coercive behavior and psychological abuse, as well as for physical and sexual abuse (Smith, Earp, & DeVellis, 1995).

All these instruments can be self-administered or read to patients. Some researchers have found that face-to-face screening increases disclosure. However, evidence also shows that this varies by ethnicity (Torres et al., 2000). Ideally, women would have the opportunity to complete both a written screening and a face-to-face screening by a health care provider. Regardless of how the screening is conducted, the client should be ensured privacy while answering the questions. No one should accompany the client when the questions are asked, including children older than 3 years. This is also an ideal time to ask questions about other sensitive topics such as history of pregnancies, abortions, and miscarriages; sexually transmitted infections; and mental health diagnoses and treatments.

Some women may not disclose abuse but nevertheless have signs that suggest it to the nurse. A client may present with injuries that are not consistent with the explanation of how they occurred. Multiple injuries in various stages of healing, especially when they appear on the head, trunk, or genitals, can also indicate abuse. In such cases, the nurse can gently confront the inconsistency, making statements such as, "In my experience, this kind of injury doesn't usually happen from what you've described."

Other clients present with less clear-cut sets of signs and symptoms. A pattern of somatic symptoms of unknown origin (e.g., chronic pelvic and other pain, neurological symptoms, gastrointestinal symptoms, frequent sexually transmitted diseases), a pattern of difficulty in keeping appointments, increased anxiety when the partner is present, or a partner's refusal to allow the client private time with the provider can all indicate IPV. A provider can always document that IPV was not disclosed, note "injuries consistent with abuse" or "IPV suspected," and provide the client with written information on abuse "to share with a friend." The nurse should inform the client that she is available if needed in the future. If possible, a follow-up visit should be scheduled.

Although providers are often concerned that women will be offended by routine IPV screening, research has shown that both abused and nonabused women support routine screening in health care settings (Glass et al., 2001; Renker & Tonkin, 2006). A variety of studies have found that abused women supported screening and believed that such screening would make obtaining help easier for women when needed (Gielen et al., 2000; Rodriguez, McLoughlin, Nah, & Campbell, 2001; Sachs, Koziol-McLain, Glass, Webster, & Campbell, 2002).

☀ After a Positive Screen

When clients disclose abuse, the nurse's first response should be to listen empathetically and nonjudgmentally. The woman may never have previously disclosed abuse or may not have been believed in the past. Statements such as "I believe you" and "The abuse is not your fault" are helpful and supportive. Women often believe that they have no choices or that their only choice is to leave the abuser. Women can contact the police and press charges, contact police and obtain a restraining order, engage in safety planning around staying or leaving at a future date, contact a shelter or a hotline, attend support groups related to domestic violence, try to get her partner into a program for abusers, or any combination of these activities. The woman should hear that she does have options and that people will help her. Findings should be documented; the records can be used in court for criminal and civil proceedings.

Assess the client's immediate safety by asking, "Are you safe to go home right now?" If the woman answers no, assist her in developing a plan. The plan should include how she will exit the office and building, who will assist her in leaving safely (e.g., security officers, police officers), and where she will go (e.g., to a friend's house, women's shelter). Available resources (e.g., police and security phone numbers, shelter hotline, social work, depending on the setting) should be identified by office staff before they are needed. The woman can be moved to another room within the setting and assisted with calling an abuse hotline while practitioners see other clients, if needed. Remember that having access to a phone where the abuser cannot hear her call or track the calls she makes and where she has some privacy can be enormously empowering for a woman in a battering relationship. Also note that although some areas do not have local hotlines, state hotline numbers are available in all areas. The national hotline, which will refer women to the appropriate local programs and provide direct assistance, is 800-799-SAFE (7233).

If the woman feels safe to leave at that time, she can be assisted in identifying her current level of safety and developing an appropriate safety plan. This can be done in several ways, depending on the setting. At a minimum, the nurse should let the client know that she has options to help her stay safer while in an abusive relationship, encourage her to think about her safety and that of her children, and provide her with the appropriate hotline numbers and other local resources so that she can discuss safety planning. The nurse should ask whether the client has a safe place from which to make the calls, and if not, provide her with a phone in the health care facility from which she can make private phone calls. If the nurse is in a setting where more elaborate safety planning can be done, information is provided below.

Finally, offer information on local resources. Know the local shelter hotline number and the state hotline number and provide these to the client. Most programs have informational cards small enough to be slipped into a shoe. If possible, offer the woman a phone from which to make the call.

Ideally, in addition to the minimum interventions discussed above, the nurse should obtain a thorough history of the abuse; perform a physical examination focusing on the injuries; document thoroughly; and make referrals to social service, criminal justice, mental health, and specialty medical services as needed. A critical pathway for IPV has been developed and can serve as a guide for assessment and interdisciplinary referrals (Dienemann, Campbell, Wiederhorn, Laughon, & Jordan, 2003). Consensus guidelines for assessing and intervening for IPV have been developed, including forms and assessment tools, and can be accessed online (http://endabuse.org/programs/healthcare).

SUMMARY

Violence against women is a serious health problem. Women who live with violence experience a range of poor physical and mental health problems and are at risk for femicide. Children living in the home are also at direct and indirect risk. Nurses have an essential role to play in assessing women for violence and providing competent, empathic, and thorough intervention. Nursing interventions, which have been shown to be effective, are an essential part of making the health care system an empowerment zone for "battered women and their children to find safety, to find respite, and affirmations for their strengths" (Campbell, Rose, Kub, & Nedd, 1998, p. 744).

KEY POINTS

- Sexual assault nurse examiners (SANEs) are specially trained forensic nurses who provide health evaluations, treatment, and evidence collection to victims of sexual and intimate partner violence.
- Intimate partners are current and former husbands and wives, same-sex partners, boyfriends, and girlfriends. IPV is either physical or sexual violence, both physical and sexual violence, or threats of either.
- A wide range of health consequences are associated with IPV, including injuries, death, headaches, fainting, chronic pain syndromes, upper respiratory problems, sexually transmitted infections, urinary tract infections, and pelvic pain.
- The prevalence of depression in abused women is two to four times higher than the rate of depression in the general population.
- PTSD is present in 64% of battered women. PTSD symptoms include intrusive thoughts, avoidance behaviors, exaggerated startle responses, and insomnia.
- Death from IPV is the seventh most common cause of premature death for women overall in the United States and the second leading cause of death in African American women aged 15 to 34 years.
- Women can successfully be screened for IPV by using tools such as the AAS. The AAS is reliable and valid in white, African American, and Hispanic women.
- Nurses can facilitate disclosure of abuse through therapeutic interactions with the client, provision of a safe environment, use of valid screening tools, and referral to available resources.
- In the event of a disclosure of IPV, the nurse should listen empathetically, offer options available to the client, document all findings, perform a safety assessment, and assist the client in developing a safety plan.

CRITICAL THINKING EXERCISES

1. Role-playing with a peer, practice therapeutic communication techniques that you would use during an assessment in which you suspect IPV.
2. Identify opportunities to screen for abuse in your clinical setting. Identify "safe" areas in your clinical setting for abuse assessment screening and resources (e.g., telephones, security) available in the event of disclosure of abuse.
3. Investigate local resources available in your community to assist victims of IPV.
4. Print the Abuse Assessment Screen brochure found at www.nnvawi.org. Become familiar with screening questions and interventions for IPV.
5. Formulate an intervention plan in the event of an abuse disclosure in your clinical setting.

REFERENCES

Campbell, J., & Lewendowski, L. (1997). Mental and physical health effects of intimate partner violence on women and children. *Psychiatric Clinics of North America, 20*, 353–374.

Campbell, J., Webster, D., Koziol-McLain, J., Block, C., Campbell, D., Curry., M. A., et al. (2003). Risk factors for femicide in abusive relationships: results from a multisite case control study. *American Journal of Public Health, 93*(7), 1089–1097.

Campbell, J. C. (2002). Violence against women and health consequences. *The Lancet, 359*, 1331–1336.

Campbell, J. C., Glass, N., Sharps, P. W., Laughon, K., & Bloom, T. (2007). Mortality related to intimate partner violence: A review of research and implications for the advocacy, criminal justice and health care systems. *Trauma, Violence, & Abuse, 8*(3), 246–269.

Campbell, J. C., Rose, L., Kub, J., & Nedd, D. (1998). Voices of strength and resistance: A contextual and longitudinal analysis of women's responses to battering. *Journal of Interpersonal Violence, 13*, 743–762.

Campbell, J. C., & Soeken, K. L. (1999). Women responses to battering over time: An analysis of change. *Journal of Interpersonal Violence, 14*, 21–40.

Centers for Disease Control and Prevention. (2005). Web-based injury statistics query and reporting system (WISQARS) [Online]. Retrieved from http://www.cdc.gov/ncipc/wisqars

Dienemann, J., Campbell, J., Wiederhorn, N., Laughon, K., & Jordan, E. (2003). A critical pathway for intimate partner violence across the continuum of care. *Journal of Obstetric, Gynecologic, and Neonatal Nursing, 32*, 594–603.

Dube, S. R., Felitti, V. J., Dong, M., Giles, W. H., & Anda, R. F. (2003). The impact of adverse childhood experiences on health problems: evidence from four birth cohorts dating back to 1900. *Preventive Medicine, 37*, 268–277.

El-Bassel, N., Fontdevila, J., Gilbert, L., Voisin, D., Richman, B. L., & Pitchell, P. (2001). HIV risks of men in methadone maintenance treatment programs who abuse their intimate partners: A forgotten issue. *Journal of Substance Abuse, 13*, 29–43.

El Kady, D., Gilbert, W. M., Xing, G., & Smith, L. H. (2005). Maternal and neonatal outcomes of assaults during pregnancy. *Obstetrics & Gynecology, 105*, 357–363.

Gielen, A. C., O'Campo, P. J., Campbell, J. C., Schollenberger, J., Woods, A. B., Jones, A. S., et al. (2000). Women's opinions about domestic violence screening and mandatory reporting. *American Journal of Preventative Medicine, 19*(4), 279–285.

Glass, N., Dearwater, S., & Campbell, J. (2001). Intimate partner violence screening and intervention: Data from eleven Pennsylvania and California community hospital emergency departments. *Journal of Emergency Nursing, 27*(2), 141–149.

Hathaway, J. E., Mucci, L., Silverman, J. G., Brooks, D. R., Mathews, R., & Pavlos, C. A. (2000). Health status and health care use of Massachusetts women reporting partner abuse. *American Journal of Preventive Medicine, 19*(4), 302–307.

Kaysen, D., Resick, P. A., & Wise, D. (2003). Living in danger: The impact of chronic traumatization and the traumatic context on posttraumatic stress disorder. *Trauma, Violence, & Abuse, 4*, 247–264.

Kernic, M. A., Holt, V. L., Wolf, M. E., McKnight, B., Huebner, C. E., & Rivara, F. P. (2002). Academic and school health issues among children exposed to maternal intimate partner abuse. *Archives of Pediatric and Adolescent Medicine, 156*, 549–555.

Koziol-McLain, J., Coates, C. J., & Lowenstein, S. R. (2001). Predictive validity of a screen for partner violence against women. *American Journal of Preventive Medicine, 21*, 93–100.

Krulewitch, C. J., Pierre-Louis, M. L., de Leon-Gomez, R., Guy, R., & Green, R. (2001). Hidden from view: Violent deaths among pregnant women in the District of Columbia, 1988-1996. *Journal of Midwifery and Women's Health, 46*, 4–10.

Krulewitch, C. J., Roberts, D. W., & Thompson, L. S. (2003). Adolescent pregnancy and homicide: Findings for the Maryland Office of the Chief Medical Examiner, 1994-1998. *Child Maltreatment, 8*, 122–128.

Langford, L., Isaac, N., & Kabat, S. (1998). Homicides related to intimate partner violence in Massachusetts: Examining case ascertainment and validity of the SHR. *Homicide Studies, 2*, 353–377.

Laughon, K., Renker, P., Glass, N., & Parker, B. (2008). Revision of the Abuse Assessment Screen to address non-lethal strangulation, *Journal of Obstetric Gynecologic, & Neonatal Nursing, 37*(4), 502–7.

Laughon, K., Steeves, R., Parker, B., Sawin, E., & Knopp, A. (2008). Forgiveness, and other themes, in women whose fathers killed their mothers. *Advances in Nursing Science*, PMID: 18497591.

McFarlane, J., Campbell, J. C., Sharps, P., & Watson, K. (2002). Abuse during pregnancy and femicide: Urgent implications for women's health. *Obstetrics & Gynecology, 100*, 27–36.

McFarlane, J. M., Groff, J. Y., O'Brien, J. A., & Watson, K. (2003). Behaviors of children who are exposed and not exposed to intimate partner violence: An analysis of 330 black, white, and Hispanic children. *Pediatrics, 112*(3), E202–E207.

McFarlane, J., Malecha, A., Gist, J., Watson, K., Batten, E., Hall, I., et al. (2004). Increasing the safety-promoting behaviors of abused women. *American Journal of Nursing, 104*, 40–50.

Neighbors, C. J., O'Leary, A., & Labouvie, E. (1999). Domestically violent and nonviolent male inmates' responses to their partners' requests for condom use: Testing a social-information processing model. *Health Psychology, 18*, 427–431.

Parker, B., McFarlane, J., Silva, C., Soeken, K., & Reel, S. (1999). Testing an intervention to prevent further abuse to pregnant women. *Research in Nursing and Health, 22*, 59–66.

Plichta, S. (1997). Violence, health and the use of health services. In M. Falik, & K. Collins (Eds.), *Women's health: The Commonwealth Fund survey* (pp. 237–272). Baltimore: Johns Hopkins University Press.

Renker, P. R., & Tonkin, P. (2006). Women's views of prenatal violence screening: Acceptability and confidentiality issues. *Obstetrics & Gynecology, 107*(2), 348–354.

Rennison, C., & Welchens, S. (2000). *Intimate partner violence (Rep. No. Publication NCJ 183781)*. Washington, DC: U.S. Department of Justice.

Renzetti, C. M. (1998). Violence and abuse in lesbian relationships: Theoretical and empirical issues. In R. K. Bergen (Ed.), *Issues in intimate violence* (pp. 117–127). Thousand Oaks, CA: Sage.

Rodriguez, M. A., McLoughlin, E., Nah, G., & Campbell, J. C. (2001). Mandatory reporting of domestic violence injuries to the police: What do emergency department patients think? *Journal of the American Medical Association, 286*, 580–583.

Sachs, C. J., Koziol-McLain, J., Glass, N., Webster, D., & Campbell, J. (2002). A population-based survey assessing support for mandatory domestic violence reporting by health care personnel. *Women & Health, 35*(2-3), 121–133.

Saltzman, L. E., Fanslow, J. L., McMahon, P. M., & Shelley, G. A. (1999). *Intimate partner violence surveillance: Uniform definitions and recommended data elements.* Atlanta, GA: Centers for Disease Control and Prevention.

Sato-DiLorenzo, A., & Sharps, P. W. (2007). Dangerous intimate partner relationships and women's mental health and health behaviors. *Issues in Mental Health Nursing, 28*(8), 837–48.

Sharps, P. W., Koziol-McLain, J., Campbell, J., McFarlane, J., Sachs, C., & Xu, X. (2001). Health care providers' missed opportunities for preventing femicide. *Preventive Medicine, 33,* 373–380.

Sharps, P. W., Laughon, K., Giangrande S. K. (2007). Intimate partner violence and the childbearing year: Maternal and infant health consequences. *Trauma, Violence, & Abuse, 8*(2); 105–116.

Silva, C., McFarlane, J., Soeken, K., Parker, B., & Reel, S. (1997). Symptoms of post-traumatic stress disorder in abused women in a primary care setting. *Journal of Women's Health, 6,* 543–552.

Silverman, J. G., Decker, M. R., Reed, E., & Raj, A. (2006). Intimate partner violence around the time of pregnancy and breastfeeding behavior among U.S. women. *Journal of Women's Health, 15,* 934–940.

Smith, P. H., Earp, J. A., & DeVellis, R. (1995). Development and validation of the Women's Experience with Battering (WEB) scale. *Women's Health, 1,* 273–288.

Soeken, K., McFarlane, J., Parker, B., & Lominack, M. C. (1998). The Abuse Assessment Screen: A clinical instrument to measure frequency, severity, and perpetrator of abuse against women. In J. C. Campbell (Ed.), *Empowering survivors of abuse: Healthcare for battered women and their children* (pp. 195–203). Thousand Oaks, CA: Sage.

Tjaden, P., & Thoennes, N. (2000). Full report of the prevalence, incidence, and consequences of violence against women (Rep. No. NCJ 183781). Washington, DC: U.S. Department of Justice, Office of Justice Programs.

Torres, S., Campbell, J., Campbell, D. W., Ryan, J., King, C., Price, P., et al. (2000). Abuse during and before pregnancy: Prevalence and cultural correlates. *Violence & Victims, 15*(3), 303–21.

Wadman, M. C., & Muelleman, R. L. (1999). Domestic violence homicides: ED use before victimization. *American Journal of Emergency Medicine, 17*(7), 689–691.

Wingood, G. M., & DiClemente, R. J. (1997). Effects of having a physically abusive partner on the condom: Use and sexual negotiation rates of young adult African American women. *American Journal of Public Health, 2,* 53–60.

Woods, S. J. (2005). Intimate partner violence and post-traumatic stress disorder symptoms in women: What we know and need to know. *Journal of Interpersonal Violence, 20,* 394–402.

Yost, N. P., Bloom, S. L., McIntire, D. D., & Leveno, K. J. (2005). A prospective observational study of domestic violence during pregnancy. *Obstetrics Gynecology, 106,* 61–65.

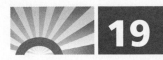

19

Vulnerable Populations

MARILYN GRACE O'ROURKE, DNP, APHN-BC

OBJECTIVES

At the completion of this chapter, the reader will be able to:

- Define the concepts of vulnerability, risk, cumulative risk, relative risk, social determinants of health, social equity, and health disparities.
- Discuss individual and societal factors that contribute to vulnerability.
- Discuss the roles of *Healthy People 2010* and *Healthy People 2020* in reducing health disparities.
- Recognize current critical issues contributing to vulnerability.
- Describe nursing strategies at the individual, family, group, and societal levels to reduce health disparities in vulnerable populations.

PROFILE IN PRACTICE: VULNERABLE ADOLESCENTS

Carol Wardlaw, MSN, APRN
Rush University Medical Center, College of Nursing, Chicago, Illinois

I am a family nurse practitioner in a school-based health center located in an inner-city high school. I have worked in this health center for 14 years. What I have learned is that I cannot begin to know what some of the young people's lives are like, and so I listen to them. Gang recruitment, drug dealing (going on right outside the school windows), mothers and fathers in prison, and mothers and fathers on drugs are often part of their experience. In some cases the students "don't know, don't care" where their parents are. In this setting, physical health is not the only type of health I deal with. Sometimes the problems are about emotional and mental health. Thus I have learned that it is important to ask questions and let the young person tell his or her story. Poverty, depression, and

disappointment are bound to affect a young person's ability to learn and are often underlying factors for the headaches and stomach aches that bring the adolescents into the health center. I am waiting there—someone who is willing to listen and who wants to listen.

Sometimes the stories are painful for me to hear. Once I asked a young man, as gently as I could, why he had body odor and why his clothes smelled. Without asking, I could have just assumed that he had poor hygiene and was too lazy to care for himself or his clothes. Because I asked, I heard his story. He proceeded to tell me about the financial problems facing his mother and siblings. Their utilities had been disconnected because his mother was unable to pay the bills. He asked me not to tell anyone his situation. He did not want anyone to know. He said he had a plan. He would get a summer job and pay the bills and have all the utilities reconnected. In the fall when school started, he returned to the health center to tell me he had done exactly what he said he would. I smiled but thought to myself, "Why should a 16-year-old have to bear this burden? Why should his summer be spent working to pay the water and gas bills?"

One question that I frequently ask is, "Have you ever had sex?" Later in the conversation I will ask, "Have you ever been raped?" Too often the answer is yes. Recently, a 16-year-old girl reported going to spend the night with her aunt and female cousin. At some point during the night, her cousin's drunken boyfriend came into her room and raped her. She did not tell anyone

about the rape except her 14-year-old sister. But she did not want to tell her mother—especially not her mother. She wanted to protect her mother from this stress because she and her mother were facing eviction at the end of the week, and her mother did not know where the family was going to live.

"Ms. Wardlaw, come and see what we want. You know you got to take care of your girls," said one young lady who came into the health center, interrupting my paperwork. She wanted me to come and address the pressing concerns of the group in the waiting area. I smiled because I wanted her to feel that I was here for her and her friends. I want to help them graduate and go on to live healthy and successful lives.

PROFILE IN PRACTICE: HOMELESS MEN

Elizabeth Herzan-Taylor, MS, APRN
Rush University Medical Center, College of Nursing, Chicago, Illinois

I work as a family nurse practitioner in a small urban shelter for homeless men. When I was considering taking the position, my introduction consisted of a morning spent observing the nurse practitioner who was covering the shelter on a somewhat irregular basis. The shelter's health program had been founded several years before, but the nurse who created it had retired out of state, and the program had been dormant for lack of funding to hire a replacement. Now they were ready for a new nurse. Was I the right person for the job? My nursing background was in home care. I enjoyed the opportunity to work with a patient one on one, on his or her own turf, really individualizing the care. After becoming a family nurse practitioner, I had most recently worked in a small geriatric clinic serving a mostly poor, minority population. If nothing else, I was used to figuring out what was "doable," knowing that although economic considerations should not be a deciding factor, all too often they do limit the options.

So I was used to working largely independently, individualizing care to a patient's situation, finding cost-effective, practical solutions, and especially advocating for the patients to ensure their needs were met.

I found all these experiences had prepared me pretty well for working in the field of homeless health care. As I watched, I thought, "Yes, I can do this. I want to do this." I saw that there was much that could be done despite limited resources. I consider it an extra blessing to have a job where I really feel like I can make a difference. Still, I had a lot to learn, and I am still learning.

For each new client, I perform a basic assessment of health needs and develop an initial plan to help meet those needs. I know that I may have the opportunity to work with a homeless person over a period of time during his stay at the shelter. Or I may get only this one chance, depending on how long he is able or willing to remain. Since time and resources are both limited, it is necessary to focus on the client's immediate priorities. Sometimes I cannot do everything I would like to do. But for someone who has completely lost contact with the health care system, even little things such as over-the-counter cold medication and simple foot care mean a lot.

I would characterize my experience thus far in terms of satisfactions and frustrations. For example, it is very satisfying to care for a client with an aching, abscessed tooth and be able to prescribe the pain medication and penicillin that will result in grateful relief. It is not so satisfying to realize that, despite having dealt with his immediate problem, I cannot offer him the long-term solution (he needs to see a dentist!) because the only clinic I know that treats homeless, uninsured people is so heavily overbooked that it is not taking new patients for at least 2 to 3 months. Where will he be then?

I remember John, who came to me with uncontrolled diabetes. He had not had any medication in weeks. His blood sugar was quite elevated, but he felt "okay." I tried oral medications first, not expecting him to be able to manage insulin in his current circumstances, though he reluctantly admitted he had been on it before. His blood glucose did not budge, so eventually, after consulting with my collaborating physician, I put him on insulin anyway. After several weeks his diabetes was finally under somewhat better control. Then he left the shelter one weekend and did not return. His insulin is still in my refrigerator. In a few days or weeks, he will be right back where he started.

Of course, I also have many clients who are success stories. They leave with medication they did not have before, better control of and understanding of their health issues, and resources to continue obtaining primary care after they are no longer under my care. Finding and cultivating relationships with other resources in the community are essential parts of my practice. Ours is an emergency shelter. The intent is to help the men move on to something more permanent. I do what I can, knowing that sometimes the best I can do is to help these men who have fallen between the cracks of the health care system get plugged back into the system.

To be homeless is to be in survival mode. Finding somewhere to fill a prescription for free, and likely waiting a very long time for it, falls somewhere way behind having a meal and a place to sleep that night. Part of helping these men get their lives on track is showing them that they do not have to just survive day to day—that they can begin to make plans again and can be part of a society in which all too often they have become invisible. The shelter prides itself on respecting the dignity of each individual. We care about them, so they can again begin caring about themselves.

Introduction

On any given day, the waiting room in a family practice physician's office might include a variety of people who seem to have nothing in common: an infant in the arms of his mother awaiting a well-baby check-up, an elderly woman with edematous feet, an African American man concerned about a persistent cough, and a young woman diagnosed with HIV. Yet all these individuals do have something in common. They all fit the definition of belonging to a vulnerable group.

Key Concepts

DEFINITION OF VULNERABILITY

Why should nurses study the concept of vulnerability and the needs of vulnerable populations? Shi and Stevens (2005) give the following five reasons:

1. Vulnerable populations have greater health needs than the general public.
2. The prevalence of vulnerability is increasing in the United States.
3. Vulnerability is influenced by social forces, so societal forces rather than individual effort are required to remedy it.
4. Vulnerability is fundamentally linked to the overall health and resources of the United States.
5. Interest in ensuring that health care is delivered in a fair and equitable manner is increasing.

VULNERABILITY

What is meant by *vulnerability*, and what are *vulnerable populations?* To be vulnerable means to be susceptible to wounding or injury. Certainly, the infant and elderly woman in the waiting room fit this definition by virtue of their ages. But what about the others? What makes them vulnerable? Flaskerud and Winslow (1998) say that vulnerable populations are groups of people who have limited resources and are at increased risk for developing poor health. They list the poor, persons subject to discrimination or intolerance, those who are politically marginalized, women and children, ethnic people of color, immigrants, gays and lesbians, the homeless, and the elderly as vulnerable groups. Aday (2001) indicates that high-risk mothers and infants, the chronically ill and disabled, persons living with HIV/AIDS, the mentally ill and disabled, alcohol and substance abusers, the suicide and homicide prone, abusing families, homeless persons, racial and ethnic minorities, and immigrants and refugees fit into such groups. She divides these groups into three categories on the basis of where their principal needs lie: *physical* needs, *psychological* needs, or *social* needs. For example, Aday places homeless persons in the category of primarily having social needs, such as housing and employment. Depending on the circumstances involved, an individual could fit into multiple categories. For example, consider a person with a chronic illness who loses his employment because of absenteeism, begins drinking excessively, and becomes abusive toward his spouse; this person would fit into all three categories. Most literature says that anyone who is of low socioeconomic status (SES) as measured by education, occupation, and income is vulnerable to poorer health.

Aday gives the following reasons for placing the individuals she selected into vulnerable groups (2001):

- Their needs are serious or even debilitating and life-threatening.
- They require significant medical and nonmedical services.
- Their needs place increasing demands on the medical, public health, and service sectors.
- Their needs are complex and not adequately met through existing services and financing mechanisms.

Given these criteria, additional groups might be considered vulnerable: veterans returning from combat duty, victims of natural disasters, prisoners, migrant workers, pregnant teenagers, and the uninsured or underinsured. See Box 19-1 for a list of potential vulnerable groups of people.

RISK, CUMULATIVE RISK, AND RELATIVE RISK

To understand the challenges faced by vulnerable populations, an understanding of the concept of risk is helpful. *Risk* refers to the probability that some event

---

BOX 19-1	Potentially Vulnerable Groups of People

Children
Chronically ill individuals
Combat veterans
Disaster victims
Older adults
Lesbian, gay, bisexual, and transgender (LGBT) individuals
High-risk mothers and infants
Homeless individuals
Immigrants or refugees
Mentally ill individuals
Migrant workers
Politically marginalized individuals
Prisoners
Racial or ethnic minorities
Substance abusers
Suicide-prone or homicide-prone individuals
Unemployed individuals
Uninsured or underinsured (health insurance) individuals
Victims of domestic violence
Victims of stigmatized infections (e.g., HIV/AIDS)

---

or outcome will occur within a given time frame. Individuals vary as to how much they are at risk for a given health problem. Some risks reside within the individual, such as gender and state of wellness, whereas other risks exist in the environment, such as violence and pollutants. Women with a family history of breast cancer and polycystic breast disease are at higher risk for getting breast cancer. Multiple factors in a woman's life may affect whether she gets breast cancer, such as her age at menarche, her age at her first pregnancy, and her history of using hormones.

Vulnerable populations are at increased risk for disease because of the interplay of the risk factors they face. If the woman described above has not received education regarding early detection, is homeless, and is uninsured with no regular source of health care, her risk for advanced breast cancer increases. Vulnerable populations are especially prone to these *cumulative risks*. Shi and Stevens (2005) describe these additional risks as not just adding to the probability of disease but

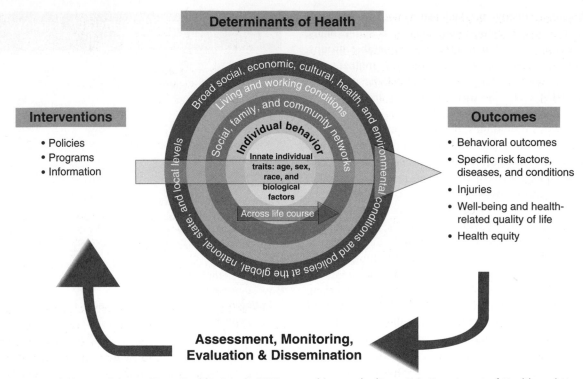

FIGURE 19-1 Action model to achieve *Healthy People 2020* overarching goals. (From U.S. Department of Health and Human Services. [2008b]. Secretary's Advisory Committee on National Health Promotion and Disease Prevention Objectives for 2020. Developing *Healthy People 2020*: Phase I report: Recommendations for the framework and format of *Healthy People 2020* [p. 22]. [Online]. Retrieved from www.healthypeople.gov/hp2020/advisory/PhaseI/PhaseI.pdf.)

multiplying the probability of becoming ill. As Rogers (1997) states, those who have a combination of high-risk factors are the most vulnerable.

Healthy People 2020 graphically depicts how these internal and external factors interplay to determine the health of individuals (Figure 19-1). For example, discriminatory policies, substandard health care, lack of access to health care, environmental pollution, unsafe occupations, poverty, lack of social support, lack of education, unhealthy behaviors, and other factors can all be accommodated by the model.

Relative risk is a ratio used in epidemiology to compare the risk for poor health among groups exposed to a risk factor versus those who are not exposed. Some will get the disease, and others will be more resilient and remain healthy. Members of vulnerable groups have been shown to have higher rates of disease

than others and to have worse health outcomes. Perhaps their nutrition is not as good, or they are sleep deprived from working two jobs, or they have significant depression and fail to seek medical care. As a result, they are exposed to more risks and are likely to suffer more from a given risk than the general public. Flaskerud and Winslow (1998) say that a lack of resources increases relative risk, reduces the ability to avoid risks, and reduces the capacity to minimize any disease that may result.

SOCIAL DETERMINANTS OF HEALTH

Some may ask, "Why do these individuals not protect themselves better and make better choices?" Some studies on vulnerability examine personal factors that contribute to vulnerability (Lessick, Woodring, Naber,

& Halstead, 1992; Rogers, 1997), but there are also very influential social factors involved. These are called the *social determinants of health*. They are defined as "the circumstances in which people are born, grow up, live, work, and age, as well as the systems put in place to deal with illness. These circumstances are in turn shaped by a wider set of forces: economics, social policies, and politics." (World Health Organization, 2010).

Social determinants of health can be divided into three main categories:

- Social institutions—for example, cultural and educational institutions, religious institutions, economic systems, political structures
- Surroundings—for example, neighborhoods, housing, workplaces, towns and cities
- Social relationships—for example, position in social hierarchy, social networks, differential treatment of social groups

Geiger (2006) also lists income levels, rates of employment, educational opportunities, workplace safety, safe water, nutritious food, clean air, good sanitation, and uncontaminated soil as important factors. See Box 19-2 for some examples of social determinants of health.

In contrast, factors that are internal to the individual are not modifiable (age, gender, race, ethnicity, genetic makeup). However, individual factors in the environment (social support, education, income, lifestyle choices, adaptation, and coping) are potentially modifiable. Examples of efforts to affect these social conditions include:

- Improving housing
- Increasing neighborhood safety
- Ensuring quality and equitable education opportunities
- Eliminating environmental hazards
- Employment opportunities that provide a living wage

A closer look at these lists indicates that most of these determinants and remedies are not in the total control of the individual involved.

Individuals vary regarding how they respond to internal and environmental stressors. Their degree of

| BOX 19-2 | Examples of Social Determinants of Health |

- Socioeconomic status
- Rates of employment
- Educational opportunities
- Transportation
- Housing
- Access to services
- Discrimination
- Social or environmental stressors
- Workplace safety

Data from National Center for Chronic Disease Prevention and Health Promotion, CDC/Social Determinants of Health Working Group. (2005). Social determinants of health. Retrieved from www.cdc.gov/sdoh; and Geiger, H. J. (2006). Medical care. In B. S. Levy, & V. W. Sidel (Eds.). Social injustice and public health (pp. 208–209). New York: Oxford University Press.

vulnerability is influenced by their perception of the situation, the degree of control they feel, and the situation itself (Rogers, 1997). For example, a recent immigrant who is looking forward to living in the United States, chooses where to live and with whom to live, and is surrounded by some prized possessions and other supportive immigrants would be less vulnerable than someone who is returning from combat in Iraq, is suffering from posttraumatic stress disorder, and feels alienated from civilians and unable to find employment. Lessick and colleagues (1992) propose that people have a vulnerability threshold that varies among individuals. When a person's internal resources are exceeded by external stressors, illness is likely to occur.

Vulnerability can extend from one generation to the next. McNaughton, Cowell, Gross, Fogg, & Ailey (2004) studied Mexican-American immigrant women and their children. They found that 51% of children with high scores on scales measuring depression also had a mother with high depression and anxiety scores.

Although vulnerability results from the interplay of personal and environmental factors, what poses the strongest influence? Shi and Stevens (2005) state that although personal behaviors contribute to health, they "explain only a modest portion of health disparities" (p. 10). Social determinants of health are believed to play a much greater role. Some would argue that the lack of socioeconomic resources and exposure to risk factors in the environment reduce a person's ability to avoid risks and minimize disease (Aday, 2001; Flaskerud & Winslow, 1998). There is evidence that vulnerable groups bear a greater burden of illness because of social (not personal) factors and have poorer access to care. When they receive health care, it is of a poorer quality (Gornick, 2003; Shi & Stevens, 2005). Geiger (2006) states that at no time in the history of the United States has the health status of its minority groups equaled or approximated that of the white majority. He summarizes the problem as follows: "These minority and poor populations thus bear a triple burden: they live, on average, in the most dangerous biological and physical environments and are exposed to the worst social determinants of health status; they have the least access to care; and, when care is provided, it tends to be of poorer quality" (p. 209).

HEALTHY PEOPLE 2010 AND HEALTHY PEOPLE 2020

Every 10 years since 1980, the U.S. Department of Health and Human Services (USDHHS) has developed a plan to improve the health of the nation and direct its efforts in health promotion and disease prevention. A document is developed called *Healthy People,* based on the belief that setting priorities, developing measurable objectives, and tracking progress toward those objectives will "motivate, guide, and focus action" (USDHHS, *Healthy People 2020*). Using the best evidence and scientific expertise available, the plan consists of a vision, goals, and multiple objectives. It also guides federal agencies in providing funding and support to organizations that align their efforts with the objectives in the plan.

Healthy People 2010 (USDHHS, *Healthy People 2010*) included two goals: (1) to increase quality and years of healthy life and (2) eliminate health disparities. To achieve these goals, 498 very specific and measurable objectives were developed. However, the plan was considered too cumbersome and difficult to use. In some cases, lack of access to care resulted in the objectives and their targets for accomplishment being unrealistic.

Healthy People 2020 attempts to learn from these lessons with a simplified vision, four goals, and fewer objectives to meet those goals. When it is published in

early 2010, it will be readily accessible online using an interactive, searchable, multilevel interface. The planners want to avoid developing a print-based document that sits on a shelf for the 10-year period. See Table 19-1 for more information about *Healthy People 2020*.

Healthy People 2020 also distinguishes between health equity and health disparities. *Health equity* means striving:

- For fairness in efforts to achieve the best possible health for everyone
- To eliminate remediable disparities in health and health care
- To eliminate disparities in social conditions that lead to disparities in health

Health disparities are defined in different ways by different groups and governmental bodies (Carter-Porras & Baquet, 2002). In 2004 the National Institutes of Health defined it as the "differences in the incidence, prevalence, mortality, and burden of diseases and other adverse health conditions that exist among specific population groups in the United States (Prevention Institute, 2004). The Minority Health and Health Disparities Research and Education Act of 2000 also applies the term to populations for whom there is disparity in the quality, outcomes, cost, use of, access to, or satisfaction with health care services as compared with the general population (Carter-Porras & Baquet, 2002). There is research support for this expanded definition. The Institute of Medicine (2003) report found that disparities cannot be totally explained by SES, insurance status, or patient preference. This report came to the disturbing conclusion that some health disparities are a result of provider bias and stereotypical beliefs that influence clinical decision making.

The literature examining health disparities and their possible causes is extensive. In 2004, Woolf, Johnson, Fryer, Rust, and Satcher compared the number of lives saved from 1991 to 2000 by medical advances with the number of lives that could have been saved by equalizing the mortality rate between whites and African Americans. They determined that medical technology averted 176,633 deaths, but achieving equity would have averted five times this number (886,202 deaths). The authors acknowledge the formidable task of reducing disparities, but they wanted policymakers to be aware of

TABLE 19-1	*Healthy People 2020* Vision and Goals	
Vision	**Mission**	**Goals**
A society in which all people live long, healthy lives	To improve health through strengthening policy and practice, *Healthy People* will identify nationwide health improvement priorities; increase public awareness and understanding of the determinants of health, disease, and disability and the opportunities for progress; provide measurable objectives and goals that can be used at the national, state, and local levels; engage multiple sectors to take actions that are driven by the best available evidence and knowledge; and identify critical research and data collection needs.	• Eliminate preventable disease, disability, injury, and premature death. • Achieve health equity, eliminate disparities, and improve the health of all groups. • Create social and physical environments that promote good health for all. • Promote healthy development and healthy behaviors across every stage of life.

Data from U.S. Department of Health and Human Services. (2008c). Secretary's Advisory Committee on National Health Promotion and Disease Prevention Objectives for 2020. Executive summary. Developing *Healthy People 2020*: Phase I report: recommendations for the framework and format of *Healthy People 2020*. [Online]. Retrieved from www.healthypeople.gov/hp2020/advisory/PhaseI/summary.htm.

the benefits of addressing these challenges as opposed to continued investment in the technology of care.

In 2007 the Agency for Healthcare Research and Quality (AHRQ) released a National Healthcare Disparities Report. This report stated, "Overall, disparities in quality and access for minority groups and poor populations have not been reduced since the first NHDR ... the number of measures on which disparities have gotten significantly worse or have remained unchanged since the first NHDR is higher than the number of measures on which they have gotten significantly better for blacks, Hispanics, American Indians and Alaska Natives, Asians, and poor populations" (AHRQ, 2007, para. 2). See Table 19-2 for some examples of health disparities documented by *Healthy People 2020*.

Current Challenges to Health Equity

POVERTY

Socioeconomic status is determined by income, occupation, educational attainment, and housing. More than any other, this factor has an impact on health.

Poverty is defined as living below a certain level established each year by two different entities of the federal government. The Census Bureau establishes *poverty thresholds,* which are used to calculate the number of people living in poverty. The Department of Health and Human Services determines *poverty guidelines,* which are used to determine eligibility for certain federal programs of support. For instance, in 2009/2010, the poverty guideline for a family of four was $22,050. Poverty is defined as having less than this amount of household income. *Extreme poverty* is defined as income that is half or less of the poverty guideline—$11,025 or less for a family of four in 2009 (U.S. Department of Health and Human Services, 2010). In 2007 the overall percentage of Americans living in poverty was 12.5%, as the number of people living in poverty rose to 37.3 million in 2007, an increase of 2.2 million since 2006. The number of people living in extreme poverty remained at 15.6 million people for the third consecutive year—the highest level since the data became available in 1975 (U.S. Conference of Catholic Bishops, n.d.).

Since that time the economy in the United States has deteriorated even further as the country entered a recession in December 2007 and an economic crisis involving financial markets, financial institutions, large and

TABLE 19-2	Examples of Health Disparities and Disparities in Health Care
Condition	**Disparity**
Infant mortality	Black infants have higher mortality than white infants.
Life expectancy	Blacks, Hispanics, Native Americans, and those with lower incomes and educational level have shorter life expectancy, as calculated at age 26.
Obesity	Obesity is more prevalent in adults with sensory, physical, and mental health conditions.
Disability in older adults	Disability rates in older adults go up as income goes down (inverse relationship).
Breast cancer	Black women are more likely than white women to die of breast cancer.
Pain control	Latinos are less likely than whites to receive pain medication for major fractures in a large emergency department (not due to language barrier).
Cardiovascular disease	Blacks and women receive less appropriate care for cardiovascular disease than white men with the same clinical presentation.

Data from U.S. Department of Health and Human Services. (2008a). Secretary's Advisory Committee on National Health Promotion and Disease Prevention Objectives for 2020. Appendix 10: Clarification and examples of health disparities and health equity. Developing *Healthy People 2020:* Phase I Report: Recommendations for the framework and format of *Healthy People 2020.* [Online]. Retrieved from www.healthypeople.gov/hp2020/advisory/PhaseI/appendix10.htm.

small businesses, and currencies spread throughout the world. The poverty rates for 2008 will be available online (http://census.gov), and it is likely that they will increase significantly and involve more sectors of the country because of this crisis. In addition, some of the safety net programs and agencies that assist in cushioning the blow of difficult economic times are being challenged by reduced contributions from donors and delayed funding from financially strapped local, state, and federal governmental agencies.

UNEMPLOYMENT

Employment not only provides needed income but also determines the social class to which a person belongs. In 2008 the United States lost 2.6 million jobs, and another 2 million are forecast to disappear in 2009. As of August 2009, nonfarm unemployment in the United States measured 9.4% with 14.5 million people unemployed. Of those individuals, 5 million are considered "long-term unemployed" (U.S. Bureau of Labor Statistics, 2009).

New people are joining the ranks of the unemployed at an increasing rate. Michigan's unemployment soared to 15% in July of 2009, related to problems with the automobile industry, while the Rhode Island rate jumped to 12.9%, the highest since 1976. Other states dependent on textile, recreational

vehicle, and retail industries also suffered significant losses. According to Aversa (2009), on January 26, 2009, approximately 40,000 job cuts were announced in a single day by companies as varied as Pfizer (pharmaceuticals), Caterpillar (heavy equipment manufacturing), and Home Depot (home improvement and construction materials).

In the United States, employment also plays a major role in whether an individual has health insurance. Small business workers, self-employed people, and people working in low-paying service jobs are often not covered by group health insurance. Buying health insurance outside a group plan is prohibitively expensive for many people. In addition, the percentage of people (workers and dependents) with employment-based health insurance dropped from 70% in 1987 to 62% in 2007—the lowest level of employment-based insurance coverage in more than a decade (National Coalition on Health Care, n.d.).

HOUSING

Housing is considered affordable if it costs no more than 30% of annual income. This allows sufficient money to purchase food, clothing, transportation, medical care, and other necessities. In 2006, the U.S. Department of Housing and Urban Development

(HUD) estimated that 12 million renter and home-owner households were paying more than 50% of their annual income for housing.

In 2008, 2.3 million American homeowners faced foreclosure proceedings on their homes, an 81% increase from 2007 (Associated Press, 2009). This was caused not only by homeowners being overextended, but also by faulty lending practices and decreasing home values. For example, some homeowners did not have sufficient income to pay the mortgages they were given. Other homeowners, who hoped to borrow the increased equity on their home to finance higher adjustable mortgage rates or other expenses, found that they owed more on their home than it was currently valued.

Williams (1999) states that the single most important factor that contributes to lower SES and poor health in minority groups is *residential segregation,* which he attributes to beliefs about inferiority and a desire to avoid social contact. Although laws have been passed against discriminatory lending and real estate practices, minority people disproportionately live in the least desirable areas.

One of the factors in such neighborhoods contributing to poorer health is a lack of access to healthy foods. Larson, Story, and Nelson (2009) reviewed 54 studies published between 1985 and 2008 and found that people living in poorer neighborhoods have less access to supermarkets with a variety of healthy foods at lower prices. These communities are referred to as *food deserts.* For example, predominately African American neighborhoods had half as many supermarket chains, and Hispanic neighborhoods had one third as many as white neighborhoods. People who have better access to a supermarket have a reduced risk for obesity, whereas those with easy access only to convenience stores and energy-dense food from fast-food restaurants have an increased obesity risk.

Working with Vulnerable Populations

NURSING CONSIDERATIONS FOR CARE

When working with individuals, families, and groups, the nurse should start by attempting to bring into consciousness any *biases* or *stereotypes* that might affect the nurse-patient interaction. Stereotypes can be challenged by gathering new information and actively listening to the stories of clients, as exemplified by Carol Wardlaw's Profile in Practice at the beginning of this chapter. Biases and stereotypes are also discussed in the chapter on diversity (see chapter 14).

Other strategies the nurse can use when working with vulnerable individuals, families, and groups include the following:

- Establish a relationship of mutual respect and trust. The client may have had previous negative experiences with the health care system.
- Adopt a nonjudgmental attitude. Recognize the obstacles in the person's life that make adherence to health recommendations a challenge.
- Determine the client's priorities and start there. The client's main concern may not seem the most important, but once it is addressed, the nurse and patient can build on that success to work on other issues.
- Address primary prevention as much as possible; although this may not be uppermost in the client's mind, it prevents acute illness in those financially ill-prepared to deal with it. Primary prevention includes activities that promote health *before* illness occurs or prevents disease or injury from occurring, such as good nutrition, adequate exercise, and up-to-date immunizations.
- Follow clinical practice guidelines to ensure that care is delivered in an equitable manner. For example, follow screening guidelines for mammography to ensure that vulnerable women receive early detection and treatment.
- Deliver care that is culturally competent. Recognize that the client's cultural values and behaviors may be counter to mainstream culture.
- Ensure that translation services, translated documents, and health information at the appropriate literacy level are available to clients.
- Eliminate as many "hassles" and barriers to care as possible in the delivery of health services. These can include long wait times, inconvenient hours, lack of child care, inaccessibility by public transportation, fragmented services, and inflexible payment options (Box 19-3).

BOX 19-3	Case Study: Daily Hassles

Janet is a single mother with two school-age children. She lives in a subsidized apartment composed of 10 units. She works as a teacher's aide at her children's school. This morning Janet noticed that there were cockroaches in her apartment related to the spraying the building manager did in the neighboring apartment yesterday. Although she is careful about food storage, it looks like her neighbor's roaches are looking for a new place to get a meal. Her oldest daughter has asthma, and both roach droppings and roach sprays are triggers to be avoided. Janet prepares breakfast with the remaining food in the apartment, but she will need to get groceries (food, milk, laundry detergent, bleach) on the way home. She will have to be frugal because it is the end of the month and money is running low. The kids keep complaining that they are tired of oatmeal, soup, and macaroni and cheese. Janet is tired of their complaining.

After everyone is dressed, the family piles into Janet's old car. She turns on the ignition, but only gets a "click click click." The engine refuses to turn over. She looks at her watch. Even if her neighbor is home with his car, they will still be late. Janet was late for work earlier in the month when she had to take her daughter to the emergency department in the middle of the night with an asthma attack. She also was late another day when the building had no power and her alarm did not go off. She received a verbal warning not to be late again, and now she is worried about losing her job. The kids do not like being late for school, which means getting reprimanded and having to stay in for recess. Both children begin to cry. It is too far to get to school by walking, and Janet does not like her children walking past the group of men hanging out on the corner. The school bus has already made its rounds. The city bus stop is three blocks away. Janet will use some grocery money for the bus if her neighbor cannot drive her and the kids to school. She feels very tired, and she knows she is also getting another cold.

- Use community resources and consider factors such as cost, eligibility, and access.
- Serve as an advocate. People who are vulnerable often do not have the social connections, power, and collective voice needed to advocate for themselves.
- Teach skills related to accessing the health care system, actively participating in care planning, using community resources, and advocating for one's self.
- Identify, or even develop, social supports for the client. Social isolation is common among vulnerable groups. Social support has been shown to alleviate some of the problems associated with vulnerability.
- Collaborate with other health professionals and agencies to secure what is needed for vulnerable people, families, and groups.
- Identify ways to nurture and support yourself when working with vulnerable populations to decrease frustration and burnout.
- Assist in the recruitment and retention of more racially and ethnically diverse nurses in the profession.

SOCIAL AND POLITICAL ACTIVISM

Because many of the factors contributing to vulnerability involve social determinants of health, a change in social or political policy is required to address these factors. Professional nurses need to become politically involved in issues that affect health. Social injustice is at the core of many of the conditions that contribute to vulnerability. Levy and Sidel (2006) define *social injustice* as "denial or violation of economic, sociocultural, political, civil, or human rights of specific populations or groups in the society based on the perception of their inferiority by those with more power or influence" (p. 6). They also say that policies and actions that adversely affect the societal conditions in which people can be healthy constitute social injustice. They list the following as examples of such policies and actions: war, violence, global warming, environmental damage, lack of essential public health services, lack of access to medical services, governmental corruption, erosion of civil liberties, and restrictions on education, research, and free speech.

President Obama attributed his successful bid for election to the grassroots campaign and support he received throughout the country. He is calling upon all citizens to participate in a similar way to rebuild the systems and structures in this country. These efforts have the potential to contribute directly and indirectly to improved health for all.

SUMMARY

Nurses play a key role in bridging the gap between vulnerable populations and other parts of the health care system. Because nurses are educated to deliver holistic care that is client centered, they are in a good position to work effectively with vulnerable populations. Because of the challenges vulnerable clients face, nurses will feel equally challenged by what seem, in many cases, to be insurmountable problems. By drawing on and further developing their nursing skills, collaborating with others, using community resources, and maintaining personal hope through self-care, nurses can make a significant difference in the lives of society's neediest citizens.

KEY POINTS

- Vulnerability is an important factor for nurses to consider when working with clients across the life span.
- Vulnerability is a result of uncontrollable individual factors over which the client has no influence, modifiable individual factors that the client can change, and societal factors that require social or political action to address.
- *Healthy People 2010* sought the elimination of health disparities as one of its two goals and achieved some gains by 2005.
- *Healthy People 2020* has four goals: (1) Eliminate preventable disease, disability, injury, and premature death; (2) achieve health equity, eliminate disparities, and improve the health of all groups; (3) create social and physical environments that promote good health for all; and (4) promote healthy development and healthy behaviors across every stage of life.
- Nurses need to recognize the social and political factors contributing to the vulnerability of the clients with whom they work to avoid blaming the victim for conditions beyond one's control.
- Poverty, low socioeconomic status, and lack of access to health care have a large and negative impact on health.
- Unemployment and underemployment, lack of affordable housing, and lack of access to quality education directly contribute to poverty.
- Chronic stress and exposure to adverse environmental conditions increase the risk for poor health.
- Racism and discrimination contribute to health disparities and are modifiable risks on the part of health care professionals.

- Nurses can work effectively with vulnerable populations by building skills in nursing care delivery.
- Nurses need to become politically informed and active to advocate for social justice and health equity.

CRITICAL THINKING EXERCISES

1. Access the following site regarding health literacy: www.AskMe3.org. Using the information at the site, how would you counsel a member of a vulnerable group who is planning a visit to a primary care provider?
2. What factors do you think contribute the most to homelessness in the United States? Check your perceptions against the information provided by The National Alliance to End Homelessness (www.endhomelessness.org/index.htm).
3. Have you experienced any instances of members of vulnerable groups receiving differential treatment? Why do you think this happened? Was bias or racism involved? Visit www.kff.org/whythedifference to learn more about health disparities.
4. What social conditions in your local community contribute to the vulnerability of its residents? What national trends are you aware of that negatively affect health? Identify two or three things that you can do to address societal or political policy on either a local or national level that might address the issue(s) you identified.
5. Pick one vulnerable group in your local community. What resources are available to assist its members? Pick one resource in the community that addresses a need of this group. Determine what it provides, how much it costs, who qualifies for service, and how easy it is to access.

REFERENCES

Aday, L. A. (2001). *At risk in America: The health and health care needs of vulnerable populations in the United States.* San Francisco: Jossey-Bass.

Agency for Healthcare Research and Quality. (n.d.). 2007 National healthcare disparities report. Retrieved from http://www.ahrq.gov/qual/nhdr07/Glance.htm

Associated Press. (2009). Housing crisis: U.S. foreclosure Findings jump a record 81% in 2008. Retrieved from http://www.nydailynews.com/money/2009/01/15/2009-01-15_housing_crisis_us_foreclosure_filings_ju.html?print=1&page=all

Aversa, J. (2009). Unemployment rate hits double digits in Michigan, Rhode Island: Every state saw rise in Dec. Retrieved from http://www.chicagotribune.com/business/sns-ap-state-unemployment,05401002,print.story

Carter-Porras, O., & Baquet, C. (2002). What is a "health disparity"? *Public Health Reports, 117*, 426–434.

Flaskerud, J. H., & Winslow, B. J. (1998). Conceptualizing vulnerable populations health-related research. *Nursing Research, 47*(2), 69–78.

Geiger, H. J. (2006). Medical care. In B. S. Levy, & V. W. Sidel (Eds.). *Social injustice and public health* (pp. 208–209). New York: Oxford University Press.

Gornick, M. A. (2003). A decade of research on disparities in Medicare utilization: Lessons for the health and health care of vulnerable men. *American Journal of Public Health, 93*(5), 753–759.

Institute of Medicine. (2003). *Unequal treatment: Confronting racial and ethnic disparities in healthcare.* Washington, DC: National Academies Press.

Larson, N. I., Story, M. I., & Nelson, M. C. (2009). Neighborhood environments: Disparities in access to healthy foods in the U.S. *American Journal of Preventive Medicine, 36*(1), 74–81.

Lessick, M., Woodring, B. C., Naber, S., & Halstead, L. (1992). Vulnerability: A conceptual model applied to perinatal and neonatal nursing. *Journal of Perinatal Neonatal Nursing, 6*(3), 1–14.

Levy, B. S., & Sidel, V. W. (2006). The nature of social injustice and its impact on public health. In B. S. Levy, & V. W. Sidel (Eds.). *Social injustice and public health* (pp. 6–8). New York: Oxford University Press.

McNaughton, D. B., Cowell, J. M., Gross, D., Fogg, L., & Ailey, S. H. (2004). The relationship between maternal and child mental health in Mexican immigrant families. *Research and Theory in Nursing Practice: An International Journal, 18*(2/3), 229–242.

National Center for Chronic Disease Prevention and Health Promotion, CDC/Social Determinants of Health Working Group. (2005). Social determinants of health. Retrieved from http://www.cdc.gov/sdoh

National Coalition on Health Care. (n.d.). Health insurance coverage. [Online]. Retrieved from http://www.nchc.org/facts/coverage.shtml

Prevention Institute. (2004). [Online]. Retrieved from http://www.preventioninstitute.org/healthdis.html

Rogers, A. C. (1997). Vulnerability, health, and health care. *Journal of Advanced Nursing, 26*, 65–72.

Shi, L., & Stevens, G. D. (2005). *Vulnerable populations in the United States.* San Francisco: Jossey-Bass.

U.S. Bureau of Labor Statistics. (2009). Current unemployment rates for states and historical highs/lows. [Online]. Available at http://www.bls.gov/web/lauhsthl.htm

U.S. Conference of Catholic Bishops. (n.d.). Poverty U.S.A: The state of poverty in America. [Online]. Retrieved from http://www.usccb.org/cchd/povertyusa/povfacts.shtml

U. S. Department of Health and Human Services. (2010). The 2009 U.S. Poverty Guidelines. Retrieved from http://aspe.hhs.gov/poverty/09poverty.shtml

U.S. Department of Health and Human Services. (n.d.). Healthy People 2010. [Online]. Retrieved from http://www.healthypeople.gov/Default.htm

U.S. Department of Health and Human Services. (n.d.). Healthy People 2020. [Online]. Retrieved from http://www.healthypeople.gov/HP2020

U.S. Department of Health and Human Services. (2008a). Secretary's Advisory Committee on National Health Promotion and Disease Prevention Objectives for 2020. Appendix 10: Clarification and examples of health disparities and health equity. Developing *Healthy People 2020*: Phase I report: Recommendations for the framework and format of *Healthy People 2020*. [Online]. Retrieved from http://www.healthypeople.gov/hp2020/advisory/PhaseI/summary.htm

U.S. Department of Health and Human Services. (2008b). Secretary's Advisory Committee on National Health Promotion and Disease Prevention Objectives for 2020. Developing *Healthy People 2020*: Phase I report: Recommendations for the framework and format of *Healthy People 2020* (p. 22). [Online]. Retrieved from http://www.healthypeople.gov/hp2020/advisory/PhaseI/PhaseI.pdf

U.S. Department of Health and Human Services. (2008c). Secretary's Advisory Committee on National Health Promotion and Disease Prevention Objectives for 2020. Executive summary. Developing *Healthy People 2020*: Phase I report: Recommendations for the framework and format of *Healthy People 2020*. [Online]. Retrieved from http://www.healthypeople.gov/hp2020/advisory/PhaseI/summary.htm

Williams, D. R. (1999). Race, socioeconomic status, and health: The added effects of racism and discrimination. *Annals of the New York Academy of Sciences, 896*, 173–188.

Woolf, S. H., Johnson, R. E., Fryer, G. E., Rust, G., & Satcher, D. (2004). The health impact of resolving racial disparities: An analysis of U.S. mortality data. *American Journal of Public Health, 94*(12), 2078–2080.

World Health Organization. (2010). What are the 'social determinants' of health? Retrieved from http://www.who.int/social_determinants/thecommission/finalreport/key_concepts/en/index.html

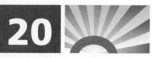

20

Patient Safety

VICKI S. GOOD, MSN, RN, CCNS, CENP

OBJECTIVES

At the completion of this chapter, the reader will be able to:

- Describe the RN's central role in patient safety.
- Illustrate the regulatory requirements specific to patient safety.
- Characterize a "just culture."
- Explain the role of a healthy work environment and culture on patient safety.
- Demonstrate the utilization of key tools to enhance patient safety.

PROFILE IN PRACTICE

Sonya A. Flanders, MSN, RN, ACNS-BS, CCRN
Clinical Nurse Specialist for Internal Medicine Services, Baylor University Medical Center, Dallas, Texas

As a nurse with over 20 years of clinical and leadership experience in critical care, administration, cardiovascular services, care coordination, patient safety, and internal medicine, I have seen many examples of the dedication exhibited by professional nurses in providing safe patient care. I have also come to recognize the necessity to mitigate threats to patient safety inherent to the complex environments in which nurses, physicians, and other health care team members work.

Although the concept of patient safety has always been embedded in my clinical and leadership work, patient safety became my primary area of focus a few years ago. Because ineffective communication is a known threat to patient safety, my earliest formal patient safety work was to help design a standardized educational presentation and tools for nurses to learn and apply the Situation-Background-Assessment-Recommendation (SBAR) standardized communication

method. SBAR communication guides nurses to articulate a patient situation or problem to a physician or other health care professional in a clear, concise, and assertive way. Developing SBAR education and tools (such as pocket cards and posters placed near telephones) that all nurses in the organization could use was a step aimed at fostering consistent and effective interdisciplinary communication. SBAR not only helps nurses convey information more effectively, but also provides a framework for the receiver to get the information necessary to act on a patient problem. The recommendation step in SBAR encourages nurses to state what they think the patient may need to address a problem, a step some nurses may omit without this structured communication method. Examples of recommendations include requesting a new medication order, suggesting transfer to a higher level of care, or asking a physician to assess the patient. A recent survey of a sample of physicians within our organization indicated many prefer receiving patient information in SBAR format.

Building on the SBAR work, next steps were to collaborate with other patient safety nurses, physicians, and team members to train our peers and interdisciplinary colleagues about the value of teamwork and the ways in which effective teamwork and communication contribute to building a culture of patient safety. Together, we developed a training program that included general concepts about patient safety, human factors, characteristics of high-reliability organizations, and SBAR. Over time, new content has been added to include other patient safety practices and concepts. During the training, a variety of examples are used to convey this very critical message: Patient safety is everyone's responsibility. Regardless of education level, job title, or position within the organization, everyone has the right to speak up about patient safety concerns and is supported when doing so. A culture that supports excellent teamwork and communication gives patients and caregivers alike an added layer of protection because there are more eyes and ears working synergistically to identify and eliminate patient safety risks. Nurses are in an ideal position to contribute to this positive patient safety culture as we are often at the hub of patient care and interdisciplinary communication.

Another patient safety activity I worked on involved implementing a multi-hospital program focused on The Joint Commission's National Patient Safety Goals (NPSG). The goals of the program have been to enhance overall awareness of the NPSG, ensure a shared understanding of what the expectations are for each goal, clarify how each goal applies in clinical practice, measure performance, and act on opportunities to improve patient safety processes. A complementary part of the NPSG program has been to enhance patient, family, and visitor awareness of the NPSG by placing posters and cards explaining the goals in public areas of the hospitals. This is one way to encourage patients and families to ask questions and speak up about patient safety concerns—as we know, involving them is another valuable patient safety strategy.

My career path has continued to evolve, and I now practice as a clinical nurse specialist in a large acute care hospital, but patient safety is still very much a part of my work. As nurses and steadfast patient advocates, almost everything we do involves a component of providing safe care. From performing appropriate infection prevention measures, to correctly identifying every patient before administering every medication, to participating in a "time out" before a surgical or invasive procedure, nurses are on the front lines of patient safety. As the science of patient safety matures, I think nurses in all practice environments have an opportunity to take an active role in patient safety activities and programs. Nurses have the ability and responsibility to continually assess and identify actual and potential threats to patient safety, develop plans and processes to eliminate or minimize risks, evaluate effectiveness of patient safety activities, and act as role models and entrepreneurs in the area of patient safety. Together with our colleagues, patients, and families, we must be leaders in achieving the goal of providing patients the safest possible care.

Introduction

Ten years have passed since the Institute of Medicine (IOM) published *To Err Is Human: Building a Safer Health System*, a report that is considered a milestone in the history of patient safety (Ilan & Fowler, 2005). The report estimated that as many as 98,000 hospitalized patients die each year from errors in hospital care (IOM, 2000). It also illustrated that although human beings are not perfect and will continue to make errors, the responsibility lies with health care systems to identify processes leading to errors and design improvements to decrease errors, with the ultimate goal of mitigating and eliminating health care errors. Because professional nurses have the greatest amount of interaction with patients throughout the hospital stay, they are in a key position to identify and implement process improvements to enhance patient safety. Professional nurses have the ability to intercept medical errors as much as 90% of the time due to the frequency of interaction nurses have with patients (Lin & Liang, 2007; Tregunno, Jeffs, & McGillis Hall, 2009).

Patients across the United States continue to advocate for a safer health care delivery system, and practitioners continue to struggle with the provision of a safe health care delivery system. This chapter will focus on the central role of the nurse on regulatory requirements for patient safety, establishing and sustaining a culture of patient safety, and defining key processes to enhance patient safety.

Regulatory Overview

THE JOINT COMMISSION

As the *To Err Is Human* report was being released by the IOM, The Joint Commission (TJC) began its journey toward providing a safer health care system. In 1999, TJC's mission statement (Box 20-1) was revised to explicitly reference patient safety as a key initiative (TJC, 2009a, 2009b; TJC Online, 2009).

The Joint Commission continued pursuing patient safety by introducing the National Patient Safety Goals (NPSG) in 2002. The purpose of the NPSG is to promote patient safety improvements based on recommendations made from sentinel event alerts, the Sentinel Event Advisory Group, and review of current patient safety literature. NPSGs address the complex health care environment by providing specific requirements for a variety of settings, including ambulatory, behavioral health care, critical access hospitals, home care, hospital, laboratory, long-term care, and office-based surgery centers.

In 2002, the initial hospital goals consisted of six goals focused on patient identification; improvement of communication among caregivers; medication safety; elimination of wrong-site, wrong-patient, wrong-procedure surgery; safety of infusion pumps; and effectiveness of clinical alarm systems. Each year the goals are analyzed based on current trends in patient safety, and recommendations are made for goals to be retained, be revised, or moved to TJC standards (TJC, 2006). Accredited health care organizations are required to demonstrate ongoing NPSG compliance using specific requirements established by TJC. NPSG requirements are more prescriptive than TJC standards, but they do allow facilities flexibility

---

BOX 20-1	The Joint Commission Mission Statements

Mission Statement 1999
To continuously improve the safety and quality of care provided to the public through the provision of health care accreditation and related services that support performance improvement in health care organizations.

Mission Statement 2009
To continuously improve health care for the public, in collaboration with other stakeholders, by evaluating health care organizations and inspiring them to excel in providing safe and effective care of the highest quality and value.

in process implementation to meet the requirements (TJC, 2006).

In addition to NPSG requirements, TJC demonstrates its commitment to patient safety by providing guidance to health care delivery systems in a variety of efforts. These efforts include sentinel event policy, sentinel event alerts, patient safety advisory groups, universal protocol, office of quality monitoring, patient safety research, patient safety education, and Speak Up Initiative. Although TJC takes a multidisciplinary view of patient care, the professional nurse plays the central role in implementing many of the safety programs as the primary coordinator of patient care. Health care organizations rely on the professional nurse as a team leader to design process improvement with colleagues (e.g., pharmacy, respiratory therapy) to continuously meet NPSG requirements. Information on TJC's patient safety initiatives can be found at www.jointcommission.org/PatientSafety

U.S. DEPARTMENT OF HEALTH AND HUMAN SERVICES

The U.S. Department of Health and Human Services (DHHS) is the agency charged with protecting the health of all Americans and providing services for

TABLE 20-1	Department of Health and Human Services Resources for Patient Safety
Resource	**Website**
Agency for Healthcare Research and Quality (AHRQ)	www.ahrq.gov
Agency for Toxic Substances and Disease Registry (ATSDR)	www.atsdr.cdc.gov
Centers for Disease Control and Prevention (CDC)	www.cdc.gov
Centers for Medicare and Medicaid Services (CMS)	www.cms.hhs.gov
Food and Drug Administration (FDA)	www.fda.gov
Health Resources Services Administration (HRSA)	www.hrsa.gov
National Institutes of Health (NIH)	www.nih.gov
Substance Abuse and Mental Health Services Administration (SAMHSA)	www.samhsa.gov

those that cannot provide for themselves. As a part of this responsibility, the DHHS has initiated several programs with the specific goal of improving patient safety. Table 20-1 outlines agencies within DHHS that play key roles in defining and regulating patient safety initiatives. DHHS agencies work with the health care team to coordinate and collaborate on initiatives to improve the health and safety of Americans. The Agency for Healthcare Research and Quality (AHRQ) serves as the lead organization for quality of care and patient safety research (both the provision of research and the synthesis of published research evidence). One of the goals of AHRQ is to promote the use of evidence-based practice in everyday care. Therefore AHRQ partners with key regulatory agencies such as the Centers for Medicare and Medicaid (CMS), TJC, and other partners such as the National Quality Forum to move research into health care practice (Couig, 2005).

PATIENT SAFETY AND QUALITY IMPROVEMENT ACT OF 2005

Learning from health care errors is a foundational principle to mitigate and prevent future occurrences of errors. A key way of learning from errors is for practitioners and organizations to share information with others. Unfortunately, providers remain cautious about sharing information regarding errors and the lessons learned from those errors. This caution arises out of

fear of litigation, potential professional sanctions, and potential damage to professional reputations (Catalano, 2008). Recognizing the importance of designing systems to mitigate errors, the Patient Safety and Quality Improvement Act of 2005 was signed into law on July 29, 2005. The primary purpose of the act was to amend Title IX of the Public Health Service Act, encouraging a culture of safety by facilitating the sharing of information through patient safety organizations (PSOs) that are administered through AHRQ. PSOs create a secure environment where information can be shared, aggregated, and analyzed, thus improving patient care by identifying trends and patterns amenable to risk prevention and reduction and program improvement. Participation in a PSO is highly encouraged; in fact, many states require participation in a PSO in order to strengthen the state patient safety program.

The Patient Safety and Quality Improvement Act of 2005 is divided into three distinct divisions. First, all PSOs must be certified and meet patient safety criteria in order to influence the learning from numerous patient safety events. Second, PSOs must maintain strict confidentiality of patient safety work products. Patient safety work products are protected from any proceedings and legal actions against providers and health care facilities. Finally, PSOs report to the Secretary of Health and Human Services, who is then responsible to report to Congress all successful strategies that have reduced medical errors, thus increasing patient safety across the United States (Catalano, 2008).

The professional nurse is the primary advocate for the patient and is responsible for ensuring that all regulatory requirements are met during patient care activities. The professional nurse can identify key patient care process improvements to meet and exceed regulatory requirements. When key processes are not carried out as intended, the professional nurse has been described as the clinician on the "sharp end" of patient care or the clinician closest to the patient care delivery—thus often the last line of defense to potentially mitigate or avoid medical errors (Hughes, 2008).

Patient Safety Culture

Many industries have demonstrated success in reducing and preventing errors, not by changing processes but by changing the culture to maintain vigilance for detection of potential errors, analysis of actual errors when they occur, and addressing those errors. In organizations with a high focus on patient safety culture, the administrative team demonstrates an unyielding commitment to a safety culture by ensuring that appropriate organizational resources are dedicated to patient safety, including training, human resource policies, budget, and personnel (Feng, Bobay, & Weiss, 2008; IOM, 2000). The nurses in these organizations demonstrate a sense of personal responsibility and shared ownership for promoting a work environment supportive of patient safety (Armstrong, Laschinger, & Wong, 2009; Hughes, Chang, & Mark, 2009). Applying principles from industry partners such as aviation and nuclear power, health care has identified many key concepts fundamental to ensuring a culture of patient safety. Concepts central to the role of the professional nurse that will be explored in this chapter include establishing a just culture, building and sustaining a healthy work environment, and facilitating teamwork among colleagues (Leonard, Graham, & Taggart, 2004).

JUST CULTURE

Human factors science, simply stated, is the science of determining how human beings interact with the environment (e.g., devices, policies and procedures,

work space). Human factors research has assisted health care practitioners to shift focus when medical errors occur, from the individual person to the system or processes that led to the error. Despite several years working on human factors in health care, health care organizations continue to lack progress toward an error-free care delivery system. Many argue that this is a result of the fact that most organizations have not devoted adequate resources and attention to analyzing organizational and system processes but have continued to focus on the individual (Henriksen, Dayton, Keyes, Carayon, & Hughes, 2008; Kaissi, 2006). Focusing on the individual creates a culture of blame in which practitioners become more reluctant to report errors and failures of the system. To overcome the culture of blame and to increase organizational learning from health care errors, *just culture* philosophies are increasing across health care. Just culture philosophy encourages open and active reporting of errors and learning from mistakes, while holding practitioners and organizations accountable as indicated (Gorzeman, 2008; IOM, 2000).

There are two primary types of failures or errors within the health care literature. First is an *active failure,* which is an unsafe act committed by a clinician who is in direct contact with the patient—"the sharp end." The second type is a *latent failure,* which is a system problem that is not within the direct control of the clinician—for instance, poor system design, organizational structure, and policies and procedures, often referred to as the "blunt end" (Henriksen et al., 2008). Latent failures lead to organizational accidents or medical errors more often than do active failures. Latent failures in health care may include building design, communication, management/leadership, policies and procedures, and bypassed defenses or safeguards (Kaissi, 2006).

The fundamental challenge for health care organizations and nurses, in particular, is to move prevention of medical errors from a system focusing on active failures or the individual to a system approach focusing on latent failures or the organization. Organizations that have achieved inspiring safety records are referred to as *high reliability organizations* (HROs). An HRO is an organization that recommends systems to produce consistent results and to quickly detect deviations and/or potential errors within the system before the error reaches the patient (Hughes, 2008). A defining factor for an HRO is mindfulness, keeping all practitioners acutely aware of all processes that could potentially go wrong and ways to quickly identify and recover from errors when they occur.

There are five mindful processes that comprise the core of an HRO. As a key member of the health care team, the professional nurse has a key role in all five processes. First, the nurse must have a constant preoccupation with failure. Nurses must confidently share their inner voice of concern with the rest of the health care team. Often, prior to a patient becoming extremely unstable, a nurse has reported "a feeling" that something is not right with the patient. Unfortunately, many nurses do not confidently act on these concerns (Henriksen et al., 2008; Weick & Sutcliffe, 2001). Second, nurses must be reluctant to simplify interpretations and not accept conventional explanations that are obvious. The professional nurse who has strong collaborative relationships is in a position to facilitate the health care team's performance of thorough investigations when errors occur. Third, nurses must maintain situational awareness during all clinical exchanges. *Situational awareness,* term commonly used in the airline industry, means that the entire team demonstrates an understanding of all people's roles and responsibilities and of the progress the team is making toward the ultimate outcome. Nurses have a full understanding of the complex roles outside of their own role; therefore they serve as "clinical glue," helping the team maintain situational awareness. Fourth, nurses must be committed to resilience. *Resilience* is the ability to quickly recover when an error does occur, thus mitigating any adverse consequences of the error. Nurses continuously demonstrate their commitment to resilience in numerous ways—for example, maintaining supplies and equipment in key locations and maintaining continual competency in using such devices for the safety of their patients. Fifth, nurses in HROs show deference to expertise, allowing decisions to be made by those clinicians with the expertise, resources, and ability to assist the patient. HROs that demonstrate deference to expertise have less rigid hierarchical structure, and team members are treated with mutual respect. Typically, nurses can cite several examples of how misplaced deference is granted

to physicians; on the other hand, it is not uncommon for nurses to automatically assume that those with "less experience" are unable to make decisions for patients (Henriksen et al., 2008; Weick & Sutcliffe, 2001).

High reliability organizations place emphasis on strategies to develop a just culture where practitioners are encouraged to report errors and concerns free from blame, humiliation, and retaliation. Recently, critics have raised the concern that a blame-free culture is risky and could lead to unsafe clinical practice. However, the purpose of a just culture is to balance the need to learn from mistakes with the need to hold practitioners accountable (Marx, 2001). In a just culture, nurses are protected from disciplinary action both within the facility and within regulatory agencies when reporting injuries, errors, and near misses in which they are personally involved (Gorzeman, 2008). Such protection should not be granted in three important exceptions. These exceptions are criminal behavior (e.g., a nurse who treats a patient while under the influence of drugs or alcohol), active malfeasance (e.g., a nurse who actively or purposely violates safety protocols), and an injury or incident that has not been reported in a timely manner (IOM, 2004b).

HEALTHY WORK ENVIRONMENT

Fundamental to any patient safety culture is the work environment in which the nurse practices. Nursing literature supports the fact that unhealthy work environments lead to decreased quality outcomes of patient care and decreased nursing satisfaction, which can result in challenges to recruitment and retention of staff nurses (Aiken, Clarke, Sloane, Lake, & Cheney, 2008; Browne, 2009). Ironically, although patients come to health care facilities seeking an environment in which to heal, that very environment can often be toxic to the extent that patient safety is in jeopardy. Recognizing these concerns, after the release of the IOM's *To Err Is Human* report, the American Association of Critical-Care Nurses (AACN) began landmark work exploring the work environment of nursing staffs. As a result of the exploration, the AACN Healthy Work Environment Standards were introduced (AACN, 2005; Browne, 2009).

The AACN Healthy Work Environment Standards are divided into six areas (Table 20-2): skilled

TABLE 20-2	AACN Standards for Establishing and Sustaining Healthy Work Environments
Skilled communication	Nurses must be as proficient in communication skills as they are in clinical skills.
True collaboration	Nurses must be relentless in pursuing and fostering collaboration.
Effective decision making	Nurses must be valued and committed parties in making policy, directing and evaluating clinical care, and leading organizational operations.
Appropriate staffing	Staffing must ensure an effective match between patient needs and nurse competencies.
Meaningful recognition	Nurses must be recognized and must recognize others for the value each brings to the work of the organization.
Authentic leadership	Nurse leaders must fully embrace the imperative of a healthy work environment, authentically live it, and engage others in the achievement.

American Association of Critical-Care Nurses. (2005). AACN standards for establishing and sustaining healthy work environments: a journey to excellence. *American Journal of Critical Care, 14(3)*, 187–197.

communication, true collaboration, effective decision making, appropriate staffing, meaningful recognition, and authentic leadership. The standards provide a framework for nurses to establish and sustain a healthy work environment. They are not all-inclusive, and other factors such as regulatory requirements, unique clinical needs, and patient outcomes must be considered. The standards are interdependent; for example, in order for the environment to provide meaningful recognition, nurses must posses both skilled communication and authentic leadership (Good, 2009).

Key Processes

Once a healthy work environment and culture are established, nurses must engage key processes that are fundamental to patient safety. Depending on the maturity of the clinical practice environment, processes can range from basic to advanced concepts. For example, an immature environment/culture may need to focus first on basic teamwork and basic communication processes, whereas a mature environment may choose to focus on more advanced communication processes. An example of a more advanced concept is "Stop the Line," a communication process that has been adopted from the Toyota Production System into health care. In this process, all staff members are empowered to draw attention to any potential error. At Toyota, at the time a potential error is identified, any employee has

the authority to stop the production line; in the case of health care, all staff members have the authority to stop the procedure until clarification is sought and corrective action is taken if applicable. "Stop the Line" means more than merely stopping a procedure. The goal of this process is to establish a culture in which it is every team member's responsibility to speak up in order to identify and mitigate errors effectively (Liker & Meier, 2006; Leonard et al., 2004). Although this chapter will only focus on the processes of teamwork, communication, and clinical tools to support these processes, numerous processes exist and continue to be developed to enhance patient safety. Many of these tools can be found on the websites identified in Table 20-1, especially those of the AHRQ, CMS, and TJC.

TEAMWORK

The complexity and diversity of the health care team continue to transform at a rapid rate. Previously, the health care team consisted of the physician and the nurse; now a health care team may consist of the physician, nurse, pharmacists, therapists, dietitian, social workers, care coordinators, and others. Often, there is an automatic belief that when a group of individuals is referred to as a *team,* they will function as a team (i.e., communicating, collaborating) but this simply is not reality. The majority of traditional health care educational programs (nursing and medical alike) do not teach teamwork or collaboration in the basic curriculum or in postgraduate residencies and/or internships. Patient safety experts have demonstrated that patient safety increases when teamwork and collaboration skills are taught and empowered; when teamwork and collaboration are not present, medical errors will result (Leonard et al., 2004). Nursing leadership must take an active role in promoting a collaborative work environment where the nurse feels comfortable participating as an equal partner on the health care team (Clark, 2009; Hughes, 2008; Leonard et al., 2004). When nurses accept this responsibility, the patient will benefit from the teamwork and collaboration.

One of the more successful models for teamwork training was developed by the Agency for Healthcare Research and Quality (AHRQ) in partnership with the Department of Defense. Team Strategies and Tools to Enhance Performance and Patient Safety (TeamSTEPPS) is an evidence-based curriculum that integrates teamwork principles and skills in the entire health care team. TeamSTEPPS involves a three-phase approach to creating and sustaining a culture of safety. In Phase I, the institution conducts a pretraining assessment to determine readiness for the training. During Phase 2, the institution trains members of the health care team to become the onsite trainers for the curriculum. Phase 3 consists of the implementation and sustainment of the teamwork training across the institution. Teamwork training should begin initially in high-risk departments such as obstetrics, intensive care, or the operating room, and then progress to other departments until the entire organization has been trained. The initial departments should become leaders and role models to other areas and serve as change agents, promoting and sustaining the teamwork model of care delivery. The TeamSTEPPS curriculum is a flexible system that allows customization of materials to the institution or departmental needs. The curriculum consists of presentations, pocket guides, video vignettes, workshop materials, and a variety of case studies, all available on DVD/CD-ROM.

Beyond TeamSTEPPS, other teamwork training programs exist, each offering advantages and disadvantages to individual programs. For any teamwork training program, the primary element of success is the full support of nursing leadership, physician leadership, administration, and other informal change agents within the facility. Without this network of support, teamwork training will not be successful (Clark, 2009; Leonard et al., 2004).

COMMUNICATION

One of the primary trainable teamwork skills is communication, a foundational element to a healthy work environment and patient safety. Failures in communication continue to be the leading cause of preventable patient injuries and death according to TJC (2005). Common communication mistakes in health care include providing patient care with incomplete or missing information; poor patient hand-offs among nurses, physicians, and other clinical staff; failing to share known information; and making assumptions regarding patient outcomes and safety (Leonard et al., 2004). Communication is as critical to patient safety as having trained, competent staff; unfortunately, many clinicians, including nurses, struggle with this skill. The reasons for the challenges nurses experience with communication are numerous; one problem is inadequate education for staff nurses on how to communicate with other health care professionals. Despite efforts to remove hierarchical communication patterns, power struggles and hierarchy continue to exist, while the ever-changing health care environment becomes increasingly complex.

On a basic level, *communication* can be defined as the exchange of information from one individual to another; this exchange can be verbal or nonverbal. Nurses and physicians are educated to communicate in very different styles. Physicians are taught and expected to communicate in brief, succinct, problem-oriented styles. On the other hand, nurses are taught to communicate in narrative styles, describing an event or condition rather than using a focused approach. This has led to frustrations and miscommunications among nurses and physicians, putting the patient at risk for receiving suboptimal care (IOM, 2004a; Leonard et al., 2004; Nadzam, 2009; Scalise, 2006; Shojania, Fletcher, & Saint, 2006).

Enhancing communication among the health care team requires a systematic approach, beginning with establishing a health care culture that emphasizes open communication and proceeding with intentional training on communication strategies. As part of TJC's

TABLE 20-3	Structured Communication Strategies		
Strategy	**Key Features**	**Techniques**	**Uses**
Briefings	Briefings are structured interactions in which the team shares the goals of the procedure or shift to ensure all members have the current information regarding the patient's care.	When utilizing a briefing, always be concise in message delivery, involve the entire team, use first names, and make eye contact facing the individual(s) communicating.	This tool can be used in a variety of circumstances, including procedural areas, ambulatory care to develop a plan for the day's activities, as situations change, and during hand-offs. A "time-out" is one example of a briefing.
SBAR	SBAR represents a particular type of briefing by defining the specific information that is to be communicated during each patient interaction.	*Situation*—What is going on with the patient? *Background*—What is the clinical background? *Assessment*—What are the current patient assessment data? *Recommendation*—What should be done or what is needed?	This technique is especially helpful during nurse-to-physician interactions by assisting to bridge any potential communication style gaps. Other uses include hand-offs of patient information during critical times (i.e., after a rapid response call or code), interdisciplinary communication, and hand-offs post procedures.
Debriefing	Debriefings are constructive conversations held after an event or procedure in which the team can analyze activities to enhance organizational learning.	During the debriefing, utilize the following questions to guide the discussion: What went well? What should be done differently next time? Where there any system issues that impeded the success of the event, such as equipment, incomplete data, policies, and/or procedures? What did the team learn from the event? Who will accept the responsibility for following up on any system problems or other issues that need follow-up?	Debriefing conversations should be positive in nature, while maintaining specific focus to ensure that lessons learned can be identified.

Data from Institute of Medicine, 2004a; Leonard, Graham, & Taggard, 2004; Nadzam, 2009; and Simpson, James, & Knox, 2006.

National Patient Safety Goals, health care organizations are required to establish consistent processes and strategies to improve the effectiveness of communication. Each organization can choose to meet minimum requirements or elect to maximize communication opportunities to provide optimal patient safety.

Because of the variability in practitioner training, cultural issues, hierarchical concerns, and the critical nature of health care, utilization of structured communication techniques becomes essential to enhance the consistency of communication. *Structured communication techniques* offer the benefit of the entire team having a shared model through which to communicate, thus helping to reduce incidents of miscommunication. Table 20-3 outlines proven structured communication techniques to enhance communication among the health care team. In each of these techniques the professional nurse plays an essential role in the dialogue as both a facilitator and participator (IOM, 2004a; Leonard et al., 2004; Nadzam, 2009; Simpson, James, & Knox, 2006).

SUMMARY

Patients enter the hospital or other health care organizations at a time of great vulnerability. These patients expect safe, high-quality care from the health care team, whether the ultimate goal is being healed or being provided a dignified end-of-life experience. As a key member of the health care team, the professional nurse has the most interaction with a patient during the course of treatment. The nurse's ability to assess, identify problems, and plan, implement, and evaluate the care rendered to a patient has been shown to be directly linked to the outcomes the patient achieves. This places the professional nurse in a central role to keep patients safe.

In order for any health care worker to successfully keep patients safe, a culture of safety must exist in the organization. If an organization maintains a culture of safety, that organization is constantly examining existing and new processes to enhance patient safety through prevention, mitigation, and process improvement. The organization does this not because of regulatory requirements, but because of a desire to achieve the safest environment possible for its patients. The professional nurse is the essential advocate for the patient, continually examining all processes for improvements, identifying potential and actual errors to mitigate potential harm to the patient, and maintaining a just culture that offers the opportunity to learn from *any* event.

KEY POINTS

- The Joint Commission (TJC) introduced National Patient Safety Goals (NPSG) in 2002 to promote patient safety, addressing the complex health care environment by defining key safety requirements for all accredited organizations.
- The Agency for Healthcare Research and Quality (AHRQ) serves as the lead organization within the Department of Health and Human Services for research for quality of care and patient safety.

- Patient safety organizations (PSO) were created by the "Patient Safety and Quality Improvement Act of 2005 to provide a secure environment to share information surrounding adverse events to facilitate a safer health care environment.
- Just culture philosophy and practice encourages open and active reporting of errors and learning from mistakes, while holding practitioners and organizations accountable.
- Healthy work environment standards (HWE) are fundamental to a patient safety culture. HWE standards includes skilled communication, true collaboration, effective decision making, appropriate staffing, meaningful recognition, and authentic leadership.
- Teamwork skills must be taught just as any other clinical skill.
- Common communication mistakes in health care include incomplete or missing information, poor patient hand-offs among clinicians, and making assumptions regarding patients.

CRITICAL THINKING EXERCISES

1. As a charge nurse you are working with a team of nurses, patient care assistants (PCAs), and a secretary on a busy 3:00 to 11:00 PM shift on a 36-bed medical-surgical floor. During the shift, a new graduate RN reports to you that one of her patients is going to radiology for a CT scan with contrast. The patient has had periods of confusion, history of renal insufficiency, and is a high fall risk according to the hospital fall-risk scale. The graduate nurse reports that radiology is calling for the patient to come to the department. The graduate nurse states, "Why can't they just read the chart; the hand-off transfer document is too time consuming."

   a. Why is utilization of a hand-off process crucial to patient safety?
   b. How would you respond to this graduate nurse's concerns?

2. A 56-year-old patient was admitted to 2-West from PACU after an emergency appendectomy. The patient has a BMI of 42, prior history of sleep apnea treated with CPAP device at night, COPD, and diabetes mellitus. Approximately 1 hour after admission to the floor, the patients Spo_2 is 67%, HR is 102, BP is 96/40, and RR 42. The RN calls for the rapid response team (RRT) and crash cart. The ICU RRT RN reports to the patient's bedside.

a. What communication methods would be beneficial for the 2-West RN to use when giving "report" to the RRT RN?

b. After the patient is stabilized, discuss the benefits of the team participating in a debriefing.

3. Recognizing the importance of an HWE for patient safety, Kim RN approaches her unit-based shared leadership team with the idea to implement the HWE standards as outlined by AACN. Many of the team recognizes the important role that these standards have in improving the health of the unit, but others remain skeptical.

a. Discuss the importance of engaging a multidisciplinary team in the implementation of HWE.

b. Which standard do you feel would be most important to begin with on the journey?

4. During two separate root cause analysis meetings on a high-risk obstetrics unit, lack of teamwork, specifically communication, was identified as the root cause for two adverse patient events. The medical director, patient safety officer, and nurse manager begin discussions on how to improve communication and teamwork in this highly complex environment.

a. What initial steps should this team consider to assess the team and environment?

b. Describe key learning points from TeamSTEPPS and/or crew resource management that would be beneficial for this team to implement.

c. What additional resources would be needed by this team?

REFERENCES

Agency for Healthcare Research and Quality. (n.d.) TeamSTEPPS National Implementation. [Online]. Retrieved December 19, 2009, from http://teamstepps.ahrq.gov/index.htm

Aiken, L. H., Clarke, S. P., Sloane, D. M., Lake, E. T., & Cheney, T. (2008). Effects of hospital care environment on patient mortality and nurse outcomes. *Journal of Nursing Administration*, 38(5), 223–229.

American Association of Critical-Care Nurses. (2005). AACN standards for establishing and sustaining healthy work environments: a journey to excellence. *American Journal of Critical Care*, 14(3), 187–197.

Armstrong, K., Laschinger, H., & Wong, C. (2009). Workplace empowerment and magnet hospital characteristics as predictors of patient safety climate. *Journal of Nursing Care Quality*, 24(1), 55–62.

Browne, J. A. (2009). Healthy workplaces and ethical environments: a staff nurse's perspective. *Critical Care Nursing Quarterly*, 32(3), 253–261.

Catalano, K. (2008). Proposed regulations for enforcement of the patient safety and quality improvement act of 2005. *Plastic Surgical Nursing*, 28(2), 96–98.

Clark, P. R. (2009). Teamwork: building healthier workplaces and providing safer patient care. *Critical Care Nursing Quarterly*, 32(3), 221–231.

Couig, M. P. (2005). Patient safety: A priority in the US Department of Health and Human Services. *Nursing Administration Quarterly*, 29(1), 88–96.

Feng, X., Bobay, K., & Weiss, M. (2008). Patient safety culture in nursing: a dimensional concept analysis. *Journal of Advanced Nursing*, 63(3), 310–319.

Good, V. S. (2009). The critical care environment. In K. Carlson (Ed.), *Advanced critical care nursing*. St. Louis: Saunders.

Gorzeman, J. (2008). Balancing just culture with regulatory standards. *Nursing Administration Quarterly*, 32(4), 308–311.

Henriksen, K., Dayton, E., Keyes, M. A., Carayon, P., & Hughes, R. (2008). Understanding adverse events: A human factors framework. In R. G. Hughes (Ed.), *Patient safety and quality: An evidence-based handbook for nurses*. (Vol.#1 AHRQ Publication NO. 08-0043). Rockville, MD: Agency for Healthcare Research and Quality.

Hughes, L. C., Chang, Y., & Mark, B. A. (2009). Quality and strength of patient safety climate on medical-surgical units. *Health Care Management Review*, 34(1), 19–28.

Hughes, R. G. (2008). Nurses at the 'Sharp End' of patient care. (pp. 1–7-1–35). In R. G. Hughes, (Ed.), *Patient safety and quality: An evidence-based handbook for nurses*. AHRQ (Vol. 1). Publication No. 08-0043. Rockville, MD: Agency for Healthcare Research and Quality.

Ilan, R., & Fowler, R. (2005). Brief history of patient safety culture and science. *Journal of Critical Care*, 20(1), 2–5.

Institute of Medicine. (2000). *To err is human: Building a safer health system*. Washington, DC: National Academy Press.

Institute of Medicine. (2004a). *Keeping patients safe: Transforming the work environment of nurses*. Washington, DC: National Academy Press.

Institute of Medicine. (2004b). *Patient safety: Achieving a new standard for care*. Washington, DC: National Academy Press.

The Joint Commission. (2006). Introduction to National Patient Safety Goals. [Online]. Retrieved December 8, 2009, from http://www.jointcommission.org/PatientSafety/NationalPatientSafetyGoals/npsg_intro.htm

The Joint Commission. (2009a). A journey through the history of the Joint Commission. [online]. Retrived December 8, 2009, from http://www.jointcommission.org/AboutUs/joint_commission_history.htm

The Joint Commission. (2009b). Facts about patient safety. [online]. Retrived December 8, 2009, from http://www.jointcommission.org/GeneralPublic/PatientSafety.

The Joint Commission on Accreditation of Healthcare Organizations. (2005). *Sentinel event statistics*. Oak Brook, IL: Author.

The Joint Commission Online. (2009). The Joint Commission updates its mission, creates vision statement. Retrieved December 8, 2009, from http://www.jointcommission.org/NR/rdonlyres/2F04C126-906D-4155-B16F-1F1A6570C387/0/jconlineAug1209.pdf

Kaissi, A. (2006). An organizational approach to understanding patient safety and medical errors. *Health Care Manager*, 25(4), 292–305.

Leonard, M., Graham, S., & Taggart, B. (2004). The human factor: Effective teamwork and communication in patient strategy. In M. Leonard, et al.(Eds.). *Achieving safe and reliable healthcare: Strategies and solutions.* Chicago: Healthcare Administration Press.

Liker, J. K., & Meier, D. (2006). *The Toyota way fieldbook: A practical guide for implementing Toyota's 4Ps*. New York: McGraw-Hill.

Lin, L., & Liang, B. A. (2007). Addressing the nursing work environment to promote patient safety. *Nursing Forum*, 42(1), 20–30.

Marx, D. (2001). *Patient safety and the "Just Culture": A Primer for health care executives.* Funded by a grant from the National Heart, Lung, and Blood Institute, National Institutes of Health (Grant RO1 HL 53772, Harold S. Kaplan, M.D., Principle Investigator). New York, NY: Trustees of Columbia University.

Nadzam, D. M. (2009). Nurses' role in communication and patient safety. *Journal of Nursing Care Quality*, 24(3), 184–188.

Scalise, D. (2006). Clinical communication and patient safety. *Hospitals & Health Networks*, 80(8), 49–54.

Shojania, K. G., Fletcher, K. E., & Saint, S. (2006). Graduate medical education and patient safety: A busy—and occasionally hazardous—intersection. *Annals of Internal Medicine*, 145(8), 592–598.

Simpson, K. R., James, D. C., & Knox, G. E. (2006). Nurse-physician communication during labor and birth: Implications for patient safety. *Journal of Obstetric, Gynecologic, & Neonatal Nursing*, 35(4), 547–556.

Tregunno, D., Jeffs, L., & McGillis Hall, L. (2009). On the ball: Leadership for patient safety and learning in critical care. *Journal of Nursing Administration*, 39(7/8), 334–339.

Weick, K., & Sutcliffe, K. (2001). *Managing the unexpected: assuring high performance in an age of complexity.* San Francisco: Jossey-Bass.

Index

A

Abstraction level, of theories, 100
Abuse Assessment Screen (AAS), 389
Abuse. *See also* Domestic violence
Accessibility, of nursing program, 35
Accident, as cause of death, 374
Accountability
  attributes of, 274
  of nurses, 53
Accreditation
  definition of, 33–34
  master's degree and, 34
Acquired immunodeficiency syndrome (AIDS), 256
Active failure, 411
Active learning, 226
Active listening
  focus of, 190
  selective attention and habituation in, 190
  silence and, 190
  therapeutic responses and, 190
Acute care nurse practitioner (ACNP) program, 17
Acute care nurse specialist, 16–17
Adaptation, 104
Adaptation model, 103–104
  assumptions about the individual, 104
  concepts of, 104
    adaptative system, 104
    adaptive level, 104
    adaptive modes, 104
  environment and, 104
  health and illness, 104
  nursing and, 104
  overview of, 103
  theoretical perspectives, comparison of, 111t
Adaptive level, determination of
  contextual stimuli, 104
  focal stimulus, 104
  residual stimuli, 104
Adaptive model, 331–332

Adaptive modes
  physiological as, 104
  role function as, 104
  self-concept as, 104
Adaptive system, control process of
  cognator subsystem, 104
  regulator subsystem, 104
Adjourning phase, of groups, 196
Adjudicatory power, 246
Administrative law, 243
  in nursing, 243–247
Administrative model, 63
Adolescent
  human papilloma virus vaccine in
    benefits of, 282–283
    in boys, 283
  sleep need in, 340
  smoking in, 338–340
  tobacco advertisements for, 131
  as vulnerable population, 394
Adult learner, adragogy and, 55
Advance directive, 283
Advanced nurse specialist, 82
  advanced practice nurse as, 82–83
Advanced practice nursing
  in clinical setting, 16–18
  critical elements of, 82f
  laws governing, 245
  role of, 82–83
  as specialist, 82–83
Advocacy
  definition of, 273
  economic concepts for, 161–173
  importance of, 80
  nursing and, 80–81, 143–144
  nursing ethics and, 273–274
  for patient safety, 409
  purpose of, 80
  values-based decision model for, 273–274

Page numbers followed by b, t, and f indicate boxes, tables, and figures, respectively.

Advocate, nurse as, 80–81
Aesthetics, 47
Affective learning objective, 235
African American
    HIV in, 320–321
    respecting authority, 234
African American nurse, 8, 13f
    ANA membership and, 13
    in Cadet Nurse Corps, 12
    education for, 12
Agency for Healthcare Research and Quality, 132
    National Healthcare Disparities Report by, 401
    teamwork training by, 414
Aggregated information resources, 304
Agriculture. *See* Department of Agriculture
Allan, Janet, 132
Allele, 357b
Allostasis, 344–345
Allostatic load, 344–345
Altruism, 50
America' Health Insurance Plans (AHIP), 81
American, diversification in, 322–323
American Association of Colleges of Nursing (AACN)
    clinical nurse leader and, 17–18, 81
    membership in, 66
    mission of, 66
    origin of, 66
    programs through, 66
    role of, 11
American Association of Critical Care Nurses (AACCN)
    healthy work environment and, 412, 413t
    nursing education and, 133
    role of, 16–17
American Civil War, 7–8
American Dental Association (ADA), expert testimony by, 133
American Diabetes Association (ADA), tele-educational unit and, 295
American Medical Association (AMA), 10
    expert testimony by, 133
American Nurses Association
    accountability interpretation by, 274
    African American nurse membership in, 13
    code of ethics for, 45, 49, 264b, 267, 363
    expert testimony by, 133
    health policy and, 118–119
    informatics and, 290
    membership in, 64
    mission of, 64
    nurse recruitment/retention, 159
    nursing process and, 206
    nursing roles, expanding, 179
    online resources by, 306–307
    origin of, 64
    political action committees for, 121
    programs through, 64
    Social Policy Statement of, 269

American Nurses Credentialing Center (ANCC), 133
American Psychological Association (APA), 308
American Public Health Association (APHA), expert testimony by, 133
American Red Cross
    disaster nursing through, 255–256
    volunteer nurses' aides program and, 11–12
Americans with Disabilities Act (ADA), 247
Analysis/diagnosis, nursing process and, 206, 206t, 208
Analyticity, 214
Andragogy, 55
Anger
    management of, 341
    suppression of, 341
    wellness and, 340–341
Applied ethics, 262
Apprenticeship model of nursing, 4
Appropriation bill, 127–128
Asian population, "saving face," 234
ASKED, 325, 325b
Assault, 251–253
    against women, 386
Assessment, nursing process and, 206
    data
        sources of, 207
        types of, 207
    data collection
        instruments for, 207–208
        techniques for, 207
    nurse-client/nurse-family relationship, 208
Associate degree in nursing (ADN), 26, 31t–32t
    focus of, 81
    recommendations for, 36
    strengths of, 36
    weaknesses of, 36
Association for Women's Health (AWH), 133
Asynchronous learning, 232
Attitude, critical thinking competency, 211
Australian Triage Scale (ATS), 295–296
Authorization bill, 127
Autonomous nursing practice, 62
Autonomy
    children and, 272
    definition of, 47, 53
    as ethical principle, 270–272
    factors limiting, 48
    internal/external constraints on, 271
    in nursing, 53
    as self-determination, 271
Autonomy struggle, 196
Avatar, 239

B

Baccalaureate nursing program, 14, 31t–32t
    accelerated program for, 25
    competency areas for, 52–53

Baccalaureate nursing program (Continued)
  faculty for, 25
  focus of, 81
  history of, 25
  length and components of, 25
  NCNAC and CCNE, 133
  recommendations for, 37
  RN-BSN track for, 25
  strengths of, 36–37
  weaknesses of, 37
Background information, 299–300
Balanced Budget Act, 127
  purpose of, 129
  SCHIP and, 136
Bandura, Albert, 113
Barrier
  to health care, 324b
  to professionalism, 47–49
Battery, 251–253
Beck, Dr. Cornelia, 141–142
Behavior
  contract for change in, 343f, 343b
  for disease prevention, 332
  interventions promoting change in, 341–343
  knowledge changing, 228–229
  modification of, 332–341
  values guiding, 88–89
Behavioral outcome, as measurable, 209t
Behaviorism, 225
Behaviorist theory
  learning principles/teaching applications relating
      to, 225t
  teaching and, 225
Beneficence
  definition of, 269–270
  principle of, application of, 269
Benner's novice-to-expert model, 59
Bergstrom, Nancy, 132, 142
Betts, Virginia Trotter, 132
Bias
  definition of, 320
  management of, 320
Bibliographical database, 301t
  links to full texts in, 304
Bibliographical management tool, 308
Biculturalism, 56
Bill
  authorization, 127
  passing and killing, 123
Biobehavioral intervention, 141–142
Biological age, chronological age
      versus, 342
Biomedical information, 304
Black nurses, 8
Blind, Johari window as, 188–189

Blue Cross health plan
  AMA opposition of, 10
  development of, 9–10
Bolton, Frances Payne, 12
Brady Bill gun control legislation, 127
Breach of duty, 251
Breaux, Senator John, 131–132
Brewster, Mary, 7
Briefing, 415t
Broad-purpose association, 63
Brooten, Dorothy, 132
Budget
  crisis management for, 126–127
  fund appropriation for, 126–127
  process for, 126
Budget bill
  federal government and, 127–128
  House of Representatives and, 125
Buerhaus, Peter, 132
Bureau of Census, 130
Bureau of Health and Medicaid Services (BHP), 128
Bureaucracy, nurse and, 59
Bureaucratic organization
  characteristics of, 61t
  conflict in, 59

C
Cadet Nurse Corps
  African American nurses in, 12
  establishment of, 12
  World War II and, 11–12
California Critical Thinking Disposition Inventory (CCTDI), 216
Campaign, financing for, 122
Campinha-Bacote, Dr. Josepha, 326
Campinha-Bacote Model of cultural competence, 317
Capital inputs, 153
Capitated cost, under Medicare, 136–138
Capps, Lois, 143
Care sphere, 205–206
Career development
  Dalton's longitudinal model of, 59
  socialization and, 58–59
Caregiver, 75–77
Caregiving, 49–50
Caring
  cultural care theory and, 109
  ethics of, 275
  Watson's philosophy and science of, 105–106
    assumptions about the individual, 106
    concepts of, 106
    environment and, 106
    health and illness, 106
    nursing and, 106
    overview of, 106
    theoretical perspectives, comparison of, 111t

Caritas processes, 106
Carmona, Dr. Richard H., 131
Carpenito, Lynda, 342
Carrier testing, 361
Causation, 251
Census Bureau, 130
  rural classification by, 370–371
Centers for Disease Control (CDC), 141
Centers for Medicare and Medicaid Services (CMS), 128, 130
Centura St. Anthony Hospital North, 256
Certification
  purpose of, 34–35
  types of, 34
Change theory, 226
Charting, rules of, 252b
Children
  autonomy and, 272
  dental health in, 374
  immunization rates for, 374
  intimate partner violence and, 388
  obesity in, 338
  sleep need in, 340
Children's Bureau, 7
Children's Health Insurance Program, 129
Chromosome
  definition of, 357b
  inherited disease and, 357
Chronological age, biological age versus, 342
CINAHL database
  clinical practice guidelines in, 304
  information in, 300
  MeSH and, 300–301
  sample record in, 302b
  sample search in, 303f
  search strategies for, 302–304
Citation, of database, 300–301
Clarification, 191, 191b
Clinical autonomy, 62
Clinical Care Classification (CCC), 297–298
Clinical decision support system (CDSS), 295–296
Clinical documentation, 292–293
Clinical judgment
  case analysis for, 275–279
  critical thinking model for, 211–212
  nursing process and, 200
Clinical model/medical model, 331
Clinical nurse, health system quality of care and, 169
Clinical nurse leader (CNL), 17–18
  AACN and, 81
  education for, 17–18
    concept for, 28
  role of, 28
Clinical practice guidelines
  in CINAHL database, 304
  critical appraisal and, 304–305

Clinical practice guidelines (Continued)
  on Internet, 304
  links to full texts in, 304
Closed information processing, 321f
Closure, 190
Clothing style, professionalism and, 48
Coaching, 57
Code of ethics
  AMA and, 49
  provisions and concepts for, 51
Cognator subsystem, 104
Cognitive competency, 211
Cognitive dissonance theory, 226
Cognitive learning objective, 235
Cognitive theory, 226
  learning principles/teaching applications relating to, 226t
Collaboration
  definition of, 77, 274
  lessons in, 77
Collaborative learning, 228
Colleague
  collaboration with, 77
  nurse as, 77
Collective bargaining, 248–249
Collegiate nursing education, 11
  Florence Nightingale and, 23–24
Colorblind, 320–322
Colorectal cancer screening, 143
Columbia University Teachers College, nursing theory birth at,
  15–16
Commission on Collegiate Nursing Education (CCNE), 33
Committee for Disaster Medicine Reform (CDMR), 256–257
Common law, 243, 251–252
Communication
  active listening and, 190
  adverse factors affecting, 195
    autonomy struggles as, 196
    interprofessional understanding, lack of, 196
    role stress as, 195–196
  clarification and, 191, 191b
  cultural barriers to, 284
  definition of, 187, 414
  dose of, 193
  interpersonal, 189–194
  interprofessional understanding, lack of, 196
  intrapersonal, 188–189
  Johari window and, 188–189, 188t
  nonverbal behavior as, 192
  organizational, 194–198
  patient entrusting and, 194
  pragmatic competence in, 188
  professional-to-professional, 195
  questioning in, 192
  reflection and, 191, 191b
  restatement and, 191, 191b

Communication *(Continued)*
  silence and, 190
  skills and techniques for, 186
  structured strategies for, 415–416, 415t
  summarization in, 191–192
  teamwork training and, 414
  therapeutic responses in, 190–192
  timing for, 193–194
  validation in, 191
Communication theory, 187
Community college nursing program, 14–15
Community decision-making model, 380
Community health nursing
  development of, 7
  social reform through, 7
Community health promotion, 346–347
Community intervention, 346
Compassion, 75
Competency
  critical thinking model and, 211
  in genetic testing, 279–280
Competition, restrictions on, 155
Complement
  definition of, 159
  nurse as, 159–161
Complexity, principle of, 175
Compliance program, 249
Computers on wheels (COW), 292
Concept
  definition of, 97
  nursing theory and, 97–100
Conceptual theory, 100
Cone of experience theory, 228t
Cone of learning theory, 228
Confidentiality
  breach of, 255
  electronic health record and, 293–294
  HIPAA and, 192–193
  in rural populations, 379
Conflict resolution, 56
Congress
  Balanced Budget Act and, 127
  committee structure for, 125
  rules for administration and governance in, 123
  sessions for, 125
  Social Security Trust Fund and, 128
Congressional model, 63
Consensus, in groups, 196
Consideration, 247–248
Constitutional directive, 125
Constitutional law, 243
Constructivism, 226
Consumer health information, 305
Consumerism, 177–178
Continuous creation, principle of, 175

Contract
  for behavior change, 343b
  consideration in, 247–248
  definition of, 247
  example of, 343f
  for exercise, 342–343
  statute of frauds for, 248
Contract law, 243
  nursing and, 247–248
Cooperation, 274
Cooperative learning, 228
Co-payment, 162
Core sphere, 205–206
Cornell Critical Thinking Test (CCTT), 216
Coronary care unit (CCU), 16
Cost, of nursing education, 30
Cost agreement, 136–138
Cost containment, quality of care and, 168–169
Cost-benefit analysis, 172b–173b
Cost-consequence analysis, 172b–173b
Cost-effectiveness analysis, 172b–173b
Cost-minimization analysis, 172b–173b
Cost-utility analysis, 172b–173b
Councilor model, 63
Crime, 256
Crimean War, 3–4
Criminal law, 243
Crisis management, for budget achievement,
    126–127
Critical access hospital (CAH), 377
Critical reflection, 215
Critical thinker
  characteristics of, 213
  traits of, 213
Critical thinking
  application of, 217–218
  characteristics of, 205
  cognitive skills/subskills for, 204
  curriculum for teaching, 215
  definition of, 202–204, 205t
  disposition toward, 213–214
  functions of, 202–203
  levels of, 212–213
  in nursing, 204–205
  nursing process and, 200, 204–205, 206t
  requirements for, 212–213
  research in, 216–217
  skills for, 203
  strategies to enhance, 214
Critical thinking measures, 216
Critical thinking model, 205f
  components of, 211–212
    attitude, 211
    competency, 211
    experience, 211

Critical thinking model *(Continued)*
    knowledge, 211
    standards, 211–212, 212f
Cross-sectional study, in critical thinking, 217
Cultural assessment, 324
    aspects of, 325
Cultural care, 109
    approaches for, 325b
Cultural care accommodation, 109
Cultural care diversity, 109
Cultural care preservation/maintenance, 109
Cultural care repatterning/restructuring, 109
Cultural care theory, 108–109
    assumptions about the individual, 108
    concepts of, 109
        care, 109
        caring, 109
        cultural care, 109
        cultural-congruent care, 109
        culture, 109
    environment and, 108–109
    health and illness, 109
    nursing and, 109
    overview of, 108
    theoretical perspectives, comparison of, 111t
Cultural care universality, 109
Cultural competence
    ASKED and, 325, 325b
    Campinha-Bacote Model of, 317
Cultural diversity
    in health care plan, 316
    in language, 188
    sensitivity in, 316
Cultural assessment strategies, 325–326
Cultural-congruent care, 109
Culturally Competent Nursing Modules, 323–324
Culture, 109
    wellness and, 344
Cumulative risk, 397–398
Cure sphere, 205–206

D

Dale, Edgar, 228, 228t
Dalton's longitudinal model, 59
Damages, 251
Data
    sources of, 207
    types of, 207
Data collection
    instruments for, 207–208
    techniques for, 207
Database
    bibliographical, types and descriptions of, 301t
    CINAHL as, 300
    citation of, 300–301

Death
    femicide and, 387–388
    leading cause of, 332b
    unintentional injuries/accidents as cause of, 374
Debriefing, 87–88, 415t
Decision-making tool
    definition of, 268
    as ethical, 268
    as frameworks, 268
Deductible, 162
Delano, Jane, 8
Delphi research project
    critical thinking and, 203
        definition of, 215
        for nurses, 204
    ideal critical thinker, 213
Demand, 156
Demonstration, as teaching format, 236
Dental health, in rural communities, 374
Deoxyribonucleic acid (DNA), 357b
Department of Agriculture, 130
Department of Veterans Affairs, 132
Depression. *See* Economic depression
Descriptive practice theory, 100
Developmental theory, 113
Diagnostic testing, 361
Diagnostic-related group (DRG), 136–138
Dilemma, 263
Diploma nursing program, 31t–32t
    history of, 23–24
    length of, 24
    number of, 24
    recommendations for, 36
    strengths of, 36
    weaknesses of, 36
Directing, 57
Direct-to-consumer genetic testing, 362–363
Direct-to-consumer marketing (DTCM), of drugs and tests, 280b
Disaster Medicine Reform, Committee for, 256–257
Disaster nursing, 255–256
Discretionary health care program, 128–129
Disease, vulnerable populations and, 397–398
Disease prevention, health promotion and, 332
Distance education, for nursing, 35
Diversity
    in America, 322–323
    definition of, 315–316
    in health, 315–322
    in health and illness, 312
    in health care providers, 319
    management of, 320
Doctor of nursing practice, 17–18
Doctoral education in nursing
    disciplines for, 28–29
    pathways for, 29

Doctoral education in nursing *(Continued)*
  practice-focused program for, 29–30
  recommendations for, 37
  research-focused program for, 29
  strengths of, 37
  weaknesses of, 37
Documentation
  purpose of, 252–253
  rules of, 252b
  types of, 292–293
Doe v. Roe, 255
Domain-specific knowledge, 211
Domestic violence. *See also* Intimate partner violence
  history of, 386
  in rural communities, 374
Double helix, 357b
Downward communication, 195
Drama, as role-playing, 231
Drug discount card, 136
Drugs
  direct-to-consumer marketing of, 280b
  response to, 362
Dual decision making, 296
Due process, 246
Dunn, Halpert, 330–331
Duty, 250–251
Duty-based ethics, 264
Dyad, 75

E
Economic depression
  Blue Cross and, 10
  effects of, 9–10
Economic theory
  application of, 174
  concepts of, 153
  supply and demand, 156
Economics, 128
  definition of, 153
  nurses and principles of, 152
  principles of, 154b
  scarce resources, distribution of, 155
Education. *See also* Nursing education
  accreditation of, 140–141
  socialization through, 54–56
Educator, nurse as, 78–79
EDUCAUSE Center for Applied Research (ECAR), 232
Electronic health record
  implementation of, 293
  information in, 292
  issues in, 293
  key standards for, 293
  laboratory/pharmacy systems and, 292–293
  privacy, confidentiality and security in, 293–294
Emergency spending, 127

Emergent competition, principle of, 175
Emotion management, 340–341
Empathy
  caring and, 76–77
  nurse educator and, 78
Empirics, 47
Employer-sponsored group insurance, 163
Employment
  compliance programs in, 249
  government employee, 249
  of graduate nurse, 6
  in health care, 156
  healthy environment for, 412–413
  labor law, 248–249
  nurse flexibility in, 156
  of private duty nurse, 5–6
  of registered nurse, 6
  in rural communities, 372
  social class and, 402
Employment at will, 248
Employment law, 247–249
  contract law, 247–248
Empowerment, 69
Energy field
  characteristics of, 102
  types of
    environmental, 102
    human, 102
Enforceable contract, 247–248
Entitlement health care program
  budget for, 128
  types of, 129
Environment
  definition of, 97–100
  as infection source, 100
  for learning, 228–229
  science of unitary human beings and, 101
Environmental energy field, 102
Environmental theory
  assumptions about the individual, 100
  concepts of, 101
  Florence Nightingale and, 100–101
  health and illness, 101
  nursing and, 101
  overview of, 100
  theoretical perspectives, comparison of, 111t
Erikson, Erik, 113
Error
  in health care literature, 411
  reduction/prevention of, 411
  resilience to, 412
Esprit de corps, 196
Essential Nursing Resource list, 299–300
Ethical, Legal and Social Implications (ELSI) program, 363–364
Ethical judgment, 275–279

Ethical nursing practice, 265–279
Ethical organizational culture
    recommendations for, 90b
    role incongruity and, 89–90
Ethical principle
    accountability as, 274
    autonomy as, 270–272
    beneficence as, 269–270
    communication and, 284
    cooperation and collaboration as, 274–275
    definition of, 268–269
    issues and problems in, 279–284
    justice as, 270
    in problem-solving process, 269
    reasoning and, 269
    veracity as, 272–273
Ethics, 47
    American Nurses Association and, 49, 264, 264b, 267, 363
    applied, 262
    of caring, 275
    decision-making tools as, 268
    International Council of Nurses (ICN) and, 264
    in nursing, 263–265
    overview of, 261–262
    preventive, 283–284
    professional, 262–263
    steps in decision-making, 276t
    virtue-based versus duty-based, 264
Ethnic diversity, 322–323
Ethnic minority enrollment, in nursing education, 38
Ethnicity, 320
Eudaemonistic model, 332
Eunice Kennedy Shriver NICHD, 141
Euthanasia, nurses charged with, 256
Evaluation
    methods of
        formative, 237
        peer, 237
        summative, 237
    nursing process and, 206, 206t
        definition of, 210
        guidelines for, 211
        occurrence of, 210
    of teaching-learning experience, 237
Evidence, 251
Evidence-based nursing, 305
Exercise
    as role-playing, 237
    wellness and, 337–338
    writing prescription/contract for, 342–343
Experience, critical thinking model and, 211
Experience theory, cone of, 228t
Experiential knowledge, 211
Expert testimony, 133
Express contract, 247

External constraints, on autonomy, 271
External evidence, 305
External locus of control, 334
Extrapersonal stressor, 105
Extreme poverty, 401
Eye contact
    meaning of, 192
    as nonverbal behavior, 192

F
Facial expression, 192
Failure to rescue, 170
Faith Clinic, 256
Faith in reason, 213
False imprisonment, 254–255
Familial status, in rural communities, 372
Family history
    for genetics and genomics, 359–360
    pedigree/standardized symbols for, 360, 360f
Family Medical Leave Act (FMLA), 85
Family Violence Prevention Fund, 389
Federal agency, 130
Federal Elections Commissions (FEC), 122
Federal Funding Accountability and Transparency Act, 129
Federal government
    appropriation/budget bills and, 127–128
    health care, role in, 129
Federal health care program, 128–129
Federally Qualified Health Center (FQHC), 377
Femicide, 387–388
Fiduciary, nurse-patient relationship as, 267
Financial assistance, for nursing education, 30
Financing, legislation and, 122–123
Follower, directing and coaching of, 57
Fontaine, Dorrie, 77
Food and Drug Administration (FDA), health policy and, 118–119
Food Pyramid Guide, 338
Ford, Loretta, 17
Forecasting model, 157b, 158f
Formal teaching-learning, 228
Formative evaluation, 237
Forming phase, of groups, 196
Foundation, health policy and planning, 132
Framework, 100
    decision-making tools as, 268
Frances Payne Bolton School of Nursing, 29–30
Frist, Senator Bill, 131–132
Frontier, 370–371
Frontier Nursing Service, 17
Fugate-Woods, Nancy, 132
Funding
    appropriation of, 126–127
    legislation and, 121–122
    modes of, 122–123
    for states, types of, 125–126

G

Gatekeeper, nurse as, 324
Gene
    definition of, 357b
    role of, 357–358
General adaptation syndrome, 113
General critical thinking competency, 211
General systems theory, 112
Generation Y, 232
Genetic counseling, referral for, 361–362
Genetic disorder
    definition of, 357b
    family history and, 360
Genetic Information Nondiscrimination Act (GINA), 136
    limitations of, 365
    purpose of, 365
Genetic literacy, 279
Genetic nursing
    categories of, 358
    competency strategies for, 358–359
    development of, 358
    educational resources for, 359b
Genetic specialist
    resources for, 362
    role of, 361
Genetic testing, 279–280, 281b–282b
    availability for, 361
    direct-to-consumer, 362–363
    Internet and, 362–363
    nurse role in, 361
    personalized medicine and, 362–363
    purpose of, 357–358
    types of
        carrier testing, 361
        diagnostic testing, 361
Genetics
    definition of, 357b
    discrimination based on, 365
    ethical issues in, 363–365
    history of, 357
    in nursing, 354, 359–362
    resources for, 364b
Genomic health care, 356
Genomic medicine, 136
Genomic nursing
    categories of, 358
    competency strategies for, 358–359
    development of, 358
    educational resources for, 359b
Genomic research, 362–363
    social, cultural and religious issues in, 363–364
Genomic testing, personalized medicine and, 362–363
Genomics
    definition of, 357b
    discrimination based on, 365

Genomics *(Continued)*
    ethical issues in, 363–365
    in nursing, 354, 359–362
    resources for, 364b
Gesture, arm and hand, 192
Gettis, Debbie, 132
Gilligan, Carol, 75
Goal attainment theory, 107–108
    assumptions about the individual, 107
    concepts of, 108
        nurse-client relationship, 108
    environment and, 107
    health and illness, 108
    nursing and, 108
    overview of, 107
    theoretical perspectives, comparison of, 111t
Goal-directed interpersonal model, 107
"Good" nurse
    characteristics of, 263
    concept of, 263
Good Samaritan Acts, 255–256
Goodrich, Annie, 5
Government employee, 249
Government Performance and Results Act, 129
Government subsidies, in health care, 155–156
Government-sponsored insurance, 164
Graduate nurse
    employment of, 6
    professional identity of, 55
Graduate nurse. *See also* Registered nurse
Graduate nursing program, 15–16
Gramm-Rudman-Hollings law, 127
Grand theory, 100–106
Great War, 8
Gross domestic product (GDP), 128
Group discussion, 236
Group. *See also* Special group
    advantages/disadvantages of, 196
    functions of, 196–198
    maintenance behaviors in, 197t
    phases of, 196
    task behaviors in, 197t
Gunderson Lutheran's Respecting Choices Organization & Community Advance Care Planning Course, 283–284

H

Habituation, 190
Hampton, Isabel
    nursing education and, 4–5
    nursing registration and, 5
Harris County Hospital District v. Estrada, 250b
Health
    concept of, 330–331
    conceptions of, 331–332
        adaptive model as, 331–332

Health *(Continued)*
  clinical model as, 331
  eudaemonistic model as, 332
  role performance model as, 331
  diversity in, 312, 315–322
  health policy affecting, 137t
  as investment, 178–179
  models of, 331t
  of rural residents, 372–373
  social determinants of, 398–400
    categories of, 399
    examples of, 399
    factors improving, 399
    social/political activism, 404
Health and Human Services. *See* U.S. Department of Health and
    Human Services (USDHHS)
Health attitude, 332–341
Health behavior
  modification of, 332–341
  wellness and, 335–341
Health behavior model, 337
Health Belief Model (HBM), 226, 335
  for smoking cessation, 340t
Health care
  barriers to, 167f, 323, 324b
  competition in, 174–175
    positive-sum, 175, 176b–177b
    zero-sum, 174–175, 176b–177b
  consumer costs of, 162
  cost agreement for, 136–138
  criminalization in, 256
  cultural decisions in, 323
  demand for, 162
  disparities in, 402t
  economic analysis of, 174b
  economic issues in, 151, 180t
  employment opportunities in, 156
  ethical dimensions of, 260
  financial barriers affecting, 164–165
  financial burden of, 166f
  government intervention in, 155–156
  health policy affecting, 134t–135t
  insurance and third-party payment for, 153
  market-based model in, 174
  minority access to, 321–322
  nanotechnology in, 290
  need for, 153
  paying for, 161–163
  as public good, 155
  in rural Appalachia, 314
  statistics across nations, 170t
  terms and organizations in, 120b–121b
  uninsured/underinsured and, 167
  values shaping, 318–319
Health care access, disparities in, 81

Health care costs
  evaluation of, 172b–173b
  factors affecting, 168
  insurance premiums versus, 164
  rise in, 136–138
Health care disparity, in minorities, 320
Health Care and Education Reconciliation Act of 2010, 145–146
Health care expenditure
  decrease in, 164
  distribution by service type, 165f
  trends in, 164–168
Health care financing, by government, 164
Health care informatics, 288
  clinical decision support system as, 295
  definition of, 289–290
Health care literature, failures/errors within, 411
Health care market, 155
Health care organization
  influencing factors of, 195f
  professional-to-professional communication and, 195
Health care program, 128–129
Health care provider
  diversity in, 319
  fear of litigation and, 162
  resources for, 323–324
  in rural communities, 378–379
  teamwork of, 413–414
  unwarranted criminal allegations/lawsuits against, 256–257
Health care quality, 168–169
Health care reform 2010, 144
Health care resources
  availability of, 153
  types of, 153
Health care system
  cost evaluation of, 168
  intimate partner violence and, 388
  quality of care in, 168–169
    clinical nurses, 169
    nurse educator, 169
    nurse managers, 169
    nurse researcher, 169
  signs of ailing, 179
  technology in, 171–173
  value of, 169–171
Health care system reform, 173–181
Health care team, 413–414
Health disparity
  definition of, 400
  examples of, 402t
  health equities versus, 400
Health economics, 153
Health equity
  challenges to, 401–403
  health disparity versus, 400
Health habits, wellness and, 337

Health information, criteria for evaluating, 307t
Health Information Management Systems Society (HIMSS), 292
Health Insurance Portability and Accountability Act (HIPAA),
        131–132, 192–193, 255
    requirements for, 293
Health insurance. *See* Insurance
Health maintenance organization (HMO), 347
Health on the Net (HON), 231–232
Health on the Net (HON) Foundation, code of conduct by, 306
Health policy. *See also* Legislation
    before1990, 133–135
    from1990-2000, 135 136
    affecting nursing and health care, 134t–135t, 137t, 139
    development/implementation of, 133
    implementation and regulation of, 129
    leadership and, 131–132
    nurse as advocates for, 143–144
    nursing practice environment and, 117
    organizational impact on, 133
    politics and, 118–123
    in present day, 136
    process for, 124f
    think tanks and, 132
Health Professional Shortage Area (HPSA), 377
Health Professions Education Partnerships Act, 136
Health promotion, 329
    within community, 346–347
    disease prevention and, 332
    Healthy People2010 objectives for, 346t
    nursing interventions for, 331
    sleep hygiene and disorders, 340
Health promotion model, 336f
Health Resource and Services Administration (HRSA),
        140–141
    funding through, 143
Health risk appraisal, 342
Health technology assessment (HTA), 171
Healthcare Research and Quality, Agency for, 132
Healthy Cities initiative, 346–347
Healthy eating, 338
Healthy People 2000 Review, 345
Healthy People 2010, 346t
    goals of, 400
    outcomes research for, 142–143
Healthy People 2020, 345, 398
    action model for goals of, 398f
    goals of, 400, 401t
    health equities versus health disparities, 400
Healthy People initiative, 131
Healthy work environment, 412–413
    AACN and, 412, 413t
    key processes for, 413–416
Helicy, 102
Henry Street Settlement House, 7
Hierarchy of needs, 113

High level wellness, 330–331
High Reliability Organization (HRO)
    definition of, 411–412
    Just Culture and, 412
    processes for, 412
Higher Education Opportunity Act, 133, 143
Hill, Dr. Martha, 141–142
Hill-Burton Act, 133–135, 134t, 376
Hinshaw, Ada Sue, 132
Hispanic population
    HIV in, 320–321
    insurance coverage and, 166t
    as uninsured, 165
Holism, 330 331
Holistic, 330–331
Holzemer, Dr. William, 141–142
Homeless person
    communication and, 284
    as vulnerable population, 395
Homeodynamics, principles of, 102
Honor Society of Nursing, Sigma Theta Tau International
    membership in, 66
    mission of, 66
    origin of, 66
    programs through, 66–67
Hopper, 123
Horizontal communication, 195
Hospital
    as business, 9–10
    competing for nurses, 157
    function of, 6
    monopsony power of, 156 159
    as not-for-profit, 155
    nurse employment by, 6, 10
    training school costs and, 10
Hostility, wellness and, 340–341
House of Representatives, 125
    budget bills and, 125
    members of, 129
Housing, social class and, 402–403
Human energy field, 102
Human epidermal growth factor receptor (HER2), 362
Human factors science, 411
Human genome, 356
    mapping and sequencing of, 357–358
Human genome research, 363
Human Genomic Project, 363–364
Human immunodeficiency syndrome (HIV)
    in African Americans and Hispanics, 320–321
    revealing status of, 255
Human papilloma virus (HPV)
    in adolescent boys, 283
    benefits of, 282–283
Humanistic theory, 226–228
Humor, 193

Humor, sense of, 335
Hurricane Katrina, 256
Hypertension, 338
Hypertension intervention study, 141–142

I

Identity
    concept of, 75
    definition of, 74–75
Illness, diversity in, 312
Implementation, nursing process and, 206, 206t, 210
Implied contract, 247
Income, health care financial burden by, 166f
Indentification, 74–75
Indian Health Service (IHS), 376
Infant
    intimate partner violence and, 388
    wrongful medication of, 256
Infection, environment as source of, 100
Informal learning, 228
Informal network, 195
Information
    citing sources of, 308
    criteria for evaluating, 307t
    strategies for managing, 306–308
Information literacy, 299
Information processing, open versus closed, 321f
Information resources, for nursing practice, 299–305
Information technology (IT), 292
Informed consent, 253–254
Informed consent lawsuit, 253
Inherited genetic disorder, 360
Inquisitiveness, 214
Institute of Medicine
    expanding insurance coverage, 179
    patient safety and, 408
Instructional technology, 232–233
Instructivism, 225
Insurance, 153
    co-payment for, 162
    expanding coverage of, 178–179
        principles of, 179
        prototypes for, 179
    moral hazard in, 162
    out-of-pocket expense and, 162
    risk aversion and, 161
    trends in, 164–168
    types of, 163–164
        health care financial burden by, 166f
        population covered by, 166t
Insurance premium, health care costs versus, 164
Integrality, 102
Intellectual autonomy, 213
Intellectual courage, 213
Intellectual empathy, 213

Intellectual humility, 213
Intellectual integrity, 213
Intellectual perseverance, 213
Intellectual sense of justice, 213
Intellectual standards, 211–212, 212f
Intensive care unit (ICU)
    concept of, 16
    coronary care unit as, 16
Internal constraints, on autonomy, 271
Internal evidence, 305
Internal locus of control, 334
International Council of Nurses (ICN)
    code of ethics for, 264
    membership in, 64
    mission of, 64
    origin of, 64
    programs through, 64–65
Internet
    clinical practice guidelines on, 304
    evaluation of, 306
    genetic testing via, 362–363
    health information on, 231
    Health on the Net (HON), 231–232
    information on
        accuracy of, 231
        evaluating, 231b
        finding, 230–231
    navigation of, 305–306
    ready reference information on, 299–300
    for self-directed learning, 232
    teaching and learning, 231–232
    voice-over-IP and, 232–233
    web tools for, 233
Interpersonal communication, 188t
    closure in, 190
    noisy environment, coping with, 190
    selective attention and habituation in, 190
Interpersonal process, 106
    goal-directed, 107
Interpersonal process model
    assumptions about the individual, 107
    concepts of, 107
        exploitation, 107
        identification, 107
        orientation, 107
        resolution, 107
    environment and, 107
    health and illness, 107
    nursing and, 107
    overview of, 107
    theoretical perspectives, comparison of, 111t
Interpersonal stressor, 105
Interprofessional collaboration, 77
Interprofessional understanding, lack of, 196
Interstate RN and LPN/VN licensure compact, 138

Intervention
    in community, 346
    health maintenance organization and,
        347
    for health promotion, 331
    of Neuman systems model, 105
    promoting behavior change, 341–343
    school-based, 347
    for system stability, 105
Intimate partner violence. *See also* Domestic violence, 385
    assessment for
        guidelines for, 389
        positive screening, 390
        tools for, 389
    children and, 388
    consequences of
        femicide, 387–388
        mental health as, 387
        physical health as, 387
    health care system and, 388
    posttraumatic stress disorder from, 387
    pregnancy and, 388
    prevalence of, 386
    safety factors for, 390
    signs and symptoms of, 389
Intrapersonal communication
    context of, 188
    self-awareness in, 188–189
    translation processes of, 187
Intrapersonal stressor, 105

J
Job satisfaction, 84–85
Johari window, 188–189, 188t
Johnson, Eddie Bernice, 143
The Joint Commission (TJC), 256–257
    patient safety and, 409, 414
Jones, Cheryl, 132
Journal article database
    critical appraisal and, 304–305
    database citations and, 300–301
    links to full texts in, 304
    search strategies for, 301–304
    types of, 300–305
Just Culture
    philosophy of, 411
    purpose of, 412
"Just Culture" building, 411
Justice, 270

K
Kant, Immanuel, 270–271
Karney v. Arnott-Ogden Memorial Hospital, 250b
Key provisions of PPACA 2010, 147b
King, Imogene, 107

Knowledge
    changing behavior, 228–229
    critical thinking model and, 211
    fundamentals and patterns of, 47
    necessity of, 229–230
    of nurse, 263–264
    transfer of, 228–229
Kovas v. Kawakami, 250b
Kramer's socialization model, 56–57

L
Labor law, 248–249
Ladies' Aid societies, 7–8
Language, cultural diversity in, 188
Latent failure, 411
Law
    definition of, 243
    function of, 243
Leadership
    educating nurses for, 78–79
    health policy and, 131–132
    importance of, 62
    nurses and, 132, 141–142
    working environment and, 78
Leads, in therapeutic communication,
        191
Learner
    assessment of, 234
    characteristics of effective, 229–233
    motivation of, 229–230
Learner objective
    categories of, 235
    examples of
        affective objectives, 235
        cognitive objectives, 235
    purpose of, 235
Learning
    barriers to, 237
    behaviorist theory and, 225t
    challenges in, 223
    change theory and, 226, 227t
    cognitive theory and, 226, 226t
    environment for, 228–229
    future trends in, 239
    humanistic theory and, 226–228,
        227t
    informal ways of, 228
    nurse role in, 239
    psychomotor domain of, 235
    by reading and listening, 228
    styles and preferences of, 230
    technology influence on, 230–231
    in virtual environment, 239
Learning principle, 228–229
Learning sources, 57–58

Learning theory
  classic cone of, 228
  teaching and, 225–228
Learning transfer, 228–229
Lecture, as teaching format, 236
Legal accountability, 274
Legislation. *See also* Health policy; Politics
  administration and committees, 123–125
  Brady Bill gun control legislation, 127
  congressional sessions for, 125
  funding and, 121–122
  nurses in, 143–144
  political parties for, 119
  process of, 123–126
  state practice acts and, 139
Legislator, role of, 131–132
Leininger, Madeleine, 108
Leininger model of transcultural nursing, 318f
Leininger theoretical framework for transcultural nursing,
    316–317
Library information resources, for nursing practice,
    299–305
Library online catalogues, 299–300
Licensed practical nurse/licensed vocational nurse (LPN/LVN),
    26, 31t–32t
Licensed practical nurse/licensed vocational nurse (LPN/LVN)
    program
  recommendations for, 36
  strengths of, 36
  weaknesses of, 36
Licensure
  laws and regulations controlling, 244
  nurse practice acts and, 243
  police power and, 244
Licensure compact
  goal of, 244
  for RN and LPN/VN, 138
Literature, citing and acknowledging, 308
Litigation, fear of, 162
Local-area network, 291–292
Locus of control, 226, 334
Longitudinal study, in critical thinking, 216–217
Loveland-Cherry, Carol, 132
Lowery, Julie Ann, 143–144

M
Magnet hospital, 139
  employment at, 62
  as positive-sum competition, 177
  success of, 61–63
    leadership in, 62
    nurse attributes in, 62
Magnet Nursing Services Recognition Program
    (MNSRP), 139
Maintenance behavior, in groups, 196–197, 197t

Male nurse
  bias against, 12
  military discrimination against, 12–13
  stereotype of, 73–74
Malone, Beverly, 132
Malpractice, 250
Managed care, Medicare Choice/Advantage plans and, 136–138
Managed care organization, 136–138
Manager
  nurse as, 77–78
  role of, 78
Marion, Lucy, 132
Market failure, 163
Market-based model, 174
Maslow, Abraham, 113
Master's degree in nursing, 31t–32t
  degree designations for, 28
  enrollment in, 27
  history of, 27
  length and components of, 27
  NCNAC and CCNE, 133
  recommendations for, 37
  RN-MSN and nonnurse entry options for, 27–28
  strengths of, 37
  weaknesses of, 37
Maternal and Infant Act (Sheppard-Towner), 7
Maturity, 214
McCain, Dr. Nancy, 141–142
McCain, Senator, 122
McCarthy, Carolyn, 143
McKinney Homelessness Act, 135–136
Media, portrayal of nurse, 74
Medicaid
  creation of, 129
  FQHC and, 377
  purpose of, 155–156
  as state-funded care, 164
  universal health coverage affect on, 179
Medicaid managed care plans, 136–138
Medical error, interception of, 408
Medical reform, 35–36
Medical supplies, 153
Medicare
  capitated costs under, 136–138
  creation of, 129
  as federally-funded care, 164
  FQHC and, 377
  Part D coverage, 136
  parts of, 155–156
  rural hospitals and, 377
  universal health coverage affect on, 179
Medicare and Medicaid Services. *See* Centers for Medicare and
    Medicaid Services (CMS)
Medicare Choice/Advantage managed care plans,
    136–138

Medicare managed care plans
  consumer rights, regulation of, 138
  types of, 136–138
Medicare Modernization Act, 136
Medicare Prescription Drug Act, 377
Medicare Rural Hospital Flexibility Act, 377
Medication
  direct-to-consumer marketing of, 280b
  response to, 362
Mediterranean diet, 338
MEDLINE, 300
  clinical practice guidelines in, 304
MedlinePlus, 299–300
Mendelian inheritance, 357b
Mental disorders, in rural communities, 373
Mental health coverage, 136
Mental health, in rural communities, 373
Mentor
  identification and characteristics of, 58
  role of, 79
  in socialization process, 58
Mentoring
  features of, 58
  function of, 58
  process of, 79
  role ambiguity and, 87
  success in, 58
MeSH vocabulary, 300–301
Meta-dyad, 75
Metaphor, 193
Methamphetamine, 374
Metropolitan Life Insurance Company, 7
Metropolitan statistical area (MSA), 370
Micropolitan, 370
Midrange theory, 100
  Peplau's interpersonal process, 106–107
Mills v. Moriarty, 251–252
Minimal cues, in therapeutic communication, 191
Minority
  faculty and nursing students as, 319
  health care of, 320–322
  in rural communities, 371
Minority enrollment, in nursing education, 38
Mississippi Bd. of Nursing v. Hanson, 250b
Modern Language Association (MLA), 308
Monopsony model, 156–159
Moody, Linda, 132
Moral distress, 88–89
Moral hazard, 162
Moral outrage, 56
Moral philosophy
  definition of, 262
  ethics and, 261
  use of, 262
Moral theory, 262

Motivational enhancement counseling, 341–342
Munhall, Patricia, 79–80
Murder, of women, 387
Mutuality, trust and, 229
MyPyramid, 338

N

Nanopatterned substrate, 290
Nanotechnology, 290
National Advisory Council for Nursing (NAC), 141
National Bipartisan Commission on the Future of Medicare,
  131–132
National Center for Minority Health and Health Disparities
  (NCMHD), 141
National Council Licensure Examination (NCLEX), 138
National Council of State Boards of Nursing (NCSBN), licensure
  compact by, 138
National Guideline Clearinghouse, 304
National Health Service Corps (NHSC), 377
National Healthcare Disparities Report, 401
National Human Genome Research Institute (NHGRI), 363–364
National Institute of Health (NIH)
  health policy and, 118–119
  NINR and, 141
National Institute of Nursing Research (NINR)
  funding from, 141
  purpose of, 141
National Labor Relations Act (NLRA), 248–249
National League for Nursing
  accreditation through, 140–141
  membership in, 65
  mission of, 65
  origin of, 65
  programs through, 65
National League for Nursing Accreditation Commission
  (NLNAC), 33
  emphasis of, 133
National League for Nursing Education, 5
National Organization for Public Health Nursing (NOPHN), 7
National Student Nurses Association (NSNA)
  membership in, 65
  mission of, 65
  origin of, 65
  programs through, 65
National Weight Control Registry, 342
Negligence, 250–251
Nelson, Dr. Audrey, 141–142
Networking, 291–292
Neuman, Betty, 104
Neuman systems model, 104
  assumptions about the individual, 104–105
  concepts of, 105
    interventions, 105
    relating to client system stability, 105
  environment and, 105

Neuman systems model *(Continued)*
  health and illness, 105
  nursing and, 105
  overview of, 104
  theoretical perspectives, comparison of, 111t
Newborn nursery, 9f
Newborn screening, 361
Nightingale, Florence
  apprenticeship model for, 4
  collegiate nursing and, 23–24
  Crimean War and, 3–4
  environmental theory and, 100–101
  nursing role and, 74
Nightingale Training School for Nurses, 3–4
Noisy environment, coping with, 190
Nondiscriminatory insurance, 176b–177b
Nonmaleficence, 269
Nonmetropolitan area, 370
Nonprofit firm, role of, 155
Nonverbal behavior, 192
Noodle Tools, 308
Norming phase, of groups, 196
North American Nursing Diagnosis Association (NANDA), 297
  classification system for, 297
North Carolina Association of Nurse Anesthetists (NCANA),
  143–144
Not-for-profit, 155
Nowak v. High, 250b
Nurse
  accountability of, 53
  accreditation of, 33–34
  aggregated information resources for, 304
  attributes of, 62
  in bureaucratic environment, 59–61
  burnout and stress in, 275
  certification of, 34–35
  as complement/substitutes for physician, 159–161
  cultural bias against, 74
  as educator, 78–79
  employment opportunities for, 5–6, 156
  function of, 74
  as gatekeeper, 324
  hospitals competing for, 157
  job satisfaction of, 84–85
  leadership role of, 132, 141–142
  legal registration of, 5
  LPN/LVN, 26
  mandatory overtime for, 126
  from novice to expert, 60b–61b
  obedience to physician, 4
  organizations, membership in, 119
  portrayal of, 73
  preceptor role of, 57–58
  public stereotypes of, 48–49
  recruitment of, 8

Nurse *(Continued)*
  as researcher, 79–80
  responsibilities of, 52–53
  role dynamics of, 83
  standards/competencies for, 139–140
  supply and demand for, 156, 157b
  teaching or learning role of, 239
  torts against, 249–250
  unwarranted criminal allegations/lawsuits against, 256–257
  war, role in, 7–8
  working environment of, 83
  in World War II, 11–12
Nurse activism, 143–144
Nurse advocate, 80–81
  role of, 81
Nurse aide, in World War II, 11–12
Nurse Education Act, 127–128
Nurse educator, health system quality of care and, 169
Nurse Faculty Loan Program (NFLP), 140
Nurse leader
  characteristics of, 78
  at magnet hospital, 62
  as manager, 77–78
  passion and, 62–63
Nurse licensure compact, 244
Nurse manager, health system quality of care and, 169
Nurse Multi-State Licensure compact, 244
Nurse practice act (NPA)
  function of, 244
  licensing and, 243–244
  role of, 243
Nurse practitioner, 17
  acute care program for, 17
  pediatric program for, 17
  in rural Virginia, 17f
Nurse Reinvestment Act, 118–119
  nursing shortage and, 140
Nurse researcher, health system quality of care and, 169
Nurse Training Act, 140
Nurse-doctor relationship, 61
Nurse-led clinic, 160–161, 177
Nurse-managed care, 160
Nurse-midwifery program, 34
Nurse-patient relationship, as fiduciary, 267
Nurses' Associated Alumnae, 5
Nursing
  administrative law in, 243–247
  in American Civil War, 7–8
  apprenticeship model for, 4
  autonomy in, 53
  beneficent goal of, 269
  challenges to, 319
  competency areas for, 52–53
  critical thinking in, 204–205
  during disaster, 255–256

Nursing *(Continued)*
  in early 20th-century, 5–6
  economic issues in, 151
  employment law and, 247–249
  environmental theory and, 101
  ethical dimensions of, 260
  as female profession, 73
  genetics and genomics in, 354
  in Great War, 8
  health policy affecting, 133, 134t–135t, 137t, 139
  historical development of, 1, 3–14
  issues in, 133
  men in, 73
  patient beliefs and values, 319
  as profession, 44–45
  professionalism of, 47–49, 50f
  socialization to, 42, 53–58
  society's image of, 45
  in Spanish American War, 7–8
  studies in, 37–38
  supply and demand in, 157b
  telehealth and, 77
  tort law in, 249–256
  values shaping, 318–319
  in World War I, 8f
Nursing administrator, 62
Nursing board, 243
  regulatory/adjucatory powers of, 246
  role of, 246
Nursing database, 207–208
Nursing diagnosis
  definition of, 208–209
  prioritizing of, 209
Nursing doctorate
  concept and goal for, 29
  establishment of, 29–30
Nursing education
  accreditation of, 140–141
  associate degree for, 26
  baccalaureate programs for, 14
  community college program for, 14–15
  comparison of, 31t–32t
  considerations for, 30–35
    accessibility of, 35
    cost of, 30
    financial assistance for, 30
    quality of, 30–35
  diploma programs for, 23–25
  doctoral degree in, 28–29
  dual degree programs in, 28
  financial endowments for, 11
  future of, 38–39
  graduate program for, 15–16
  history of, 23–30
  master's degree in, 26–28

Nursing education *(Continued)*
  minority enrollment in, 38
  nursing history and, 3
  observations and analysis of, 35–37
  origination of, 140
  pathways of, 22
  for registered nurse, 24f, 33f
  relationships among, 98f
  research-focused program for, 29
  specialized accreditation in, 33–34
  standards for, evolution of, 5
  state board examination and, 81
  university programs for, 11
  vocational program for, 26
Nursing ethics. *See also* "Good" nurse, 263
  advocacy and, 273–274
  concepts in, 273
  history of, 264
  research on, 265, 266b
Nursing informatics, 290
Nursing intervention, 331
Nursing Interventions Classification (NIC), 297, 298t
Nursing judgment model, 211–213
Nursing knowledge, 47
Nursing language, 296–299
  Nursing Minimum Data Set (NMDS) as, 297
  taxonomy as, 297–299
Nursing Minimum Data Set (NMDS), 297
Nursing organization, 61–63
Nursing Outcomes Classification (NOC), 297–298
Nursing practice
  competency areas for, 59
  delegation in, 246
  doctor of, 17–18
  economic concepts for, 161–173
  as ethical, 265–279
  features of, 49
  health policy and planning, 117
  legal aspects of, 242
  library information resources for, 299–305
  moral decision/actions in, 268f
  moral philosophy of, 262
  outcomes research for, 142–143
  practice theory application to, 110–113
  reframing, challenges to, 180
  relationships among, 98f
  in rural communities, 375–376
  standards of, 52b
  theories and frameworks for, 95
  values of, 49
    altruism as, 50
    caregiving as, 49–50
    service to society as, 50
Nursing practice environment, 159

Nursing process
   approach to, 205–206
   concept of, 206
   critical thinking and, 204–205, 206t
   critical thinking, clinical judgment and, 200
   phases of
      analysis/diagnosis, 206, 206t, 208–209
      assessment, 206–208, 206t
      evaluation, 206, 206t
      implementation, 206, 206t
      planning, 206, 206t
Nursing process model, 205–206, 207f
Nursing proficiency, 59
Nursing registry, 5–6
Nursing research
   funding for, 142
   NINR and, 141
   relationships among, 98f
Nursing role
   as caregiver, 75–77
   characteristics of, 75
   as colleague, 77
   identity dyads of, 76f
   as manager, 77–78
   media portrayal versus actual, 74
   meta-dyad of, 75
   public perception of, 74
   stereotypes of, 72–74
Nursing science, 102
Nursing shortage, 8
   cause of, 156–157
   as cyclical, 156
   Nurse Reinvestment Act and, 140
Nursing student
   preceptor program and, 56–57
   socialization and, 54
Nursing Students Without Borders (NSWB), 312
Nursing superintendent, 4–5
Nursing systems, 103
   subsystems of
      interpersonal, 103
      social, 103
      technological, 103
   types of
      partly compensatory, 103
      supportive-educative, 103
      wholly compensatory, 103
Nursing taxonomy, 297–299
Nursing theory
   birth of, 15–16
   comparison of, 111t
   composition of, 97–100
   development, history of, 98t–99t
   evaluating utility of, 110–112
   frameworks and theories from other disciplines, 112–113

Nursing training program. *See also* Nursing education
   economic plight of, 9–10
   evolution of, 3
   number of, 4
Nursing Workforce Diversity (NWD) grant, 140
Nursing's Agenda for Health Care Reform, 132

O
Obama, President, 122, 404
Obedience of nurse, 4
Obesity, 338
   prevalence of, 374–375
Obstetrical and Neonatal Nursing (ONN), 133
Obstetrics, twilight sleep and, 9
Occupational injury rate, in rural communities, 374
Office of Management and Budget (OMB), 370
Omaha Problem Classification, 297–298
Omnibus Appropriations Act, 371
Omnibus Budget Reconciliation Act (OBRA),
      133–135, 134t, 271
   Federally Qualified Health Center and, 377
Oncology Nursing Society (ONS), 133
Open information processing, 321f
Open systems, 290
Open-mindedness, 214
Operating room, 4f
Opportunity cost, 168
Optimism, 335
Oral testimony, 253b
Orem, Dorothea, 102
Organ donor, speeding death of, 256
Organization
   definition of, 194
   health policy and planning, 132
Organizational autonomy, 62
Organizational communication
   definition of, 194–198
   types of, 195–196
Orientation, in therapeutic relationship, 193–194
Other-centeredness, 84
Outcome, in nursing process, 209
Outcomes research, 142–143
   technology assessment and, 171
Out-of-pocket expense, 162–163

P
Parole evidence rule, 248
Passive learning, 226
Paternalism, 271, 318–319
Patient Protection and Affordable Care Act (PPACA) of 2010,
      145–146
Patient safety, 407
   The Joint Commission (TJC) and, 409, 414
   teamwork and, 413–414
   USDHHS and, 409–410

Patient Safety and Quality Improvement Act
    divisions of, 410
    health care errors and, 410
Patient Safety Organization (PSO), 410
Patient Self-Determination Act (PSDA), 271, 271b
Patient-centered care, impediment of, 78
Paul Wellstone Mental Health and Addiction Equity Act, 136
Pediatric nurse practitioner program, 17
Pedigree symbols, of family history, 360f
Peer evaluation, 237
Pender, Nola, 336–337
Pender's health promotion model, 336–337, 336f
Peplau, Hildegard, 106
Peplau's interpersonal process model, 106–107
Performing phase, of groups, 196
Persistent vegetative state (PVS), 283
Personal knowledge, 47
    definition of, 78
Personal Responsibility and Work Opportunities Act (Welfare), 136
Personal space, 192
Personalized medicine, 362–363
Personnel, 153
Pew Charitable Trust (PCT), 132
Pharmacogenetics, 362
Pharmacogenomics, 362
Phenylketonuria (PKU), 357
Physical abuse. See also Domestic violence
    in women, 386
Physician
    fear of litigation and, 162
    nurse as complement/substitute for, 159–161
    nurse obedience to, 4
Physician-managed care, 160
Plagiarism, 308
Plaintiff, 249–250
Planning, nursing process and, 206, 206t, 209–210
Point-of-care computing, 291–292
Point-of-care resources, 299
Police power, 243
    licensure and, 244
Political action committee (PAC), 121
527 political groups, 122–123
Political parties, 119
Politics. See also Health policy; Legislation
    health policy and, 118–123
Positive-sum competition, 176b–177b
    goal of, 175
    principles of, 175
Posttraumatic stress disorder (PTSD), 387
Posture, as nonverbal behavior, 192
Poverty
    definition of, 401
    health equity and, 401–402
    in rural communities, 371–372
Poverty threshold, 401

Practice. See Nursing practice
Practice theory, 100
    characteristics of, 110
    example of, 110
    nursing practice application and, 110–113
    purpose of, 109–110
Practice-focused program for nursing, 29–30, 31t–32t
Praxis, 75
Precautionary Principle, 344
Preceptor
    benefit for, 57–58
    followers of, 57
    role and function of, 57
Preceptor program, 56–57
Pregnancy, intimate partner violence and, 388
Preorientation, in therapeutic relationship, 193
Prescription drug, direct-to-consumer marketing of, 280b
Prescriptive practice theory, 100
Presidential Election Campaign Fund (PECF), 122
Preventive ethics, 283–284
Pre-Y generation, 232
Primary care nurse practitioner, 17
    pediatric program for, 17
Primary intervention, 54–55
Privacy, electronic health record and, 293–294
Privacy issues, genetic information and, 136
Private duty nurse
    economic plight of, 6
    employment of, 5–6
Private individual insurance, 163
    percentage covered by, 164–165
Private law, 243
Problem-solving skills, 341
Prochaska's transtheoretical model of change, 339t
Profession
    characteristics of, 45, 46t
    definition of, 44–45
    nursing as, 44–45
Professional association
    classification of, 63
    definition of, 63
Professional ethics, 262–263
Professional governance
    approaches to
        administrative model, 63
        congressional model, 63
        councilor model, 63
        shared governance model, 63
    nurse and, 63
Professional identity, 55
Professional organization, 61t
Professional standards, 211–212
Professionalism
    clothing styles and, 48
    model for, 49

Professionalism *(Continued)*
  of nursing, 47–49
    wheel of, 50f
Professionalization, 47–49
Professional-to-professional communication, 195
Proposition, 97
Protein, 357b
Provider-consumer relationship, 174–177
Psychodrama, as role-playing, 237
Psychomotor skills
  learning and, 235
  objectives for, 235
PsycINFO, 300
Public good, health care as, 155
Public health nurse
  number of, 7
  role of, 7
Public law, 243
Public-sponsored insurance, 164
Purpose, sense of, 334–335

Q

Quebec Heart Health Demonstration Packet, 347
Questioning, 192

R

Race, categories for data on, 319–320
Racial disparity, 320
Racial diversity, 322–323
Racial minority enrollment, in nursing education, 38
Ready reference information, 299–300
Reality shock, 56
Reflection, 191, 191b
Reframing, 193
Registered nurse. *See also* Graduate nurse
  education for, 24f, 33f
  employment/working conditions for, 6
  evolution of, 5
  hospital loyalty and, 10
  population growth of, 156
  threat of, 10
Registry, 5–6
Regulator subsystem, 104
Regulatory power, 246
Relative risk, 397–398
Remote Evaluation of Acute Ischemic Stroke (REACH), 295
Research
  in critical thinking, 216–217
  on nursing ethics, 265, 266b
Research genetic testing, 361
Research. *See* Nursing research
Researcher, nurse as, 79–80
Research-focused program for nursing, 29, 31t–32t
Resilience, 412
Resocialization, 55–56

Resonancy, 102
Resource
  for health care providers, 323–324
  for rural health, 378b
  rural health policy and, 376–377
Restatement, 191, 191b
Retail clinic, 160
Returning nurse, 55
Ribonucleic acid (RNA), 357b
Risk, 397
Risk aversion, 161
Risk pooling, 162
Robert Wood Johnson Foundation (RWJF), 132
Rockefeller General Education Board, 11
Rogers, Martha, 101–102
Role
  concept of, 75
  definition of, 74
Role advancement program, 88
Role ambiguity
  mentoring and, 87
  role stress from, 86–87
  sources of, 86–87
  strategies for, 87
Role conflict
  occurrence of, 195–196
  sources of, 85
  strategies for, 85
Role discrepancy
  role stress and, 87
  sources of, 87–88
  strategies for
    debriefing, 87–88
    role advancement program, 88
    task analysis, 88
Role extension, 86
Role incongruity
  example of, 89
  sources of, 88
  strategies for
    empowerment, 89
    values clarification, 89
    whistle-blowing, 89–90
Role integration, 83–84
Role mastery, 86
Role model
  definition of, 57
  peers as, 57
Role overload
  cause of, 195–196
  definition of, 85
  prioritizing for, 86
  sources of, 85–86
  strategies for, 86
Role performance model, 331

Role segmentation, 83–84
Role strain, 84
   impact of, 84
Role stress
   cause of, 84, 195–196
   from role ambiguity, 86–87
   role conflict and, 85
   role discrepancy and, 87
   role incongruity and, 88–89
   role overload as source of, 85
   stepwise approach to, 90b
Role theory, 56
Role transition, 86
   example of, 86
Role-playing, 237
Rooziokh, Dr. Hooian C., 256
Rosenstock's health belief model, 226
Roy, Sister Callista, 103
Rural, classification system for, 370
Rural Appalachia, health care needs in, 314
Rural community
   characteristics of, 371–372
   childhood immunization rates in, 374
   dental health in, 374
   domestic violence in, 374
   employment in, 372
   familial status in, 372
   health care providers in, 378–379
   mental health/disorders in, 373
   minorities in, 371
   occupational injury rate in, 374
   poverty in, 371–372
   schools in, 379
   substance abuse in, 374
Rural health
   concepts of, 368
   resources for, 378b
Rural Health Clinics Act, 133–135
Rural Health Clinics Service Act, 377
Rural health policy, resources and, 376–377
Rural Healthy People 2010, 372–373
Rural hospital, Medicare payments to, 377
Rural life, characteristics of, 369
Rural nursing practice
   challenges for, 378
   characteristics of, 375–376
   implications for, 377–380
Rural nursing theory, 376
Rural population, as underinsured, 165–167
Rural resident
   communicating with, 378
   confidentiality issues in, 379
   employment of, 372
   health status of, 372–373
Ryan White Act, 135–136

S
Safety. See Patient safety
SBAR, 415t
Schiavo, Terri, 283
Schlotfeldt, Rozella, 29
School, in rural communities, 379
School-based intervention, 347
Science of unitary human beings
   assumptions about the individual, 101
   concepts of, 102
   environment and, 101
   health and illness, 101
   Martha Rogers and, 101–102
   nursing and, 102
   overview of, 101
   theoretical perspectives, comparison of, 111t
Search engine, 306
Search strategy, 301–304
Secondary intervention, 34–35
Secretary of Health, role of, 129–130
Security, electronic health record and, 293–294
Selective attention, 190
Selective Service Act draft, 12–13
Self-actualization, 332
Self-awareness, 188–189
   values clarification and, 189
Self-care, 103
Self-care agency, 103, 334
Self-care deficit, 103
Self-care deficit theory
   assumptions about the individual, 102
   concepts of, 103
   environment and, 103
   focus of, 102
   health and illness, 103
   nursing and, 103
   overview of, 102
   theoretical perspectives, comparison of, 111t
Self-care requisites
   definition of, 103
   types of
      developmental, 103
      health deviation, 103
      universal, 103
Self-concept, 333–334
Self-confidence, 214
Self-determination, autonomy as, 271
Self-directed learning, 228
   Internet for, 232
Self-efficacy, 334
Self-efficacy theory, 113, 226
Self-serving behavior, in groups, 196–197, 198t
Selye, Hans, 113
Sense of humor, 335
Sense of purpose, 334–335

Shared governance model, 63
Shortage. *See* Nursing shortage
Silence, 190
Silver, Henry, 17
Sister to Sister project, 347
Situation-specific theory, 100, 109–110
Skill/routine mastery, 56
Sleep, 340t
Smoking, 338–340
    soliciting adolescents and, 131
Smoking cessation
    health belief model for, 340t
    motivation for, 339–340
    nurse-delivered counseling for, 339
    Prochaska's transtheoretical model of change for, 339t
    Sister to Sister project for, 347
Smoking Zine, 347
Social determinants of health, 398–400
    categories of, 399
    examples of, 10019#b0015
    factors improving, 399
    social/political activism, 404
Social injustice, 404
Social integration, 56
Social learning theory, 334
Social Policy Statement, of ANA, 269
Social reform, 7
Social Security Act, 9–10, 129, 133–135, 134t
Social support, 345
Socialization
    career development and, 58–59
    definition of, 44
    environmental factors influencing, 59–63
    Kramer's socialization model, 56–57
    mentor and, 58
    to nursing, 42, 53–58
    nursing students and, 54
    process of, 44, 53
    role theory and, 56
    through education, 54–56
    to work setting, 56–57
Socializing agent, 57
Social/political activism, 404
Society of Gastroenterology Nurses and Associates (SGNA), 143
Society of Superintendents of Training Schools for Nurses of the
        United States and Canada, 5
Socioeconomic status
    employment and, 402
    housing and, 402–403
    poverty and, 401
Software spider/robot, 306
Spanish-American War, 7–8
Special group, assessment of, 234–235
    challenged populations, 234–235
    cultural considerations, 234

Specialist. *See* Advanced nurse specialist
Specialty association, 63
Specific critical thinking competency, 211
Spirituality, 335
Stakeholder cooperation, principle of, 175
Standardized symbols, of family history, 360f
Standards, critical thinking model and, 211–212
State board examination, 81
State Children's Health Insurance Program (SCHIP), 155–156
    universal health coverage affect on, 179
State legislature
    mandatory overtime for nurses, 126
    role and activities of, 125–126
    rules for administration and governance in, 123
State nurse practice acts, 138–139
State practice acts, 139
Statute of frauds, 248
Statutory law, 243
Stereotyping, of nurses, 48–49
Stierle, Linda J., 143
Stimulation game, as role-playing, 237
"Stop the Line", 413
Storming phase, of groups, 196
Stressor, 105
    extrapersonal, 105
    interpersonal, 105
    intrapersonal, 105
    wellness and, 344–345
Strickland, Ora, 132
Structured communication techniques, 415–416, 415t
Studies in nursing, impact of, 37–38
Substance Abuse and Mental Health Services Administration
        (SAMHSA), 141
Substance abuse, in rural communities, 374
Substitute
    definition of, 159
    nurse as, 159–161
Summarization, 191–192
Summative evaluation, 237
Superintendent of nursing, 4–5
Supply, 156
Surgeon General (SG), 129–131
Synchronous learning, 232
System stability
    concepts relating to, 105
    interventions for, 105
    stressors and, 105
Systematicity, 214
Systems theory, 194–195

T
Task analysis, 88
Task behavior, in groups, 196–197, 197t
Taxonomy, nursing, 297–299
Taxpayer Refund and Relief Act, 127

Teacher, effectiveness of, 78
  characteristics of, 229
Teachers College, nursing theory birth at, 15–16
Teaching
  behaviorist theory and, 225, 225t
  challenges in, 223
  change theory and, 226, 227t
  cognitive theory and, 226, 226t
  future trends in, 239
  humanistic theory and, 226–228, 227t
  learning theory and, 225–228
  nurse role in, 239
  tailoring to learner, 229
  technology influence on, 230–231
  in virtual environment, 239
Teaching identity, 76–77
Teaching principle, 228–229
Teaching-learning experience
  evaluation of, 237
  future trends in, 239
Teaching-learning material, choosing and learning, 238t
Teaching-learning plans, 233–234
Teaching-learning strategies
  demonstration as, 236
  group discussion as, 236
  lecture as, 236
  questioning technique as, 236
  role-playing and case studies, 237
  selection of, 236–237
Team Strategies and Tools to Enhance Performance and Patient
    Safety (TeamSTEPPS), 414
Teamwork
  communication and, 414–416
  patient safety and, 413–414
Technology
  in health care, 171–173
  in teaching and learning, 239
Technology assessment, 171
Tele-educational unit, 295
Telehealth, 77
  definition of, 294
  diabetes self-management system and, 295
  REACH as, 295
Temporary Assistance to Needy Families, 136
Termination phase, in therapeutic relationship, 194
Tertiary intervention, 54–55
Testimony, expert, 133
Testing, direct-to-consumer marketing of, 280b
Theoretical statement, 97
Theory
  abstraction level of, 100
  concept and, 97
  relationships among, 98f
  value and logical structure of, 110–112
Theory of caring, 76

Therapeutic communication
  minimal cues, leads, and touch in, 191
  timing and, 193
Therapeutic privilege, 254
Therapeutic relationship, phases of
  orientation as, 193–194
  preorientation as, 193
  termination phase, 194
  working phase, 194
Therapeutic response, 190–192
Therapeutic self-care demand, 103
Think Cultural Health, 324
Think tank, 132
Timing, therapeutic communication and, 193
Tissue plasminogen activator (tPA), 295
To Err Is Human report, 408, 412
Tobacco Master Settlement Agreement, 131
Tobacco use, 338–340
  intervention for, 347
  in rural communities, 374
Toowoomba Adult Triage Trauma Tool (TATTT), 295
Tort, types of, 249–250
Tort law, 243
  in nursing, 249–256
Touch, in therapeutic communication, 191
Transcultural nursing. *See* Cultural care theory
  model of, 318f
  theoretical frameworks in, 316–317
Transparent pricing, 176b–177b
Transpersonal caring, 106
Trastuzumab (Herceptin), 362
Trust, mutuality and, 229
Truth seeking, 214
Twilight sleep, 9

U
Underinsured
  characteristics of, 165–167
  health care risks/barriers for, 167
  percentage of, 167–168
Unemployment, 402
Unequal Treatment report, 141–142
Uninsured persons
  characteristics of, 165
  health care risks/barriers for, 167
  percentage of, 167–168
Unintentional error, criminalization of, 256–257
Unintentional injury, as cause of death, 374
Unintentional tort, 249–250
Unitary human beings, science of, 101–102, 111t
Universal health coverage
  employer/individual mandate for, 179
  single payer, 179
  tax credit for, 179
Unreasonable conduct, 250

Upward communication, 195
Urban, 370–371
Urgent care clinic, 160
U.S. Department of Health and Human Services (USDHHS)
    budget for, 128
    Higher Education Opportunity Act and, 133
    patient safety and, 409–410
    role of, 129–130
U.S. Sanitary Commission, 7–8

V

Vaccine
    direct-to-consumer marketing of, 280b
    efficacy and affects of, 282–283
Validation, 191
Value development, 189
Values, 334
    behavior and, 88–89
    importance of, 189
Values clarification, 89, 189b
    self-awareness and, 189
Values-based decision model, for advocacy, 273–274
Veracity, 272–273
Vertical communication, 195
Veterans Affairs, Department of, 132
Veterans Mental Health and Other Care Improvements Act,
        118–119
Videostreaming, 232
Virginia Henderson International Nursing Library, 304
Virtual environment, teaching and learning in, 239
Virtue-based ethics, 264
Visiting Nurse Association (VNA), telehealth and, 294–295
Vocational nursing program, 26
Voice-over-IP (VoIP), 232–233
Vulnerability
    definition of, 396
    factors affecting, 399–400
    throughout generations, 399
Vulnerable populationsSocioeconomic status
    adolescents as, 394
    characteristics of, 397
    definition of, 396–397
    homeless men as, 395
    nursing considerations for, 403–404
    risks for, 397–398
    types of, 397b

W

Wage control, 159
Wald, Lillian, 7
    health promotion/disease prevention by, 7
    NOPHN, founding of, 7
War. *See also* specific wars
    nurse role in, 7–8
Watson, Jean, 76
    philosophy and science of caring, 105–106

Watson-Glaser Critical Thinking Appraisal (WGCTA), 216
Web tools, 233
WebMD, 307–308
Wellness
    attitudes and characteristics of, 333–335
    comprehensive model of, 333f
    emotion management and, 340–341
    environmental factors affecting, 344
        chemicals, 344
        culture, 344
        social support, 345
        stress, 344–345
    exercise and, 337–338
    health behaviors associated with, 335–341
    health habits and, 337
    healthy eating and, 338
    locus of control and, 334
    optimism and, 335
    problem-solving skills and, 341
    self-care agency, 334
    self-concept and, 333–334
    sense of humor and, 335
    sense of purpose and, 334–335
    sleep and, 340
    spirituality and, 335
    tobacco use and, 338–340
    values and, 334
Wells, Thelma, 132, 142
Whistle-blowing, 89–90
Wide-area network, 290–292
Women. *See also* Domestic violence
    employment of, 4
    femicide in, 387–388
Women's liberation movement, 177–178
Wood, Susan, 74
Work environment
    as healthy, 412–413
    of nurse, 83
Working phase, in therapeutic relationship, 194
Workstations on wheels (WOW), 292
World Health Organization, smoking and, 338–340
World War I, 8f
World War II, 11–12
    nursing shortage after, 14
    post-war era, 13–14
World Wide Web
    evaluation of, 306
    information on
        evaluating, 231b
        finding, 230–231
    navigation of, 305–306
Wyman, Jean, 142

Z

Zero-sum competition, 174–175, 176b–177b
Zotero, 308